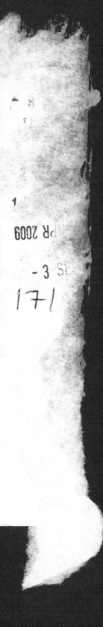

NEUROPSYCHIATRY AND BEHAVIOURAL NEUROLOGY EXPLAINED

Clinical experience reveals that many, and perhaps all, disease states are the expressions of both organic and psychic factors.

René Jules Dubos 1968
(Man, medicine, and environment.
Praeger, New York, p 65)

Commissioning Editor: Michael Parkinson

Project Development Manager: Colin Arthur

Project Manager: Helius, Frances Affleck

Designers: Andrew Jones, Sarah Russell

Illustrator: Ethan Danielson

ALEX J MITCHELL

Formerly, Lecturer in Psychiatry, University of Leeds, UK

Currently, Consultant in Liaison Psychiatry, Leicester General Hospital, UK

Neuropsychiatry and behavioural neurology explained

SAUNDERS

EDINBURGH LONDON NEW YORK PHILADELPHIA ST LOUIS SYDNEY TORONTO 2004

SAUNDERS

An imprint of Elsevier Science Limited

First published 2004

ISBN 0-7020-2688-3

British Library Cataloguing in Publication Data
A catalogue record for this book is available from the
British Library

Library of Congress Cataloging in Publication Data
A catalog record for this book is available from the
Library of Congress

Notice
Medical knowledge is constantly changing. Standard
safety precautions must be followed, but as new
research and clinical experience broaden our
knowledge, changes in treatment and drug therapy
may become necessary or appropriate. Readers are
advised to check the most current product
information provided by the manufacturer of each
drug to be administered to verify the recommended
dose, the method and duration of administration, and
contraindications. It is the responsibility of the
practitioner, relying on experience and knowledge of
the patient, to determine dosages and the best
treatment for each individual patient. Neither the
Publisher nor the author/editor/contributor (delete as
appropriate) assumes any liability for any injury
and/or damage to persons or property arising from
this publication.

The Publisher

WM 220
TL 1921

your source for books,
journals and multimedia
in the health sciences
www.elsevierhealth.com

The
Publisher's
policy is to use
**paper manufactured
from sustainable forests**

Printed in China

Preface

In attempting to answer the question 'What is neuropsychiatry?', there is a danger of falling at the first hurdle. It seems too easy to say that neuropsychiatry concerns the interface of neurology and psychiatry. After all, which neurological condition does not feature a disturbance in mood or psychological distress? By the same token, which psychiatric condition has not been shown to encompass changes in neuroanatomy or neurophysiology at some level? To make this book more useful to clinicians I will define the remit of the book by the question 'What are the psychiatric and behavioural consequences of neurological conditions that affect the brain, and how can these consequences be explained?'

Neuropsychiatry is an exciting and rapidly evolving field. Some consider neuropsychiatry to be a highly specialized and overly complicated area. Yet every psychiatrist, neurologist and primary care physician regularly has contact with patients who suffer from dementia, delirium, stroke and Parkinson's disease, to name a few common presentations. In the course of their illness, the majority of patients with inherited or acquired brain injury will develop a complication involving unwelcome changes in mood, cognition, thoughts or behaviour. For this reason clinicians must be prepared to answer difficult questions, such as: 'Is this patient depressed or is it a behavioural manifestation of their stroke?', 'Should I treat this patient's delirium with atypical antipsychotics?' and 'Why is this patient with Parkinson's disease complaining of visual hallucinations?' The primary aim of this book is to help with these everyday clinical questions and to provide essential information about less common presentations. In attempting to demystify neuropsychiatry I have made great effort to limit information to data collected from robust primary research, a method that invariably leaves some gaps.

With a myriad of unfamiliar terms, neuropsychiatry can be off-putting, especially to trainees. Yet its study is also richly rewarding. It is here that abnormalities of brain structure and function interface with powerful modifying variables such as the individual differences in adjustment to illness. An exploration of neuropsychiatry provides a valuable insight into how regional brain dysfunction influences mood, cognition, motivation and thoughts. This book looks beyond the old dichotomy of functional and organic and attempts to integrate the two components into part of a bigger picture. I hope that this book will appeal to a broad range of clinicians and trainees and particularly to liaison psychiatrists and old age psychiatrists, who are regularly asked to see patients who have underlying neurological illnesses.

Acknowledgements

A single-author textbook is anything but a solo performance. I have been encouraged by three authorities in neuropsychiatry, namely, German Berrios (Cambridge), Alwyn Lishman (London) and Richard Mindham (Leeds).

Many individuals have given material or suggestions (or, more accurately, corrections) during the 3-year production of this book. These include: in general adult psychiatry, Lian Chua (Leeds), Angelica Izquierdo DeSantiago (Leeds), Karel DePauw (Leeds), Johanna Herrod (Bristol), Mahmood Khan (Leeds), Albert Michael (Bury St. Edmonds), David Newby (Leeds), Shubulade Smith (London), Chris Williams (Glasgow); in liaison psychiatry, Manoj Kumar (Leeds), Peter Trigwell (Leeds) and, with special thanks for many years of support, Veronica O'Keane (London); in old age psychiatry, Tim Branton (Leeds), Pratibha Nirodi (Harrogate) and John O'Brien (Newcastle upon Tyne); in neurology, Julián Benito-León (Madrid) Stuart Jamieson (Leeds), Markus Reuber (Sheffield), Cord Spilker (Leeds); in neuropsychiatry, Jonathan Bird (Bristol), Peter Eames (Gwent) and Max Henderson (London); in radiology, Paul Cronin (Leeds); in rehabilitation, Vera Neumann (Leeds) and in psychology, Steven Kemp (Leeds). I am also grateful for the hard work of the production team employed by Elsevier, particularly Colin Arthur, Julie Gorman and Robert Whittle.

Alex J Mitchell

Figure Acknowledgements

Fig. 12.2 reproduced with permission of Gareth Gina, Department of Radiology, Brigham and Women's Hospital, Harvard Medical School, Boston, MA, USA

Figs 29.2, 30.5, 40.6 and 43.1 reproduced courtesy of Dr PK Chandak, Department of Radiology, Brigham and Women's Hospital, Harvard Medical School, Boston, MA, USA

Fig. 4.4 reproduced with permission from Burkitt G, Quick CRG 2001 Essential surgery, 3rd edn. Churchill Livingstone, Edinburgh

Figs 15.1, 19.3 and 29.1 reproduced with permission from Cooke RA, Stewart B 1995 Colour atlas of anatomical pathology, 2nd edn. Churchill Livingstone, Edinburgh

Figs 11.1, 17.5, 43.3 and 56.2 reproduced with permission from Fitzgerald MJT, Folan-Curran J 2001 Clinical neuroanatomy and related neuroscience, 4th edn. Saunders, Philadelphia

Figs 18.1, 18.3, 23.2 and 35.1 reproduced with permission from Haslett C 1999 Davidson's principles and practice of medicine. Churchill Livingstone, Edinburgh

Fig. 4.2 reproduced courtesy of Emma Burton and John O'Brien, Institute for Ageing and Health, University of Newcastle upon Tyne, UK

Fig. 14.2 reproduced with permission of Professor M Mesulam, Feinberg Medical School, Northwestern University, Chicago, IL, USA

Figs 19.4, 30.1 and 43.4 reproduced with permission of Peter Rochford, Museum Curator, James Vincent Duhig Pathology Museum, University of Queensland, Australia

Fig. 4.1 reproduced with permission from Kaufman DM 2001 Clinical neurology for psychiatrists, 5th edn. Mosby, Philadelphia

Fig. 16.1 reproduced with permission from Kerr JB 1999 Atlas of functional histology. Mosby, St. Louis

Figs 21.1, 21.2, 21.5, 32.2, 36.1, 40.4 and 41.1 reproduced with permission of Professor Edward C Klatt, Florida State University, College of Medicine, Tallahassee, FL, USA

Figs 26.2 and 26.3 reproduced with permission from Kumar P, Clark M 1998 Clinical medicine, 4th edn, Churchill Livingstone, Edinburgh

Figs 4.3 and 4.5 reproduced with permission of KA Johnson, Radiology and Neurology, Massachusetts General Hospital, Harvard Medical School, Boston, MA, USA

Figure on page vii reproduced with permission from Richter RW, Richter BZ 2000 Rapid reference to Alzheimer's disease. Mosby, St. Louis

Fig. 23.1 reproduced with permission of James G Smirniotopoulos, Uniformed Services University, Bethesda, MD, USA

Figs 17.1, 17.4, 17.8, 19.1, 20.1, 22.1, 27.2, 31.1, 32.1, 35.2, 40.1 and 42.1 reproduced with permission from Stevens A, Lowe J 2000 Pathology, 2nd edn. Harcourt, St Louis

Figs 20.2, 23.3, 25.1 and 29.3 reproduced with permission from Underwood JCE 2000 General and systematic pathology. Churchill Livingstone, Edinburgh

Figs 35.3 and 35.4 reproduced with permission of Professor K Hegedüs, University of Debrecen, Hungary

Figs 27.3, 29.4, 29.5 and 29.6 reproduced with permission of Professor G Baumbach, Online Virtu-al Hospital, University of Iowa, Iowa City, IA, USA

Fig. 26.6 reproduced with permission of James M Powers, Department of Neurology, University of Rochester School of Medicine and Dentistry, NY, USA

Figs 40.2 and 40.3 reproduced with permission from Schmitt B (ed) 1999 Pathologic basis of disease, 6th edn. Saunders, Philadelphia

Foreword

Neuropsychiatry, once a somewhat small and esoteric subspecialty of psychiatry, has grown tremendously in importance both clinically and as an academic discipline. In this latter guise it has acquired increasing relevance to mental illness generally, in effect bringing the brain back into psychiatry as a worthy and important object of study.

This reawakening of mind–brain relationships is largely due to the astonishing amount we have learned over recent decades in the fields of neurochemistry, neuroendocrinology, neuropharmacology, neuropsychology and neuroimaging. Brain malfunction of one sort or another is now apparent not only with regard to the classic syndromes of delirium, dementia and organic amnesic states, but also in relation to affective disorders and, increasingly, the psychoses and disorders of behaviour.

Neuropathological enquiries, using modern techniques, are beginning to clarify a range of new conditions such as frontotemporal dementia and Lewy body dementia, while HIV- and prion-related disorders have been thrust to the forefront of our attention as critical disorders of the young. In the segment of psychiatry dedicated to the mental health of the elderly, we have seen striking advances in our understanding of the complications of Alzheimer's disease, vascular dementia and Parkinson's disease.

Thus we have entered the new millennium with a 'new' neuropsychiatry, representing a fascinating growth area in which brain malfunction is clearly reinstated as warranting the attention of every practising psychiatrist and clinical psychologist. There has been a corresponding outpouring of research, both fundamental and clinical, and the appearance of several new textbooks in what was once a rather barren field.

The present book aims to review what is currently known in the arena of neuropsychiatry in a manner easily accessible to all. It is concise yet remarkably up to date. In order to make it manageable in size Dr Mitchell has sensibly opted for describing the psychiatric manifestations of common neurological disorders (and what this teaches us about the genesis of psychiatric symptoms) rather than attempting to review every possible aspect of the interface between psychiatry and neurology.

A principal virtue, obvious at the very first glance, is that the book is designed to interest, even to captivate the reader, by its wealth of illustration and tabulation and by the inclusion of summary points and clinical guidelines along the way. The accent throughout is on practical, clinically relevant material. Skilful use is made of present-day techniques in information technology to ensure that the subject is presented here in a user-friendly manner.

I have found the book appealing as well as informative. Unlike most authors of substantial medical texts, Dr Mitchell is still close enough to his own learning experience to appreciate the value of attractive presentation in holding the attention of those engaged in absorbing new and sometimes complex information. The reader can be assured that here they will encounter not only a sound and comprehensive text, but also one that will carry them on an enjoyable journey to greater understanding.

WA Lishman
Emeritus Professor of Neuropsychiatry,
Institute of Psychiatry, University of London

How to Use this Book

What style of book would you find most appealing? Clearly it is impossible to know what every reader wants, and therefore I have tried to put together a text in a format that I would most like to read.

I have tried hard to avoid the two major limitations inherent in medical textbooks. The first limitation is that textbooks tend to cover a large area too superficially. Consider how many times you have read that memory loss is a common complication of head injury or stroke. I challenge the reader not to accept these kinds of oversimplification, but to ask what type of memory loss occurs and in what circumstances. Only by questioning the status quo will progress be made in patient care. The second limitation is that textbooks are about 6 months out of date by the time they come to press. I am confident that the book is up to date as of the beginning of 2003 (see Appendix VI). In the fast-moving field of neuropsychiatry it is inevitable that new developments and discoveries will be made. The impact of which will inevitably enhance, challenge or in some cases make obsolete 'facts' as they stand today.

One of the strengths of this book is the visual aids designed to interest the reader and to enhance learning. We all have a limited attention span for novel material, but charts, figures and tables help to avoid boredom setting in. Practical clinical aspects are highlighted in clinical pointers with their own source of recommended reading. Many lists are presented as text boxes. For continuity, the reader may find it helpful to refer to the views of the brain shown in Figures II.1 and 4.7. I quote only the most important and robust of individual studies, but I am happy to provide additional references if required. I also welcome comments, suggestions or corrections at: research@doctors.org.uk.

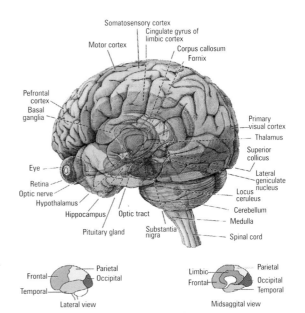

From Richter & Richter (2001).

This book is divided into five main sections. Section I discusses the foundations of neuropsychiatry and tools of clinical assessment. Section II provides of summary of the psychiatric complications of neurological disease. Where the literature allows, I have attempted to use the same format under each condition. In Section III, dementia and delirium are dealt with separately in accordance with the division of services in many countries. In Section IV important treatment trials relevant to neuropsychiatric disorders are reviewed. This section is more detailed than others, as dictated by the principles of critical appraisal. In Section V the information from the preceding chapters is brought together to give the reader a coherent overview of the mechanisms underlying the neuropsychiatric complications of neurological disease. To many this section will be the most interesting, since it provides intriguing clues to the fundamental origin of many psychiatric symptoms and signs.

Finally, consider that patients presenting with neuropsychiatric problems often do not conform to what is written in medical textbooks.

Alex J Mitchell

Abbreviations

In most cases abbreviations are defined at their first usage in a chapter. However, the following common abbreviations have not been defined in the text:

A&E	accident and emergency
AChE	acetylcholinesterase
ACTH	adrenocorticotropic hormone
AIDS	acquired immune deficiency syndrome
AMP	adenosine 3′,5′-monophosphate
BChE	butylcholinesterase
CAG	cytosine, adenine, guanine
CNS	central nervous system
CSF	cerebrospinal fluid
CT	computed tomography
DNA	deoxyribonucleic acid
DOPA	L-3,4-dihydroxyphenylalanine
DSM-III	Diagnostic and Statistical Manual, 3rd edition
DSM-IV	Diagnostic and Statistical Manual, 4th edition
ECG	electrocardiogram
ECT	electroconvulsive therapy
EEG	electroencephalograph
EMG	electromyogram
ESR	erythrocyte sedimentation ratio
GABA	γ-aminobutyric acid
HIV	human immunodeficiency virus
ICD	International Statistical Classification of Diseases
IgG	immunoglobulin G
IgM	immunoglobulin M
IQ	intelligence quotient
MRI	magnetic resonance imaging
NHS	National Health Service
PANDAS syndrome	paediatric autoimmune neuro-psychiatric disorders associated with streptococcal infections
PET	positron emission tomography
REM	rapid eye movement
SPECT	single photon emission tomography
SQUID	superconducting quantum interference device
TORCH infections	toxoplasmosis; other infections (e.g. hepatitis b, syphilis, and herpes zoster); rubella; cytomegalovirus; herpes simplex

Contents

Principles of Clinical Neuropsychiatric Assessment

This section is about the tools of clinical assessment. The most important tool is your knowledge and experience. The basic premise of the medical history is to elicit information that you evaluate for its degree of clinical significance. History-taking skills are really no different in neuropsychiatry from those in any other branch of medicine where symptoms are complex and distressing – but bear in mind two caveats. First, patients do not wish to volunteer embarrassing symptoms such as sexual dysfunction, social disability and psychiatric experiences to you, a stranger. For this reason, clinicians should be prepared to spend more time with such patients than is conventionally allocated in medicine. Secondly, the process of taking the history should reveal much about a patient's higher function, and their beliefs about and their understanding of their illness.

The approach to a patient with a suspected neuropsychiatric problem is rather like the approach to a puzzle. You begin by skilfully documenting symptoms and signs in accordance with what you know about the psychopathology of neurological and psychiatric diseases. Information about how the condition developed with time, its modifying variables (see Ch. 68, Box 68.1 and Fig. 67.1) and its previous

incarnations help to form a short differential diagnosis. Mental state and physical and neurological examinations should clarify a preferred diagnosis. Carefully considered investigations (including talk-

---

Box I.1   Ten maxims of neuropsychiatry

- Any significant lesion to the brain can cause diverse neuropsychiatric complications
- Predicting which neuropsychiatric complication(s) will develop after brain injury is difficult
- Psychological symptoms may manifest before neurological symptoms of neurological disease
- The relationship between neuropsychiatric complication(s) and health-related disability is not simple
- Most neuropsychiatric complications go unrecognized and untreated
- Treatment of secondary psychiatric complications is similar to treatment of primary psychiatric disorders
- Neuropsychiatric complications affect neurological recovery and mortality
- Neurobiological markers are the same in primary and secondary psychiatric disorders
- Neuropsychiatric complications arise from a combination of organic and non-organic factors
- Neuropsychiatric complications dramatically affect quality of life (QoL)

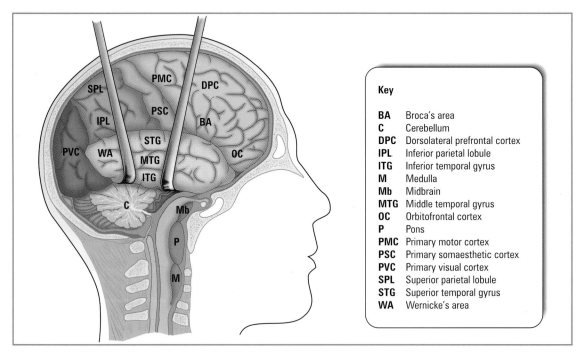

Key

BA	Broca's area
C	Cerebellum
DPC	Dorsolateral prefrontal cortex
IPL	Inferior parietal lobule
ITG	Inferior temporal gyrus
M	Medulla
Mb	Midbrain
MTG	Middle temporal gyrus
OC	Orbitofrontal cortex
P	Pons
PMC	Primary motor cortex
PSC	Primary somaesthetic cortex
PVC	Primary visual cortex
SPL	Superior parietal lobule
STG	Superior temporal gyrus
WA	Wernicke's area

Fig. I.1   Schematic view of the brain, illustrating the major subdivisions.

Table 1.1   Master overview of neuropsychiatric disorders: depression, anxiety, apathy and irritability or anger

Disorder and main region affected	Depression	Anxiety	Apathy	Irritability or anger
Frontal lobe disorders				
Motor neurone disease	+	+	+	0
Normal-pressure hydrocephalus	+	0	+	+
Classical frontotemporal dementia	+	0	+ + +	+ +
Occipital lobe disorders				
Occipital dementia	0	0	0	0
Temporal lobe disorders				
Alzheimer's disease*	+	+	+ +	+ +
Herpes simplex encephalitis	0	0	+	+ +
Temporal lobe epilepsy	+ +	+ + +	0	+
Temporal variant of frontotemporal dementia	+	0	0	+
Transient global amnesia	0	0	0	0
Diencephalon disorders				
Wernicke–Korsakoff syndrome	0	+	0	+
Substantia nigra disorders				
Parkinson's disease	+ + +	+ +	+ +	+
Caudate disorders				
Caudate infarctions	+	0	+	+
Huntington's disease	+ + +	+ +	+ +	+ + +
Neuroacanthocytosis	+ +	0	0	+ +
Progressive supranuclear palsy	+ +	+	+ + +	+
Sydenham's chorea	+	+	0	0
Wilson's disease	+ +	+ +	+	+ +
Globus pallidus disorders				
Carbon monoxide toxicity	+ +	+ +	0	+
Manganese toxicity	+ +	+ +	+ +	+
Postencephalitic parkinsonism	+	0	+ +	+
Thalamic disorders				
Familial fatal insomnia	0	0	+	0
Thalamic infarction	0	0	+ +	+
Variable anatomy				
Brain tumour*	+	+	+ +	+
Neurosyphilis*	+	+ +	+	+ +
Head injury*	+ +	+ +	+ + +	+ +
AIDS dementia*	+	+ +	+ +	+
Lewy body dementia	+	+ +	+	+ + +
Multiple sclerosis*	+ + +	+ +	+	+
Variant Creutzfeldt–Jacob disease	+ +	+ +	+ +	+ +
Stroke*	+ + +	+ +	+ +	+ +
Tourette's syndrome	+ +	+ +	+	+ +
Vascular dementia*	+ + +	+	+ +	+ + +

0, Not significant; +, mild; + +, moderate; + + +, severe
*Complications highly dependent on subtype and/or regional effects

Table 1.2 Master overview of neuropsychiatric disorders: psychosis, cognitive deficit, obsessive–compulsive disorder (OCD) and personality change

Disorder and main region affected	Psychosis	Cognitive deficit	OCD	Personality change
Frontal lobe disorders				
Motor neurone disease	0	+ +	0	+
Normal-pressure hydrocephalus	0	+ +	0	+
Classical frontotemporal dementia	+	+ + +	+	+ + +
Occipital lobe disorders				
Occipital dementia	0	+	0	+
Temporal lobe disorders				
Alzheimer's disease*	+ + +	+ + +	0	+ + +
Herpes simplex encephalitis	+ +	+ + +	0	+ +
Temporal lobe epilepsy	+ + +	+	+	0
Temporal variant of frontotemporal dementia	+	+ +	+ + +	+ +
Transient global amnesia	0	+ +	0	0
Diencephalon disorders				
Wernicke–Korsakoff syndrome	0	+ + +	0	+
Substantia nigra disorders				
Parkinson's disease	+ + +	+ +	0	+
Caudate disorders				
Caudate infarctions	0	+	+ +	+
Huntington's disease	+ +	+ + +	+	+ +
Neuroacanthocytosis	0	+ +	+	+ +
Progressive supranuclear palsy	+	+ +	+	+ +
Sydenham's chorea	0	0	+ + +	+
Wilson's disease	+	+	0	+
Globus pallidus disorders				
Carbon monoxide toxicity	0	+	+ +	+
Manganese toxicity	+	+ +	+	+ +
Postencephalitic parkinsonism	0	+	+	+ + +
Thalamic disorders				
Familial fatal insomnia	+	+	0	+ +
Thalamic infarction	0	+ +	0	+
Variable anatomy				
Brain tumour*	+	+ + +	+	+ + +
Neurosyphilis*	+	+ +	0	+ +
Head injury*	+	+ +	+	+ + +
AIDS dementia*	+	+ + +	0	+ +
Lewy body dementia	+ + +	+ + +	0	+
Multiple sclerosis*	+ +	+ +	0	+
Variant Creutzfeldt–Jacob disease	+ +	+ + +	0	+ +
Stroke*	0	+ +	0	+ +
Tourette's syndrome	0	0	+ + +	+
Vascular dementia*	+ +	+ + +	0	+

0, Not significant; +, mild; + +, moderate; + + +, severe
*Complications highly dependent on subtype and/or regional effects

Clinical Pointer I.1

Revealing a diagnosis and breaking bad news

This is one of the areas in medicine where it is frequently reported that, as clinicians, we must do better. Fortunately, old practices of giving patients misinformation or no information at all are fading. Most patients want to know a great deal about their illness, even though their initial reaction to that news may be intense distress or anger. It is often a fear of that reaction that prevents the medical professional giving an honest opinion, yet it is wise to remember that it is the patient and their family that must live with the consequences of the illness, not the doctor. It is usually not appropriate to give information solely to relatives in the hope of somehow protecting the patient from bad news (unless the patient is incapable of understanding basic information). In reality, the bad news is the suffering that the illness causes, not the diagnosis itself. Appropriate information, guidance and support will help ease suffering, and in this respect patient-led groups can be used to great advantage.

However, even with these sound principles, we can all find the practical process of breaking bad news difficult. One reason for the difficulty is that time spent with patients is often so limited that communicating important information is compressed into an unrealistically short time. Breaking bad news (such as revealing a diagnosis of motor neurone disease or dementia) should be seen as a process with the following basic steps:

- *Preparation.* What are the patient's current expectations and understanding of the situation?
- *Setting.* How can this consultation be as comfortable as possible for the patient? Is a family member present? Are you free from interruptions?
- *Disclosure.* Telling the key points in plain language, without euphemisms and with sensitivity.
- *Discussion.* Discussing the alternatives or uncertainties with the information put forward.
- *Questions.* Offering to answer questions. Patients invariably have some unrealistic, inaccurate or exaggerated health beliefs that they may be afraid to ask about.
- *Action.* The 'bad news' should not be the end of the process, but really the first step. The individual patient then needs to know where to get help (medical and non-medical) should they need it. An offer of follow-up with a member of the team is usually welcome.

In my experience, the multidisciplinary team can be invaluable in this process, but usually the medical consultant must also be involved.

Further reading Girgis A, Sansonfisher RW 1995 Breaking bad news – consensus guidelines for medical practitioners. *Journal of Clinical Oncology* 13:2449–2456
Buckman R 2001 Communication in palliative care. In: Carver A, Foley KM *Neurologic Clinics* 19(4): 989–1004

ing to carers and the primary care physician, examining the medical notes and biomedical investigations) should confirm the diagnosis in most cases. In a minority, reassessment or a second opinion will be required. Treatment begins from the moment you meet the patient, in forming a therapeutic relationship, starting the process of education and involving the patient in therapeutic options and self-help strategies.

Throughout this book, certain themes are played out repeatedly. I have attempted to collect the most con-sistent themes together in the form of ten maxims in neuropsychiatry (Box I.1). At the end of the book, I have collected together evidence that supports these statements (see Ch. 82).

REFERENCES AND FURTHER READING

Fitzgerald MJT, Folan-Curran J 2001 Clinical neuroanatomy and related neuroscience, 4th edn. Harcourt, Philadelphia

1

Neuro-psychiatric Epidemiology from a Global Perspective

It is often difficult to look at one's own situation from a truly objective point of view. A case in point is the impact of CNS disease on the population at the turn of the 21st century. It is important to recognize temporal changes in disease epidemiology that have occurred with time because this will help to predict changes in the future. It is also vital to recognize the burden of disease that exists in other parts of the world, especially in developing countries (National Academy of Sciences' Institute of Medicine 2001).

MORTALITY AND LONGEVITY

For thousands of years life expectancy was less than 40 years. This changed dramatically in the mid-19th century with improvements in housing, sewage disposal and availability of fresh food and water (Fig. 1.1). Within 100 years antibiotics were in use. Comparing 1965 with 1995 reveals some interesting findings. In 1965, about 40% of the world's population died before the age of 5 years and only 10%

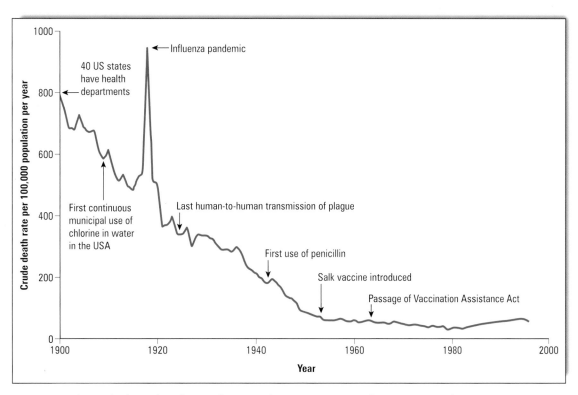

Fig. 1.1 Decline in death rate for infectious diseases in the USA since 1990. After Armstrong et al (1999).

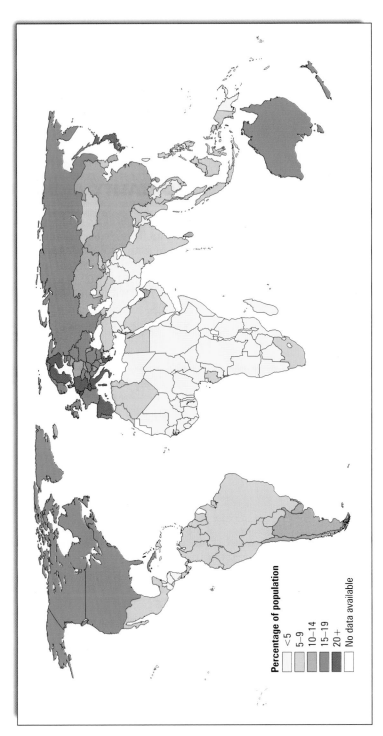

Fig. 1.2 Percentage of the population estimated to be aged above 65 years by the year 2020.

reached the age of 75 years. In 1995, the death rate up to age 5 years and the death rate at 75 years or older were 25%. The World Health Organization predicts that, by 2025, 40% of the world's population will survive to 75 years and only 10% will die before the age of 5 years – in effect a mirror image of the 1965 figures. During the 20th century, advances in perinatal care, management of the complications of labour and control of associated infectious diseases led to a reduction in infant mortality from 160 per 1000 live births in 1900 to 6 per 1000 in 1999 (UNICEF). The result of these changes has been a population explosion. Looking forward, improvements in the control of acute (infectious) diseases will continue in the developing world. This will be followed by a further increase in the proportion of people who survive to old age – an estimated 50% increase in the population of the developed world between now and 2025 and a 100% increase in the population of the developing world over the same period. Current life expectancy in developed countries is close to 84 years for women and 79 years for men. Thus, the majority of illnesses in the developed world are the chronic diseases of middle and old age.

In order to predict the impact on services, consider the number of people who are aged over 65 years. At the turn of the 20th century, 5% of the population of the USA were aged over 65 years – that is 3 million people. One hundred years later this proportion has tripled to 15%, and the raw numbers are 10-fold greater (owing to the additive effect of population growth). There are now more than 33 million people aged over 65 years in the USA. This effect will replay in the developing world during this century (see Fig. 1.2).

Table 1.1 Worldwide annual mortality figures

Cause of death	Number of deaths (millions)
Coronary heart disease	7.2
Cancer	6.3
Stroke	4.6
Acute lower respiratory infections	3.9
Tuberculosis	3.0
Chronic obstructive pulmonary disease	2.9
Diarrhoea or dysentery	2.5
Malaria	2.1
HIV infection and AIDS	1.5
Hepatitis B	1.2

DISABILITY

So what are the current major causes of illness? The first point to make is that life expectancy is not the same as health expectancy. On average, at the age of 65 years men can expect 8 years of disability-free life and women 10 years of disability-free life. Years of healthy life lost as the result of a disability represent about 18% of total life expectancy in the least developed countries and about 8% in the countries with the highest healthy life expectancies (Mathers et al 2001). In the USA the prevalence of disability in those aged over 65 years is 20% (Manton & Gu 2001). To examine the contribution of illness to disability, a recent concept is that of disability-adjusted years.

The Global Burden of Disease Study was launched in 1992 to develop an objective measure of the burden of disease. Two measures were introduced. Healthy years lost from disability (YLD) is a measure of premature poor health. Healthy years lost from disability added to years lost from mortality (years of life lost (YLL)) forms the composite measure of disability-adjusted life years (DALYs), or the total years of life lost as the result of a disease. Non-communicable diseases account for 79% of the disability-adjusted life years lost, with the single largest contributor being ischaemic heart disease (Fig. 1.3). Neuropsychiatric disorders and mental health problems account for more than 23% of DALYs and 30% of the YLDs (Schopper et al 2000).

The most informative study on the nature and frequency of chronic disease was undertaken by Dr Colin Mathers from the Australian Institute of Health and Welfare, and the two project teams who produced the Victoria Burden of Disease Study (Public Health Division, Department of Human Services 2001). This study examined disability, impairment, injury and mortality arising during 1996 from 176 common diseases in the state of Victoria (population 4.5 million). This study confirmed that mental and neurological conditions contribute more than any other category to years lost through disability (two-fifths of the total in men and one-half of the total in women). Depression is the single most common cause of years lost due to disability, followed by dementia.

Measures of disability in the developed world include rates of institutionalization and rates of required assistance, if living independently. Although only about 10% of the non-institutionalized elderly require assistance with basic activities of daily living, about one-quarter require help with more complex instrumental activities of daily living and one-quarter require help with personal activities of daily living (Steen et al 2001). Half of the oldest old (85 years or older) require daily assistance and a quarter require full-time care.

Lifestyle and risk factors

Risk factors are an important determinant of premature disability and death. In the Victoria Burden of Disease Study, smoking contributed 10% of total DALYs and physical inactivity, high blood pressure and obesity each contributed 5%. High cholesterol, poor diet and illicit drug use contributed about 2% of total DALYs. This may not sound like much, but only one disease also accounted for more than 5% of total DALYs – ischaemic heart disease (Table 1.2).

The quoted rates of institutionalization and disability are not static but in a state of flux, varying over time. On an individual basis risk factors are important modifiable variables that determine morbidity

Table 1.2   Ranked DALYs in Victoria, Australia, 1996 (both sexes)

Disease	DALYs (% total)
Ischaemic heart disease	11.96
Smoking	9.8
Physical inactivity	6.6
High blood pressure	5.8
Obesity	4.7
Dementia	3.78
Depression	3.76
Lung cancer	3.75
Poor diet	2.8
High cholesterol	2.1
Illicit drugs	1.8

Adapted from Public Health Division, Department of Human Services (2001)

and mortality. For example, in one 15-year follow-up study of 7142 healthy middle-aged men (Wannamethee et al 1998), the probability of surviving free of vascular events and diabetes ranged from 89% for a moderately active man aged 50 years with

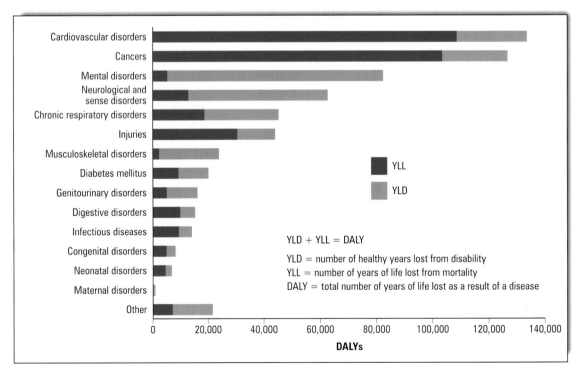

Fig. 1.3   Burden of neurological disease by sex, Victoria, Australia, 1996. Data from Public Health Division, Department of Human Services (2001).

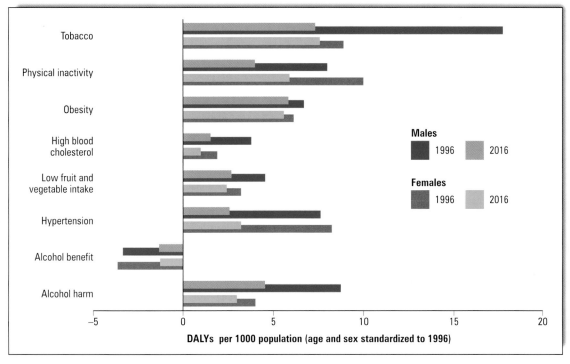

Fig. 1.4 Rates of DALYs attributed to selected risk factors in Victoria, Australia, 1996, projected to 2016. Although this study predicts an improvement in most risk factors by 2016, other studies anticipate a disturbing rise in inactivity and obesity in both the developing and the developed world.

Table 1.3 Ranked worldwide causes of disability

Disease	% of all disability	Disease	% of all disability
Acute lower respiratory infections	7	Alcohol dependence	1.3
HIV infection and AIDS	6	Bipolar affective disorder	1.1
Diarrhoeal diseases	5	Cirrhosis	1.1
Unipolar major depression	4	Osteoarthritis	1.1
Ischaemic heart disease	4	Homicide and violence	1.0
Childhood diseases	3.8	Drowning	0.9
Cerebrovascular disease	3.5	Tropical diseases	0.9
Malaria	3.1	Asthma	0.9
Road traffic accidents	2.8	Psychoses	0.8
Chronic obstructive pulmonary disease	2.6	Tetanus	0.8
Tuberculosis	2.3	Obsessive–compulsive disorder	0.8
Falls	2.1	Diseases of the trachea, bronchus or lung	0.8
Measles	2.0	Nephritis or nephrosis	0.8
Anaemias	1.8	Pertussis	0.8
Self-inflicted injuries	1.7	Fires	0.7
Unintentional injuries	1.4	Alzheimer's disease and other dementias	0.7
Sexually transmitted diseases (excluding HIV infection)	1.4		

a body mass index of 20–24 kg/m^2 who had never smoked to 42% for an inactive smoker with a body mass index of more than 30 kg/m^2.

Projected burden

The influence of a reduction in infant mortality and an increase in longevity upon current disease burden has already been mentioned. What pattern is predicted in developed economies? Such estimates are extrapolations of existing trends and therefore are not 'written in stone'. Nevertheless, these projections make fascinating reading. The Melbourne group predict a 32% drop in total mortality and a smaller 7% drop in morbidity over the next 20 years. This is largely as a result of improvements in care of ischaemic heart disease and stroke, and may also result from improvements in reversible risk factors (Fig. 1.4). Contrary to this trend, dementia DALYs are predicted to rise by a massive 68% in women (although only 4% in men). This will take dementia into the lead as the largest single cause of ill health by the year 2016.

REFERENCES AND FURTHER READING

Armstrong GL, Conn LA, Pinner RW 1999 Trends in infectious disease mortality in the United States during the 20th century. JAMA 281:61–66

Mathers CD, Sadana R, Salomon JA et al 2001 Healthy life expectancy in 191 countries, 1999. Lancet 357:1685–1691

Manton KG, Gu XL 2001 Changes in the prevalence of chronic disability in the United States black and nonblack population above age 65 from 1982 to 1999. Proceedings of the National Academy of Sciences USA 98:6354–6359

Murray CJL, Lopez AD 1977 Global mortality, disability and the contribution of risk factors: global burden of disease study. Lancet 349:1463–1442

National Academy of Sciences' Institute of Medicine 2001 Neurological, psychiatric, and developmental disorders: meeting the challenge in the developing world. Available: http://www.iom.edu/iom/iomhome.nsf/WFiles/Nervous4pager5–1/$file/Nervous4pager5–1.pdf

Public Health Division, Department of Human Services 2001 Victoria burden of disease study: morbidity. Department of Human Services, Melbourne. Available: http://www.dhs.vic.gov.au/phd/9909065/index.htm

Schopper D, Pereira J, Torres A et al 2000 Estimating the burden of disease in one Swiss canton: what do disability adjusted life years (DALY) tell us? International Journal of Epidemiology 29:871–877

Steen G, Sonn U, Hanson AB et al 2001 Cognitive function and functional ability. A cross-sectional and longitudinal study at ages 85 and 95 in a non-demented population. Aging: Clinical and Experimental Research 13:68–77

Wannamethee SG, Shaper AG, Walker M et al 1998 Lifestyle and 15-year survival free of heart attack, stroke, and diabetes in middle-aged British men. Archives of Internal Medicine 158:2433–2440

World Health Organization 1977 Conquering suffering, enriching humanity. World Health Organization, Geneva

2

Mental State Examination

Clinical assessment requires skills from general medicine, neurology and psychiatry. Examination of higher function and, in particular, psychiatric symptoms and signs is known as the mental state examination. It is not immediately obvious how 'higher function' should be classified (Fig. 2.1). *Cognition* concerns the largely conscious process of thinking and information manipulation in order to alter responses in the light of environmental experiences. *Mood* describes prevailing emotions associated with certain basic responses (such as defeat, attack, defence and reward) that act as a feedback mechanism to reinforce associated behaviours. Mood disorders are too often discussed rather simplistically in terms of depression, euphoria and anxiety – with other emotions (such as irritability, anger, disgust, jealousy and surprise) almost totally ignored. In close proximity to changes in mood lie changes in drive or *motivation*. Excess drive is sometimes seen in combination with high mood (mania), but more often low drive and lack of emotional interest is seen in depression. Changes in motivation are usually represented by changes in interaction with the environment. This could be referred to as *complex behaviour*. Intact, logical thought processes are taken for granted, but problems at the interface between the concept of self and one's interpretation of the world can give rise to the dramatic presentation of *psychosis*, with its delusions, hallucinations and breakdown of logical thought form.

As with the neurological examination, it takes practice to carry out a competent mental state examina-

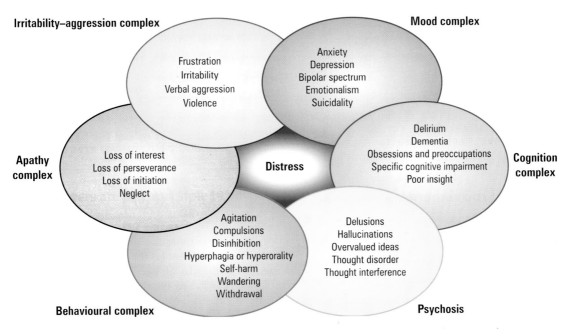

Fig. 2.1 Schema of neuropsychiatric symptoms and syndromes. This figure presents a conceptual overview of common presenting problems in neuropsychiatry. Certain symptoms tend to occur together and can be grouped in syndromes or clusters. Symptoms have particular importance in neuropsychiatry because even specific symptoms occurring in isolation following acquired brain injury can still cause significant distress or dysfunction.

tion. Nevertheless, the clinician's instincts about a patient's prevailing mood or level of behavioural disturbance is often accurate. A clinical assessment can and should be performed even if the patient is unco-operative or has reduced consciousness.

Whilst making the assessment it is wise to keep in mind these key questions:

- What are the current symptoms and signs?
- Why is the person presenting today with these problems?
- What are the most likely causes for this presentation?
- How can I help?

APPEARANCE AND BEHAVIOUR IN PATIENTS WITH ORGANIC ILLNESS

A surprising amount can be gained by taking the time to inspect the appearance of a patient for a few seconds. The demeanour of a patient with severe depression is unmistakable. Similarly, patients with mania, anxiety, delirium and dementia all present with their own characteristic appearances. A poor level of self-care is an important indicator of the inability to manage activities of daily living. This is particularly apparent in depression and dementia. Disturbances in behaviour may be categorized using the dimensions of neglect, agitation and apathy (see Fig. 40.10). Agitation refers to overactivity, restlessness and often hostility associated with anxious, irritable or aggressive mood. Apathy also has a strong mood component. Changes in activity (e.g. abnormal movements) are usually described using the term 'behaviour', as are more complex changes which merge with changes in personality.

Abnormal movements

Abnormal movements are a vital clue to underlying pathology. By convention they are often included in the mental state examination. They can be classified into volitional or non-volitional and purposeful or non-purposeful (Fig. 2.2). Most focal abnormal movements arise from disorders of the basal ganglia and related structures. Exceptions include myoclonus, tics and some types of tremor (Box 2.1).

Chorea is an involuntary irregular jerky movement that follows a random, changing pattern. *Athetosis* is slow, writhing (serpentine-like) movements, often

---

Box 2.1   Anatomical associations of abnormal movements

- Ballism: subthalamic nucleus
- Bradykinesia: substantia nigra
- Chorea: caudate nucleus
- Dysmetria: cerebellum
- Dystonia: putamen
- Intention tremor: cerebellum
- Myoclonus: cortex, brainstem, spinal cord
- Rest tremor: substantia nigra

---

in the upper limbs. Chorea and athetosis are worsened by anxiety and alleviated by sleep, a pattern also seen in patients with psychomotor agitation. Chorea can sometimes be recognized by failure to sustain a contraction (motor impersistence). Chorea is caused by any condition that affects the caudate nucleus of the basal ganglia. Presentation in childhood with a history of arthritis or carditis would suggest Sydenham's chorea. In mid-life, a presentation with no previous family history suggests a drug-induced cause or an undiagnosed medical illness such as AIDS, systemic lupus erythematosus, hyperthyroidism or Wilson's disease. In the elderly senile chorea or basal ganglia infarction are possibilities. Occasionally, it has been found that Huntington's disease presents without a family history. These are cases in which the father of the patient had a subclinical premutation.

Dystonia refers to the tonic contraction of a muscle group leading to sustained uncomfortable posture. Dystonia may be focal, involving a single body part (e.g. torticollis, scoliosis), segmental, involving adjacent body parts, or generalized (opisthotonus). Dystonia is most commonly seen as a consequence of an adverse drug event, but persistent dystonia can occur with a wide variety of inherited and degenerative disorders (Box 2.2). Dystonia associated with degenerative disease is more likely if there is dystonia at rest, hemidystonia and accompanying neurological signs.

Myoclonus is a muscular jerk that may be localized or diffuse. It is seen on the EMG as a brief burst of activity lasting 10–50 ms. It can arise from lesions in the cortex (cortical myoclonus), brainstem (palatal and ocular myoclonus) or spinal cord (segmental and propriospinal myoclonus). Cortical myoclonus is usually betrayed by the presence of giant somatosensory evoked potentials. It can occur in isolation in the form of either essential myoclonus or physiological myoclonus, although it

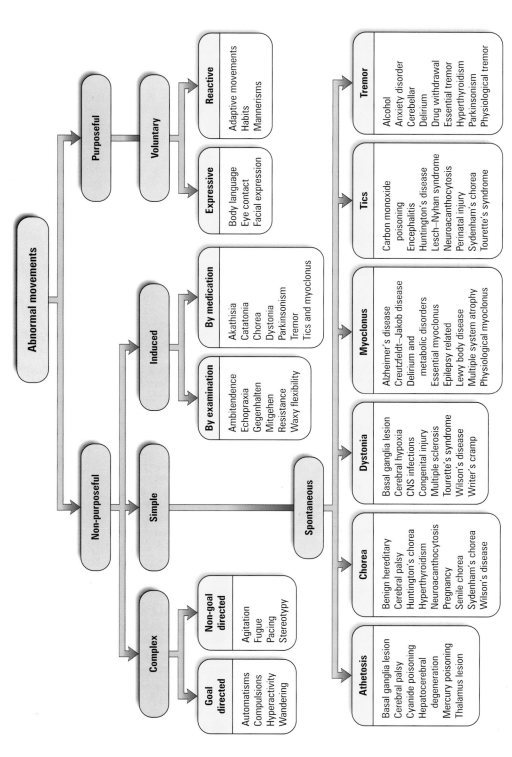

Fig. 2.2 Schema of abnormal movements. Detailed examination of patients presenting with unusual movements helps narrow the differential diagnosis to a handful of likely disorders.

is most commonly encountered in delirium, particularly in the metabolic encephalopathies. More unusually, a brief absence period of electrical activity can occur, typically causing flexion of outstretched wrists. This is known as asterixis or negative myoclonus. Dementia with myoclonus raises several important differential diagnoses, including Creutzfeldt–Jakob disease and late stages of dialysis dementia, AIDS dementia and Alzheimer's disease. Myoclonus and parkinsonism occurs in about 20–30% of patients with Lewy body dementia and also in multiple system atrophy, but not in idiopathic Parkinson's disease. At the other end of the age spectrum, myoclonus occurs in progressive myoclonic epilepsy and in several childhood epilepsy syndromes.

Parkinsonism refers to a triad of tremor, rigidity and bradykinesia (slowed movements). Three important additional symptoms are poor initiation (akinesia), slowed thoughts (bradyphrenia) and autonomic instability. The causes of parkinsonism are diverse and include degenerative diseases that involve the basal ganglia, metabolic disorders, toxins and drugs (Box 2.3).

Tics are sudden interruptions to normal activity characterized by simple or complex motor or vocal outbursts. Simple tics include blinking, shrugging and twitching. Complex tics include hitting, kicking, jumping and waving. Tics are not always pathological. In childhood, the majority of tics are transient. However, less benign disorders, such as Huntington's disease, head injury, stroke, perinatal injury and carbon monoxide poisoning, can produce tics. Tics also accompany various learning disabilities, including Down's syndrome, fragile X syndrome and the pervasive developmental disorders (see Box 24.1). Tics can be distinguished from vol-

---

Box 2.2   Causes of secondary dystonia

Congenital and perinatal
Kernicterus
Miscellaneous congenital malformations
Perinatal anoxia

Acquired CNS lesions
Basal ganglia infarct or haemorrhage
Head trauma
Hypoxia
Multiple sclerosis
Spinal cord or peripheral nerve injury

Infectious or inflammatory causes
Creutzfeldt–Jakob disease
Reye's syndrome
Systematic lupus erythematosus and antiphospholipid
   syndrome
Subacute sclerosing panencephalitis
Syphilis
Tuberculosis
Viral encephalitis and HIV infection

Neurotoxins
Carbon disulphide
Carbon monoxide
Manganese
Methanol

Adapted from Friedman & Standaert (2001)

Box 2.3   Causes of parkinsonism

Basal ganglia diseases
Tumours
Vascular parkinsonism

Genetic Parkinson's disease
Autosomal-dominant synuclein mutation
Autosomal-dominant UCHL1 (ubiquitin carboxy-terminal
   hydrolase 1) mutations
Autosomal-recessive parkin mutations

Lewy bodies
Idiopathic Parkinson's disease
Lewy body dementia

Degenerative diseases
Alzheimer's disease
Corticobasal degeneration
Hallervorden–Spatz disease
Huntington's disease
Multiple system atrophy
Progressive supranuclear palsy

Infections
Creutzfeldt–Jakob disease
Encephalitis lethargica

Metabolic disorders
Fahr's syndrome
Hypoparathyroidism
Wilson's disease

Drugs and toxins
Antidopaminergic agents
Carbon disulphide
Carbon monoxide
Manganese
MPTP (1-methyl-4-phenyl-1,2,3,6-tetrahydropyridine)
Solvents

Box 2.4 Movement disorders in children and adolescents

Infancy
Childhood athetosis
Lesch–Nyhan syndrome

Childhood
Dopa-responsive dystonia
Dystonia associated with DYT1 gene
Myoclonus from subacute sclerosing panencephalitis
Parkinson's disease
Sydenham's chorea
Tourette's syndrome
Withdrawal emergent dyskinesia

Adolescence
Drug-induced movement disorder
Essential tremor
Juvenile Huntington's disease
Tardive dyskinesia
Wilson's disease

Adapted from Kaufman (2001)

untary movements using electrophysiology, since there is an absence of the pre-voluntary negative potential (Bereitschaftspotential) in true tics.

Tremor is probably the most commonly encountered movement abnormality and is characterized by rhythmic oscillation of a body part. Tremor can occur at rest (a rest tremor) or upon voluntary muscle contraction, usually when resisting gravity (a postural tremor) or upon carrying out a specific action (an intention tremor). A very fast fine tremor (10–14 Hz) is either physiological (i.e. anxiety and stress related) or postural (e.g. in thyrotoxicosis, substance withdrawal, hypoglycaemia, encephalopathy). A slower tremor (5–10 Hz) may be indicative of an essential tremor or senile tremor. A parkinsonian tremor is usually described as a coarse (3–7 Hz) 'pill-rolling' tremor present at rest. The occurrence of tremor at the onset of illness increases the likelihood of Parkinson's disease over the parkinsonian syndromes. The cerebellar tremor is made worse with extremes of movement (rather like the effect of alcohol).

Drug-induced movement disorders

Akathisia is an increasingly recognized and particularly unpleasant adverse effect of antipsychotic drugs. It consists of subjective feelings of inner restlessness and the urge to move, with the need for continuous movements of the legs, pacing and rocking. Antipsychotic-induced akathisia can be classified according to the time of onset in the course of antipsychotic treatment – acute, tardive, chronic or related to withdrawal. Some evidence links akathisia with low serum iron (Clinical Pointer 2.1).

Drug-induced chorea is seen with stimulants, oral contraceptives, levodopa, phenytoin and lithium intoxication (Table 2.1). Tardive dyskinesia (see below) is a form of chorea caused by chronic use of typical antipsychotics, but it is usually distinguished from primary chorea by its orofacial and repetitive pattern.

Dystonia is a frequent acute side effect of treatment with high-potency dopaminergic agents, such as haloperidol, droperidol and levodopa. It can also be

Clinical Pointer 2.1

Distinguishing akathisia and anxiety

Akathisia is one of the most unpleasant movement disorders that occurs (usually) within the first 3 months of drug treatment. The disorder may predispose to tardive akathisia, tardive dyskinesia and higher rates of suicide. There is usually an unpleasant sense of inner restlessness accompanied by a drive to move. By this definition it is clear that akathisia is as much a disorder of mood accompanied by tension-relieving voluntary movements as a movement disorder. It overlaps greatly with the presentation of anxiety disorders. Distinguishing the two conditions is extremely difficult, and this is no doubt one reason why the rate of akathisia has been hard to estimate. Akathisia almost always occurs after an increase in dopamine antagonists. Unlike anxiety, it is often focused on the lower legs (with a description of abnormal sensation) and is not accompanied by a clear set of psychological worries. Patients with akathisia often describe an 'alien' drive to move, despite their ability and desire and suppress it. Asking the patient to move an unaffected body part (activation procedure) has been found by some researchers to improve akathisia and exacerbate agitation, but results are mixed. Ultimately, treatment of 'probable akathisia' may be required to confirm the diagnosis.

Further reading *Cunningham Owens DG 1999 A guide to the extrapyramidal side-effects of antipsychotic drugs. Cambridge University Press, Cambridge*

Table 2.1 Drug-induced movement disorders

Drug	Movement disorder							
	Parkinsonism	Tremor	Ataxia	Chorea	Dystonia	Tics	Myoclonus	Akathisia
Amioderone	+							
Amphetamine (illicit drug)				++				
Antihistamines			+	++				
Antimalarials			+					
Antipsychotics	+++			+	+++	+		+++
Barbiturates		+	+					
Bromocriptine				+	+		+	
Bronchodilators	++							
Caffeine	++							
Calcium channel blockers	+							
Carbamazepine			+	+	+	+		+
Cimetidine	+		++	++	++			+
Cocaine (illicit drug)	++		++	++	++		++	
Ethosuximide							+	
Hypoglycaemic drugs	+							
Levodopa	+		++	+	+	+	+	
Lithium	+	++		++	++		+	
Methyldopa	+			++				
Metoclopramide	++				+++	+		++
Monoamine oxidase inhibitors								
MPTP (illicit drug)	+++							
Oral contraceptive			+					
Pemoline			+					
Phenytoin	+		+	+				
Reserpine	++				++			
Sodium valproate	++				++	+		
Selective serotonin reuptake inhibitors	+	+				++	+	+
Thyroxine	++	++						+
Tricyclic antidepressants	+				+	+	+	

MPTP, 1-methyl-4-phenyl-1,2,3,6-tetrahydropyridine

+, Infrequent; ++, common; +++, very common

caused by anticonvulsants, antidepressants, flecainide and cocaine. The term 'dyskinesia' is often used, meaning a generic movement disorder (including dystonia and chorea). It is noteworthy that 25% of people developed dyskinesia while taking part in long-term trials of levodopa.

Myoclonus can result from treatment with cardiovascular drugs such as calcium channel blockers, drugs with an endocrine action such as bromocriptine and levodopa, anticonvulsants, antidepressants and antipsychotics, opioid narcotics and other miscellaneous compounds, including tryptophan, metoclopramide, bismuth salts and lithium. In psychiatry, myoclonus is an important warning sign of the neuroleptic malignant syndrome and severe forms of the serotonin syndrome.

Parkinsonism is the most common drug-related extrapyramidal side effect and is linearly related to dopamine blockage in the nigrostriatal system. Like akathisia, it has a gradual onset over days or weeks in most people. The features of drug-induced parkinsonism may be slightly different from idiopathic Parkinson's disease – it usually begins with bradykinesia and a postural tremor rather than a resting tremor. There are likely to be cognitive and behavioural effects of drug-induced parkinsonism, but these are poorly described and often clinically overlooked.

Tardive dyskinesia is one of the most important drug-induced movement disorders. It is usually irreversible, but is almost certainly preventable. It is thought to be related to the cumulative burden of antidopaminergic medication and is most often seen after treatment with typical antipsychotics. Doubt has been expressed as to whether 'drug holidays' (i.e. intermittent treatment) positively alters the rate of tardive dyskinesia. Movements are choreiform and involve the face, shoulders and trunk. Sometimes dystonic and tic-like movements appear. Increasing recognition of tardive dyskinesia followed the publication of two large-scale studies of drug-treated patients, showing an unexpectedly high prevalence of tardive dyskinesia (Muscettola et al 1993, Woerner et al 1991). Woerner et al (1991), using the Abnormal Involuntary Movement Scale (see Appendix V) detected a rate of tardive dyskinesia of 1.3% in the healthy elderly without antipsychotic exposure, 5% in the medically ill elderly (again without antipsychotic exposure), but almost 25% in young patients exposed to antipsychotics for varying periods. In a second study of 261 patients

over 55 years of age, Woerner et al (1998) found a rate of tardive dyskinesia of 25% after 1 year of treatment and 53% after 3 years of treatment. Predictors included early extrapyramidal side effects, highlighting a possible means of prevention. From their original study, Woerner et al have published estimates of the risk of tardive dyskinesia given previous lack of exposure. In effect, the longer that tardive dyskinesia has not developed in a person exposed to antipsychotics, the less likely it is to develop. Nevertheless, after 25 years of antipsychotic exposure, the authors estimate that the risk of tardive dyskinesia is 65% (Glazer et al 1993).

Tics can be caused by stimulants and antipsychotics. This is relevant to the treatment of Tourette's syndrome (see Ch. 53). Rarely, tics have been linked with SSRIs and opioids.

Tremor is induced by various psychotropics, the most problematic being lithium and sodium valproate. A special type of tremor of the jaw induced by antipsychotics is called the 'rabbit syndrome'. Other drugs well known to cause tremor include beta-agonists (e.g. salbutamol), theophylline, thyroxine, hypoglycaemics and amiodarone. Abuse of alcohol, amphetamines, caffeine, cocaine and nicotine causes or exacerbates tremor.

PERSONALITY CHANGE IN PATIENTS WITH ORGANIC ILLNESS

To understand personality change one must first understand what is meant by personality. A conventional definition is that personality refers to stable patterns of behaviour that determine the way one relates to the environment. Changes in personality in response to illness are usually first noted by family and friends. Relatives of patients expect that their loved one will behave somewhat differently during a period of acute illness. However, they are not prepared for the enduring changes that result from chronic illness, including impairments in independence, stability, social function and contentment. Relatives may describe these as personality change, but changes in personality are taken to mean more than reversible difficulties in adjustment and coping (see Clinical Pointer 44.2). There is a difference between change in personality traits and the development of an acquired 'personality disorder' with clear associated social dysfunction.

Often it is difficult to single out one particular trait that has changed in response to an acquired brain insult. Indeed, it is usually a combination of changes in mood, cognition and social behaviour that are described crudely as personality change. In recognition of this, DSM-IV has dropped the category of organic personality disorder and replaced it with personality change due to a general medical condition that represents a change from the individual's previous characteristic personality pattern.

MOOD IN PATIENTS WITH ORGANIC ILLNESS

Mood refers to our emotional evaluation of the environment and also that internal milieu which mediates motivation and action. Mood state can be described by its subjective components – tone (character), intensity, duration, reactivity – and by its objective components – associated behaviour and demeanour. Mood is not just low (dysphoric) or high (euphoric), but can be neutral (euthymic), angry, apathetic, apprehensive, anxious, labile, fear-

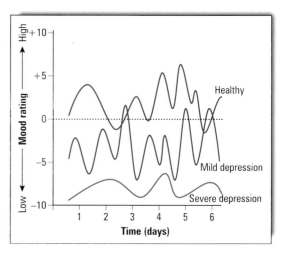

Fig. 2.3 Mood variation in three individuals with depressed mood of different severities.

ful or irritable, often in complex combinations. In depression, mood reactivity is a particularly useful observation (Fig. 2.3). In mild depression, patients are low in mood most days, but can improve with

Table 2.2 Terminology for emotional problems in neuropsychiatry	
Term	Definition
Apathy*	Loss of interest (including emotional interest) and motivation
Alexithymia	Difficulty describing one's emotional state
Anhedonia	Inability to experience pleasure
Catastrophic reaction	Extreme negative emotional and behavioural reaction to a specific stimulus
Dysthymia*	Persistent low mood, often of moderate intensity
Dysphoria	Feeling upset and demoralized, often as a transient reaction to stressful circumstances
Anxiety*	Disabling fearful mood, which is usually recurrent and persistent
Irritability and anger	Feelings of frustration and aggression, usually directed towards family and carers
Mania*	Sustained high mood associated with typical somatic symptoms and overactive behaviour
Pathological laughing or crying (emotionalism)	Sudden intense, unpredictable and uncontrollable laughing or crying, of short duration, and not entirely appropriate to the stimulus
Pseudobulbar affect	Abnormally intense, labile emotion with uncontrollable facial expression in association with lesion of corticobulbar pathways
Depression*	Sustained low mood and/or lack of interest associated with negatively biased cognitions and somatic symptoms

*Refers to both a symptom (e.g. depressed mood) and a syndrome (e.g. depressive disorder)

positive stimuli. In severe depression, even positive experiences cannot pull mood up to a neutral state.

Rapidly changing emotional tone (sometimes defined as *affect*) should be separated from emotions over hours or days (*mood*).

For more than a century many eminent researchers, including Darwin, James, Cannon and Papez, have attempted to find the anatomical substrate of emotion (Arciniegas & Topkoff 2000). This has proven to be an elusive goal, for good reason. It is become clear that emotions do not reside in one discrete anatomical area. Sensory inputs must be evaluated in the context of previous experiences to generate an appropriate emotional output. The amygdala and related limbic areas have an important role in processing sensory information. The most rapid emotional reactions (such as fear, rage or surprise) are integrated with the autonomic 'flight or flight' response, which is reliant on hypothalamus and insular cortex. More complex emotional reactions (such as dysphoria, jealousy or disgust) almost certainly involve cortical areas. Examination of lesions in patients with acquired emotional disorders provides further clues. In 1914, Babinski denoted unawareness of illness or anosognosia in patients with non-dominant (right) hemisphere lesions. This is sometimes called the *indifference reaction*. Patients with non-dominant lesions (and limbic lesions) have been found to be less emotionally expressive when judged by facial expressions, although voluntary facial movement may be preserved (*hypomimia*). They also perform poorly in comprehending or expressing emotionally toned language. In contrast, Goldstein (1952) noted that patients with left-sided lesions were suddenly sad or anxious in response to early signs of failure, a phenomenon he named the *catastrophic reaction*. This reaction is most commonly encountered in patients with Alzheimer's disease (see Ch. 40). Patients with stroke or head injury may also suffer an inability to control anger or dysphoria. This 'impulsivity of mood' has a recognized link with damage to the frontal lobes that causes disinhibition of emotions or a *pseudobulbar affect*. Damage to the orbital surface may produce callous disregard for social convention or emotional blunting. Bitemporal lesions can cause the *Klüver–Bucy syndrome*, with placidity (loss of fear), visual agnosia, hypersexuality and hyperorality (Klüver & Bucy 1937). In humans, one of the best lessons in the role of the temporal lobe in emotion comes from temporal lobe epilepsy, in which ictal changes include fear, anger, aggression, sexual feelings and, occasionally, pathological laughing (gelastic epilepsy) or crying (dacrystic epilepsy).

Apathy is usually considered to be a loss of motivation but this is a simplification of what is a complex problem for many patients (Box 2.5). There is usually a reduction in function (goal-directed behaviour), loss of drive (effort and enthusiasm), loss of attentiveness (goal-directed cognition) and a loss of emotional interest (goal-directed mood). It is not due directly to loss in consciousness, cognition or mood (although these can be major influences). It might be noticed by others as a problem in starting new activities (initiative), with or without a problem in continuing tasks (perseverance). The syndrome of apathy is sometimes referred to as an 'avolitional state' or an *amotivational syndrome*. When severe loss of action occurs, the term *abulia* is used (see Ch. 73). The most extreme form of abulia is akinetic mutism. Neither apathy nor depression are synonymous with fatigue, which implies a limitation in perseverance due to the sensation of tiredness or weakness. However, the boundaries may be blurred in people who do not initiate activities because they have become fatigued in the past (conceptually a form of learned helplessness) (see Ch. 20).

Drug-induced mood disorder

A large number of prescribed drugs have been associated with both depression and mania. Common suspects in depression are anabolic steroids, corticosteroids, calcium channel blockers, cytotoxics, digoxin, and isotretinoin. Reserpine, which depletes monoamines, is of particular note because it is purported to support a monoamine theory of depression. However, the association between reserpine and depressive disorder is being re-evaluated. Mania

---

Box 2.5   Definition of apathy

- Lack of motivation
- One of the following:
  - reduction in goal-directed behaviour (shown by lack of effort or dependency on others)
  - reduction in goal-directed cognition (shown by lack of interest or lack of concern)
  - associated features (blunted affect or anhedonia)
- Symptoms cause problems
- Symptoms not due to impaired consciousness

After Marin (1991)

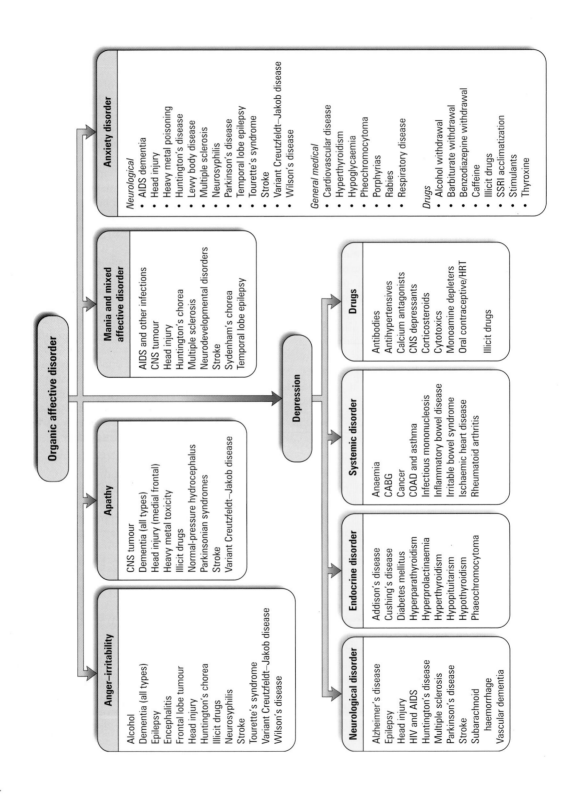

Organic affective disorder

Anxiety disorder

Neurological
• AIDS dementia
• Head injury
• Heavy metal poisoning
• Huntington's disease
• Lewy body disease
• Multiple sclerosis
• Neurosyphilis
• Parkinson's disease
• Temporal lobe epilepsy
• Tourette's syndrome
• Stroke
• Variant Creutzfeldt–Jakob disease
• Wilson's disease

General medical
• Cardiovascular disease
• Hyperthyroidism
• Hypoglycaemia
• Pheochromocytoma
• Porphyrias
• Rabies
• Respiratory disease

Drugs
• Alcohol withdrawal
• Barbiturate withdrawal
• Benzodiazepine withdrawal
• Caffeine
• Illicit drugs
• SSRI acclimatization
• Stimulants
• Thyroxine

Mania and mixed affective disorder

AIDS and other infections
CNS tumour
Head injury
Huntington's chorea
Multiple sclerosis
Neurodevelopmental disorders
Stroke
Sydenham's chorea
Temporal lobe epilepsy

Apathy

CNS tumour
Dementia (all types)
Head injury (medial frontal)
Heavy metal toxicity
Illicit drugs
Normal-pressure hydrocephalus
Parkinsonian syndromes
Stroke
Variant Creutzfeldt–Jakob disease

Anger–irritability

Alcohol
Dementia (all types)
Epilepsy
Encephalitis
Frontal lobe tumour
Head injury
Huntington's chorea
Illicit drugs
Neurosyphilis
Stroke
Tourette's syndrome
Variant Creutzfeldt–Jakob disease
Wilson's disease

Depression

Drugs

Antibodies
Antihypertensives
Calcium antagonists
CNS depressants
Corticosteroids
Cytotoxics
Monoamine depleters
Oral contraceptive/HRT

Illicit drugs

Systemic disorder

Anaemia
CABG
Cancer
COAD and asthma
Infectious mononucleosis
Inflammatory bowel disease
Irritable bowel syndrome
Ischaemic heart disease
Rheumatoid arthritis

Endocrine disorder

Addison's disease
Cushing's disease
Diabetes mellitus
Hyperparathyroidism
Hyperprolactinaemia
Hyperthyroidism
Hypopituitarism
Hypothyroidism
Phaeochromocytoma

Neurological disorder

Alzheimer's disease
Epilepsy
Head injury
HIV and AIDS
Huntington's disease
Multiple sclerosis
Parkinson's disease
Stroke
Subarachnoid
  haemorrhage
Vascular dementia

can be caused by several of the same drugs, including anabolic steroids and corticosteroids. Antidepressant-induced mania and mania associated with stimulant drugs of abuse are also well described. Anxiety is a symptom associated with levodopa, amantadine, sympathomimetics, yohimbine and naltrexone.

PSYCHOSIS IN PATIENTS WITH ORGANIC ILLNESS

Psychosis refers to the presence of one or more the following experiences:

- a fixed, erroneous belief of morbid origin (a delusion)
- a perception without a stimulus (an hallucination)
- disorganized thinking with loosening of logical associations (formal thought disorder).

When psychosis occurs acutely, psychotic symptoms are often florid but superficial (unsystematized) and unstable, and are associated with grossly disturbed behaviour. This is typical of psychosis presenting as a symptom of delirium. Unsystematized delusions and simple hallucinations are also a feature of degenerative disease, although in this case they tend to be relatively stable and integrated into a poor understanding of the environment. Phenomenologically, psychosis occurring in the absence of cognitive impairment may take the form of pure hallucinations or a more complex schizophreniform or affective psychosis (Fig. 2.5).

Fig. 2.4 (opposite) Overview of organic affective disorder. Disorders of affect include depression, mania, apathy, anger–irritability and anxiety. Classification systems have not agreed on the status of mood symptoms that occur secondary to organic disease. DSM-IV includes the category of mood disorder due to a general medical condition (293.83), but for some reason excludes disturbance during the course of delirium or dementia. Such presentations may be much shorter and more unstable than their non-organic counterparts. It is important not to overlook the possibility of disorders of anger, apathy and mania (including mixed affective disorder and hypomania), which have been less intensively studied than depression. CABG, coronary artery bypass graft; COAD, chronic obstructive airways disease; HRT, hormone replacement therapy; SSRI, selective serotonin reuptake inhibitor.

Hallucinations

Hallucinations in the visual, olfactory and gustatory sensory modalities may occur as a direct result of CNS disease. Hallucinations in migraine vary from simple light flashes through scintillating scotomata to fully formed complex visions. The classic hallucination of migraine precedes the headache and may be the dominant aspect of the migrainous attack. The hallucinations are recognized as odd by the patient (i.e. insight is preserved). Patients sometimes describe the classical 'fortification spectra' that looks like a jagged ridge. In narcolepsy, hypnagogic and hypnopompic hallucinations occur. These may be due to an alteration in REM sleep and should be distinguished from other types of hallucinations. Focal seizures may produce hallucinations. Occipital seizures tend to produce simple hallucinations, whereas parietal and temporal foci produce formed hallucinations. Complex partial seizures of temporal lobe, insula or opercular areas can also cause the sensation of odd smells or tastes known as uncinate fits. Ictal hallucinations are typically brief and stereotyped and not lateralized in the visual field. Visual anomalies can occur, such as objects looking small and far away (micropsia), objects looking large and close (macropsia), and visual distortions (metamorphopsia). Three special types of organic hallucinations are of particular interest:

- *Charles Bonnet syndrome*, in which complex visual hallucinations occur in a person with impaired vision but with normal emotional and intellectual functions. Usually, a sharply focused image appears suddenly and involuntarily, without any apparent trigger or voluntary control, then suddenly vanishes (Schultz et al 1996). This was described by Charles Bonnet in 1760 (see Appendix I).
- *Peduncular hallucinosis*, originally described by Lhermitte (1922) and Van Bogaert (1927), in which patients with upper midbrain lesions experience bizarre hallucinations that may have an amusing quality (e.g. of small people in the room – Lilliputian hallucinations); the hallucinations occur in association with sleep disturbance (often in a dream-like oneroid state).
- *Visual release hallucinations*, which occur when damage to the visual pathways results in hallucinations of variable quality that can be influenced by the environmental conditions. Vitreous traction and inflammation of the optic nerves can cause phosphenes or unformed flashes of light.

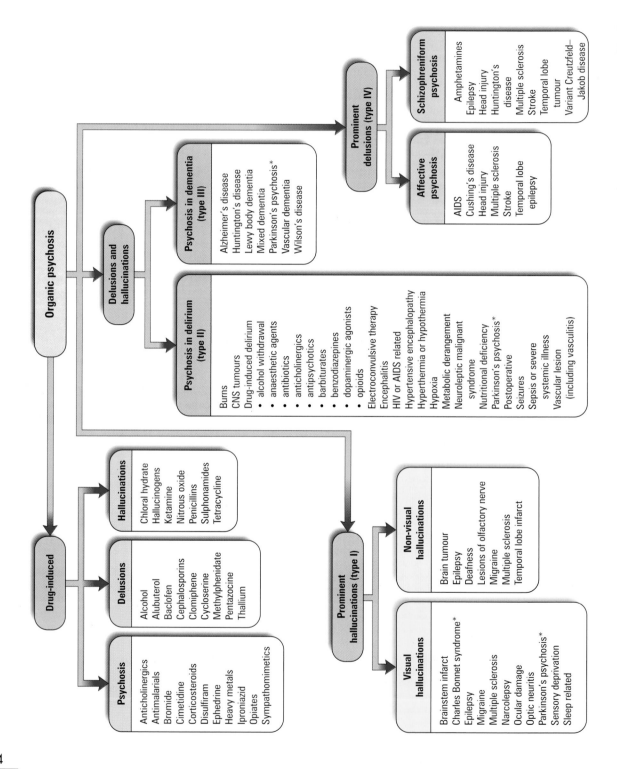

Organic psychosis

Drug-induced

Psychosis
Anticholinergics
Antimalarials
Bromide
Cimetidine
Corticosteroids
Disulfiram
Ephedrine
Heavy metals
Iproniazid
Opiates
Sympathomimetics

Delusions
Alcohol
Alubuterol
Baclofen
Cephalosporins
Clomiphene
Cycloserine
Methylphenidate
Pentazocine
Thallium

Hallucinations
Chloral hydrate
Hallucinogens
Ketamine
Nitrous oxide
Penicillins
Sulphonamides
Tetracycline

Delusions and hallucinations

Psychosis in delirium (type II)
Burns
CNS tumours
Drug-induced delirium
• alcohol withdrawal
• anaesthetic agents
• antibiotics
• anticholinergics
• antipsychotics
• barbiturates
• benzodiazepines
• dopaminergic agonists
• opioids
Electroconvulsive therapy
Encephalitis
HIV or AIDS related
Hypertensive encephalopathy
Hyperthermia or hypothermia
Hypoxia
Metabolic derangement
Neuroleptic malignant syndrome
Nutritional deficiency
Parkinson's psychosis*
Postoperative
Seizures
Sepsis or severe systemic illness
Vascular lesion (including vasculitis)

Psychosis in dementia (type III)
Alzheimer's disease
Huntington's disease
Lewy body dementia
Mixed dementia
Parkinson's psychosis*
Vascular dementia
Wilson's disease

Prominent delusions (type IV)

Affective psychosis
AIDS
Cushing's disease
Head injury
Multiple sclerosis
Stroke
Temporal lobe epilepsy

Schizophreniform psychosis
Amphetamines
Epilepsy
Head injury
Huntington's disease
Multiple sclerosis
Stroke
Temporal lobe tumour
Variant Creutzfeld–Jakob disease

Prominent hallucinations (type I)

Visual hallucinations
Brainstem infarct
Charles Bonnet syndrome*
Epilepsy
Migraine
Multiple sclerosis
Narcolepsy
Ocular damage
Optic neuritis
Parkinson's psychosis*
Sensory deprivation
Sleep related

Non-visual hallucinations
Brain tumour
Epilepsy
Deafness
Lesions of olfactory nerve
Migraine
Multiple sclerosis
Temporal lobe infarct

Delusions

Delusions occur in a variety of neuropsychiatric disorders. In contrast to primary psychiatric illness, these are often isolated experiences with preserved insight. The phenomenology of delusions in organic disease has not been well studied. By convention, delusions are usually classified by content, although the validity of this has never been tested. Delusions of persecution and delusions of ill health are probably the most commonly encountered and in most cases there is no obvious relationship to the nature of the underlying disease. There may be a few exceptions to this rule. In *Anton's syndrome* (see Ch. 15), patients with bilateral occipital pole lesions may be blind, but describe fictitious visual images and deny their blindness. In the neglect syndromes, patients with non-dominant parietal lobe damage may deny hemiparesis (Cummings 1985).

Drug-induced delusions or hallucinations

Perhaps the best example of organic psychosis in the presence of clear consciousness is drug-induced psychosis. Although persistent psychotic experiences after illicit drug use can occur, it is much more common to experience acute intoxication (and to a lesser extent acute withdrawal) psychosis (see Table 36.2). Intoxication is usually associated with high doses of stimulants in young people who are well aware of the psychotic effect. It is important not to overlook unpleasant psychotic experiences induced by prescribed drugs, often in the elderly.

Fig. 2.5 *(opposite)* Overview of organic psychoses. Psychosis can take many forms, but may be broadly divided into those presentations with pure hallucinations, those with pure delusions and those with both delusions and hallucinations. In the context of brain disease, patients with pure hallucinations (type I psychosis) tend to have good insight and often good prognosis. Conversely, mixed delusions and hallucinations can be symptoms of delirium (type II psychosis) or dementia (type III psychosis) and this usually reflects underlying cognitive deficits. Pure delusions in patients without cognitive impairment are suggestive of schizophreniform or affective psychoses. DSM-IV includes the category of a psychotic disorder due to a general medical condition (293.8), but excludes cases in which psychosis occurs exclusively during the course of a delirium.

*See text for details.

Illicit drugs are associated with types of perceptions that are unusual in CNS disease, such as synaesthesia (an hallucination in a different perceptual modality from the stimulus), bizarre illusions involving perceptual distortions, somatic hallucinations such as the sensation that insects are crawling under the skin (formication) or alterations in the sense of time.

COGNITION IN PATIENTS WITH ORGANIC ILLNESS

Cognition is the ability to process (largely subconsciously) and manipulate (largely consciously) information in order to adapt best to changes in the environment. Impaired cognition may be restricted to a specific area, as in amnesia, or include global aspects of cognition, as in dementia. Impaired cognition may also be usefully divided into reversible and non-reversible causes and by those that run an acute versus chronic course. These divisions are an oversimplification of what patients actually suffer in clinical practice (for further discussion see Section III, Introduction).

Cognitive impairment may be broadly divided into four types:

- delirium – global cognitive impairment with an acute onset and impairment of attention or consciousness
- dementia – global cognitive impairment with a gradual onset and a progressive course
- learning disability – cognitive impairment with an onset in early life
- specific cognitive impairment and mild cognitive impairment – neuropsychological impairment insufficient to cause dementia.

Table 2.3 Terminology of cognitive impairment

	Focal	Diffuse
Acute	Amnesia*	Delirium
Chronic, early onset	Specific learning disability	Learning disability
Chronic, late onset	Focal dementia	Classical dementia

*Where memory is involved

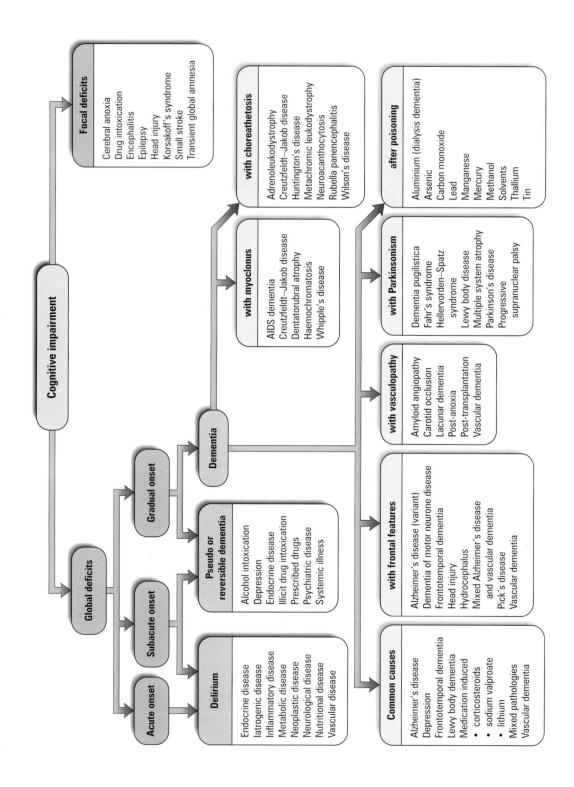

Cognitive impairment

Focal deficits
- Cerebral anoxia
- Drug intoxication
- Encephalitis
- Epilepsy
- Head injury
- Korsakoff's syndrome
- Small stroke
- Transient global amnesia

Global deficits

Acute onset

Subacute onset

Gradual onset

Delirium
- Endocrine disease
- Iatrogenic disease
- Inflammatory disease
- Metabolic disease
- Neoplastic disease
- Neurological disease
- Nutritional disease
- Vascular disease

Pseudo or reversible dementia
- Alcohol intoxication
- Depression
- Endocrine disease
- Illicit drug intoxication
- Prescribed drugs
- Psychiatric disease
- Systemic illness

Dementia

with choreathetosis
- Adrenoleukodystrophy
- Creutzfeldt–Jakob disease
- Huntington's disease
- Metachromic leukodystrophy
- Neuroacanthocytosis
- Rubella panencephalitis
- Wilson's disease

with myoclonus
- AIDS dementia
- Creutzfeldt–Jakob disease
- Dentatorubral atrophy
- Haemochromatosis
- Whipple's disease

after poisoning
- Aluminium (dialysis dementia)
- Arsenic
- Carbon monoxide
- Lead
- Manganese
- Mercury
- Methanol
- Solvents
- Thallium
- Tin

with Parkinsonism
- Dementia pugilistica
- Fahr's syndrome
- Hellervorden–Spatz syndrome
- Lewy body disease
- Multiple system atrophy
- Parkinson's disease
- Progressive supranuclear palsy

with vasculopathy
- Amyloid angiopathy
- Carotid occlusion
- Lacunar dementia
- Post-anoxia
- Post-transplantation
- Vascular dementia

with frontal features
- Alzheimer's disease (variant)
- Dementia of motor neurone disease
- Frontotemporal dementia
- Head injury
- Hydrocephalus
- Mixed Alzheimer's disease and vascular dementia
- Pick's disease
- Vascular dementia

Common causes
- Alzheimer's disease
- Depression
- Frontotemporal dementia
- Lewy body dementia
- Medication induced
  - corticosteroids
  - sodium valproate
  - lithium
- Mixed pathologies
- Vascular dementia

Delirium

The cognitive impairment of delirium is difficult to characterize because it encompasses several overlapping areas, including poor attention and concentration as well as difficulty with registration and retention of knowledge. Clues to the presence of delirium come from the course of the disorder and the presence of likely aetiological factors (e.g. a recent surgical procedure). Cognition in delirium is extremely difficult to assess accurately, owing to lack of cooperation and consent from the patient and the inherently fluctuating course (see Ch. 38).

Dementia

In dementia, as in delirium, the character of the cognitive impairment rarely allows a specific diagnosis to be made. In other words, the underlying cause tends to influence onset and course more than the nature of the cognitive deficits. The majority of causes of dementia are identified through associated features and further investigations. That said, broad patterns of dementia can be delineated, including frontotemporal dementia, cortical temporal–parietal dementia, subcortical dementia and dementia involving multiple regions (multifocal dementia). Certain clinical features should point the clinician towards likely differential diagnoses (see Figs 2.6 and 9.2). For example, the presence of systemic vascular disease and dementia raises the possibility of not only vascular dementia, but also of systemic lupus erythematosus, cranial arteritis, polyarteritis nodosa, vascular Parkinson's disease, cerebral amyloid angiopathy, bilateral carotid occlusion, the MELAS syndrome (mitochondrial ence-phalopathy with lactic acidosis and stroke-like episodes) and the CADASIL syndrome (cerebral autosomal dominant arteriopathy with subcortical infarcts and leukoencephalopathy).

Fig. 2.6 (opposite) Overview of cognitive impairment. Cognitive impairment may be subdivided in a number of ways. Conventionally, conditions causing deficits in isolated domains (such as memory, language, knowledge) are separated from those that eventually impact on every domain (the dementias). In all significant brain disorders, clinicians should specify what specific domains are affected and to what extent. The term 'pseudodementia' is controversial as many causes of pseudo-dementia are not fully reversible. Whether mild cognitive impairment should be classified as a prodrome of dementia or an independent category is not yet clear.

A presentation of dementia with parkinsonism raises the differential diagnoses of idiopathic Parkinson's disease, dementia with Lewy bodies and other rarer parkinsonian syndromes, including intoxication with carbon monoxide, manganese or methanol.

A presentation of dementia and myoclonus should ring warning bells as to the possibility of Creutzfeldt–Jakob disease, dialysis dementia, dementia with Lewy bodies and multiple system atrophy. In childhood, subacute sclerosing panencephalitis, juvenile Huntington's disease and detatorubropallidoluysian atrophy can also present with myoclonus and dementia.

Dementia and ataxia have a differential diagnosis that includes multiple system atrophy, Creutzfeldt–Jakob disease, dementia pugilistica, alcoholic dementia (acquired hepatocerebral degeneration) and intoxication with solvents, lithium or mercury.

Finally, dementia associated with chorea suggests Huntington's disease, Wilson's disease, neuroacanthocytosis or unusual variants of Creutzfeldt–Jakob disease.

Associated clinical features and investigations help distinguish between these possibilities, although in the absence of more specific information – common things occur commonly.

Learning disability

Learning disabilities are much more than cognitive disorders. In most cases the cognitive deficits will be insignificant compared with the social handicap that is often exacerbated by others. Unfortunately the focus of this book must be on the neuropsychiatric aspects. The cognitive impairment seen in people with learning disability (also known as mental retardation) is usually acquired congenitally. In the majority of cases of mild learning disability (an IQ in the range 50–70), no identifiable cause is found (Fig. 2.7 and Box 2.6). There is, however, a familial clustering, suggesting that mild intellectual impairment is largely polygenetically determined.

People with mild learning disability can usually live independently with a normal quality of life. At the other end of the spectrum, there is compelling evidence that people with severe learning disability (an IQ below 35) almost always have acquired a clear insult to the CNS during early development. A specific cause is identified in about 80% of cases, but it is rarely reversible. People with severe learning difficulties are often dependent on carers and have a restricted range of communication, social skills and neurological function. Sufferers with mild or moderate learning disability develop psychiatric complications that are broadly similar to the remainder of the population, although symptoms (more than syndromes) of anxiety, dysthymia and agression are more common. Those with severe learning disability appear less likely to develop (or express) psychosis, obsessions or ruminations, due to restricted symbolic capacity. However, behavioural complications, such as stereotypies, self-injury and hyper-

orality, are common. Sufferers also have problems with adaptive behaviours (difficulty with environmental change) and social functioning. There is the additional psychological impact of living with a learning disability and constantly dealing with prejudice, misunderstanding or discrimination from other people. Consequently, many sufferers report feelings of dependence, low self-esteem, poor coping skills and sensitivity to criticism. Several authors have been developing the theory that individual neurodevelopmental diseases of early life cause recognizable disturbances in personality beyond their effects on cognition alone. This area of research is of considerable interest to those wishing to understand brain– behaviour relationships (see Ch. 77).

People with learning disability are more likely to develop neurodegenerative disease (i.e. very early onset dementia). An example of this is the Alzheimer's dementia that almost invariably develops in sufferers of Down's syndrome who survive to middle age. However, even excluding cases of Down's syndrome, pathologically confirmed dementia is much more common in people with learning disability – reaching over 50% in 50–65 year olds and 75% in 66–75 year olds (Popovitch et al 1990). Examination of clinicopathological relationships in these accelerated degenerative disor-

---

Box 2.6 The ten most frequent causes of learning disability

- Non-syndromal polygenic inheritance
- Down's syndrome
- Perinatal injury (cerebral palsy)
- Unknown intrauterine insult
- Obstetric complication
- Fragile X syndrome
- Foetal alcohol syndrome
- Prematurity
- Intrauterine rubella
- Unknown factors

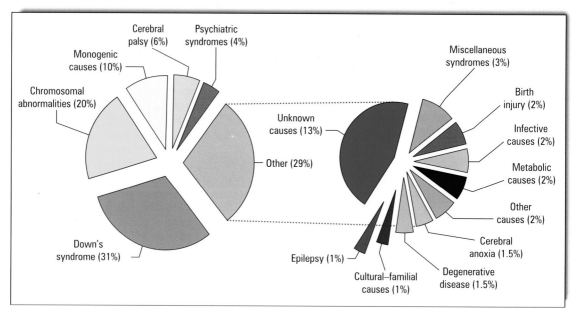

Fig. 2.7 Common causes of severe learning disability in children aged under 16 years. The causes of learning disability are extremely diverse and differ in their age of onset, cognitive profile and, often, behavioural manifestations ('behavioural phenotypes'). Data from Fraser (1997).

Clinical Pointer 2.2

What is paramnesia?

Paramnesia is not memory loss, but false or distorted memory. False memories have recently acquired a bad name, owing to the practice by some psychoanalysts of reconstructing memories for events that never occurred (typically childhood sexual abuse) – of course, there are two sides to this observation. However, there are also a group of paramnesias that are clearly organic in origin. An example is Picks' reduplicative paramnesia in which a person believes that an exact double of a person or object exists somewhere else. In a sense, they have a false memory of having seen this place before, similar to the déjà vu phenomenon but more concrete. More accurate terminology is déjà vu (meaning 'seen it before'), déjà entendu ('heard it before'), déjà pensé ('thought it before') and déjà vécu ('experienced it before'). The opposite phenomenon is jamais vu (or jamais vécu), or the sense of unfamiliarity.

Another example is confabulation in which a person fills in lost details with false memories. Fischer (1995) divided those with confabulation into spontaneous and provoked subtypes, although the supportive evidence for this distinction is weak. But are these disorders of memory (noetic consciousness), belief (a delusion) or affect (sense of familiarity)? Indeed, is it necessary to classify these experiences into one category of psychopathology alone? Whatever their description, patients with temporal lobe or limbic area lesions (possibly more often on the right than left), often in the context of clouded consciousness or arousal, are more likely to describe these experiences.

Further reading   Berrios GE, Hodges JR 2000 Memory disorders in psychiatric practice. Cambridge University Press, Cambridge
Fischer RS, Alexander MP, Desposito M et al 1995 Neuropsychological and neuroanatomical correlates of confabulation. Journal of Clinical and Experimental Neuropsychology 17:20–28

Box 2.7   Childhood-onset learning disabilities that cause dementia in adult life

- Adrenoleukodystrophy (adult form)
- Alexander's disease
- Fabry's disease
- Gangliosidosis 1iii and 2
- Gaucher's disease
- Krabbe's leukodystrophy
- Kuf's disease (adult Batten's disease)
- Lafora's disease
- MELAS (mitochondrial encephalopathy with lactic acidosis and stroke-like episodes)
- MERRF (mitochondrial encephalopathy with ragged-red fibres)
- Metachromatic leukodystrophy
- Neimann–Pick disease, types I and II
- Neuraminidase and β-galactosidase deficiency (Sanfilippo's disease)
- Wilson's disease

ders may have important implications for more mainstream conditions.

Specific and mild cognitive impairment

Certain conditions can cause localized cognitive deficits. Where there is a specific disorder of memory the term *amnestic disorder* is often used. A classic example is *transient global amnesia*, in which an elderly patient suddenly experiences memory loss with difficulty retaining new information and some loss of recent past events along with a sense of bewilderment. This may be precipitated by various types of stress. The amnesia occurs in clear consciousness with preserved non-memory cognitive functions (Box 2.8). An ischaemic interruption to the hippocampus is a possible culprit, even though no association with transient ischaemic attacks has been shown. This presentation differs from a transient ischaemic attack in that there is no alteration in consciousness and there are no neurological signs. The condition is considered benign since recurrence is about 3% a year. Other causes of isolated amnestic episodes are alcohol-related blackouts, concussion after closed head injury and temporary intoxication with drugs such as benzodiazepines (see below). Epilepsy (and electroconvulsive therapy) can cause sudden and brief periods of amnesia even when consciousness is not impaired. This has been labelled *transient epileptic amnesia*.

Many other causes of the amnesic syndrome do not spontaneously remit, and thus leave the sufferer with long-term memory deficits. Herpes simplex encephalitis causes haemorrhages in the medial (and to a lesser extent lateral) temporal lobes, sometimes resulting in permanent amnesia or global dementia (see Ch. 29). Cerebral anoxia affects some vulnerable areas of the brain more than others, with the result of post-anoxic amnesia, dementia or leukoencephalopathy. Carbon monoxide poisoning, attempted hanging, cardiac arrest and anaesthetic complications can all cause cerebral hypoxia. The pathology differs from that seen in stroke, although stroke can cause a relatively isolated amnesia when the lesion affects critical areas such as hippocampus or thalamus. Of course, the classic syndrome associated with a persistent deficit in anterograde memory is the Korsakoff's syndrome, caused by thiamine deficiency (see Ch. 35).

Elderly people who present with subjective memory complaints and evidence of memory decline 1.5 standard deviations (or more) lower than predicted, yet with preserved function, have mild cognitive impairment. As a rule of thumb, their prognosis and pathology lie between the normal elderly and dementia populations (see Clinical Pointer 39.2). Cognitively, this group tends to score borderline on the Mini-Mental State Examination and 0.5 on the Clinical Dementia Rating Scale. Deficits in memory, language and executive function tend to be worse than in patients with age-associated memory impairment (Bartrés-Faz et al 2001).

Drug-induced cognitive dysfunction

Drugs are more commonly responsible for delirium than dementia. In studies of elderly hospital patients, drugs have been reported as the cause of delirium in about 1 in 5 cases and dementia in per-haps 1 in 20 cases. Frequently, a specific agent is not identified, but rather deteriorating higher functions are noted in patients taking a combination of medications. When drugs cause a mild or moderate deterioration in cognitive function, the responsible agent is often overlooked. This is important because memory impairment caused by prescribed medication frequently progresses to dementia if treatment continues unaltered.

Drug-induced delirium

The use of opioid analgesics such as pethidine and morphine are one of the most commonly overlooked causes of delirium in postoperative patients. Hypoxia is probably the other major cause. The actual percentage of patients who experience transient drug-induced delirium postoperatively can only be estimated, but is likely to be at least 30%. A list of drugs implicated in delirium is given in Chapter 38 (see Box 38.3).

Drug-induced dementia

Medication is a contributing variable in small number of patients presenting with dementia. Authors of one study of 308 elderly patients with suspected dementia found that 35 cases were probably drug induced (Larson et al 1987). Drug-induced dementia has special significance because the cause is iatrogenic and reversible. Long-acting steroids and psychotropics are the commonest drugs to cause or

---

Box 2.8   Characteristics of transient amnesias

Transient global amnesia
Sudden onset amnesia lasting 5–10 hours
No loss of consciousness and no focal features
Slow but complete (or near complete) recovery
Severe anterograde amnesia
Variable retrograde amnesia
PET shows hypoperfusion of medial temporal lobes for
    some days
EEG normal

Transient epileptic amnesia
Amnesia occurs following a seizure, but seizure may go
    unnoticed
Amnesia lasts minutes not hours
Moderate anterograde amnesia
Moderate retrograde amnesia
Associated with progressive loss of retrograde
    memory
Routine EEG may be normal, but sleep EEG may be
    abnormal

Box 2.9   Prescribed medication that can cause dementia

High risk
Alcohol
Anticholinergics
Benzodiazepines
Corticosteroids*
Cytotoxics
Opioid analgesics*
Sedating typical antipsychotic drugs

Medium risk
Antiepileptic drugs*
Antihypertensive agents
Dopamine-activating drugs*
Histamine H_2 receptor blockers
Tricyclic antidepressants (high dose)

*Tremendous variability for individual drugs

Clinical Pointer 2.3

The effect of electroconvulsive therapy on memory

Memory difficulties are the most commonly cited problem by patients after ECT. This should not be surprising given that an effect of ECT on memory was recognized over 50 years ago in a series of studies by Irving Janis. Yet this area is still subject to a considerable debate. The argument has become polarized into those who believe ECT is a dangerous treatment causing permanent brain damage and those who believe ECT is an innocuous treatment with no persisting adverse effects at all. Close examination of the evidence shows that neither position is correct. One reason for this controversy is that subjective memory deficits are particularly difficult to measure as the time since ECT increases. The second reason for the controversy is that patients who undergo ECT are already at high risk of cognitive deficits by virtue of their age, psychiatric diagnosis, psychotropic medication and the effect of being acutely unwell. The third reason for the confusion is that clinicians want a simple answer to the simple question of whether ECT affects memory. Unfortunately, a simple yes or no answer is liable to be inaccurate, since amnesic effects depend on the definition used and the time period studied

If one considers the effect of one single seizure upon memory, the argument that ECT causes no memory difficulties is quickly dispelled. Being rendered unconscious, undergoing a generalized seizure and experiencing a period of disorientation interrupts consolidation of memories for at least several hours. Not inconceivably, a relatively brief period of interrupted memory consolidation may translate into a longer period of perceived amnesia. If tested within hours of a seizure, patients have difficulty remembering new information. That is, they have temporary anterograde amnesia. When most people ask whether ECT causes memory difficulties, they are asking whether ECT causes persisting problems in remembering new information. Given that persistent anterograde amnesia has not been clearly associated with ECT, the answer to this question is no. In fact, many persistent memory deficits associated with depression are expected to resolve with effective treatment, and thus anterograde amnesia can actually improve after ECT. When tested later, long after disorientation has passed, patients' memory for personal and impersonal experiences, particularly those that occurred at the time of the treatment, is affected. Their recall is inferior to depressed controls, whose recall is, in turn, inferior to healthy subjects. This is retrograde amnesia. Most patients who stop having ECT and recover from depression note a gradual improvement in recall of past experiences, but some never remember what they did not consolidate properly at the time. This is akin to patients who do not remember a significant family event because they were unwell in hospital at the time, and is quite different from the memory problems in amnesic syndrome, in which the patient is unable to lay down new memories.

There are several predictors of post-ECT amnesia, including pre-ECT cognitive impairment, prolonged post-ictal disorientation, high-dose bilateral ECT and multiple courses of treatment (Sobin et al 1995). In order to elicit informed consent, clinicians must inform patients that, although ECT does not cause a permanent difficulty in committing things to memory, it is likely to cause gaps in their recollection of events close to the time of the ECT. Most people admit that this is a small price to pay in return for the high success rate of ECT when it is appropriately used.

Further reading   *Janis I 1948 Memory loss following electric convulsive treatments. Journal of Personality 17:29–32*
Sackheim H 2000 Memory and ECT: from polarization to reconciliation. Journal of ECT 16:87–96
Sobin C, Sackheim HA, Prudic J et al 1995 Predictors of retrograde amnesia following ECT. American Journal of Psychiatry 152:995–1001

exacerbate dementia. Predisposing factors in drug-induced dementia are old age, pre-existing brain disease, low educational achievement and illicit substance abuse. The elderly are at particular risk because of the likelihood of multiple diseases, polypharmacy and alterations of drug metabolism associated with age.

Whereas drug-induced dementia can often be considered to be a form of dose-dependent CNS toxicity, drug-induced delirium is more likely to reflect either an idiosyncratic response or over-rapid dose titration. Even when there is gradual dose escalation, a reversible dementia may occur. For example, patients may develop tolerance to sedation or constipation induced by typical antipsychotics, but accumulate cognitive impairment with time. Therapeutically, a good rule of thumb is to suggest a medication review and, possibly, a drug-free period if there are subjective side-effects accompanied by any evidence of residual symptoms.

REFERENCES AND FURTHER READING

Arciniegas DB, Topkoff J 2000 The neuropsychiatry of pathologic affect: an approach to evaluation and treatment. Seminars in Clinical Neuropsychiatry 5:290–306

Batrés-Faz D, Jungúe C, López-Alomar A et al 2001 Neuropsychological and genetic difference between age-associated memory impairment and mild cognitive impairment entities. Journal of the American Geriatric Society 49:985–990

Babinski MJ 1914 Contribution à l'étude des troubles mentaux dans l'hémiplégie organique cérébrale (anosognosie). Revue Neurologique 12:845–848

Coker SB 1991 The diagnosis of childhood neurodegenerative disorders presenting as dementia in adults. Neurology 41:794–798

Cummings JL 1985 Organic delusions: phenomenology, anatomical correlations and review. British Journal of Psychiatry 146:184–197

Fraser WI 1997 The psychiatry of learning disability. In: Murray R, Hill P, McGuffin P (eds) The essentials of postgraduate psychiatry, 3rd edn, pp 429–445. Cambridge University Press, Cambridge

Friedman J, Standaert DG 2001 Dystonia and its disorders. Neurologic Clinics 19:681–706

Glazer WM, Morgenstern H, Doucette JT 1993 Predicting the long-term risk of tardive dyskinesia in outpatients maintained on neuroleptic medications. Journal of Clinical Psychiatry 54:133–139

Goldstein K 1952 The effect of brain damage on the personality. Psychiatry 15:245–260

Hodges JR 2001 Amnestic syndromes. Presented at the XVII World Congress of Neurology, Göttingen. Available: http://www.wfneurology.org/wfn/doc/pdf/hodges.pdf

Jain KK 2001 Drug induced neuropsychiatric disorders, 2nd edn. Hogrefe & Huber, Gottingen

Kaufman DM 2001 Clinical neurology for psychiatrists, 5th edn. WB Saunders, Philadelphia

Klüver H, Bucy PC 1937 'Psychic blindness' and other symptoms following bilateral temporal lobe lobectomy in Rhesus monkeys. American Journal of Physiology 119:353–353

Larson EB, Kukull WA, Buchner D et al 1987 Adverse drug reactions associated with global cognitive impairment in elderly persons. Annals of Internal Medicine 107:169–173

Lhermitte J 1922 Syndrome de la calotte pédoncule cérébral. Less troubles psycho-sensoriels dans less lésions du mésoncépahle. Revue Neurologique 38:1359–1365

Marin RS 1991 Apathy: a neuropsychiatric syndrome. Journal of Neuropsychiatry and Clinical Neuroscience 3:243–254

Moore AR, O'Keeffe ST 1999 Drug-induced cognitive impairment in the elderly. Drugs and Aging 15:15–28

Muscettola G, Pampallona S, Barbato G et al 1993 Persistent tardive dyskinesia: demographic and pharmacological risk-factors. Acta Psychiatrica Scandinavica 87:29–36

Popovitch ER, Wisniewski HM, Barcikowska M et al 1990 Alzheimer neuropathology in non-Down's syndrome mentally retarded adults. Acta Neuropathologica 80:362–367

Rutter M, Taylor E, Hersov L 1995 Child and adolescent psychiatry, 3rd edn. Blackwell, Oxford

Schultz G, Needham W, Taylor R et al 1996 Properties of complex hallucinations associated with deficits in vision. Perception 25:715–726

Van Bogaert L 1927 L'hallucinose pédonculaire. Revue Neurologique 47:608–617

Woerner MG, Kane JM, Lieberman JA et al 1991 The prevalence of tardive dyskinesia. Journal of Clinical Psychopharmacology 11:34–42

Woerner MG, Alvir JMJ, Saltz BL et al 1998 Prospective study of tardive dyskinesia in the elderly: rates and risk factors. American Journal of Psychiatry 155:1521–1528

3

Physical Examination

The physical examination is an essential part of clinical assessment. In one large UK postal survey, 50% of old-age psychiatrists reported that they always performed a neurological examination in cases of early-onset dementia (Cordery et al 2002). Psychiatrists should be able (and willing) to perform a competent neurological examination, as a clinician will only discover abnormalities that are looked for in the first place! Research has shown that some psychiatrists apply inappropriate or unhelpful examination techniques to patients with suspected organic disease, a mistake that they rarely make with the mental state examination. An example is the over-reliance on assessments of sensory discrimination, concentration, orientation and long-term recall. Taken in isolation these have a high false-negative detection rate. Signs more sensitive to diffuse cerebral pathology include primitive reflexes, gaze abnormalities, pyramidal abnormalities, name and address recall, and digit span (Jenkyn et al 1977). The neurological examination is particularly relevant in elderly patients, those with first-onset disease, those with suspected medical disease, those with changes in consciousness and those taking psychotropic drugs (see Table 13.1). For example, unexpected structural lesions are found in approximately 5% of patients presenting with dementia.

In assessing neuropsychiatric patients, emphasis may be placed on:

- assessment of higher cognition (see Chs 5–11)
- localizing and non-localizing signs
- extrapyramidal signs
- assessment of gait
- signs of vascular disease.

Sometimes it is difficult or impossible to perform an adequate neurological examination when the patient is behaviourally disturbed. In the author's opinion it is better to delay the neurological examination until a meaningful attempt can be made.

LOCALIZING AND NON-LOCALIZING SIGNS

Neurological soft signs

Neurological soft signs refer to non-localizing (or, more accurately, difficult-to-localize) signs of neurological disease. These signs may be a manifestation of subtle brain damage, but can also (along with localizing signs) result from significant brain lesions. In addition, new soft signs may represent accumulating CNS damage. Neurological soft signs are also recognized in primary psychiatric conditions, including schizophrenia, bipolar affective disorder, psychopathic personality disorder, obsessive–compulsive disorder and, of course, childhood developmental disorders. There is no standard list, but soft signs typically include subtle deficits in motor coordination, sensory integration, primitive reflexes and sequencing of complex motor function (Box 3.2). They are of significance because neurological soft signs are rarely found in healthy controls. At least two scales to assess soft signs are available: the Cambridge Neurological Inventory (Chen et al 1995) and the Physical and Neurologic Examination of Subtle Signs (PANESS) (Denckla 1985).

Localizing signs and pathological reflexes

Certain signs may help to pinpoint the anatomical basis of neurological disease and thus have special significance in neurology. The most obvious is weakness, which may suggest a lesion in the opposite cerebral hemisphere. Such signs are associated with vascular dementia, CNS tumours, infections of the CNS and, less commonly, degenerative disorders. Primitive reflexes (grasp, snout, sucking) are present in frontal lobe disease and may point towards an undiagnosed frontotemporal dementia. They are not diagnostic of frontal lobe damage, since they can occur in the healthy elderly; however, their presence has been correlated with neuropsychiatric complications. The *grasp reflex* is the involuntary gripping of objects in patient's hand or feet

Table 3.1 Physical examination pointers in neuropsychiatry

Anatomical area/sign	Neuropsychiatric pointer
General appearance	
Café-au-lait spots	Neurofibromatosis
Hyperventilation	Anxiety, fever, metabolic acidosis, brainstem lesion
Incontinence	Epilepsy, dementia, Parkinson's disease
Mask-like facies	Parkinson's disease, parkinsonism
Sweating	Anxiety, adverse drug effects, endocrine disease
Pupil and eye signs	
Arcus senilis	Alcohol, old age, hyperlipidaemia
Argyll–Robertson pupil (unreactive to light, but reacts to accommodation)	Tertiary syphilis
Hemianopia	CNS infiltration, stroke, space-occupying lesion
Kayser–Fleischer ring	Wilson's disease
Mydriasis	Holmes–Adie (slowly reactive) pupil, cocaine, mydriatics, midbrain lesions
Miosis	Horner's syndrome, organophosphates, pontine lesions, opiates, miotics
Nystagmus	Blindness; cerebellar, midbrain and pontine lesions; drugs
Oculocephalic (Doll's eye) reflex	Brainstem lesion or severe metabolic coma
Optic atrophy	Multiple sclerosis, frontal tumours, syphilis, optic nerve compression
Poor acuity	Old age; lesion of eye, retina or visual pathway; Parkinson's disease
Ptosis	Cranial nerve III lesion, Horner's syndrome, myasthenia
Skin	
Callus on knuckles (Russell's sign)	Eating disorder
Excoriation	Obsessive–compulsive disorder (e.g. hand washing)
Forearm scars	Self-harm
Kaposi's sarcoma	AIDS
Lanugo hair	Anorexia nervosa, starvation
Needle marks	Intravenous drug use
Palmar erythema	Alcohol, anxiety
Piloerection	Drug withdrawal
Rash	Systemic lupus erythematosus, meningitis
Striae, purpura	Endogenous or exogenous steroid excess
Cardiovascular system	
Carotid bruit	Carotid stenosis
Hypertension	Vascular disease, endocrine disease, adverse drug effects
Hypotension	Anorexia nervosa, endocrine disease, adverse drug effects, hypovolaemia, Parkinson's disease, multiple system atrophy

Contd

Table 3.1 *Contd*

Anatomical area/sign	Neuropsychiatric pointer
Gastrointestinal and urogenital system	
Chancre	Syphilis
Gynaecomastia	Alcohol, adverse drug effect
Hepatomegaly	Alcohol, Wilson's disease, malignancy, heart failure, infections
Reduced sexual characteristics	Alcohol, genetic disorders, anorexia
Neurological system	
Anosmia	Alzheimer's disease, Parkinson's disease, head injury, multiple sclerosis, CNS tumour, viral infection, cocaine abuse, toxic causes, variant Creutzfeldt–Jakob disease
Chorea	Cerebrovascular disease, Huntington's chorea, Sydenham's chorea, Wilson's disease, senile chorea, pregnancy, hyperthyroidism, benign chorea
Dementia + ataxia	Alcoholic dementia, Wernicke's encephalopathy, spinocerebellar degeneration, hydrocephalus, variant Creutzfeldt–Jakob disease
Dementia + focal signs	Vascular dementia, brain tumour, brain infiltration, haematoma, multiple sclerosis, Creutzfeldt–Jakob disease, MELAS, motor neurone disease
Dementia + myoclonus	Alzheimer's disease, Creutzfeldt–Jakob disease, AIDS dementia, uraemic encephalopathy, progressive myoclonic epilepsy, Whipple's disease
Dementia + parkinsonism	Lewy body dementia, Alzheimer's disease, progressive supranuclear palsy, Huntington's disease, corticobasal degeneration, Creutzfeldt–Jakob disease, Wilson's disease, heavy metal poisoning, dementia pugilistica
Dementia + peripheral neuropathy	Alcoholism, vitamin B_{12} deficiency, pellagra, hypothyroidism, vasculitis, renal failure, paraneoplastic syndrome, porphyria, toxins
Dementia + seizures	Alzheimer's disease, CNS tumours, meningitis, DRPLA, poisoning
Dysarthria	Spastic dysarthria, ataxic dysarthria, hypokinetic dysarthria, flaccid dysarthria, paretic (flaccid) dysarthria
Extrapyramidal signs	Parkinson's disease, normal ageing, Lewy body dementia, Alzheimer's disease, adverse drug effects
Focal signs	Multiple sclerosis, motor neurone disease, stroke, vascular dementia
Gait	Parkinsonian, cerebellar, spastic, paretic, apraxic, myopathic, sensory gait
Myoclonus	Epilepsy, delirium and metabolic, Creutzfeldt–Jakob disease, Lewy body dementia
Neck stiffness + Kernig's sign	Encephalitis, meningitis, subarachnoid haemorrhage
Papilloedema	Tumour, subarachnoid haemorrhage, hydrocephalus, hypertension
Primitive reflexes	Frontal lobe lesion, Alzheimer's disease, miscellaneous dementias
Soft signs	Schizophrenia, bipolar affective disorder, personality disorder, obsessive–compulsive disorder, minimal brain injury, attention deficit/hyperactivity disorder, autism, Tourette's syndrome
Tics	Tourette's syndrome, Huntington's chorea, Sydenham's chorea, carbon monoxide poisoning, Lesch–Nyhan syndrome, Hallervorden–Spatz disease, adverse drug effects
Tremor	Physiological or essential, hyperthyroidism, drug intoxication or withdrawal, parkinsonism, cerebellar disease, delirium

DRPLA, dentatorubralpallidoluysian atrophy; MELAS, mitochondrial encephalopathy with lactic acidosis and stroke-like episodes

(thumb flexion elicited by briskly flexing the distal phalanx of the middle finger while holding the digits in a dorsiflexed position) may be used to assess hyper-reflexia in the upper extremities. The *glabella tap reflex* (Myerson's sign) refers to blinking (four or more times) on continuous tapping of the glabellar region. This is associated with extrapyramidal dysfunction; it is seen in Parkinson's disease and drug-induced parkinsonism and is not a primitive reflex. Primitive reflexes sometimes occur in association with *imitation behaviour*, in which the patient automatically imitates the examiner, *utilization behaviour*, in which the patient uses anything that is placed in their hand, and *catatonic symptoms*, which are inappropriate motor abnormalities – suggesting these have their origin in the frontal lobes. It was Lhermittte (1986) who described utilization behaviour as a milder form of the 'environmental dependency syndrome'.

EXTRAPYRAMIDAL SIGNS

Some degree of parkinsonism (not Parkinson's disease) is present in one-third of the population aged above 75 years and half of the population aged above 85 years (Bennett et al 1996). Parkinsonism is a modest risk factor for mortality both in the healthy elderly and in the elderly with dementia. In the context of dementia, the presence of parkinsonism suggests a non-Alzheimer dementia (even though there is a recognized overlap between Alzheimer's disease and parkinsonsim. Also, in the late stages of Alzheimer's disease paratonic rigidity may simulate rigidity of parkinsonism). Extrapyramidal signs are

and is most often seen after medial frontal lobe lesions. The *snout reflex* is characterized by puckering of the lips in response to tapping of the upper or lower lip. The *palmomental reflex* features ipsilateral contraction of the mentalis muscle in response to stroking of the thenar eminence of the hand. This reflex can be seen in normal elderly patients and may be regarded as pathological when it is unilateral or when it does not expire with repeated stimulation. *Babinski's sign* (dorsiflexion of the great toe after stroking the plantar surface of the foot) is produced by upper motor neurone lesions and is a remnant of a protective flexion reflex. *Hoffmann's sign*

also extremely common with most traditional psychotropic medications. Parkinsonian symptoms are associated with distress and discomfort and often herald a more rapidly progressive condition. With this in mind, the early recognition and treatment of parkinsonian symptoms is essential. In addition, tardive dyskinesia is a major hazard for those on long-term antipsychotics. Patients should be warned of the risk, and a systematic assessment recorded in the medical notes (ideally using a structured scale such as the Abnormal Involuntary Movements Scale).

GAIT

An examination of a person's style of locomotion is a simple but easily overlooked part of the neurological examination. Not only do gait abnormalities have diagnostic significance, they may have prognostic significance – 30% of people aged over 65 years fall each year and one-quarter of these are seriously injured. Examination of gait includes assessment of the patient's standing posture (trunk, stance, postural reflexes) and assessment of the walking ability (initiation, stepping, associated limb movements). Gait disturbance can result from peripheral as well

---

Box 3.3 Classification of gait disorders

Lowest-level gait disorders
Peripheral musculoskeletal problems:
- arthritic gait
- myopathic gait
- peripheral neuropathic gait

Peripheral sensory problems:
- sensory ataxic gait
- vestibular ataxic gait
- visual ataxic gait

Middle-level gait disorders
Hemiplegic gait
Paraplegic gait
Cerebellar ataxic gait
Parkinsonian gait
Choreic gait
Dystonic gait

Higher level gait disorders
Cautious gait
Subcortical dysequilibrium
Frontal dysequilibrium
Isolated gait ignition failure
Frontal gait disorder
Psychogenic gait disorder

After Nutt et al (1993)

Table 3.2 Recognizable gait disorders in neuropsychiatry

Gait	Examples	Description of gait abnormality
Festinating	Parkinson's	Slow, shuffling steps taken with acceleration on leaning forward. Stooped posture and reduced arm swing
Cerebellar/ataxic	Cerebellar disorder*	Unsteady, wide-based and unstable, possibly veering to the side of a unilateral lesion
Hemiparetic	Upper motor neurone lesion	Slow and stiff with circumduction of the affected limb
High stepping	Lower motor neurone/sensory loss	The knee is raised excessively high in order that the foot clears the floor (often in association with foot drop) The gait is slow and careful with visual guidance
Apraxic	Normal-pressure hydrocephalus	Problems initiating and making fine adjustments to gait produces slow, broad-based steps in mild cases and complete loss of organization of leg movements in severe cases
Myopathic	Muscular dystrophy	Weak pelvic and hip muscles cause exaggerated lordosis and hip instability or a waddling gait
Sensory	Tabes dorsalis	Unsteady, wide-based, trunk instability and exaggerated steps

*Gait varies according to type of cerebellar lesion: lesions of the flocculonodular lobe produce marked disequilibrium causing postural ataxia and severe gait ataxia; lesions of the anterior vermis produce a wide-based gait with a slow and irregular cadence and superimposed lurching without incoordination; lesions of the lateral cerebellar hemispheres produce limb ataxia and secondary gait incoordination

as central problems (see Box 3.3). Involuntary movements and postures may be elicited by asking the patient to walk. At least a quarter of elderly patients who present to neurologists with gait problems have a treatable cause for their difficulty. Difficulties in locomotion form part of a complete functional assessment and give an indication of the likely independence of the patient. Orthopaedic and rheumatological problems may disturb gait, but these are easily identified by the patient. Weakness might be due to a peripheral muscle or nerve problem or to a central lesion. Other causes of disturbed gait include parkinsonism, cerebellar disorder, a proprioceptive deficit, an intracranial mass or vascular lesion and, more rarely, hydrocephalus, multiple sclerosis or a neurodegenerative disorder (Table 3.2).

VASCULAR AND SYSTEMIC SIGNS

Vascular disease is a risk factor for most major neuropsychiatric complications and an influence on mortality in its own right. In dementia, vascular disease is the most important common modifiable variable, not just in vascular dementia but also in Alzheimer's disease and cases of mixed dementia. Systemic signs of vascular disease may include skin discolouration, xanthelasma and an arcus senilis. Abnormal blood pressure and pulse are 'vital signs' of vascular disease. Blood pressure problems are well described in the parkinsonian syndromes, and also in several types of dementia. About one-third of cases of Alzheimer's disease are liable to orthostatic falls in blood pressure. An even greater percentage

of those with frontotemporal dementia also have this finding. Signs of heart failure should be sought, and examination of the fundi, peripheral pulses and carotid (carotid bruit) should not be overlooked.

REFERENCES AND FURTHER READING

Bennett DA, Beckett LA, Murray AM et al 1996 Prevalence of Parkinsonian signs and associated mortality in a community population of older people. New England Journal of Medicine 334:71–76

Chen EYH, Shapleske J, Luque R et al 1995 The Cambridge Neurological Inventory: a clinical instrument for assessment of soft neurological signs in psychiatric patients. Psychiatry Research 56:183–204

Cordery R, Harvey R, Frost C et al 2002 National survey to assess current practices in the diagnosis and management of young people with dementia. International Journal of Geriatric Psychiatry 17:124–127

Denckla MB 1985 Revised PANESS. Psychopharmacology Bulletin 21:773–800

Donaghy M, Ropper A 2001 Useful neurological tips: clinical assessment of neurological patients. Presented at the XVII World Congress of Neurology. Available: http://www.wfneurology.org/wfn/doc/pdf/donaghy_ropper.pdf

Jenkyn LR, Walsh DB, Culver CM et al 1977 Clinical signs of diffuse cerebral dysfunction. Journal of Neurology, Neurosurgery and Psychiatry 40:956–966

Lhermittte F 1986 Human autonomy and the frontal lobes. Part II. Patients' behavior in complex social situations: the environmental dependency syndrome. Annals of Neurology 19:335–343

Nutt JG, Marsden CD, Thompson PD 1993. Human walking and higher-level gait disorders, particularly in the elderly. Neurology 43:268–279

4

Neuro-psychiatric Investigations

Neurologists and psychiatrists differ in their attitudes to clinical investigation. Neurologists nearly always attempt to find neurobiological evidence to support the presence of a suspected disease. Psychiatrists often assume that there is little to be gained by investigating patients who present with typical disorders. Retrospective and prospective studies show that the detection rate of medical disorders in general adult psychiatry based on investigation alone is very low (approximately 2%), but the prevalence of occult medical disease in acute psychiatric inpatients, based on clinical examination, is significant (between 20% and 50%) (Anfinson & Stoudemire 1999). About half the cases of disease are due to previously undiagnosed disorders. The implication is that medical investigations should be used in conjunction with clinical skills and that the cost of negative tests is acceptable because the consequences of overlooking even one case of hypothyroidism or Wilson's disease would be severe.

The most important investigations when considering the psychiatric complications of neurological disease are lumbar puncture, EEG, brain neuroimaging and neuropsychological testing (see Chs 5 to 11). Acceptability and availability are also involved. Other investigations occasionally need to be considered (Box 4.1)

GENERAL INVESTIGATIONS

The importance of general medical investigations is essentially that they may identify medical causes of the current presentation. This is particularly the case for patients presenting with delirium, dementia or movement disorder (Table 4.1).

Lumbar puncture

Examination of the CSF is mandatory in cases of suspected meningitis or encephalitis. A lumbar puncture may also be useful in cases where Creutzfeldt–Jakob disease, multiple sclerosis or normal-pressure hydrocephalus requires confirma-

---

Box 4.1   Specialized tests in neuropsychiatry

Test	Indication
Acetylcholine receptor antibodies	Myasthenia gravis
Antiphospholipid antibodies	Early onset stroke
CAG repeat DNA analysis	Huntington's disease
Clotting studies	Early onset stroke
Evoked potentials	Multiple sclerosis
Urine sulfatide levels	Metachromatic leukodystrophy
Notch 3 DNA analysis	CADASIL
Serum and urinary copper	Wilson's disease
Serum long-chain fatty acids	Adrenoleukodystrophy
Skeletal muscle biopsy	Mitochondrial disorders
Tau gene DNA analysis	Familial frontotemporal dementia
Tensilon test	Myasthenia gravis
Vacuolated lymphocytes	Lysosomal storage disorders

CADASIL, cerebral autosomal-dominant arteriopathy with subcortical infarcts and leukoencephalopathy

39

Table 4.1 Recommended investigations for common neuropsychiatric presentations

Investigations for movement disorder of uncertain origin	Investigations for dementias of uncertain origin	Investigations for delirium of uncertain origin	Investigations for suspected organic psychosis or affective disorder
Background History and physical examination	*Background* History and physical examination	*Background* History and physical examination	*Background* History and physical examination
Standard Full blood count with differential Blood urea and electrolytes Plasma viscosity (ESR, CRP) Liver function and renal function Antinuclear antibodies Thyroid function tests Serum ceruloplasmin CT or MRI of the brain	*Standard* Full blood count Plasma viscosity (ESR, CRP) Blood urea and electrolytes Plasma glucose (ideally fasting) Liver function and renal function Calcium Thyroid function tests Vitamin B_{12} and red cell folate CT or MRI of the brain	*Standard* Body temperature Full blood count Plasma glucose (ideally fasting) Blood urea and electrolytes Liver function and renal function Calcium and magnesium levels Vitamin B_{12} and red cell folate Urinalysis (protein, glucose) Plasma viscosity (ESR, CRP) Thyroid function tests Plasma viscosity Chest X-ray Blood gases ECG	*Standard* Full blood count Blood urea and electrolytes Liver function and renal function* Urine drug screen Thyroid function tests* ECG* EEG Plasma glucose (ideally fasting)*
Guided by clinical features 24 hour urinary copper Slit lamp examination Chest X-ray Antistreptolysin O titres Urine toxicology and heavy metal screen DNA mutation analysis HIV antibody test Lumbar puncture Electrophysiological studies Liver, muscle and, rarely, brain biopsy	*Guided by clinical features* Syphilis serology Protein electrophoresis Chest X-ray Urine toxicology and heavy metal screen Doppler ultrasound of the carotid arteries Echocardiography Coagulation studies Antiphospholipid antibodies Proteins C and S, and antithrombin III ECG Serial blood pressure monitoring SPECT Lumbar puncture	*Guided by clinical features* Blood or breath alcohol Cardiac enzymes Paraneoplastic markers Urine drug screen EEG Lumbar puncture	*Guided by clinical features* Blood or breath alcohol Dexamethasone suppression test TRH stimulation test Syphilis serology Plasma viscosity (ESR, CRP) Prolactin* Urine toxicology and heavy metal screen HIV test
	CRP, C-reactive protein		*May be relevant to prescribed medication

tion (Box 4.2). Several groups are investigating whether biochemical analysis of CSF can be used as a diagnostic test of Alzheimer's disease or vascular dementia. The interpretation of CSF parameters is covered in any neurological reference text.

EEG

With the advent of neuroimaging, EEG recording has fallen out of fashion, to the point where this investigation is now underutilized. The recording is performed for about 30 minutes and should incorporate, where possible, periods of hyperventilation, photic stimulation and sleep. It is the electrical activity from inhibitory and excitatory postsynaptic potentials of cortical pyramidal neurones near to the scalp that are captured in EEG recordings. These signals are about one-hundredth the strength of ECG recordings. The normal wakening EEG contains an α-rhythm and β-rhythm. The sleep EEG has an REM phase and four non-REM phases. Discharges from deep brain areas may not be reflected in surface EEG recordings. For this reason, deep electrode recordings are used before surgery for intractable epilepsy. The diagnostic yield in unselected cases, based on epileptiform discharges, is somewhere between 2%

> **Box 4.2 The ten most frequent indications for a lumbar puncture**
>
> - Suspected meningitis
> - Suspected multiple sclerosis
> - Encephalitis of unknown cause
> - Suspected Creutzfeldt–Jakob disease
> - Subarachnoid haemorrhage
> - Suspected paraneoplastic syndrome
> - Stroke in the young
> - Normal-pressure hydrocephalus
> - Pseudotumour cerebri
> - Intrathecal therapy

and 8%. The majority of these represent cerebral disorders, although in the absence of a clinical history of seizures, seizures will ensue in only a small fraction of cases (Sam & So 2001).

Applied EEG in neuropsychiatry

EEG slowing into θ or δ frequencies is generally indicative of neuronal dysfunction. This can occur in a focal pattern after a seizure or in relation to a tumour, or in a generalized pattern as a result of dementia or delirium (but not in withdrawal states). Localized slow-wave disturbances are more likely to

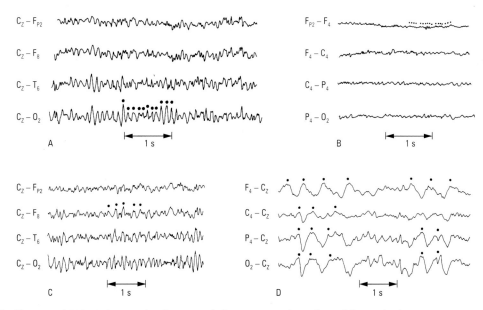

Fig. 4.1 The normal EEG. EEGs record a short period of activity near the surface of the cerebral cortex. Unsurprisingly, it can miss paroxysmal and deep abnormal electrical activity. Occasionally, special electrode placements (nasopharyngeal or ethmoid) are used. A, Alpha activity is the regular 11-Hz activity overlying the occipital lobe. B, Beta activity is the low-voltage, irregular, 17-Hz activity overlying the frontal lobe. C, Theta activity is the 5-Hz activity overlying the frontal lobe. D, Delta activity is the high-voltage, 3-Hz activity present over the entire hemisphere. From Kaufman (2001).

occur in vascular dementia than in Alzheimer's dementia, and this can be used in differential diagnosis. In these conditions reduction of wave amplitude is often seen (see also Clinical Pointer 38.1). One provocative study recently reported that subjects with mild cognitive impairment which progressed to Alzheimer's disease had more θ- and less α-activity than those whose impairment remained stable (Huang et al 2000). Anatomically, diffuse slow waves may arise from cortical or subcortical structures. Focal slow waves are purported by some authors to represent involvement of white matter.

Paroxysmal transients (spikes and sharp waves) – bursts of spikes or sharp waves often occur interictally, as well as ictally in epilepsy. Partial seizures are associated with localized abnormal discharges that may or may not generalize. Photic stimulation and sleep may precipitate epileptiform activity (see also Clinical Pointer 18.1).

Periodic complexes refer to the combination of sharp waves and slow waves that are recurrent every few seconds. Generalized background slowing may occur. The conditions responsible include subacute sclerosing panencephalitis (4–15 s complexes, usually synchronous and symmetrical) and Creutzfeldt–Jakob disease (0.5–1 s biphasic or triphasic complexes). Triphasic waves (slow waves with a triphasic appearance) are associated with metabolic delirium, especially hepatic encephalopathy and uraemia.

PRINCIPLES OF NEUROIMAGING

Neuroimaging has promised much for the understanding of neuropsychiatric disorders – but has it delivered on this promise? Before we get too swept up in the current wave of imaging enthusiasm, it is worth remembering that there is no such thing as the perfect investigation. Most psychiatric conditions feature such subtle anatomical features that, for the foreseeable future, no technique could hope to demonstrate them. Consider this – what imaging study could reveal a diagnosis of schizophrenia, depression, post-traumatic stress disorder or complicated grief? That is not to say that the ventricular enlargement or hippocampal–amygdaloid atrophy reported in some of these conditions is invalid, just that it does not aid the clinician dealing with this problem (Clinical Pointer 4.1). At this point, it is worth summarizing the techniques of neuroimaging as well as the most robust findings.

Structural imaging methodology

Computed tomography (CT) scanning is the reconstruction of conventional X-rays in a three-dimensional model. High-density tissue attenuates X-rays and appears white on the image. Intravenous iodinated contrast can be used to enhance the images. The advantages of CT are in acute haemorrhagic infarction, in calcification and in patients with medical implants.

Magnetic resonance imaging (MRI) has its roots in spectroscopy, which enables the concentration of individual elements and brain metabolites to be measured accurately. Magnetic resonance spectroscopy is now being investigated for its ability to provide detailed chemical information of brain regions in neuropsychiatric disease. The atomic nuclei studied are hydrogen-1, phosphorus-31, chlorine-13, fluorine-19 and sodium-23. MRI uses a different system from that of CT, and it employs the ingenious observation that atomic nuclei are paramagnetic. Hydrogen protons in the body (attached to oxygen in the form of water) will align their spin axis in one direction when subject to a large, uniform magnetic field. When that field is removed, energy is released in the radiofrequency range as the atoms return to their normal axis. A radiofrequency (magnetic) pulse at a different angle is then applied. Tissue has a relaxation time of atoms in a longitudinal plane (T1) or transverse plane (T2). MRI can be enhanced by injection of a paramagnetic substance such as gadolinium. The advantages of MRI are in the investigation of new-onset seizures, hydrocephalus, white matter lesions, lesions in the posterior fossa, spinal cord and medial temporal lobe and detection of blood–brain barrier breakdown.

Box 4.3   The ten most frequent indications for an EEG

- Suspected epilepsy or non-epileptic seizures
- Investigation of sleep disorders
- Differential diagnosis in early onset dementia
- Suspected encephalitis
- Diagnosis of delirium
- Suspected CNS tumour
- Investigation of persistent loss of consciousness
- Investigation of dementia with neurological signs
- Suspected Creutzfeldt–Jakob disease
- First onset of psychosis or nocturnal panic attacks

Clinical Pointer 4.1

What does neuroimaging add to clinical diagnosis?

This is a hot topic among neurologists, psychiatrists and radiologists alike, and a difficult question to answer succinctly. A handful of neurological and neuropsychiatric conditions warrant a structural scan in order to confirm or refute the diagnosis. These include head trauma (with suspected haemorrhage or fracture), temporal lobe epilepsy (is there an anatomical focus?), CNS tumour (where and what is the tumour?), suspected multiple sclerosis (is the diagnosis correct?), stroke (is it embolic or haemorrhagic?), Huntington's disease (what is the size of the caudate nucleus?) and suspected hydrocephalus (what is the ratio of cortical to ventricular enlargement?). Most clinicians would also add vascular depression and vascular dementia to this list (looking for the severity of white matter changes). Unless one of these diagnoses needs to be ruled out there is little clinical indication for ordering a structural scan in delirium, Lewy body dementia, Parkinson's disease or motor neurone disease without dementia (i.e. it will not alter management). Patients with some suspected diagnoses might benefit from a scan in that the result will alter the balance of probabilities, although the result is very unlikely to be clearly diagnostic. Examples are Alzheimer's disease, frontotemporal dementia, Wilson's disease, Tourette's syndrome and Creutzfeldt–Jakob disease. Functional imaging has a particular role in early dementias, particularly Alzheimer's disease where, again, it adds to the balance of probabilities rather than being a gold standard. Specialist techniques such as proton magnetic resonance spectroscopy and functional MRI are still experimental, but may find a role in Alzheimer's disease and HIV dementia.

Further reading *Ames D, Chiu E 1997 Neuroimaging and the psychiatry of late life. Cambridge University Press, Cambridge*
Lewis S 1996 Brain imaging in psychiatry. Blackwell, Oxford

Functional imaging methodology

Single photon emission tomography (SPECT) uses radioactive tracers that, once injected peripherally, cross the blood–brain barrier and are held within functioning cells. Examples of tracers are technetium-99m (which serves as a measure of blood flow) and iodine-123 (which serves as a measure of receptor binding). SPECT has low resolution and a slow capture of images.

Positron emission tomography (PET) measures radioactivity emitted from injected isotopes with a short half-life (fluorine-18, carbon-11). The difference compared with SPECT is that these isotopes must be generated in a cyclotron, which is costly. Positrons and electrons are annihilated in local tissue with the release of two high-energy γ-rays. PET has higher resolution than SPECT, but still very much lower resolution than CT or MRI.

Both SPECT and PET can be used to image brain receptors using ligands such as methylspiperone (which binds to serotonin and dopamine receptors). Functional MRI utilizes the fact that an increased blood supply (in an active region) changes haemoglobin concentrations. The oxygen content of haemoglobin affects magnetic field strength.

Magnetoencephalography uses a superconducting quantum interference device (SQUID) magne-tometer, the supercooled detection coil of which detects fields of 10^{-10} to 10^{5} gauss, to ascertain electrical brain activity. Using this technique, functional images of brain activity are possible with an acquisition time measured in seconds or less, rather than minutes.

APPLIED NEUROIMAGING IN NEUROPSYCHIATRY

Alcohol and drug abuse

Definite cortical atrophy and ventricular enlargement is seen on CT and MRI in the majority of patients with a history of chronic alcohol consumption. This may in part be due to white matter loss and in part due to neuronal loss. Areas most affected include the cerebral cortex, hypothalamus and cerebellum. Hippocampal atrophy is also seen, but it does not appear to be disproportionately affected or to be influenced by psychiatric symptomatology (Agartz et al 1999). There is a correlation with extent and duration of alcohol use, although a certain threshold of consumption appears to be necessary (Kubota et al 2001). In fact, moderate alcohol consumption is associated with lower rates of cardiovascular disease and associated white matter brain lesions (Mukamal et al 2001). Quite apart from the secondary influence of nutritional compromise and liver damage, it seems increasingly likely that alcohol is directly neurotoxic.

Cocaine use is associated with abnormalities in cerebral blood flow demonstrated on functional imaging, thought to be due to cocaine-induced vasoconstriction, which can lead to tissue ischaemia and, if severe, infarction. The perfusion abnormalities are predominant in the frontal cortices.

Structural and functional brain changes have been reported in cannabis users, but it is premature to lend too much weight to these findings until further work is forthcoming.

Alzheimer's disease

The distribution of the pathology determines the clinical characteristics of Alzheimer's disease (see Fig. 40.8). Some patients with early Alzheimer's disease do not demonstrate atrophy and some normal elderly persons show definite brain atrophy. Older age and poorer cognition both correlate with cortical atrophy, ventricular enlargement and total CSF space. Thus, it is not possible to confirm the diagnosis of early Alzheimer's disease on the basis of an atrophic scan. Even in moderate or late-stage

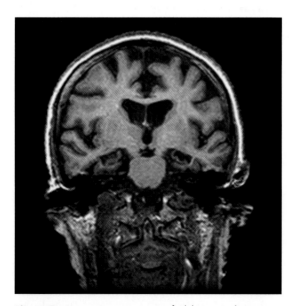

Fig. 4.2 Post-mortem specimen of Alzheimer's disease, showing cortical atrophy. From Emma Burton & John O'Brien, Institute for Ageing and Health, University of Newcastle upon Tyne.

Alzheimer's disease, a diagnosis based on neuroimaging alone is not completely accurate (Diaz-Guzman et al 2002). Progressive atrophy seen on successive scans using co-registration is more useful, but clearly more time consuming (Fox et al 1996). Recent work suggests that atrophy of the hippocampus may be an early sign of Alzheimer's disease, although this is probably too insensitive a sign to be used as a preclinical predictor. Reduced volume of the neighbouring entorhinal cortex may be even better for distinguishing patients with mild cognitive impairment from those with Alzheimer's disease (Du et al 2001). Some researchers hope that functional imaging might have added value here. Delayed recall is also associated with hippocampal atrophy in Alzheimer's disease. Studies of PET-based cerebral glucose metabolism ([^{18}F]fluoro-deoxyglucose PET) in Alzheimer's disease have revealed a decline in this metabolism in early Alzheimer's disease and possibly preclinically. The first area to show a metabolic reduction may not be the cell bodies in the hippocampus, but their synapses in mammillary bodies and secondary projections to the posterior cingulate cortex (Nestor et al 2002). More practically, temporal–parietal hypoperfusion on SPECT has some diagnostic accuracy in early Alzheimer's disease (see Ch. 40). This may be a reflection of the reduced protein synthesis and reduced mitochondrial energy metabolism in neurones seen before neuronal death. Beyond atrophy and hypoperfusion, white matter lesions are seen in Alzheimer's disease and may represent more than simple age-related changes (Clinical Pointer 4.2). Magnetic resonance spectroscopy demonstrates decreases in N-acetylaspartate and increases in myoinositol levels at an early stage. An intermediate level of change is seen in age-associated memory impairment. Changes correlate with dementia severity and may predict future cognitive decline (Clinical Pointer 4.3).

Delirium

Unless structural lesions are suspected, neuroimaging has little value in delirium at the present time.

Frontotemporal and focal dementias

Frontotemporal dementia involves the anterior temporal and frontal lobes and spares the temporoparietal regions, although CT or MRI studies are often

Clinical Pointer 4.2

The significance of white matter lesions on MRI

White matter lesions (WMLs) are found in Alzheimer's disease, multiple sclerosis and normal-pressure hydrocephalus as well as in recognized vascular brain diseases. They increase with age in all groups, from about 5% in the fourth decade to roughly 20% in the sixth decade. WMLs may result from different pathologies, including demyelination, amyloid angiopathy and gliosis; however, the principal pathogenesis of WMLs is probably ischaemic. WMLs are conventionally divided into those around the ventricular system (periventricular lesions (PVLs)) and those elsewhere (deep white matter lesions (DWMLs) or leukoaraiosis). DWMLs but not PVLs may be associated with neurological dysfunction. PVLs may be more common in Alzheimer's disease than elderly controls or depressed patients. Severe WMLs are a risk factor for later stroke and myocardial infarction. In the largest community-based MRI study of over 3000 subjects, WMLs correlated with age, silent strokes and systolic blood pressure. Large, as opposed to small, clinically insignificant PVLs were related to cognitive impairment and gait abnormalities. The association of both periventricular and subcortical WMLs with subjective memory complaints and mild cognitive impairment has been replicated. WMLs (especially DWMLs) are more prevalent in the depressed elderly, and appear to predict poor response to treatment and higher mortality. This association may be stronger in individuals carrying the ApoE4 allele.

Further reading de Groot JC, de Leeuw FE et al 2001 Cerebral white matter lesions and subjective cognitive dysfunction: the Rotterdam Scan Study. Neurology 56:1539–1545
Longstreth WT, Manolio TA, Arnold A et al 1996 Clinical correlates of white matter findings on cranial magnetic resonance imaging of 3301 elderly people the cardiovascular health study. Stroke 27:1274–1282
Pantoni L, Garcia JH 1997 Pathogenesis of leukoaraiosis: a review. Stroke 28:652–659

Clinical Pointer 4.3

What value is MRS in neuropsychiatry?

Proton magnetic resonance spectroscopy (MRS) is a non-invasive technique that has been used to study various types of dementia, multiple sclerosis, schizophrenia, autism and depression. Although several nuclei can be observed, the most investigated are phosphorus (^{31}P) and hydrogen (^{1}H). Low levels of N-acetylaspartate (NAA) appear to be a good indicator of neuronal loss and neuronal density. Increased choline may be a marker of increased neuronal turnover.

Low levels of NAA and increased levels of myoinositol are seen in the occipital, temporal, parietal and frontal regions of patients with Alzheimer's disease, even at the early stages of the disease. This diffuse NAA decline is independent of regional atrophy and probably reflects a decrease in neurocellular viability. In HIV dementia, there is a reduction in the NAA/creatine ratio and the NAA/choline ratio, the latter being a better marker of disease than MRI alone. In Parkinson's dementia, a study from one group suggests that reductions in NAA concentrations in the occipital lobes correlates with the severity of cognitive deficits. Other studies have shown that reductions in the NAA/creatine ratio in the putamen correlate with the severity of parkinsonism. In schizophrenia, studies suggest altered membrane phospholipid metabolism at the early stage of illness and reduced NAA, a measure of neuronal volume/viability. Similar studies in autism suggest excess neuronal density (failure of brain maturation). Studies employing ^{31}P-MRS and ^{1}H-MRS have indicated possible abnormalities in membrane phospholipid metabolism, high-energy phosphate metabolism, and intracellular pH in affective disorders.

Future developments in MRS may include prediction of decline in mild cognitive impairment and early Alzheimer's disease and evaluating clinical response to antidementia agents.

Further reading Kato T, Inubushi T, Kato N 1998 Magnetic resonance spectroscopy in affective disorders. Journal of Neuropsychiatry and Clinical Neuroscience 10:133–147
Rudkin TM, Arnold DL 1999 Proton magnetic resonance spectroscopy for the diagnosis and management of cerebral disorders. Archives of Neurology 56:919–926
Summerfield C, Anson BG, Tolosa E et al 2002 Dementia in Parkinson's disease – a proton magnetic resonance spectroscopy study. Archives of Neurology 59:1415–1420
Valenzuela MJ, Sachdev P 2001 Magnetic resonance spectroscopy in AD. Neurology 56:592–598

normal in the early stages. PET usually reveals frontal and anterior temporal hypometabolism with sparing of other brain regions. Like temporoparietal hypoperfusion, frontal hypoperfusion is not specific to Pick's disease or frontotemporal dementia, and patients with motor neurone disease, progressive supranuclear palsy, schizophrenia or depressive disorder have all been found to exhibit reduced perfusion of the frontal lobes. At post-mortem the pathology of the cortex may be more widespread, involving the amygdala, basal ganglia and locus ceruleus. Focal atrophy may be seen in semantic dementia (progressive fluent aphasia), progressive non-fluent aphasia, corticobasal degeneration and posterior cortical atrophy.

Lewy body dementia

Structural and functional neuroimaging of patients with Lewy body dementia has so far failed to find convincing differences from findings in Alzheimer's disease. However, one provisional finding is that the temporal lobes are relatively preserved, and another is a reduction in metabolic activity in the occipital cortex (Minoshima et al 2001).

Vascular dementia and depression

Early studies suggested that the loss of the critical volume of 100 ml of tissue was necessary for vascular dementia and that the occurrence of intellectual decline was more variable in patients with smaller volumes of infarcted tissue. PET studies have shown that this is an oversimplification and that the site of the lesion may be of critical importance (e.g. in thalamic dementia). Furthermore, hippocampal atrophy may be a feature common to both Alzheimer's disease and vascular dementia. Binswanger's disease, described by Otto Binswanger in 1894, before Alzheimer's histopathological description in 1902, is characterized by large areas of demyelination in the centrum semiovale. MRI shows that one-quarter or more of elderly persons have detectable abnormalities within their white matter. These white matter lesions occur in patients with established vascular risk factors and are thought to represent small-vessel ischaemia. The lesions have a predilection for the periventricular regions and commonly surround the lateral ventricles as a halo, or appear as scattered small punctuate lesions in the deep hemispheric white matter. The periventricular area is a watershed zone and may be more susceptible to

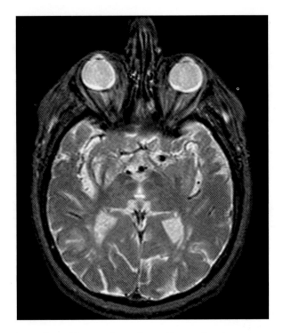

Fig. 4.3 MRI scan of a patient with vascular dementia. Diffuse areas of vascular damage may be seen as hyperintense lesions on this T2-weighted image. White matter lesions thought to result from occlusion of white matter arterioles. However, even after complete occlusion the small lacunes may be invisible macroscopically. From KA Johnson, Radiology and Neurology, Massachusetts General Hospital, Harvard Medical School.

ischaemia in the elderly. When these white matter lesions are large, there is a risk of cognitive impairment and depression. Evidence of small-vessel disease is seen in the majority of patients with vascular dementia. In addition, lacunar infarcts and solitary cortical infarcts are seen in 70% and 20%, respectively, of those with vascular dementia. Recently, magnetic resonance spectroscopy has been investigated as a method of distinguishing vascular dementia from Alzheimer's disease and healthy controls. There are reductions in N-acetylaspartate and in the N-acetylaspartate/creatinine ratio in both cortical and subcortical regions, although the hippocampus may be relatively spared, in contrast with Alzheimer's disease.

AIDS dementia

Neuroimaging is valuable in AIDS dementia to exclude other causes of cognitive impairment such as a mass lesion. Patients with AIDS dementia show severe generalized brain atrophy and extensive sub-cortical white matter changes on CT and MRI. Microscopically there is neuronal loss and atrophy of dendritic spines, especially in the frontal cortex. PET studies have found hypermetabolism in the basal ganglia early in HIV disease, followed by global cortical hypometabolism in the later stages. Treatment with zidovudine may improve the PET changes. Magnetic resonance spectroscopy has been found to have superior ability to detect the early changes of AIDS dementia (Avison et al 2003).

Dementia due to Creutzfeldt–Jakob disease

Creutzfeldt–Jakob disease is sufficiently rare that it is impossible to be certain about the neuroimaging characteristics. CT scans show either atrophy or hypodense regions. MRI studies to date show areas of hyperintensity in the basal ganglia on T2-weighted images (Barboriak et al 1994). PET scans reported to date suggest hypometabolism in diverse cortical areas.

Epilepsy

Patients with partial seizures require investigation to exclude an underlying structural lesion. Patients who experienced the first onset of complex partial seizures in early adulthood are most likely to have a normal scan. Nevertheless, there are a number of pathological processes accounting for *cryptogenic epilepsy*.

The most common pathological entity is hippocampal sclerosis, although focal trauma, cortical dysgenesis, gliomas, arteriovenous malformations and hamartomas are also candidates. Partial seizures occurring during the fourth to sixth decade are more likely to be caused by a neoplasm, trauma or a cerebrovascular disorder than by congenital lesions, such as hippocampal sclerosis or cortical dysgenesis. In the seventh, eighth, and ninth decades vascular and degenerative brain diseases become the major aetiology for focal seizures, with tumours accounting for a small percentage. A focal seizure in an adult warrants a contrast CT scan or an MRI scan. MRI is the investigation of choice (where available). MRI in patients with mesial temporal sclerosis demonstrates hippocampal atrophy, hippocampal hyperintensity on T2-weighted scans and, sometimes, atrophy of the temporal lobe and dilata-

tion of the ipsilateral temporal horn. The technique is exquisitely sensitive for detecting small gliomas, malformations (migrational disorders) and areas of cortical dysgenesis that lead to refractory complex partial seizures. PET imaging may demonstrate a zone of decreased cerebral blood flow at the site of a seizure focus, which correlates well with the extent of the epileptogenic zone on EEG, but less well with pathological findings – the area of hypometabolism is often larger than the actual area of structural abnormality.

Head injury

In the A&E setting, the introduction of CT scanning made it possible to detect lesions that required acute surgical intervention, such as extradural, subdural and intracerebral haematomas. Extradural (epidural) haematomas appear as a unilateral area of increased density in the space between the brain and the skull. They are usually biconvex (football shaped), and there is a shift of brain substance away

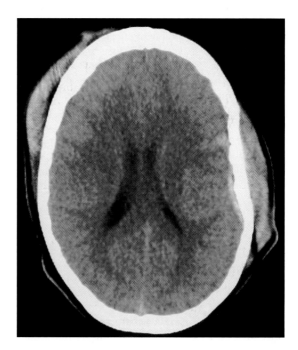

Fig. 4.4 CT scan of a patient with head injury. There are signs of external injury in the left temporal region and right frontoparietal region. There is a depressed segment of skull bone in the left temporal region and signs of intracerebral contusion beneath both areas of injury. From Burkitt & Quick (2001).

from the side of the haematoma and compression of adjacent brain. In contrast, acute subdural haematomas spread over the cortex, are crescent shaped and may be bilateral. Shifts of brain substance and acute hydrocephalus may occur. Head trauma produces parenchymal or subarachnoid blood, which can lead to the development of communicating hydrocephalus. Common sites for contusions are the frontal and anterior temporal lobes. After head trauma the carotid or vertebral arteries may be injured, leading to superimposed cerebrovascular disorders. Herniation may compress the anterior or posterior cerebral arteries, producing ischaemic deficits. Both CT and MRI detect intra- and extracerebral haematomas, although more subtle injuries can be missed.

In the years following a head injury there is reabsorbtion and remodelling of brain tissue, and all that may remain as a remnant of an old injury is mild atrophy or even a normal appearance on CT or MRI. High-resolution MRI using T2 gradient echo techniques can detect residual haemosiderin deposition after microvascular shearing injuries to small white matter tracts (known as *Strich lesions* or *diffuse axonal injury*). Nevertheless, in many patients with behavioural complications following head injury, structural imaging is normal, partly because microscopic tissue damage is beyond the sensitivity of the MRI technique. These shearing lesions tend to occur in the white matter of cerebral cortex (grade I diffuse axonal injury), posterior corpus callosum (grade II diffuse axonal injury) and dorsolateral midbrain (grade III diffuse axonal injury). Very recent research hints that MRS changes in normal-appearing white matter may be of clinical significance (Garnett et al 2000). It is not clear how valuable neuroimaging findings are in predicting functional or cognitive outcome of head injury at the rehabilitation stage, but this is a hot topic of research.

Huntington's disease

On CT and MRI, flattening of the round head of caudate nuclei, which projects into the anterior horn of the lateral ventricles, is a characteristic sign when present. Structural changes (caudate and putamen volumes) are most marked once the disease is clinically apparent, but they may manifest themselves preclinically close to the onset of the disorder (Harris et al 1999). Even in the presymptomatic stages of Huntington's disease, glucose metabolism studies with SPECT and PET show caudate hypome-

tabolism. Huntington's disease is one of the few neurological diseases in which an imaging technique can detect a progressive degenerative brain disease before it is clinically apparent.

Motor neurone disease (amyotrophic lateral sclerosis)

T2-weighted MRI shows signal changes in the corticospinal tract and cortical hypointensities ('ribbon-like bands') in a minority of patients. Cortical atrophy on CT or MRI is a late and non-specific finding. PET studies have shown reduced metabolism in the sensorimotor cortex and the basal ganglia; in patients with neuropsychological changes there is often demonstrable frontal involvement. Magnetic resonance spectroscopy has the potential to detect upper motor neurone dysfunction, with reduced *N*-acetylaspartate found in cortex and brainstem.

Normal-pressure hydrocephalus

The ventricles enlarge beginning with the lateral, third and then fourth ventricle. There is periventricular oedema, confined to the white matter. Blockage of CSF absorption over the cerebral convexities is thought to be responsible for the dilatation of the ventricles. Vascular and degenerative dementia can mimic the clinical and imaging features of the syndrome (see Clinical Pointer 31.1). Unlike Alzheimer's disease, in which the ventricles and sulci are all diffusely enlarged, the sulci appear normal or compressed in normal-pressure hydrocephalus. (Also, executive deficits appear early in the course of hydrocephalus and late in the course of Alzheimer's disease.) Caution is needed as there is a higher than expected rate of white matter lesions (see Clinical Pointer 4.2) in both normal-pressure hydrocephalus and Alzheimer's disease. Similarly, cerebral blood flow is reduced in both conditions. MRI can be useful for ruling out a fourth ventricular mass as the cause of the hydrocephalus.

Multiple sclerosis

Structural imaging can aid in the evaluation of patients with multiple sclerosis. With CT, both old and new large white matter lesions are seen as lucencies. Acute demyelination has a predilection for the regions surrounding the lateral ventricles and, with contrast, is detected as an enhancing area.

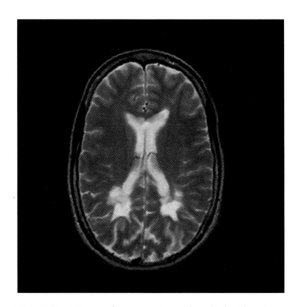

Fig. 4.5 MRI scan from a patient with multiple sclerosis. From KA Johnson, Radiology and Neurology, Massachusetts General Hospital, Harvard Medical School.

MRI is more sensitive to white matter lesions than is CT, and the T2-weighted 'flair' (fluid-attenuated inversion recovery) scan is excellent for showing multiple sclerosis plaques. MRI is also good for detecting lesions in the brainstem and spinal cord. The age of a plaque can be estimated with gadolinium, which detects the breakdown of the blood–brain barrier associated with acute inflammation. Enhancement is seen with gadolinium for 8 weeks after an acute attack. Repeat scans are used to track the course of the disease, since lesion load should reduce with successful treatment. An important recent development is the ability to analyse subtle changes in normal-appearing white matter and grey matter. New quantitative magnetic resonance approaches, such as magnetization transfer imaging and diffusion-weighted imaging, show additional structural changes occurring within and beyond T2-visible lesions.

Parkinson's disease

Structural imaging of Parkinson's disease is not diagnostic. Where CT or MRI shows multiple white matter lesions a diagnosis of parkinsonism resulting from basal ganglia infarction is suggested (vascular parkinsonism). Large lucencies on CT scanning or hyperintensity on MRI in the basal ganglia may suggest other causes for the parkinsonian syndrome, including Wilson's disease, Hallervorden–Spatz disease, carbon monoxide intoxication, striatonigral degeneration, Leigh's disease or adult aminoaciduria. Atrophy of the dorsal midbrain is a feature of supranuclear palsy and olivopontocerebellar degeneration. The latter is characterized by atrophy of the medulla, pons and cerebellum, with variable increases in lucency in the basal ganglia.

A role for functional imaging in Parkinson's disease is currently uncertain, since SPECT cerebral blood flow and PET images of glucose metabolism are often normal in idiopathic Parkinson's disease. That said, several investigators have found decreased uptake of radiolabelled compounds that are markers of presynaptic dopamine, dopamine turnover or dopamine receptors in patients with Parkinson's disease. These include 6-fluoro-dopa radiolabelled with fluoride ions (which is metabolized peripherally to fluorodopamine) and radiolabelled *m*-tyrosine (which is a substitute for the enzyme aromatic amino acid decarboxylase, which is responsible for the conversion of DOPA to dopamine). Recently, studies have suggested that hypoperfusion of the temporal and, perhaps, the frontal lobes in Parkinson's dementia may correlate with cognitive impairment. Interestingly, progressive supranuclear palsy also shows hypoperfusion in the frontal lobes with SPECT and PET scanning, which may be linked with reductions in executive function.

Stroke

The main types of stroke are thrombotic stroke, embolic stroke, intracerebral haemorrhage and subarachnoid haemorrhage (see Fig. 17.2). In the setting of an acute event, CT is performed to exclude cerebral haemorrhage. In most patients who have sustained a subarachnoid haemorrhage, CT and MRI show blood in the subarachnoid space. CT is usually unable to detect any change in the first 24–48 hours after an acute ischaemic injury, during which time hypoxic damage progresses from oedema to necrosis. Functional imaging is more sensitive and shows a disproportionate decrease in regional cerebral blood flow (rCBF) compared with the decreases in regional cerebral metabolic rate for oxygen and glucose. This uncoupling is termed *misery perfusion*, because rCBF is inadequate to supply the metabolic demand for oxygen and glucose. By 1 week after an infarction this pattern reverses, with increased rCBF associated with decreased (or unchanged) glucose utilization, a reverse uncoupling known as 'luxury perfusion'. By 1 month after an infarction, a matched decrease in rCBF, regional oxygen metabolism and glucose metabolism is seen,

indicating irreversibly infarcted tissue. Lacunar disorders in the brainstem and basal ganglia follow a similar pattern of enhancement and reabsorption, but brain haemorrhage is seen as an area of increased intensity with surrounding lucency secondary to oedema. The haematoma is gradually resorbed, leaving lucency at the site of the haemorrhage. Lacunar infarcts are caused by occlusion of small lateral and medial lenticulostriate arteries. Small arteriovenous malformations, angiomas and capillary telangiectasias are well visualized on MRI, but are often missed with CT.

Systemic lupus erythematosus

Several authors have investigated the value of structural and functional neuroimaging in systemic lupus erythematosus with CNS involvement. Lin et al (1997) reported that SPECT was more useful than MRI in identifying patients with broadly defined cerebral systemic lupus erythematosus, owing to the higher sensitivity of SPECT. However, Waterloo et al (2001) reported the opposite findings using more sensitive neuropsychological tests. They reported that several neuropsychological functions were influenced by the presence of cerebral infarcts demonstrated on MRI, but not by SPECT or immunological markers. The utility of both PET and MRI in systemic lupus erythematosus is currently being investigated.

Cerebral tumours

The most common cerebral tumours are glioblastoma multiforme, astrocytoma and meningioma. CNS lymphomas occur in the context of AIDS, and metastases from the lung, breast and gastrointestinal tract are also common. MRI is generally preferred to CT, and both are used with enhancement, since some tumours may only be visible with enhancement.

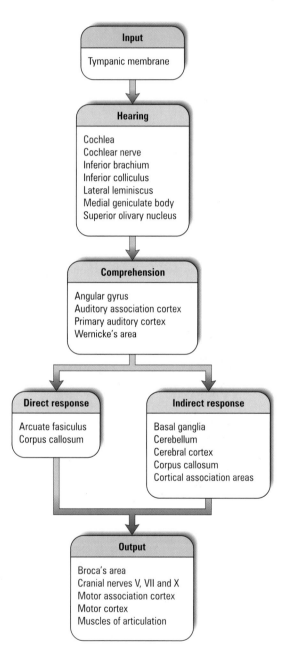

Fig. 4.6 Pathways involved in speech processing. Complex brain functions, such as generating speech, involve many interlinked areas. It is not always possible to discover which path or paths are faulty during life.

PRINCIPLES OF COGNITIVE ASSESSMENT

Cognitive testing is a vital and often poorly performed part of both the psychiatric and neurological investigations. Cognitive impairment is the hallmark of most neuropsychiatric disorders and is the aspect of higher function most accurately correlated with

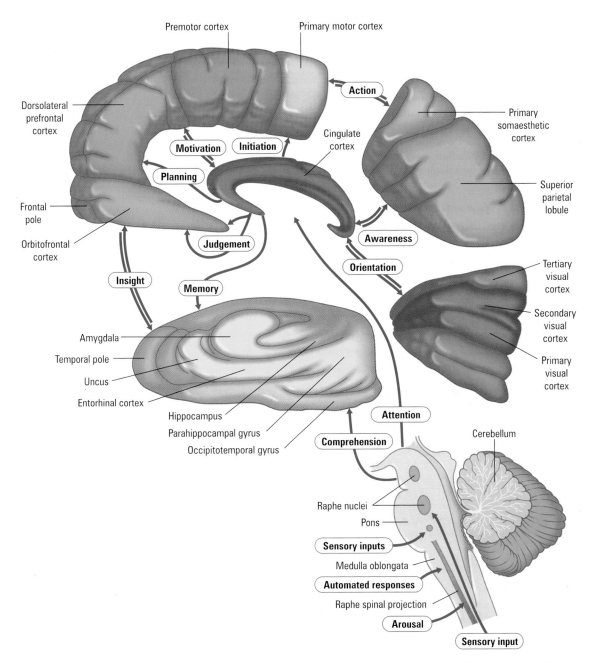

Fig. 4.7 Hierarchy of cognitive functions. Exploded sagittal view of right hemisphere illustrating a hierarchy of cognitive functions. Inputs from lower centres are largely processed unconsciously and priority is given to information of immediate significance (via attention and orientation). Although different areas of the brain are responsible for specific aspects of higher function, there is considerable interdependency.

regional brain injury. Historically, neuropsychological testing was performed to decide whether impairment was due to an organic or functional cause and also to help to localize the suspected lesion. Although these reasons remain relevant, with the advent of neuroimaging, neuropsychology is used more often to quantify the severity and rate of progression of deficits. There is considerable interpretation necessary in these tests. The effect of normative standards, premorbid function, motivation, medication effects, practice effects, compensation (malingering), physical impairment and fatigue must all be taken into account. There is no single best method of cognitive testing – rather it must be applied as clinically appropriate. Brief cognitive screening or bedside cognitive examination is very different from quantitative neuropsychological assessment.

Accounting for a hierarchy of cognitive abilities

There has been considerable effort expended in attempting to formulate neuropsychological tests that reveal specific regional dysfunction. Although partially successful (see Table 7.1), it would be wrong to assume that localization based on neuropsychological testing is entirely accurate, just as localization based on CT or MRI is not entirely accurate. One explanation for this is that the specialized areas of the brain concerned with specific functions are heavily interconnected with related areas. For example, expressive speech is the end result of a sequence of events that begins with an environmental stimulus and ends in the articulation of a response (Fig. 4.6). Lesions to any part of this chain could interfere with speech.

This hierarchy of higher functions applies not only to speech but also to every complex response. Areas of the brain responsible for perception, arousal and attention will always be involved in testing of 'higher' functions (Fig. 4.7).

Assessment of cognitive function is discussed in Chapters 5–11.

REFERENCES AND FURTHER READING

Agartz I, Momenan R, Rawlings RR et al 1999 Hippocampal volume in patients with alcohol dependence. Archives of General Psychiatry 56:356–363

Anfinson TJ, Stoudemire A 1999 Laboratory and neuroendocrine assessment in medical–psychiatric patients. In: Stoudemire A, Fogel BS, Greenberg DB (eds) Psychiatric care of the medical patient, 2nd edn. Oxford University Press, Oxford, p 120–148

Avison MJ, Nath A, Berger JR 2003 Understanding pathogenesis and teatment of HIV dementia: a role for magnetic resonance? Trends in Neurosciences 25:468–473

Barboriak DP, Provencale JM, Boyko OB 1994 MR diagnosis of Creutzfeldt–Jacob disease: significance of high signal intensity of the basal ganglia. American Journal of Roentgenology 162:137–140

Burkitt G, Quick CRG 2001 Essential surgery, 3rd edn. Churchill Livingstone, Edinburgh

Buckman R 2001 Communication in palliative care. Neurologic Clinics 19:989–1004

De Groot JC, de Leeuw FE, Oudkerk M et al 2001 Cerebral white matter lesions and subjective cognitive dysfunction: the Rotterdam scan study. Neurology 56:1539–1545

Diaz-Guzman J, Millan JM, Munoz DG et al 2002 Utility of CT scanning in diagnosing dementia. In: Qizilbash N, Broadaty H, Chiu H et al (eds) Evidence-based dementia practice. Blackwell, Oxford, p 138–154

Du AT, Schuff N, Amend D et al 2001 Magnetic resonance imaging of the entorhinal cortex and hippocampus in mild cognitive impairment and Alzheimer's disease. Journal of Neurology, Neurosurgery and Psychiatry 71:441–447

Fox NC, Freeborough PA, Rossor MN 1996 Visualisation and quantification of rates of atrophy in Alzheimer's disease. Lancet 348:94–97

Friedman J, Standaert DG 2001 Dystonia and its disorders. Neurologic Clinics 19:681–706

Garnett MR, Blamire AM, Corkill RG et al 2000 Early proton magnetic resonance spectroscopy in normal-appearing brain correlates with outcome in patients following traumatic brain injury. Brain 123:2046–2054

Harris GJ, Codori AM, Lewis RF et al 1999 Reduced basal ganglia blood flow and volume in pre-symptomatic, gene-tested persons at-risk for Huntington's disease. Brain 122:1667–1678

Huang C, Wahlund LO, Dierks T et al 2000 Discrimination of Alzheimer's disease and mild cognitive impairment by equivalent EEG sources: a cross-sectional and longitudinal study. Clinical Neurophysiology 111:1961–1967

Kaufman DM 2001 Clinical neurology for psychiatrists, 5th edn. Mosby, Philadelphia

Kubota M, Nakazaki S, Hirai S et al 2001 Alcohol consumption and frontal lobe shrinkage: study of 1432 non-alcoholic subjects. Journal of Neurology, Neurosurgery and Psychiatry 71:104–106

Lewis S 1996 Brain imaging in psychiatry. Blackwell, Oxford

Lin WY, Wang SJ, Yen TC et al 1997 Technetium-99m-HMPAO brain SPECT in systemic lupus erythematosus with CNS involvement. Journal of Nuclear Medicine 38:1112–1115

Minoshima S, Foster NL, Sima AAF et al 2001 Alzheimer's disease versus dementia with Lewy bodies: cerebral metabolic distinction with autopsy confirmation. Annals of Neurology 50:358–365

Mukamal KJ, Longstreth WT, Mittleman MA et al 2001 Alcohol consumption and subclinical findings on magnetic resonance imaging of the brain in older adults: the Cardiovascular Health Study. Stroke 32:1939–1945

Nestor P, Fryer T, Smielewski P et al 2002 Dysfunction of a

common neural network in Alzheimer's disease and mild cognitive impairment: a partial volume corrected region of interest [18]fluorodeoxyglucose-positron emission tomography study. 8th International Conference on Alzheimer's Disease and Related Disorders, Stockholm, 20–25 July

Quality Standards Subcommittee of the American Academy of Neurology 1994 Practice parameter for diagnosis and evaluation of dementia. Neurology 44:2203–2206

Sam MC, So EL 2001 Significance of epileptiform discharges in patients without epilepsy in the community. Epilepsia 42:1273–1278

Stevens A, Lowe J 2000 Pathology. Mosby, St. Louis

Waterloo K, Omdal R, Sjoholm H et al 2001 Neuropsychological dysfunction in systemic lupus erythematosus is not associated with changes in cerebral blood flow. Journal of Neurology 248:595–602

5

Assessment of Consciousness

PRINCIPLES OF ASSESSMENT

Assessment of consciousness

Assessment of consciousness is also an essential part of the clinical examination. Level of consciousness or arousal lies on a continuum, where fully alert and unconscious are at opposite ends. It is helpful to stratify consciousness into six levels (Fig. 5.1).

COMA

Coma can result from brainstem stroke (often the result of infarction of the basilar artery causing a midpontine lesion in the tegmentum), midbrain transection, lesions to the pons or thalamus (bilateral dorsal paramedian lesions) and extensive damage to the cortex (see Box 5.3). Damage to the cortex causes bilateral hemiplegia with primitive reflexes and was labelled the 'apallic state' by Kretschmer (1940). Causes of coma can be divided into abnormalities of brain structure and abnormalities of brain function, and these causes of coma can essentially also cause delirium when they manifest in milder form.

PERSISTENT VEGETATIVE STATE

In comatose patients, acute coma may give way to a chronic coma-like condition (persistent vegetative state). In this condition the sleep–wake cycle is re-established along with primitive reflexes. Thus, the patient is not continually comatose, but gives no indication of awareness. Although the eyes may open and food may be swallowed, there are no cog-

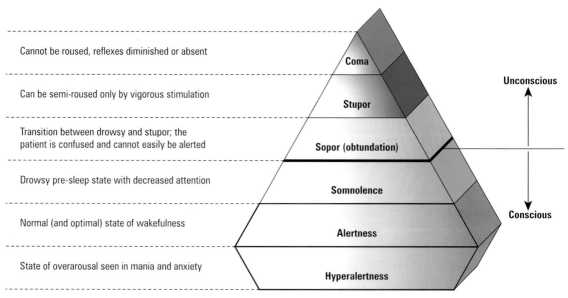

Cannot be roused, reflexes diminished or absent	**Coma**
Can be semi-roused only by vigorous stimulation	**Stupor**
Transition between drowsy and stupor; the patient is confused and cannot easily be alerted	**Sopor (obtundation)**
Drowsy pre-sleep state with decreased attention	**Somnolence**
Normal (and optimal) state of wakefulness	**Alertness**
State of overarousal seen in mania and anxiety	**Hyperalertness**

Unconscious

Conscious

Fig. 5.1 Stages of arousal.

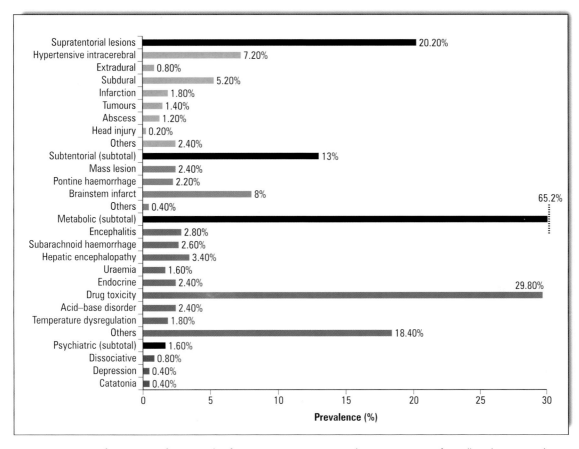

Fig. 5.2 Causes of coma. Data from a study of 500 patients presenting with coma or stupor of initially unknown aetiology. Data from Plum & Posner (1980).

Box 5.1 Definition of coma

- The patient's eyes do not open either spontaneously or to external stimulation; and
- the patient does not follow any commands; and
- the patient does not mouth or utter recognizable words; and
- the patient does not demonstrate intentional movement (may show reflexive movement such as posturing, withdrawal from pain or involuntary smiling); and
- the patient cannot sustain visual pursuit movement of the eyes through a 45° arc in any direction when the eyes are held open manually.

Note that the above criteria are not secondary to use of paralytic agents.

Adapted from American Congress of Rehabilitation Medicine (1995)

Box 5.2 Predictors of prognosis in coma

Poor prognosis:
- absent corneal or pupillary responses
- long duration of coma
- stroke
- subarachnoid haemorrhage

Good prognosis:
- early eye opening
- early motor response
- early vocalization
- infective causes
- metabolic causes
- nystagmus on oculovestibular testing

Adapted from Bates (2001)

Box 5.3   Classification of causes of coma

Coma with focal neurology:
- brain tumour
- cerebral abscess
- encephalitis*
- head injury
- hypertensive encephalopathy
- intracerebral haemorrhage
- meningitis*
- stroke
- subdural or extradural haematoma
- subarachnoid haemorrhage*

Coma without focal neurology:
- alcohol intoxication
- anoxia and carbon monoxide poisoning
- cardiovascular causes
- diabetic ketoacidosis
- drug intoxication
- epilepsy
- hypoglycaemia

*Presents with meningism, but often without focal neurology

Table 5.1   The Glasgow Coma Scale

Test	Response	Score
Eyes open	Spontaneously	4
	To command	3
	To pain	2
	None	1
Best motor response	To verbal command	6
	Localizes pain	5
	Withdrawal	4
	Abnormal (decorticate)	3
	Extension (decerebrate)	2
	No response	1
Best verbal response	Orientated	5
	Disorientated	4
	Inappropriate words	3
	Incomprehensible sounds	2
	None	1
Maximum possible total		15

Clinical Pointer 5.1

Assessment of the unconscious patient

- Emergency action may be needed to stabilize the patient (airway, breathing, respiration, spinal immobilization). The Glasgow Coma Scale is usually used to assess the level of consciousness.
- General inspection covers appearance (signs of injury, needle marks, haemorrhage, CSF leakage, fractures) and respiratory pattern (Cheyne–Stokes, respiratory arrest, central hyperventilation).
- The odour of the breath may reveal indications of alcohol, ketones, fetor hepaticus or other poisoning.
- Pyrexia suggests systemic infection or meningitis.
- Observation of the pupils for size and reaction to light is an essential for coning, drug toxicity and brainstem death.
- There may be skin discolouration – petechia (thrombocytopenic purpura, meningococcaemia, bacterial endocarditis, rickettsial infection), bruises (trauma, nutritional deficiency, purpura) and cyanosis (hypoxia, carboxyhaemoglobinaemia).
- Hypertension can be due to cerebral haemorrhage or hypertensive crisis, whereas hypotension is seen with sedatives, alcohol, myocardial infarction, septicaemia and Addison's disease.
- Examine neurologically for signs of meningeal irritation (neck stiffness, Kerning's sign, photosensitivity) and brainstem function (pupillary light reflex, corneal response, doll's eye reflex and vestibulo-ocular reflex). Fundoscopy is important – think of raised intracranial pressure, hypertensive encephalopathy, subarachnoid haemorrhage, diabetes mellitus and subacute bacterial endocarditis.
- Observe posture. A decorticate posture is flexion to pain, indicating a lesion immediately below the cortex; a decerebrate posture is extension to pain, indicating a lesion in the brainstem.
- Investigations should include biochemical profile, blood gases, blood alcohol, toxicology screen, blood glucose and, if doubt still remains, lumbar puncture and neuroimaging.
- Some clinicians administer the opiate antagonist naloxone to the newly comatose patient, along with dextrose in case of opiate poisoning and hypoglycaemia.
- The most common cause of sudden unconsciousness in the elderly is stroke and in the young is alcohol.

Further reading   Walker MC, O'Brien MD 1999 Neurological examination of the unconscious patient. Journal of the Royal Society of Medicine 92:353–355

Clinical Pointer 5.2

Causes of impaired consciousness

Consciousness is characteristically impaired by cardiovascular disease (e.g. arrhythmias, vasovagal, postural hypotension, mechanical causes), neurological disease (e.g. transient ischaemic attack, stroke, epilepsy, severe head injury, subclavian steal) or metabolic disease (hypoxia, hypoglycaemia, electrolyte imbalance, hypothermia). However, several psychiatric disorders can also be associated with loss of consciousness, including delirium and severe panic attacks (hyperventilation). Patients intoxicated with alcohol or drugs (especially benzodiazepines) complain of 'blackouts', meaning a failure to register new episodic memories during that period rather than loss of consciousness. Adequate information about the blackout really requires an informant who witnessed the event. It is relevant to ask: Was there a warning? Was the onset sudden? Was there altered mental state before? Was there a fall? Was there incontinence or tongue biting, any evidence of seizure, any pallor or flushing?

Further reading Hemphill III JC 2001 Disorders of consciousness in systemic diseases. In: MJ Aminoff (ed) Neurology and general medicine, 3rd edn. Churchill Livingstone, Edinburgh, p 1053–1068

nitive or affective functions (Howard & Miller 1995). Physiological markers of depth of coma include papillary responses, ocular movements and respiration. Bedside tests of eye opening, motor response and verbal responses have been adopted in the Glasgow Coma Scale (Teasdale & Jennett 1974) (Table 5.1). The prognosis of the persistent vegetative state is discussed in Chapter 19.

Two neurological conditions must be distinguished from coma. These are akinetic mutism and the locked-in syndrome.

AKINETIC MUTISM

In akinetic mutism, the patient appears alert and can follow the examiner with his or her eyes. There is a preserved sleep–wake cycle, but no voluntary spontaneous motor or verbal responses (Cairns et al 1941). In the full syndrome there is also incontinence. It has been described most commonly following frontal lobe lesions and lesions of the reticular formation of the midbrain (the latter is likely to impair consciousness).

LOCKED-IN SYNDROME

In the locked-in syndrome, lesions in the upper tegmentum of the ventral pons (or occasionally the midbrain) cause de-efferentation of the lower cranial nerves and the peripheral motor system (cortcospinal and corticobulbar fibres), usually at the level of the facial nuclei. Occasionally, lateral gaze is also paralysed. Such patients are self-aware, but are reduced to communicating by eye movements alone.

REFERENCES AND FURTHER READING

American Congress of Rehabilitation Medicine 1995 Recommendations for use of uniform nomenclature pertinent to patients with severe alterations in consciousness. Archives of Physical Medicine and Rehabilitation 76:205–209

Baddeley A, Hinch G 1997 Recent advances in learning and motivation, vol 8. Academic Press, New York

Baddeley A, Wilson BA, Watts F (eds) 1995 Handbook of memory disorders. Wiley, Chichester

Bates D 2001 The prognosis of medical coma. Journal of Neurology, Neurosurgery and Psychiatry 71(suppl I): I20–I23

Cairns H, Oldfield RC, Pennybacker JB et al 1941 Akinetic mutism with an epidermoid cyst of the third ventricle. Brain 64:273–290

Hemphill JC 2001 Disorders of consciousness in systemic diseases. In: Aminoff MJ (ed) Neurology and general medicine, 3rd edn. Churchill Livingstone, Edinburgh, p 1053–1068

Howard RS, Miller DH 1995 The persistent vegetative state. Information on prognosis allows decisions to made on management. BMJ 310:341–342

Kretschmer E 1940 Das apallische Syndrom. Zeitschrift für die gesamte Neurologie und Psychiatrie, Berlin 169:576–579

Plum F, Posner JB 1980 The diagnosis of stupor and coma. Davis, Philadelphia

Teasdale G, Jennett B 1974 Assessment of coma and impaired consciousness: a practical scale. Lancet 2:81–84

Tulving E 1972 Episodic and semantic memory. In: Tulving E, Donaldson W (eds) Organization of memory. Academic Press, New York, p 381–403

6

Intelligence and Cerebral Dominance

ance IQ, but in 5% of cases the opposite may occur. Verbal IQ is often used as an estimate of premorbid IQ because it is an overlearned skill (i.e. one that is rehearsed many times) that is resistant to deterioration. Experience has shown that this method is not completely accurate and that deterioration can occur, particularly with severe cognitive impairment. Other methods of estimating premorbid IQ include examination of education and occupational records. The NART was developed by Nelson (Nelson & Wilson 1991) and is similar to the vocabulary test of the WAIS, but is thought to be a more accurate estimate of premorbid IQ. Again, studies show that scores of the NART do change with substantial cognitive impairment, albeit slowly. The NART is not applicable to all patients. For example, it can be misleading in those with poor literacy skills or dyslexia and in those with dementia that disturbs language abilities.

INTELLIGENCE

Intelligence testing is at the root of neuropsychological assessment. Measures of intelligence are composite scores of performance across several individual tasks. In 1912, William Stern introduced the concept of an intelligence quotient (IQ). This is the ratio of mental age to chronological age expressed as a percentage. The mean is 100 and the standard deviation is 15. Sixty-eight per cent of the population have an IQ within one standard deviation of the mean (IQ 85–115), and 95% of the population have an IQ within two standard deviations of the mean (IQ 70–130). Learning disability is usually defined by an IQ less than 70, which corresponds to the lowest 2.2% of the population.

The most common test of intelligence is the Wechsler Adult Intelligence Scale (WAIS). This measures current intelligence, that is, intelligence as affected by the prevailing neuropsychiatric condition (Table 6.1). This test is most usefully combined with a premorbid estimate of IQ such as the National Adult Reading Test (NART).

Each group of subtests estimates a different aspect of IQ. *Verbal IQ* is associated with dominant hemisphere function and *performance IQ* is linked to non-dominant hemisphere function. A greater than 10-point difference between the two subscales is said to be suggestive of acquired pathology. Diffuse damage usually causes a greater loss in perform-

Table 6.1 Components of the Wechsler Adult Intelligence Scale, revised (WAIS-R)

Component	Example
Verbal	
Information	Who wrote *Hamlet*?
Comprehension	Why are child-labour laws needed?
Arithmetic*	How many hours does it take to walk 24 miles at 3 miles per hour?
Similarities	How are a banana and an orange alike?
Digit span*	Remember a series of numbers in forward and reverse order
Vocabulary	Meaning of difficult words (e.g. travesty)
Performance (perceptual organization)	
Picture completion	What part is missing from familiar scenes?
Block design	Reproduction of designs with coloured blocks
Picture arrangement	A set of 10 cartoon pictures must be arranged to tell a story
Object assembly	Four jigsaw-like puzzles of familiar objects must be put together
Digit symbol*	Symbols must be matched to digits using a code

*These items together may rate distractibility, which is impaired in many neurological disorders

CEREBRAL DOMINANCE

Although there is considerable individual variation, experiments with intracarotid injections of sodium amytal demonstrate that the left hemisphere is largely responsible for language in 90% or more of right-handers and 70% of left-handers. In 10% of left-handers there is mixed hemisphere dominance. Thus aphasia can occur (albeit rarely) after right hemisphere lesions in right-handed people. By convention, the hemisphere responsible for language is called the *dominant hemisphere*. It also subserves mathematical ability. The *non-dominant hemisphere* does have responsibility for some higher brain functions, including certain visuospatial abilities, music comprehension and appreciation of emotions in language and faces. Interesting and some-times surprising patterns of function are evident in patients with damage to the corpus callosum, the main pathway between the two hemispheres (see Ch. 11). Dominance may be established by using unilateral intracarotid injections of sodium amytal (the Wada technique), by using dichotic listening and visual half-field techniques or by using unilateral electroconvulsive therapy and observing the effect on language.

REFERENCES AND FURTHER READING

Nelson HE, Wilson JR 1991 The National Adult Reading Test (NART): test manual, 2nd edn. NEFR-Nelson, Windsor

7

Cognitive Assessment Scales

NEUROPSYCHOLOGICAL BATTERIES

Batteries are combinations of tests designed to assess different domains. Examples include the Halstead–Reitan battery and the Luria–Nebraska battery. The *Halstead–Reitan battery* is long (taking up to 6 hours to complete) and tends to underemphasize language and memory. Aspects of this battery that seem most sensitive to acquired brain injury include the Category Test, the Tactual Performance Test, the Trail Making Test and the Wechsler Digit Symbol Test. The *Luria–Nebraska battery* has been criticised for psychometric errors. Many psychology departments use their own collection of individual tests. Folstein, Folstein and McHugh's *Mini-Mental State Examination* (MMSE) is a widely used (but limited) mini-test battery, useful in patients with moderate to severe dementia (see Clinical Pointer 40.5 and Table 40.4). A cut-off score of 24 is on the lower 10th percentile for those aged over 65 years. The MMSE is insensitive to subtle recent memory problems seen in early dementia (ceiling effect) and there are also problems in using this test in patients with severe dementia (floor effect). Some batteries developed specifically for dementia incorporate the MMSE. An example is the test for the Consortium to Establish a Registry for Alzheimer's Disease (CERAD). Several batteries, including the Behavioral Assessment of the Dysexecutive Syndrome (BADS) (Wilson et al 1998) and the Executive Interview (EXIT) (Royall et al 1992), aim to detect specific executive deficits.

Computerized tests are increasingly used because they are objective and can measure minute differences in completion and recall times, but they can overlook strategic errors. In the Cambridge Neuropsychological Test Automated Battery (CANTAB), patients are tested with a touch-sensitive screen that determines motor response time, spatial recognition and working memory. It also includes an electronic version of the famous Shallice Tower of London Test (Fig. 7.1). This is essentially a test of planning using increasingly complicated puzzles. An alternative computerized battery is Wesnes' Cognitive Drug Research Battery, which requires subjects to react using an input button or paddle (Wesnes 2002).

NEUROPSYCHIATRIC BATTERIES

Questionnaires that assess various neuropsychiatric domains are beginning to appear. The *Neurobehavioural Rating Scale* was developed by Levin et al (1987) at the University of Texas to assess behaviour

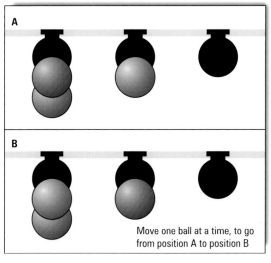

Fig. 7.1 The Tower of London Test in the Cambridge Neuropsychological Test Automated Battery (CANTAB). In a test derived from the Tower of Hanoi puzzle, subjects are asked to move the coloured spheres between three holes in the least number of moves.

Move one ball at a time, to go from position A to position B

Table 7.1 Localization of common neuropsychological tests

Test	Function	Frontal DLPFC and Broca's area	Frontal primary and premotor area	Temporal Wernicke's area	Parietal primary sensory area	Parietal superior and inferior area	Occipital	General or poorly localized	Hemisphere
Tests focusing on memory									
WAIS-R:									
digit span	Repetition	✓			✓				Dominant
digit symbol	Organization	✓	✓					✓	Non-dominant
block design	Praxis	✓	✓			✓	✓	✓	Non-dominant
object assembly	Praxis	✓	✓			✓	✓	✓	Non-dominant
Wechsler Memory Scale (3rd edn):									
logical memory	Memory			✓				✓	Dominant
visual reproduction:	Memory			✓				✓	Non-dominant
– immediate	Attention			✓			✓	✓	Bilateral
– delayed	Memory			✓		✓	✓		Bilateral
California Verbal Learning Test:									
immediate	Memory			✓					Dominant
delayed	Memory			✓					Dominant
Benton Visual Retention Test:									
figures	Memory			✓		✓	✓		Non-dominant
faces	Memory			✓		✓	✓		Non-dominant
Rey–Osterrieth Complex Figure:									
copying	Praxis					✓	✓		Bilateral
recall	Memory			✓			✓		Non-dominant
Bender Gestalt Test:									
copying	Praxis					✓	✓		Non-dominant
recall	Memory			✓		✓	✓		Non-dominant

Contd

Table 7.1 Contd

Test	Function	Frontal DLPFC and Broca's area	Frontal primary and premotor area	Temporal Wernicke's area	Parietal primary sensory area	Parietal superior and inferior area	Occipital	General or poorly localized	Hemisphere
Tests focusing on executive function									
Wisconsin Card Sorting Test	Executive	✓							
Trails Making Test – A	Visuospatial	✓					✓	✓	
Trails Making Test – B	Executive	✓					✓	✓	
Stroop Colour and Word Test	Executive	✓					✓	✓	
Halstead–Reitan Category Test	Executive	✓				✓	✓	✓	Non-dominant
Tests focusing on language									
Boston Diagnostic Aphasia Exam	Language	✓		✓		✓		✓	Dominant
Multilingual Aphasia Exam:									
sentence repetition	Language	✓		✓	✓				Dominant
calculation	Language				✓				Dominant
reading	Language		✓	✓	✓		✓		Dominant
Boston Naming Test	Language	✓	✓	✓	✓			✓	Dominant
Controlled Oral Word Association Test	Language	✓		✓				✓	Dominant
Miscellaneous tests									
Finger Tapping Test	Motor		✓		✓	✓			Dominant
Purdue Pegboard Test	Visuospatial		✓		✓		✓	✓	Non-dominant
Lezak Cancellation Test	Attention	✓		✓			✓	✓	Bilateral

DLPFC, dorsolateral prefrontal cortex; WAIS-R, Weschler Adult Intelligence Scale, Revised
Adapted from Calev et al (1999)

in patients with head injury. It is a 28-item observer-rated instrument that measures a broad range of cognitive and non-cognitive symptoms. The examiner rates each aspect on a seven-point Likert scale from 'not present' to 'extremely severe'. To date, the scale has been evaluated in large groups of patients with head injury and in small groups of patients with dementia.

The *Neuropsychiatric Inventory* (NPI) was created by Cummings et al (1994) at the University of Los Angeles. The NPI was developed to assess psychopathology in dementia patients. It evaluates 10 (or 12, depending on the version) neuropsychiatric disturbances common in dementia, with both a frequency and severity score: delusions, hallucinations, agitation, depression, anxiety, apathy, irritability, euphoria, disinhibition, aberrant motor behaviour, night-time behaviour disturbances and appetite or eating abnormalities. The NPI can also be used to assess the amount of carer distress engendered by each of the neuropsychiatric disorders. The NPI is being applied to a variety of neuropsychiatric conditions. The inventory is now available in a short, user-friendly form (Kaufer et al 2000).

The *Mini International Neuropsychiatric Interview* is a short diagnostic structured interview exploring aspects from 17 disorders of the DSM-III-R diagnostic criteria. It takes about 20 minutes to administer. It was developed by Lecrubier et al (1997) and was initially piloted on 346 patients. It is designed to allow interview by non-specialist physicians and focuses on current problems.

The *Neuropsychology Behaviour and Affect Profile* is a scale that consists of 106 randomly ordered statements encompassing five domains: inappropriateness, indifference, depression, pragnosia (communication problems) and mania.

GLOBAL ASSESSMENT SCALES

Questionnaires that assess function are often a better measure of well-being than cognitive scales alone. Unfortunately, few have been validated in patients with cognitive impairment (Riemsma et al 2001). Individual abilities show a correlation of about 0.5 with cognitive test scores in Alzheimer's disease. Basic activities of daily living include eating, dressing and toileting. More advanced 'instrumental' activities include shopping, cooking and handling money. Measures of function such as the

Progressive Deterioration Scale overlap with measures of quality of life (DeJong et al 1989). The Medical Outcomes Study Short Form Health survey (SF-36) is one of the most popular quality-of-life scales. It comprises eight health domains: physical functions, role limitations (physical), role limitations (emotional), bodily pain, general health, vitality, social functioning and mental health. The validity of the SF-36 has been assessed in at least four studies in stroke and two in multiple sclerosis (Riemsma et al 2001). Some quality-of-life scales have been tailored to assess the impact of a disease on well-being. One of the best examples is the Sickness Impact Profile (see Appendix V). The Sickness Impact Profile has been validated in five studies in head injury, three in stroke and two in multiple sclerosis (Riemsma et al 2001).

REFERENCES AND FURTHER READING

Cummings JL, Mega M, Gray K et al 1994 The neuropsychiatric inventory: comprehensive assessment of psychopathology in dementia. Neurology 44:2308–2314

DeJong R, Osterlund OW, Roy GW 1989 Measurement of quality-of-life changes in patients with Alzheimer's disease. Clinical Therapeutics 11:545–554

Kaufer DI, Cummings JL, Ketchel P et al 2000 Validation of the NPI-Q, a brief clinical form of the neuropsychiatric inventory. Journal of Neuropsychiatry and Clinical Neuroscience 12:233–239

Lecrubier Y, Sheehan DV, Weiller E et al 1997 The Mini International Neuropsychiatric Interview (MINI). A short diagnostic structured interview: reliability and validity according to the CIDI. European Psychiatry 12:224–231

Levin HS, High WM, Goethe KE et al 1987 The Neurobehavioural Rating Scale: assessment of the behavioural sequelae of head injury by the clinician. Journal of Neurology, Neurosurgery and Psychiatry 50:183–193

Riemsma RP, Forbes CA, Glanville JM et al 2001 General health status measures for people with cognitive impairment: learning disability and acquired brain injury. Health Technology Assessment 5(6). Available: http://www.hta.nhsweb.nhs.uk/fullmono/mon506.pdf

Royall DR, Mahurin RK, Gray KF 1992 Bedside assessment of executive cognitive impairment: the executive interview. Journal of the American Geriatric Society 40:1221–1226

Wesnes K 2002 Assessing cognitive function in clinical trials: latest developments and future directions. Drug Discovery Today 7:29–35

Wilson BA, Evans JJ, Emslie H et al 1998 The development of an ecologically valid test for assessing patients with a dysexecutive syndrome. Neuropsychological Rehabilitation 8:213–228

8

Orientation and Attention

ORIENTATION

There are numerous reasons why patients may respond incorrectly to questions of where they are in time and space. Assuming that a patient is able to respond (i.e. consciousness and language functions are intact), he or she may not have been given or acquired sufficient information to answer the question. This is a common scenario for chronically hospitalized patients. We place more emphasis on the failure to retain orientation information in conditions that affect arousal and memory, and less emphasis on this ability in patients with poor judgement or in those suspected of malingering. Patients will usually use environmental clues to attempt to answer correctly. When patients answer incorrectly and hold that erroneous belief with initial conviction but are amenable to persuasion, this is usually an indication of the presence of *confabulation*. The most common lesions associated with confabulation are those in the non-dominant frontal lobe, medial temporal lobe and basal forebrain. Occasionally, patients firmly and unshakably hold an erroneous belief that one real place or person is a copy of another existing somewhere else. This is a phenomenon called *reduplicative paramnesia* (see Clinical Pointer 2.2).

ATTENTION

Various terms are used to describe the ability of a person to focus on the task at hand for a sustained period without becoming distracted. The words 'attention', 'concentration' and 'vigilance' are often used interchangeably, although their scientific meanings are subtly different. *Focused attention* refers to the search and location of stimuli. *Sustained attention* (vigilance) refers to monitoring of stimuli over an extended period. *Divided attention* means the ability to perform two tasks at the same time. It is particularly important in psychiatric patients to assess, first, the level of alertness and, secondly, the level of concentration. These poorly localized cognitive functions will certainly interfere with further tests. There is also the related function of speed of processing. A handy test of attention and processing speed is the *Trail Making Test* (Armitage 1946). Part A of this test requires connection of a randomly placed numbered sequence; part B requires connection of alternative numbers and letters. The average time to complete part A is 30 s; the average time for part B is 75 s. Times longer than 80 s and 4 minutes, respectively, suggest a deficit. Other tests of processing speed include the Paced Serial Addition Test (PASAT), Map Search and Telephone Search (looking for specific symbols on a page). Implicit or reflexic aspects of attention can be tested. Complex selective attention overlaps with executive function, for example in the Stroop Test.

Neuroanatomy of attention

Attention depends on primitive brain functions such as arousal being intact. The reticular formation (responsible for arousal) relays information via ascending monoaminergic tracts to the thalamus. Almost every major sensory and arousal path routes through the thalamus on its way to the cortex (the olfactory system is the exception). The thalamus receives an equivalent number of descending pathways, which suggests that its main role is to modulate chaotic ascending information into more manageable chunks. Concentration and attention appear to be mediated via the cortex in diffuse areas, particularly the large areas of 'multimodal association

---

Box 8.1 Tests of attention

- Trails test time B minus test A time (processing speed)
- Letter cancellation test
- Digit span – forwards and backwards
- Months of the year – backwards
- Simple serial calculations
- The continuous performance test

areas' in the prefrontal cortex, the posterior parietal cortex and the ventral temporal lobes.

Disorders of attention

There are many subtle and ill-defined disorders of attention, but the most common is the acute confusional state. (The term 'confusion' is poorly defined, but is usually taken to mean varying orientation, which is itself only indirect evidence of inattention.) Right-sided focal brain lesions can cause acute confusional states, showing that focal damage causes diffuse dysfunction. Besides delirium, many psychiatric disorders feature impairments in attention, particularly in the severe stages of illness. Obvious examples are mania, the negative syndrome of schizophrenia and melancholic depression. In patients who appear to have a localized deficit in attention, it is common to test for sensory inattention via bilateral confrontation. Commonly the cause is hemianopia or dysasthesia, but a disorder of sensory awareness is a possibility (see Ch. 14).

REFERENCES AND FURTHER READING

Armitage SG 1946 An analysis of certain psychological tests used for the evaluation of brain injury. Psychological Monographs 60:1–48

9

Memory

Memory is the ability to register (encode), retain (store) and recall (retrieve) new information. Clearly registration depends on the lower neuropsychological functions of attention and arousal. Encoding includes both the process of holding information longer than the attention span and the process of chunking information into manageable pieces. Storing is the process of consolidating memories into permanent traces, and retrieving is selectively recollecting these permanent traces. Difficulty remembering newly presented information is referred to as *anterograde amnesia*, and this implies a persistent memory problem. Difficulty in remembering past information is *retrograde amnesia*, which, in isolation, is a less sinister finding.

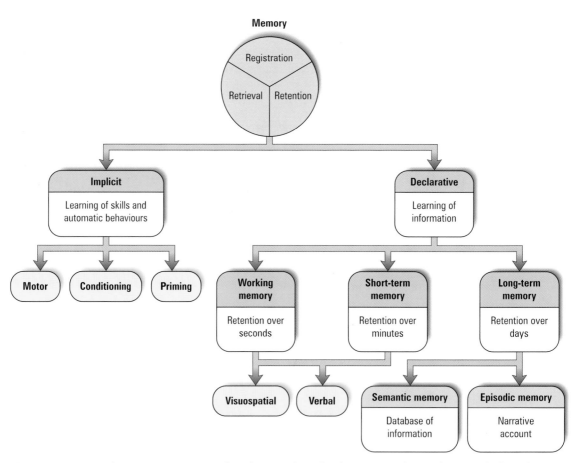

Fig. 9.1 Overview of memory. Neuroscientists have long sought to classify memory in the most legitimate biological way. There is good evidence that acquisition of information is a different process from the acquisition of skills. Learning of information can be further divided into different types of memory based on the duration of retention. Rapid developments in this field will reshape this schema.

The most biologically defined subdivision of memory divides new information into the consciously accessed and the unconsciously accessed. Unconscious access to newly learnt information (usually motor skills or reflexes) is something we all take for granted and is one of the most primitive of brain functions. This is conventionally called *implicit or procedural memory*. Memory for information that we have conscious recollection of and access to is called *explicit or declarative memory*; this is the type of memory that is assessed in routine cognitive tests. It is further subdivided into a permanent store or factual database called *semantic memory*, and a memory for day-to-day events laid down like a narrative account, called *episodic memory* (after Tulving (1972)).

A simplistic way of summarizing memory is:

- knowing how – implicit memory
- knowing what – declarative memory
- knowing when – episodic memory
- knowing about – semantic memory.

Much confusion exists about the terms 'short-term memory' and 'long-term memory'. From a physiological perspective, the *short-term memory* most accurately refers to working memory that helps to register telephone-number lengths of information over a few seconds. It may also be used to manipulate information recently retrieved from long-term stores. Working memory was divided by Baddeley & Hitch (1977) into two storage divisions – one for phonological material (words, numbers and music) and one for visuospatial material (the *visuospatial sketch pad*). Information is maintained with the aid of a rehearsal system (the *articulatory loop*) and is guided by the *central executive*.

The task of recalling previously learnt material after some delay is called *long-term memory* (see also Ch. 19). Oldest memories are usually those most resistant to erosion, a phenomenon referred to as the 'temporal gradient' (or Ribot's law, after Ribot (1882)). This effect tends to break down in Huntington's disease and cases of severe Alzheimer's disease.

NEUROANATOMY OF MEMORY

Although Papez (1898–1982; a neuroanatomist at Cornell Medical School) may not have been correct in thinking that the limbic system is responsible for emotions, it appears that the limbic system is responsible for episodic memory (Papez 1937). The hippocampus is the key component, and damage on the dominant side impairs learning of verbal material, whereas damage to the non-dominant side interferes with learning of faces and spatial information. Bilateral damage to any of part of the Papez circuit (see Figs 13.1 and 13.2) can be particularly devastating.

In contrast to the relatively localized neuroanatomy of episodic memory, semantic memory appears to be more widely distributed, largely in the neocortex. Regarding implicit memory, this primitive system has yet to be accurately localized, but evidence suggests contributions from the basal ganglia, cerebellum and spinal cord. Other areas of the brain may have specialized roles in memory (e.g. in spatial memory or memory for faces) (see also Ch. 69).

DISORDERS OF MEMORY

Disorders of working memory

Deficits in working memory are often attributed to problems in attention (deriving from lesions to the frontal lobes or the reticular activating system). Impairment in the central executive component of working memory is seen in cortical (Alzheimer's)

Box 9.1 Subjective memory complaints

Disorientation
Forgetting the time or date
Getting lost or frightened in familiar places
Losing track of current events

Disorganization
Forgetting appointments and messages
Forgetting instructions and plans
Leaving mail or finances unattended
Risking personal safety

Omission
Leaving things behind
Losing important items
Forgetting switches, locks and lights

Repetition
Asking the same question
Telling the same story
Performing the same action unnecessarily

Note: all can occur in healthy people

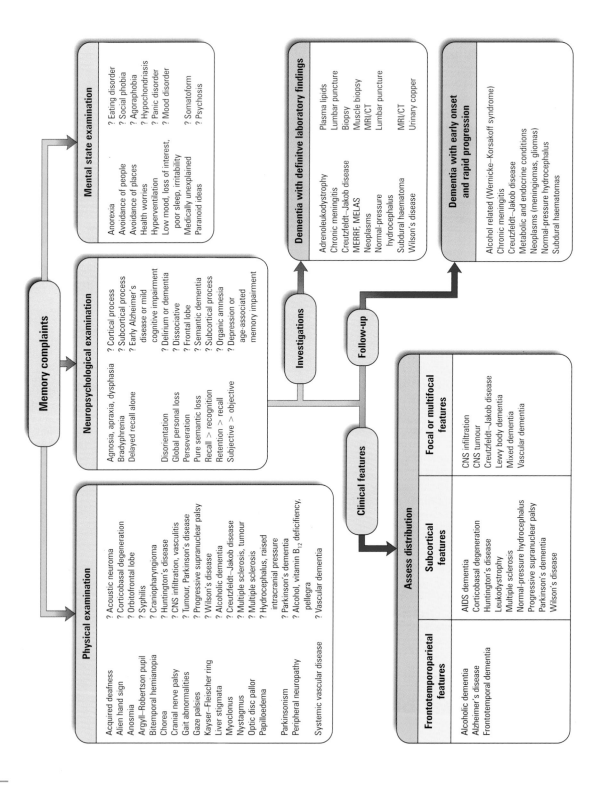

Memory complaints

Physical examination

Acquired deafness
Alien hand sign
Anosmia
Argyll–Robertson pupil
Bitemporal hemianopia
Chorea
Cranial nerve palsy
Gait abnormalities
Gaze palsies
Kayser–Fleischer ring
Liver stigmata
Myoclonus
Nystagmus
Optic disc pallor
Papilloedema

Parkinsonism
Peripheral neuropathy

Systemic vascular disease

? Acoustic neuroma
? Corticobasal degeneration
? Orbitofrontal lobe
? Syphilis
? Craniopharyngioma
? Huntington's disease
? CNS infiltration, vasculitis
? Tumour, Parkinson's disease
? Progressive supranuclear palsy
? Wilson's disease
? Alcoholic dementia
? Creutzfeldt–Jakob disease
? Multiple sclerosis, tumour
? Multiple sclerosis
? Hydrocephalus, raised
   intracranial pressure
? Parkinson's dementia
? Alcohol, vitamin B₁₂ deficiency,
   pellegra
? Vascular dementia

Neuropsychological examination

Agnosia, apraxia, dysphasia
Bradyphrenia
Delayed recall alone

Disorientation
Global personal loss
Perseveration
Pure semantic loss
Recall > recognition
Retention > recall
Subjective > objective

? Cortical process
? Subcortical process
? Early Alzheimer's
   disease or mild
   cognitive impairment
? Delirium or dementia
? Dissociative
? Frontal lobe
? Semantic dementia
? Subcortical process
? Organic amnesia
? Depression or
   age-associated
   memory impairment

Mental state examination

Anorexia
Avoidance of people
Avoidance of places
Health worries
Hyperventilation
Low mood, loss of interest,
   poor sleep, irritability
Medically unexplained
Paranoid ideas

? Eating disorder
? Social phobia
? Agoraphobia
? Hypochondriasis
? Panic disorder
? Mood disorder

? Somatoform
? Psychosis

Investigations

Dementia with definitive laboratory findings

Adrenoleukodystrophy
Chronic meningitis
Creutzfeldt–Jakob disease
MERRF, MELAS
Neoplasms
Normal-pressure
   hydrocephalus
Subdural haematoma
Wilson's disease

Plasma lipids
Lumbar puncture
Biopsy
Muscle biopsy
MRI/CT
Lumbar puncture

MRI/CT
Urinary copper

Follow-up

**Dementia with early onset
and rapid progression**

Alcohol related (Wernicke–Korsakoff syndrome)
Chronic meningitis
Creutzfeldt–Jakob disease
Metabolic and endocrine conditions
Neoplasms (meningiomas, gliomas)
Normal-pressure hydrocephalus
Subdural haematomas

Clinical features

Assess distribution

Frontotemporoparietal features	Subcortical features	Focal or multifocal features
Alcoholic dementia	AIDS dementia	CNS infiltration
Alzheimer's disease	Corticobasal degeneration	CNS tumour
Frontotemporal dementia	Huntington's disease	Creutzfeldt–Jakob disease
	Leukodystrophy	Levy body dementia
	Multiple sclerosis	Mixed dementia
	Normal-pressure hydrocephalus	Vascular dementia
	Progressive supranuclear palsy	
	Parkinson's dementia	
	Wilson's disease	

dementia and subcortical (Huntington's) dementias. Damage to the phonological system related to pathology in perisylvian language areas can also be a cause.

Disorders of episodic memory

Three classic causes of episodic memory loss (evident as an inability to retain new material for more than a few minutes) are Korsakoff's syndrome, transient global amnesia and hippocampal damage from herpes simplex encephalitis. The term *amnesia* is commonly used as a shorthand way of referring to episodic memory loss. One intriguing function of episodic memory is keeping track of a person's place in time. Patients with dense episodic memory deficits may lose the ability to associate themselves with personally significant past events or even plan for the future. In essence they become trapped in the present. This aspect of episodic memory is known as *autonoetic consciousness* (as opposed to *noetic conciousness*, which is the sense of familiarity or knowing, possibly linked with semantic memory) (see Clinical Pointer 2.2).

Amnesia can result from toxins such as alcohol, lead, mercury, carbon monoxide, organophosphates and solvents. Both the ICD and DSM-IV include the category of amnestic disorders caused by systemic medical disease that is not due to dementia or delirium. In many cases this distinction is artificial. Nevertheless, hallmarks of these conditions include potential reversibility, occurrence in clear consciousness and attribution to one clear cause identified during life. Mood and insight are often affected.

Fig. 9.2 *(opposite)* A simplified approach to memory complaints. Subjective memory complaints are usually the earliest manifestation of both psychiatric and neurological causes of cognitive impairment. However, predominant subjective complaints occur in depression and age-associated memory impairment. A careful history is vital in order to detect cultural, developmental and educational influences. Observation of the mental state will reveal current mental health difficulties. Physical examination must not be overlooked, particularly with reference to vascular disease or movement disorder. Neuropsychological examination is useful in difficult cases and also acts to benchmark performance. Results of investigations, particularly neuroimaging, should be viewed in conjunction with other clinical data. Not uncommonly, a definitive diagnosis is not possible after a single assessment and longitudinal observation is required. MELAS, mitochondrial encephalopathy with lactic acidosis and stroke-like episodes; MERRF, mitochondrial encephalopathy with ragged red fibres.

Box 9.2 Tests of memory

Working memory

Digit span

Episodic memory:
- word-list learning (verbal)
- paired associate learning (verbal)
- story recall (verbal)
- name and address recall (verbal)
- autobiographical memory (retrograde)
- complex figure recall (e.g. Rey–Osterrieth figure)
- newly presented faces (non-verbal)

Semantic memory:
- naming of familiar objects
- tests of general knowledge
- famous faces or famous scenes

Batteries:
- Wechsler Memory Scale, Revised
- Rivermead Behavioural Memory Test

Episodic memory is affected in almost every type of dementia (with the exception of early frontal lobe dementia and semantic dementia). Unlike pure organic amnesia, the episodic loss of dementia occurs in the context of a more global cognitive decline. Some literature supports the observation that, in the cortical dementias, deficits in encoding (registration) and retention as well as retrieval (recall) occur, whereas in the subcortical dementias retrieval and recall deficits occur but recognition itself is well preserved. Furthermore, a difficulty in the recall of long-term memories is said to be more prominent for recent events in the cortical dementias, but not the subcortical dementias.

Disorders of semantic memory

Semantic memory is more permanent than episodic memory, and therefore in most conditions it is less affected. A pure loss of semantic abilities suggests a semantic dementia (see Ch. 41). More commonly, semantic abilities deteriorate in the context of a more severe generalized dementia.

Disorders of metamemory

Metamemory is the ability to judge the capability of one's own memory function. Studies of patients with amnestic disorders and elderly patients have revealed low correlations between subjective memo-

Clinical Pointer 9.1

Types of memory deficits in neuropsychiatric disorders

In most situations, it is extremely difficult to diagnose a clinical syndrome on the basis of a specific memory deficit alone. This is because most neuropsychiatric disorders affect several closely located but functionally distinct anatomical areas. Localized damage to the amygdala appears to disrupt the association of threatening stimuli and the normal emotional response (usually fear) that is essential for survival. Damage to the hippocampus tends to cause problems for new learning, predominantly of verbal material. Deficits in declarative memory are seen with cortical dementias, but procedural deficits are usually more significant with subcortical dementias and also with vascular dementia.

As a rule of thumb it may be helpful to remember that deficits in registration are characteristic of degenerative dementia (Alzheimer's disease), deficits in retention are characteristic of medial temporal lobe disorders (Korsakoff's) and deficits in recall are seen in subcortical dementias.

One of the most important distinctions is between anterograde and retrograde memory loss. Patients with damage to areas responsible for memory will continue to experience difficulty dealing with new information and hence have disruption to daily living. They have *continuous anterograde amnesia*. Patchy memory loss for past events can have many explanations, including failure to register information at the time, perhaps owing to systemic illness or poor attention. In the most severe memory disorders, both anterograde and retrograde memory are affected.

Further reading   Baddeley A, Wilson BA, Watts F (eds) 1995 Handbook of memory disorders. Wiley, New York

ry complaints and objective performance on memory tasks. For example, Korsakoff's syndrome patients underestimate the severity of their memory impairment and are unable to predict performance on subsequent memory tests. Conversely, depressed patients characteristically overestimate their memory difficulties and, moreover, respond catastrophically when information about suboptimal performance is fed back in the middle of a test. Several factors influence metamemory, including severity of memory impairments, problem-solving ability, mood and feedback from others.

REFERENCES AND FURTHER READING

Baddeley AD, Hitch G 1977 Working memory. In: Bower GA (ed) Recent advances in learning and motivation, vol 8. Academic Press, New York, p 647–667

Baddeley A, Wilson BA, Watts F (eds) 1995 Handbook of memory disorders. Wiley, Chichester

Papez JW 1937 A proposed mechanism of emotion. Archives of Neurology and Pathology 38:725–743

Tulving E 1972 Episodic and semantic memory. In: Tulving E, Donaldson W (eds) Organization of memory. Academic Press, New York, p 381–403

10

Speech and Language

Disorders of speech may occur without impairments in language. Speech depends on intact cranial nerves sending signals to muscles of the jaw and pharynx. *Dysarthria* refers to a problem with articulation (more strictly, it is the misarticulation of phonemes) (Table 10.1). *Dysphonia* refers to a diminution of speech volume, usually caused by vocal cord damage.

Disorders of language are usually tested using fluency, repetition, comprehension and naming (Box 10.1). Paul Broca described non-fluent aphasia (originally labelled 'aphemia') in 1861, and this is referred to as *Broca's dysphasia* or *expressive dysphasia*. Characteristically, speech is slow and difficult (i.e. non-fluent) and, although comprehension is preserved, there are distortions of speech such as phonemic paraphasias and agrammatism. Phonemic paraphasias involve the substitution of one phoneme for another (e.g. 'look' for 'cook' or 'bink' for 'pink'). Verbal or semantic paraphasias involve

the replacement of one word with another (e.g. chair instead of 'stool'). Patients also have difficulty saying exactly what they mean and often are forced into describing an object rather than naming it (sometimes called *circumlocutory or elliptical speech*). They may substitute words of close meaning (known as *word approximation*). Simplistically, the structure of speech is grossly disturbed, but the content is relatively preserved.

Carl Wernicke, who was Professor of Neurology in Breslau, described an alternative type of communication problem in 1874. In *Wernicke's aphasia* or *receptive aphasia*, speech is spontaneous and grammatical structure is relatively good. The ability to understand written or verbal information is disturbed and speech output is increasingly senseless, with phonemic paraphasias and semantic paraphasias. In severe forms, sentences appear to follow grammatical rules but lose their meaning. This is

---

Box 10.1   Tests of language

Expressive language
- Spontaneous speech
- Word fluency: number of items named in 60 s (symbolic or semantic)
- Boston Naming Test: line drawings of increasingly difficult objects are named
- Boston Diagnostic Aphasia Examination (BDAE)
- Story-telling ability

Comprehension
- Token test: instructions are given on the manipulation of coloured shapes
- Response to bedside commands

Vocabulary
- National Adult Reading Test
- Weschler Adult Intelligence Scale, Revised, Vocabulary Test

---

Table 10.1   The dysarthrias

Type of dysarthria	Lesion	Symptom
Spastic dysarthria	Cortex or corticobulbar (upper motor neurone)	Monotonous and thick speech
Ataxic dysarthria	Cerebellar	Irregular 'scanning' speech with articulatory pauses
Hypokinetic dysarthria*	Basal ganglia	Soft, monotonous, stuttering
Flaccid dysarthria	Bulbar structures (lower motor neurone)	Nasal speech

*Hyperkinetic speech of variable rate and prolonged phonemes can occur with Huntington's disease

known as *drivelling* or *jargon agrammatism*. Simplistically, the structure of speech is preserved but the content is meaningless (as if the patient is speaking a foreign language). Patients often have reduced subjective awareness of this problem.

Several other, more unusual aphasias have also been described. In *conduction dysphasia* speech is fluent and comprehension good, but naming and repetition are severely abnormal (due to paraphasic intrusions). In *anomic aphasia* repetition is spared, but naming is poor. In patients who have features of either Broca's or Wernicke's aphasia but who are able to repeat sentences put to them, the terms *extrasylvian (transcortical) motor aphasia* or *extrasylvian (transcortical) sensory aphasia* are applied, respectively. Approximately 25% of all aphasias have shared components and these are called *global dysphasias*. Lesions to the association areas can produce unusual language impairments. Lesions of the supplemental motor region above Broca's area (known as Exner's area) causes a pure agraphia in which the patient is not aphasic but has difficulty writing and reading.

Patients with formal thought disorder often have speech patterns that are bizarre and sometimes suggestive of a Wernicke-type dysphasia. They generate words and sentences other than those expected and may respond with answers that are completely unrelated to the question (non-sequitur) and use words that are totally out of context (private word usage or out-of-class semantic paraphasia) (Box 10.2 and Fig. 10.1). The breakdown of the logical flow of thought into less and less meaningful steps is referred to by the generic term *loosening of associations*.

Perseveration of speech (and action) refers to the inappropriate continuation of a thought (or action) after its proper context has passed. This sign is highly suggestive of organic brain disease. It is most commonly seen after a stroke but is also seen in Alzheimer's disease. Similarly, intrusions (late recurrences of words taken from an earlier context) are suggestive of organic disease. Intrusions are most commonly seen in stroke patients who have Wernicke's dysphasia.

Box 10.2 Lexicon of language abnormalities

Abnormal use of words
Neologism
Verbal paraphasia (word approximation)
Private word usage

Abnormal use of sentences
Jargon speech (drivelling)
Derailment (paragrammatism)
Non-sequitur

Abnormal responses
Prolixity
Circumstantial speech
Tangential (rambling speech)

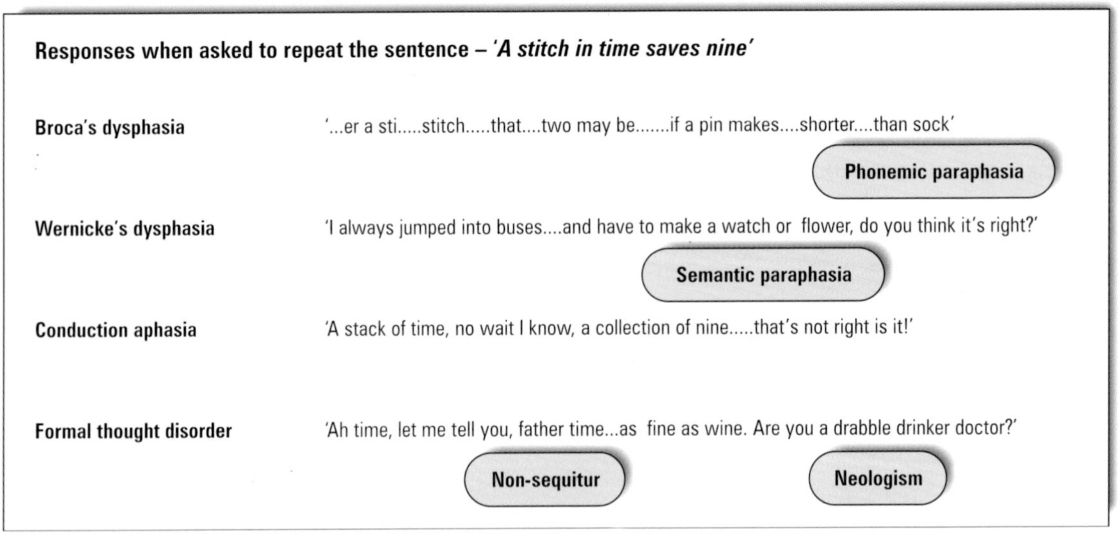

Responses when asked to repeat the sentence – *A stitch in time saves nine*

Broca's dysphasia   '...er a sti.....stitch.....that....two may be.......if a pin makes....shorter....than sock'

> **Phonemic paraphasia**

Wernicke's dysphasia   'I always jumped into buses....and have to make a watch or flower, do you think it's right?'

> **Semantic paraphasia**

Conduction aphasia   'A stack of time, no wait I know, a collection of nine.....that's not right is it!'

Formal thought disorder   'Ah time, let me tell you, father time...as fine as wine. Are you a drabble drinker doctor?'

> **Non-sequitur**   **Neologism**

Fig. 10.1 Clinical examples of language abnormalities.

NEUROANATOMY OF LANGUAGE

Broca's area lies in the inferior gyrus of the cortex in the frontal lobe. Wernicke's area lies in the posterior aspect of the superior gyrus of the temporal lobe (Fig. 10.2). Behind Wernicke's area lies the angular gyrus and lesions to this area disrupt writing. The angular gyrus has also been implicated in Gerstmann's syndrome. The pathway that links Wernicke's and Broca's areas is called the arcuate fasciculus. Lesions of this pathway cause conduction aphasia. It is also important to acknowledge the subtle role of the non-dominant hemisphere (shown best in experiments with patients who have undergone section of the corpus callosum) – melody and intonation in language are served mainly by the non-dominant hemisphere, but there is not inconsiderable comprehension ability and an auditory vocabulary located in the right hemisphere.

DISORDERS OF LANGUAGE

Meaningless fluent speech is seen in mania and schizophrenia with formal thought disorder as well as in the true Wernicke's dysphasia. However, the quality is different in each condition (see Clinical Pointer 10.1). Non-fluent hesitant speech or even aphasia may reflect a sudden neurological event (in Broca's area) but may also reflect catatonic schizophrenia, retarded depression, abulia, dissociative disorder or elective mutism. 'Mutism' refers to an inability or refusal to speak and thus has many possible explanations. 'Aphemia' refers to lesions of the frontal motor cortex (sparing Broca's area) causing pure word mutism. It could be considered as a motor disorder of speech, overlapping with apraxia of speech. Akinetic mutism was described in 1941 as a condition of alert watchfulness with no motor or verbal commands (see also Ch. 5). Some consider this an extreme form of an amotivational syndrome or abulia. Occasionally, degenerative disease of the cortex can produce a profound aphasia syndrome. The most common language deficits seen in early Alzheimer's disease are word-finding difficulties, followed by the use of increasing inaccurate terminology (circumlocutions and paraphasias) and then reductions in fluency. When the inferior and middle dominant temporal gyri temporal cortex is involved, a progressive fluent aphasia (also known as semantic dementia) occurs. When the inferior frontal perisylvian language cortex is atrophied, a progressive non-fluent aphasia results.

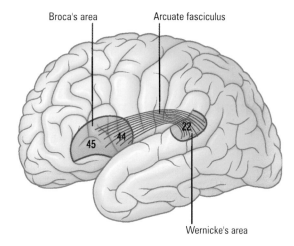

Fig. 10.2 Core regions of the brain involved in language, illustrated using Brodmann areas.

Clinical Pointer 10.1

Neurological or psychiatric cause of language problems?

Dysphasia, dysarthria and aprosody imply a focal neurological lesion, whereas derailment, echolalia, neologisms and poverty or pressure of speech imply a psychiatric cause. However, there is considerable overlap. Dysphonia and mutism occur in both psychiatric and neurological disorders. Patients with formal thought disorder present with jumbled speech that is reminiscent of a mild receptive dysphasia. However, in formal thought disorder there is often some tenuous link between disjointed phrases (e.g. rhyming or punning in the case of mania) and it also waxes and wanes across sentences, whereas in receptive dysphasia the abnormality is usually consistently present. It is advisable to test repetition, pure comprehension and use of complex words. These areas are not affected in schizophrenia. Patients with dissociative disorder can present with bizarre speech patterns. Usually these patients appear distressed, distracted and uncooperative with testing, unlike patients who have suffered a dysphasia. Patients with Alzheimer's disease who have disproportionate aphasia and patients with semantic dementia (primary progressive aphasia) have left hemispheric hypometabolism on PET scanning.

Further reading Grossman M, Mickanin J, Onishi K et al 1996 Progressive nonfluent aphasia: language, cognitive, and PET measures contrasted with probable Alzheimer's disease. Journal of Cognitive Neuroscience 8:135–154

11

Other Important Cognitive Domains

CONCEPTUAL DISORDERS OF MOVEMENT

Praxis is the ability to sequence and perform motor acts. Apraxia is a syndrome of higher motor dysfunction not due to a deficit in strength, motivation or comprehension. It implies that there is a lesion of the cerebral cortex but not the primary motor cortex. This is among the most misunderstood of higher cortical functions.

In *ideomotor apraxia* patients fail to perform motor procedures to command, despite normal dexterity. For example, they fail to imitate both symbolic and nonsense gestures and cannot reproduce pantomimes of common object use, although they can describe what they want to do (the concept of movement is intact) and given a real object can often use it appropriately (the action is intact). However, when asked to respond to a request they cannot. In contrast, patients with lesions of the motor and premotor cortices cannot perform the desired action, despite knowing what they want to do (the motor equivalent of expressive dysphasia).

Ideational (conceptual) apraxia is defined by a loss of knowledge about the idea of the movements and associated objects. Such patients may misunderstand the purpose of tools and use them inappropriately, in the real world as well as on confrontation. They may manage small components of the task in isolation but they cannot integrate these together, although they can generally follow or imitate an examiner's demonstration. Although researchers attempt to keep these concepts separate, there is considerable overlap between these types of apraxia.

In *oral (buccofacial) apraxia* patients have difficulty with movements of the mouth. This is a disorder closely affiliated with Broca's dysphasia. Lesions of the inferior frontal lobe and insula are usually responsible.

The mechanism underlying the apraxias appears to be disruption of stored complex memory engrams of skilled movements in the dominant parietal lobe plus lesions to the prefrontal cortex impairing the

---

Clinical Pointer 11

Recognizing cortical lesions

Disorders of language (dysphasia), knowledge (gnosis) and fine motor control (praxis) are indicators of lesions involving the cerebral cortex. Abnormalities of mood, cognition or behaviour are not confined to changes in the cerebral cortex. Language abnormalities are the hallmarks of cortical lesions and, in general, are easy to recognize. Cortical abnormalities of language cause dysphasia, but not dysarthria or dysphonia. Agnosia is one of the most important signs of cortical damage. Agnosia can relate to information presented in any sensory modality – hence auditory agnosia, tactile agnosia and visual agnosia. Agnosias of body awareness (neglect) are also tell-tale indicators of cortical damage. Apraxia has proven difficult to localize. Lesions to the parietal supramarginal gyrus can cause patients to have problems integrating a series of actions together (ideational apraxia). Weakness can be produced by lesions of the entire motor system. However, neurones that control the lower limbs cross into the interhemispheric fissure. Cortical lesions that cause weakness tend to be accompanied by weakness of the face and arm, but not the leg. Sensory awareness is not confined to the cortex. Thus a hemisensory loss usually implies a subcortical lesion. The cortex is more concerned with interpretation of shape and form. Cortical sensory loss is characterized by agraphaesthesia and loss of two-point discrimination ability. Visual field deficits after a stroke are more likely the be associated with subcortical than cortical disease, simply because the visual pathway runs below the cortex until the occipital lobe.

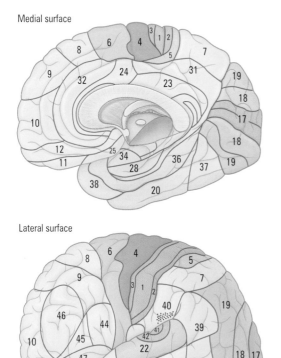

Medial surface

Lateral surface

Fig. 11.1 Cryoarchitectural areas of Brodmann. In 1901, Brodmann joined Vogt in the Neurobiological Laboratory in Berlin, where he undertook his famous studies on comparative cytoarchitectonics of mammalian cortex. Brodmann's 'areas' share similar cellular and laminar structure. He compared localization in the human cortex with that in a number of other mammals. In man, he distinguished 47 areas, each carrying an individual number, and some being further subdivided. From Fitzgerald & Folan-Curran (2001).

initiation of movement. In practice, damage to the inferior parietal lobule in Alzheimer's disease or stroke is the most common cause.

True apraxia, referring to an impairment caused by dominant hemisphere cortical lesions, should be separated from other causes of difficulty in completing tasks. *Limb-kinetic apraxia* refers to specific problems with precise movements, a condition that could be due to a number of different pathologies. *Dressing and constructional apraxias* are non-dominant functions, and are most often a result of visuospatial difficulties. Gait disorder observed in

patients with normal-pressure hydrocephalus is usually an ataxia rather than an apraxia.

PROSOPAGNOSIA

Prosopagnosia is the inability to recognize familiar faces. Patients with this condition can take in complex visual information but cannot put it together to recognize the face. It can be divided into a recent and remote recognition failure as well as agnosic and apperceptive subtypes. Apperceptive prosopagnosia is usually associated with bilateral occipitotemporal lesions. Occasionally, patients can see the details of a picture but cannot put it together as a whole, a phenomenon called *simultanagnosia*. Dominant occipital lesions may be responsible in some cases. In 1909 the Hungarian physician Rezsö Balint described simultagnosia along with optic ataxia (to which ocular pursuit and depth perception abnormalities have since been added). This is *Balint's syndrome*. In many cases bilateral posterior parietal (occipitoparietal) lesions are the cause. Rarely, such lesions appear to block the ability to generate any mental images – a phenomenon labelled the *Charcot–Wilbrand syndrome*.

THE CORPUS CALLOSUM

The hemispheres are connected by at least five separate pathways, but by far the largest is the corpus callosum. Callosal lesions (e.g. as a treatment for epilepsy) cause difficulties in motor control from one hemisphere to the *same* side of the body, because 90% of motor pathways cross in pyramidal decussations and the opposite motor cortex is required to activate the ipsilateral hand. Incidentally, ipsilateral motor actions are easier on the left side after callosal disconnection, suggesting that the left hemisphere is dominant for learned motor acts (praxis). In a series of experiments, Sperry famously showed that the left hemisphere was only aware of the right visual field and the right hemisphere was aware of the left field but could not communicate information received (due to disconnection from language centres). After section of the corpus callosum, patients often have difficulty describing emotions (presumably because there is some representation in the right hemisphere), but they do not develop neglect of the left side (showing that destruction of the right hemisphere on its own largely mediates neglect). Patients may also exhibit the alien hand sign, in which one hand interferes with the other against the patient's will. Patients may also suffer the very unusual problems of hemiagraphia and hemialexia.

VISUAL AGNOSIA

In the visual agnosias patients cannot recognize an object presented visually, but will recognize it upon description or touch. Visual agnosia has been subdivided. In *apperceptive visual agnosia* patients have full (internal) knowledge of the unrecognized object. In *associative visual agnosia* patients can copy objects they do not recognize, but usually cannot recognize the object by any modality (a reflection of disordered semantic memory). Visual neglect can occur in the Balint syndrome (see above). Ventromedial occipital or occipitoparietal lesions are thought to be the cause.

REFERENCES AND FURTHER READING

Calev A, Preston T, Samuel S et al 1999 Clinical neuropsychological assessment of psychiatric disorders. In: Calev A (ed) Assessment of neuropsychological functions in psychiatric disorders. American Psychiatric Press, Washington, DC, p 1–32

Fitzgerald MJT, Folan-Curran J 2001 Clinical neuroanatomy and related neuroscience, 4th edn. Harcourt, Philadelphia

12

The Frontal Lobes (Executive Function)

The frontal lobes are the most recent from a developmental perspective. They occupy one-third of the totality of the cortex. Despite this, there has been difficulty discovering exactly what the frontal lobes do. This is partly because interactions with other brain regions can produce apparently 'frontal'-type behaviours without frontal damage. In 1975, Benson & Blumer suggested two syndromes of frontal lobe disorder. In the pseudopsychopathic syndrome (or pseudomanic syndrome) seen with orbitofrontal lesions, the patient is often disinhibited and impulsive, with reduced empathy and judgement. Such patients are less able than normal to anticipate the future consequences of their actions, an ability described as 'future memory' by the Swedish neurobiologist David Ingvar (1985). Their mood is typically irritable or labile, with a fatuous euphoria. Inappropriate jocularity and an insensitive humour ('witzelsucht') may be seen. In the pseudodepressive state, with dorsolateral lesions, there is apathy, lack of concern and poor planning, but few other cognitive problems.

Time has shown that these presentations are quite distinct from depression and mania, and therefore the following terminology is preferred (Table 12.1). The *dorsolateral prefrontal syndrome* is the classic dysexecutive syndrome with poor cognitive function

Box 12.1 Neuropsychiatric and systemic diseases featuring frontal lobe damage

- Anterior cerebral artery stroke
- Anterior communicating artery aneurysm
- CNS infiltrations
- Encephalitis
- Frontal lobe trauma
- Frontal lobe tumours
- Frontotemporal dementias
- Hydrocephalus
- Multifocal dementias
- Motor neurone disease
- Multiple sclerosis
- Occult microvascular disease

Table 12.1 The frontal lobe syndromes (which can be defined anatomically or symptomatically)

Syndrome	Core feature	Causes
Orbitofrontal lesion	Disinhibition behaviour	Post-traumatic encephalopathy Frontal brain tumours Anterior cerebral artery occlusions or aneurysm rupture Multiple sclerosis Degenerative frontal lobe disease
Mediofrontal lesion	Amotivational behaviour	Bilateral anterior cerebral artery occlusions Trauma Hydrocephalus Bilateral thalamic infarction Tumours of thalamus, third ventricle, hypothalamus or pituitary
Dorsolateral prefrontal lesion	Dysexecutive features	Tumours Cerebrovascular trauma Frontal degeneration Dorsal caudate lesions

---

Clinical Pointer 12.1

What is the dysexecutive syndrome?

Classically, patients with frontal lobe damage to the lateral area known as the dorsolateral prefrontal cortex have a series of cognitive problems grouped together under the umbrella term 'dysexecutive syndrome'. In brief, there is a loss of flexibility in dealing with novel situations, difficulty with planning and sequencing, difficulty with multitasking, difficulty with attention and distraction, and decreased foresight and monitoring of performance. There are also related problems of reduced speech and motor fluency, and problems with abstract thought and perseveration. The disorder can be caused by basal ganglia as well as frontal lobe disorders. Response to treatment with amphetamines and MAOIs is generally better than with SSRIs.

Further reading Salloway S, Malloy PF, Duffy JD 2001 The frontal lobes and neuropsychiatric illness. American Psychiatric Press, Washington, DC

(including poor judgement and abstraction). In the *medial* (or *mesial*) *frontal syndrome* (or *anterior cingulate syndrome*) (involving the lateral hypothalamus, medial subthalamic nuclei, anterior cingulate and substantia nigra) there is an amotivational presentation (including mutism and akinesia). In the *orbitofrontal syndrome* there is disinhibition. However, clinically this distinction may not hold true, and mixed forms or form frustes (see Ch. 41) may occur. Another feature often seen in frontal lobe disorders is the tendency to erroneously repeat previous actions, called *perseveration*. It is also associated with Parkinson's disease, language disorders and damage to the non-dominant hemisphere. It is usually indicative of organic damage.

TESTS OF FRONTAL LOBE FUNCTION

In the *go–no-go test*, the examiner asks the patient to tap twice when the examiner taps the table once, and to make no response when the examiner taps twice. This is a test of perseveration. Copying multiple loops or letters is also used as a test to elicit perseveration. The execution of serial hand sequences is frequently disrupted in patients with abnormalities of the frontal–subcortical systems. To test this, the examiner demonstrates a sequence of hand positions and asks the patient to learn and to perform the sequence. If the patient is unable to do this, the examiner asks the patient to say the sequence aloud. If the patient is unable to do this, frontal dysfunction is implicated. Difficulty in maintaining a mental set and limitations in appropriately changing between tasks are typical of patients with frontal dysfunction.

Environmental dependence and poor response inhibition can be shown by the *Stroop Test*. In the Stroop

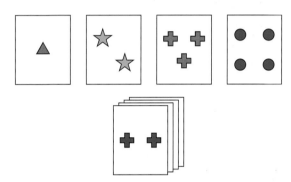

Fig. 12.1 Wisconsin Card Sorting Test. Patients are asked to sort cards according to a rule defined by the experimenter. The rule is determined by placement of the first card. The experimenter just says 'yes' or 'no'. After the subject has acquired the first rule, it is changed for another.

Test, the names of several colours are printed in random colours (e.g. the word 'green' printed in red, 'blue' in green and 'red' in blue). The patient is asked to suppress the automatic tendency to read the name of the colour and instead to say the colour of the writing. In addition, poor abstracting abilities, stimulus boundedness on clock drawing tests, poor word-list generation, and the adoption of poor strategies when asked to draw complex figures aid the examiner in concluding that a frontal–subcortical system disturbance is present.

NEUROPSYCHIATRIC CONSEQUENCES OF FRONTAL LOBE INJURY

Lishman (1968) reported that depression is a more frequent accompaniment of head injury where the frontal lobe damage is involved. Frontal hypofunctionality is seen in depressed, but not euthymic, suf-

Table 12.2 Tests of frontal lobe function

Domain	Bedside cognition	Formal neuropsychology
Response set	Verbal fluency (F, A, S, animals in 60s)	Wisconsin Card Sorting*
Problem solving	Proverb interpretation	Tower of London
Sequencing	Luria Motor Sequencing	Trails B
Similarities	Similarities	Hooper Visual Organization Test (problem solving)
Planning and impulsivity	Planning and impulsivity	Maze subtest of WISC
		Zoo Map Test
		Porteus Mazes (planning)
Set shifting	Set shifting	Card Sorting Test*
Judgement	Cognitive estimates	Tests of time estimation
Distraction	Distraction	Stroop Test, Hayling Test, Brixton Text

WISC, Weschler Intelligence Scale for Children

Many tests depend on integrity of brain areas beyond the frontal lobe. For references, see Spreen & Strauss (1997).
*The Card Sorting Test is often considered the classic test of frontal lobe function, although a specific association with frontal lobe has been called into question (see Fig. 12.1).

ferers from Parkinson's disease, Huntington's disease and temporal lobe epilepsy. The frontal lobes have been repeatedly implicated in primary psychiatric disorders, usually in the form of bifrontal ventricular enlargement, frontal cortical atrophy and hypoperfusion. When challenged by a cognitive test of frontal lobe function, patients with schizophrenia fail to activate frontal lobes as adequately as do controls. There are also microscopic neuronal abnormalities in schizophrenia, although these are not confined to the frontal lobes. Where the orbitomedial surface of the frontal lobe is damaged, disinhibition and impulsivity are core features. When these areas are overfunctioning, attention may be excessive and overpowering. It is tempting to draw a parallel with obsessive–compulsive disorder, in which hypermetabolism of the orbitofrontal cortex has been observed.

The frontal lobes are also increasingly being recognized as critical to cognitive function. This applies to the so-called executive functions and also to the reciprocal relationship with subcortical areas. Clinically, the cortical–subcortical interaction is clearly shown in patients who have suffered subcortical stroke but who develop cortical hypometabolism in the cerebral cortices, especially the frontal lobes (Kwan et al 1999). In elderly patients with lacunar infarcts and silent stroke, it may also be frontal hypometabolism that contributes to poor cognitive function (Reed et al 2001). Note that this relationship could be confounded by secondary effects on motivation and arousal. One fascinating finding discussed elsewhere (see Fig. 42.2) is that patients with mixed dementia (Alzheimer's disease pathology with frontal vascular white matter lesions) present with fluctuating cognitive performance that is often mistaken for Lewy body dementia (see Ch. 42). Frontal lobe atrophy or hypoperfusion is also seen in Parkinson's disease, progressive supranuclear palsy, Huntington's disease and motor neurone disease and, furthermore, may be correlated with cognitive deficits in these conditions. Recently, hypop-

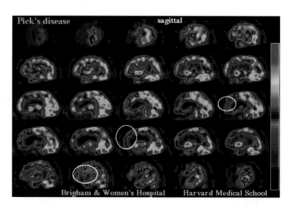

Fig. 12.2 SPECT scan in Pick's disease, illustrating frontal lobe hypoperfusion. From Gareth Gina, Department of Radiology at Brigham and Women's Hospital, Harvard Medical School.

erfusion of the orbitofrontal area has been described in association with head-injury-related behavioural disturbance (Kim & Humaran 2001). However, a word of caution is required, since these frontal deficits may be part of a more generalized fronto-temporoparietal hypoperfusion in these diseases. It will be of interest to discover whether larger functional imaging studies can elucidate consistent metabolic differences (similar to the anatomical differences) in these conditions.

REFERENCES AND FURTHER READING

Benson DF, Blumer D (eds) 1975 Psychiatric aspects of neurological disease. Grune and Stratton, New York

Ingvar DH 1985 'Memory for the future': an essay on the temporal organization of conscious awareness. Human Neurobiology 4:127–136

Kim E, Humaran TJ 2001 SPECT imaging in behavioural and psychiatric complications of acquired brain injury. Journal of Neuropsychiatry 13:141

Kwan LT, Reed BR, Eberling JL et al 1999 Effects of subcortical cerebral infarction on cortical glucose metabolism and cognitive function. Archives of Neurology 56:809–814

Lishman WA 1968 Brain damage in relation to psychiatric disability after head injury. British Journal of Psychiatry 114:373–410

Reed BR, Eberling JL, Mungas D et al 2001 Frontal lobe hypometabolism predicts cognitive decline in patients with lacunar infarcts. Archives of Neurology 58:493–497

Spreen O, Strauss E 1997 A compendium of neuropsychological tests: administration, norms and commentary, 2nd edn. Oxford University Press, New York

13

The Temporal Lobes and Limbic System

The temporal lobes are located below the lateral cerebral fissure and are divided into the superior, middle and inferior gyri on their lateral surface and the uncus and parahippocampal gyri on their medial surface. Functionally the temporal lobes are complex. Uniquely, stimulation of the temporal lobes causes complex perceptions, memories and experiences. (In 1938, whilst working at the Montréal

Neurological Institute, Wilder Penfield (1891–1976) demonstrated that electrical stimulation of the lateral surface of the temporal cortex caused awake sub-

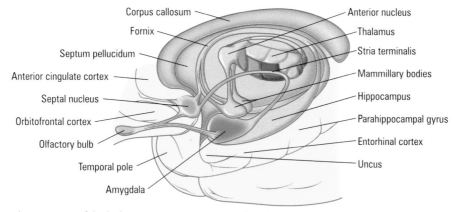

Fig. 13.1   Schematic view of the limbic system. In 1878, Broca described 'le grand lobe limbique' [the great limbic lobe] as an area of the brain bounded by the subcallosal gyrus rostrally, the parahippocampal gyrus inferiorly and the cingulate gyrus superiorly. Broca believed that the great limbic lobe was primarily involved in olfaction. In 1937, Papez published his famous work moving towards a functional description of the limbic circuit. He suggested that the hippocampi were sites that programmed emotional expression, the mamillary bodies were sites that programmed emotional expression and the cingulate cortices were the receptive areas for experiencing emotion. Fifteen years later, Paul McLean expanded the boundaries of the limbic system, adding the orbitofrontal and mediofrontal cortices, the parahippocampal gyrus and amygdala, the septum, the hypothalamus, the habenular and the anterior thalamic nuclei.

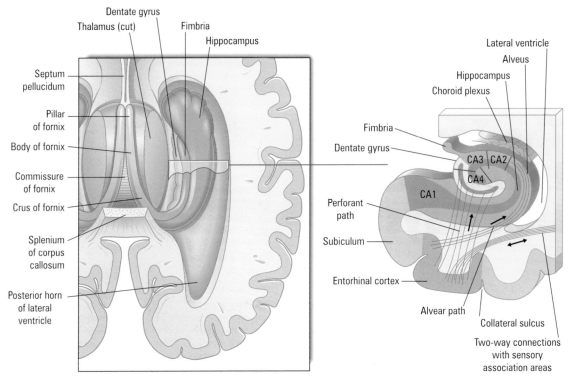

Fig. 13.2 The hippocampus and limbic system. The main output signal of the CA1 fields follows the postcommissural fornix to the chain of structures in the limbic circuit: the mammillary bodies (medial nucleus) and the anterior thalamic nuclei (mainly the anteroventral nucleus). Secondary projections pass to the cingulate limbic cortex, mainly the posterior area.

jects to relive previous experiences.) Stimulation of the anterior temporal lobe also produces panic attacks. A portion of the temporal lobes is integrated in the limbic system and has a vital role in memory (see below and Ch. 69). Destructive lesions to the temporal lobe can cause visual field defects when the optic radiation is affected. Perhaps more importantly for psychiatry, irritative lesions can cause complex visual and auditory hallucinations. The olfactory cortex is located in the uncus and related parahippocampal gyrus. Irritative lesions in this area cause uncinate fits, often as the aura of temporal lobe epilepsy. The proximity of the uncus to the medial hippocampus and the site of mesial temporal sclerosis may explain the association of temporal lobe epilepsy and olfactory aura.

AUDITORY AGNOSIA

Rarely, patients may have an inability to recognize sounds despite intact hearing. Particular aspects of

sound can cause problems – for example, speech, music and paralinguistic (prosodic) aspects of language. In *cortical deafness*, patients have problems with verbal and non-verbal material. Bilateral destruction of the primary auditory cortex (Heschl's gyrus) is usually found. In *pure word deafness*, the sufferer in unable to comprehend spoken language, but there is relative preservation of reading, writing and speech (Wernicke's and Broca's areas are intact). In its sister disorder, *auditory sound agnosia*, patients have difficulty recognizing non-verbal sounds. This may be because of a perceptive abnormality (associated with the non-dominant hemisphere) or an associative–semantic deficit (associated with lesions to the dominant hemisphere). All these disorders feature problems with musical perception, although if musical perceptual deficits occur in isolation the term *sensory amusia* is sometimes used. Finally, some patients have problems with the rhythm of speech (i.e. *aprosody*). Usually this is expressive aprosody, in which patients lose intonation in their own speech, but it can overlap with receptive aprosody, in which patients fail to grasp the significance of other people's intonation. The latter can occasionally lead to the unusual problem of the inability to recognize familiar voices (*phonagnosia*). Aprosody has been associated with non-dominant hemisphere cortical lesions in the mirror regions to Broca's and Wernicke's areas as well as subcortical lesions to the basal ganglia.

THE KLÜVER–BUCY SYNDROME

The limbic system is a perennial favourite of biological psychiatrists. Lesions in several related areas have profound effects on personality, mood and perceptions (Box 13.2). Bilateral medial temporal lobe lesions can produce the Klüver–Bucy syndrome described by Heinrich Klüver and Paul Bucy while they were working at the University of Chicago (Klüver & Bucy 1937). This syndrome is characterized by placidity, hypersexuality or altered sexual behaviour, visual agnosia, hypermetamorphosis (compulsive exploration of the environmental), hyperorality and a failure to learn from aversive stimuli. Apart from this rare, anatomically localized

> **Box 13.2   Diseases that can cause Klüver–Bucy-like syndrome in humans**
>
> - Alzheimer's disease
> - Carbon monoxide poisoning
> - Cerebral infiltrations
> - Frontotemporal dementia
> - Head injury
> - Herpes encephalitis
> - Systemic metabolic disorders
> - Temporal lobe stroke
> - Temporal lobectomy
> - Temporal lobe tumour

syndrome, abnormalities of mood and perception associated with temporal lobe lesions are more difficult to pin down.

REFERENCES AND FURTHER READING

Klüver H, Bucy PC 1937 'Psychic blindness' and other symptoms following bilateral temporal lobe lobectomy in Rhesus monkeys. American Journal of Physiology 119:352–353

14

The Parietal Lobe

Alexia without agraphia (pure alexia) is an unusual syndrome, patients can recognize words that are read to them but cannot read the words themselves. In addition, patients can write normally but cannot recognize what they have written! For more information, see Chapter 15.

In *neglect dyslexia* patients fail to read half (usually the left half) of words.

In *surface dyslexia*, patients have difficulty grasping the meanings behind irregularly spelled words (such as 'Wednesday') and try to pronounce and deduce meanings from the letters and sounds. They can read made-up non-words. An unusual type of dyslexia has also been described, which is the opposite to this in that patients cannot read non-words but can pronounce irregularly spelled words in everyday use. This is called *phonological dyslexia*.

In *deep dyslexia*, patients understand the meaning of familiar words but cannot follow the phonemic or grammatical rules of language from first principles. They rely on their semantic memory to pronounce a word such as 'house' as 'home'.

The anterior portion of the parietal lobe adjoins the central sulcus in the primary somaesthetic cortex (corresponding to Brodmann areas 3, 1 and 2). The remainder of the parietal lobe is divided into the superior parietal lobule and the inferior parietal lobule. The superior parietal lobule serves to integrate somatic sensation with visual information processed in the occipital lobe. The inferior parietal lobule consists of the supramarginal gyrus (Brodmann area 40) and the angular gyrus (Brodmann area 39) (see Figs I.1, II.1 and 11.1).

DOMINANT PARIETAL LOBE FUNCTIONS

Lesions to the dominant parietal lobule and the inferior parietal lobule can produce agnosia. *Gerstmann's syndrome* refers to the presence of dyscalculia, dysgraphia, finger agnosia and left–right confusion with angular gyrus lesions. Balint syndrome (see Ch. 11) is a consequence of bilateral inferior parietal lobule damage (involving the adjacent occipital cortex).

Disorders of reading and writing

Disorders of reading are called *dyslexias*. Problems can arise in the decoding of the written form (or visual analysis) or in deriving meaning from words (central representation). Several types of dyslexia are described.

Disorders of writing

Disorders of writing are called *dysgraphias*. In *dyspraxic dysgraphia* there is a problem with writing caused by motor control. In *neglect dysgraphia*, patients with perceptual abnormalities make characteristic errors in writing. In *surface dysgraphia*, patients cannot spell irregularly spelt words but substitute plausible alternatives. In *deep (phonological) dysgraphia*, patients characteristically cannot spell unfamiliar words based on first principles.

Disorders of calculation

Strictly, *acalculia* is the inability to comprehend or write numbers properly. The term *anarithmetria* is used for patients who cannot perform number manipulation. A rare form of calculation error, seen in patients with neglect, is spatial dyscalculia.

NON-DOMINANT PARIETAL LOBE FUNCTIONS

The so-called non-dominant (right) hemisphere is in fact dominant in certain domains (Table 14.1). Most important among these are visuospatial ability, certain praxias, topographic memory, appreciation of music, recognition of faces and appreciation of emotions in voice and gesture. It also has a greater role than the left hemisphere in moderating attention and duplicates some aspects of language and consciousness from the left hemisphere.

Unilateral neglect

In patients with extensive non-dominant hemisphere damage, there is often indifference concerning left-sided weakness known as *anosodiaphoria*. Alternatively, there may be complete denial that any impairment exists, a phenomenon called *anosognosia*. Some patients display a striking alteration in the sense of self on the affected side, so that they fail to recognize the body part as their own. This is called *asomatognosia*. Various degrees of neglect are seen in about one-quarter of stroke patients. Such patients typically neglect their reading or writing on the left side. This can be difficult to distinguish from hemianopia, although in hemianopia the loss is fixed about a vertical line at the midpoint. The cortical areas most commonly affected are the prefrontal and inferior parietal regions. Occasionally, neglect of the right arm occurs after dominant lesions. This is a separate condition from *autotopagnosia*, which refers to the inability to identify personal body parts (such as the fingers in 'finger agnosia') and is usually due to a dominant lesion. This finding is closely allied with visual neglect (spatial agnosia). Severity of neglect can be tested simply by asking the patient to draw a clock face (Fig. 14.1) or, more formally, by using the *Mesulam Cancellation Task* (Fig. 14.2). The reason why neglect occurs more commonly following right hemisphere lesions probably relates to the way dominant consciousness in the left hemisphere masks the awareness of sensory information loss perceived by the right hemisphere (see corpus callosal lesions, Ch. 11).

Table 14.1 Summary of the functions of the left and right cerebral hemispheres

Function	Left (dominant) hemisphere	Right (non-dominant) hemisphere
Vision	Visual detail	Faces Depth perception
Audition	Language sounds	Non-linguistic sounds
	Rhythm and musical order	Melody
Memory	Verbal memory	Non-verbal memory
Language	Language Arithmetic	Prosody
Spatial processes	Generation of imagery	Geometry Spatial orientation

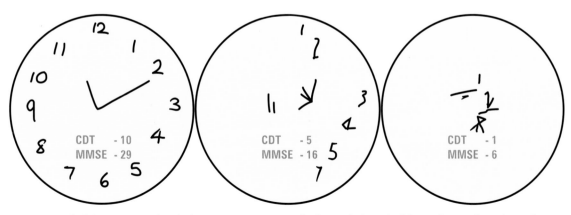

Fig. 14.1 Clock face errors in the Clock Drawing Test. A normally drawn clock on the left. A subject with moderate dementia scores 5 out of 10 and shows perseveration on the middle clock. A subject with severe dementia produces a barely recognizable attempt on the right.

Dressing apraxia

Problems with dressing can arise as a result of apraxia, paresis or neglect. Thus 'dressing apraxia' is not a very useful term, since problems with motor control (praxis) are not necessarily involved.

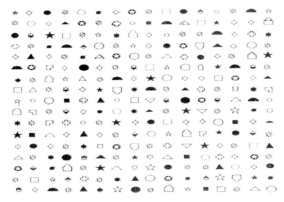

Fig. 14.2 The Mesulam Cancellation Test. This is a test of visual scanning and attention that is often used as a measure of the accuracy of selective attention. The subject is required to scan a large field of either letters or symbols for a target letter or form and to cancel all the targets as quickly as possible on the stimulus sheet. From Professor M Mesulam, Feinberg Medical School, Northwestern University.

Visuospatial ability

Both hemispheres are involved in the visual pathays but higher visual processing is largely subserved by the non-dominant hemisphere. The dominant hemisphere has a lesser role in visual detail and

---

Box 14.2   Tests of visuospatial function

Visuospatial constructional ability
WAIS-R Visual Reproduction
Benton Visual Retention Test
Simple Drawing
Rey–Osterrieth Complex Figure Reproduction

Visuospatial orientation
Personal Orientation Test
Various maze tests
Visual Object and Space Perception (VOSP) Battery

WAIS-R, Weschler Adult Intelligence Scale, Revised

Clinical Pointer 14.1

Using the Clock Drawing Test as a screening tool for dementia

There are many cognitive tests available, but the Clock Drawing Test is particularly appealing because it requires no special equipment, is non-threatening and is extremely simple. The cognitive domains tested include comprehension, motor function, visuospatial integrity, numerical knowledge and executive function. Shulman (2000) reviewed the literature concerning the validity of the Clock Drawing Test as a screening tool for dementia and found a sensitivity and specificity of 85%. One problem, however, is disagreement about how to score the test. Certain components can be scored to attempt to delineate executive performance. This is the basis for the CLOX test (Royall et al 1998). At least a dozen other methods of scoring are available. To validate and compare these, Storey et al (2001) analysed five of the most popular methods on a total of 127 consecutive new referrals to a memory clinic in Sydney. The area under the receiver operating characteristic (ROC) curve was largest for the Shulman method and Mendez method. The inter-rater and intra-rater correlation coefficients were high for all five methods.

Thus the Clock Drawing Test can be recommended as a simple screen of cognitive function, but it must be used together with a clinical assessment. It cannot be used to distinguish between dementias, and it may be affected by delirium, dysphasia and neglect. It can enhance the sensitivity of simple bedside tests such as the Mini Mental State Examination or the Short Performance Test (Syndrom–Kurztest) in the detection of dementia. This appears to hold true for early dementia (Schramm et al 2002).

Further reading   Royall DR, Cordes JA, Polk M 1998 CLOX: an executive clock drawing task. *Journal of Neurology, Neurosurgery and Psychiatry* 64:588–594
Schramm U, Berger G, Muller R et al 2002 Psychometric properties of Clock Drawing Test and MMSE or Short Performance Test (SKT) in dementia screening in a memory clinic population. *International Journal of Geriatric Psychiatry* 17:254–260
Shulman KI 2000 Clock-drawing: is it the ideal cognitive screening test? *International Journal of Geriatric Psychiatry* 156:548–561
Storey JE, Rowland JTJ, Basic D et al 2001 A comparison of five clock scoring methods using ROC (receiver operating characteristic) curve analysis. *International Journal of Geriatric Psychiatry* 16:394–399

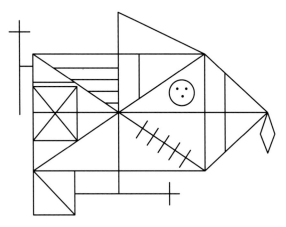

Fig. 14.3 The Rey–Osterrieth Complex Figure can be used as a test of constructional apraxia and visuospatial memory.

praxis (on drawing tests). Impaired visuospatial abilities affect visual orientation, orientation of the body, geometric design, maze performance and geographical knowledge. Typically, affected patients are unable to copy simple line drawings and are labelled with the misnomer *constructional apraxia* (even though fine motor control is intact).

REFERENCES AND FURTHER READING

Mesulam MM 1985 Principles of behavioral neurology. Davis, Philadelphia

15

The Occipital Lobes

Although the occipital lobes appear to have little role in behavioural disorders, lesions of the occipital lobe are important neuropsychiatrically and are also relatively common (posterior cerebral artery stroke accounts for about 5% of all strokes) (Fig. 15.1). The occipital lobes are largely concerned with vision. Large numbers of specialized neurones are required to process information about the form, motion, colour and depth of objects. Visual information is processed by the six layers of the primary visual cortex (corresponding to Brodmann area 17) and also in the visual association cortex (prestriate cortex, corresponding to Brodmann areas 18 and 19). Many connections link the occipital lobe with limbic, parietal, temporal and frontal lobes.

NEUROPSYCHOLOGY OF OCCIPITAL LOBE LESIONS

Deficits associated with lesions involve visual fields, visual acuity and visual recognition, and can be summarized as follows:

- Visual blind spots (scotomas) and partial blind spots (amblyopias) are caused by occipital lesions. There may be macular sparing if collateral vascular supply to the occipital pole from posterior branches of the middle cerebral artery prevents complete destruction. There may also be 'temporal crescent' sparing in that the area of the cortex responsible for vision in the most extreme contralateral temporal field may be unaffected.

- Visual field abnormalities are common, particularly with a homonymous hemianopia of the contralateral visual field (following a unilateral lesion).
- Unilateral ventromedial and occipitoparietal lesions can cause visual agnosia (in which an object can be seen but not named). Bilateral occipital cortex lesions may result in loss of vision with preserved pupillary light reflexes (*cortical blindness*), associated with denial of the loss (or *anosognosia*), often called *Anton's syndrome*. Another intriguing condition is blind sight, in which patients who are blind on conscious testing still respond to movement or changes in the environment. This is thought to be due to unconscious processing in the prestriate area following striate lesions.
- Stimulation of the cortex (after acute trauma and epilepsy) may cause warping of vision and simple (elemental) hallucinations. Elemental hallucinations are often flashes of colour or odd patterns in the contralateral visual field. More complex visual distortions (shifts in the visual axis, micropsia, macropsia and movement artefacts) are typical of irritation of the association cortex and also occipitoparietal lesions, and these are sometimes labelled *dysmorphopsia*. A similar phenomenon is visual perseveration precipitated by movement (*polyopia*) or with a hallucination-like quality (*palinopsia*).
- An inability to recognize faces (*prosopagnosia*) appears to result from a disconnection of the inferior visual association cortex of the non-dominant temporal cortex. Thus lesions to the occipital cortex or temporal cortex may be responsible. Prosopagnosia usually occurs in conjunction with more generalized visual agnosia or visual field defects. *Autoprosopagnosia*

Box 15.1 Tests of occipital lobe dysfunction

- Clinical examination: visual fields, visual acuity, eye movements and pursuit; formal perimetry (using Harms perimeter) reveals problems with visual fields and acuity
- Naming to confrontation testing for the presence of visual object agnosia
- Matching of facial pictures and identification of famous faces for suspected prosopagnosia
- Picture description for suspected simultanagnosia
- Testing with Ishihara plates and the Farnsworth–Munsell test examines colour perception

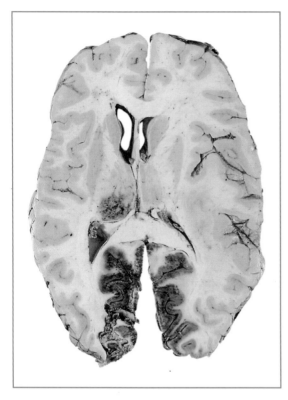

Fig. 15.1 Infarction of the occipital lobes after bilateral posterior cerebral artery occlusion. From Cooke & Stewart (1995).

(the inability to recognize one's own face in a picture or mirror) may also occur (see Ch. 40, in which the mirror sign is discussed).

- Pure alexia (without agraphia) may result from lesions to the dominant occipital cortex. A dominant occipital lesion with involvement of the splenium of the corpus callosum disconnects the visual centre from the temporal language centre. This produces a visual field deficit on the right side, and visual information can be perceived only by the right hemisphere; however, because the connection between the right occipital area and the left temporal area is lesioned, the patient cannot decode the language-related visual information and cannot read.

- Lesions of the lingual and fusiform gyri in the inferior occipital lobe may produce disorders of colour perception. Colours are often described as 'washed out' in the contralateral visual field, a condition known as *hemiachromatopsia*. Some patients perceive colours on testing but cannot name them. Lesions of the dominant occipito-temporal junction may be the cause.

REFERENCES AND FURTHER READING

Cooke RA, Stewart B 1995 Colour atlas of anatomical pathology, 2nd edn. Churchill Livingstone, Edinburgh

16

The Basal Ganglia and Subcortical Areas

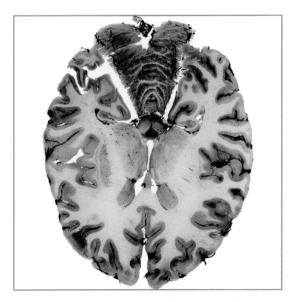

Fig. 16.1 Post-mortem coronal slice. 80% of all neurones lie within the thin 2–5 mm of cortex. They are densely packed in six horizontal layers, with approximately 150,000 neurones and 10 million synapses/mm². From Kerr (1999).

The cortex consists of only a few millimetres of grey matter. The area below the cortex (including white matter pathways, such as the corona radiata) is referred to as 'subcortical'. This term encompasses the brainstem, thalamus and basal ganglia. The basal ganglia comprise the caudate, putamen, nucleus accumbens, globus pallidus, substantia nigra and subthalamic nucleus (and, historically, the unconnected claustrum and the amygdala). 'Striatum' is a term for the caudate, putamen and nucleus accumbens, 'corpus striatum' for the striatum and globus pallidus, and 'lenticular nucleus' for the globus pallidus and putamen (Fig. 16.2).

The term 'subcortical dementia' was introduced by McHugh and Folstein in 1973 as a characteristic description of the changes seen in Huntington's disease. Independently, Albert et al (1974) described four features of subcortical disease using the model of progressive supranuclear palsy:

- forgetfulness
- slow thoughts (bradyphrenia)
- personality changes (includes apathy and depression)
- impaired manipulation of acquired knowledge.

These signs are not particularly specific and hence are of only modest clinical value. Cortical deficits of aphasia, apraxia and agnosia are absent in pure sub-cortical dementias. As these dementias progress there is thought to be difficulty in retrieval of existing memories, although on prompting recognition is usually intact. Albert et al (1974) said patients 'forget to remember'. Associated signs of motor slowness, 'lead pipe' tone and dysarthric speech are additional clues to a subcortical lesion. Neuroimaging and neuropsychological studies do not support this neat delineation of the subcortical and cortical dementias. More recent work describes impairments due to linked frontal–subcortical circuit involvement rather than pure subcortical disease.

Frontal–subcortical circuits

There are two circuits that are well described: the (lateral) orbitofrontal–subcortical circuit (associated with disinhibition) and the anterior cingulate–subcortical circuit (associated with apathy). The *lateral orbitofrontal–subcortical circuit* arises in the orbital surface of the frontal lobe and projects via the ventral caudate (ventral striatum) to the globus pallidus and substantia nigra and then on to the anteroventral and dorsomedial thalamic nuclei. The circuit completes through a thalamic connection to the lateral orbitofrontal cortex.

Table 16.1 Summary of regional neuropsychiatric syndromes

Lesion location/type	Symptoms
Frontal lobe	
Orbitofrontal	Disinhibition, poor judgement (risk-taking) and empathy, lack of insight
Dorsolateral prefrontal cortex	Executive dysfunction (planning and set-shifting)
Mediofrontal	Apathy, akinetic mutism
Precentral	Contralateral monoplegia or hemiplegia, apraxia
Paracentral	Incontinence
Broca's area	Expressive (motor) dysphasia, transcortical motor aphasia
Frontal middle gyrus	Saccadic gaze abnormality
Poorly localized	Motor perseveration, primitive reflexes, utilization/imitation behaviour, inattention
Irritative	Eye deviation, amnesia
Parietal lobe	
Post-central gyrus	Sensory loss (astereognosis, sensory inattention)
Optic radiation	Lower homonymous quadrantanopia
Non-dominant hemisphere	Dressing apraxia, anosognosia, constructional apraxia, geographical agnosia, spatial neglect
Dominant hemisphere	Finger or body agnosia, agraphia, acalculia, alexia, left–right disorientation (*Gerstmann's syndrome*)
Irritative	Somatic (haptic) hallucinations
Temporal lobe	
Wernicke's area	Receptive dysphasia, transcortical sensory aphasia
Insula (superior gyrus)	Cortical deafness and amusia
Medial temporal	Amnesia (episodic memory)
Inferior lateral	Amnesia (semantic if left-sided; faces if right-sided)
Limbic area	Hyperorality, hypersexuality, visual agnosia, metamorphosis (*Klüver–Bucy syndrome*)
Optic radiation	Upper homonymous quantrantopia
Irritative	Forced thinking, forced recall, déjà vu, jamais vu
Occipital lobe	
Cortical lesion	Homonymous hemianopia
Pole	Central (macular) hemianopia
Striate	Cortical blindness, *Anton's syndrome*
Occipitotemporal (non-dominant)	Prosopagnosia (amnesia for faces)
Association cortex	Alexia without agraphia, palinopsia (after-effects)
Irritative	Elementary visual hallucinations
Basal ganglia	
Dominant hemisphere	Impaired verbal fluency, impaired motor programming, poor concentration

Contd

Table 16.1 *Contd*

Lesion location/type	Symptoms
Basal ganglia – contd Non-dominant hemisphere	Impaired visuospatial memory, impaired visuospatial fluency
Irritative	Obsessive–compulsive disorder (?)
Corpus callosum With occipital lobe involvement	Alexia without agraphia
Without occipital lobe involvement	Left-hand agraphia and anomia, alien hand syndrome

Note: all lesions are destructive, unless otherwise noted

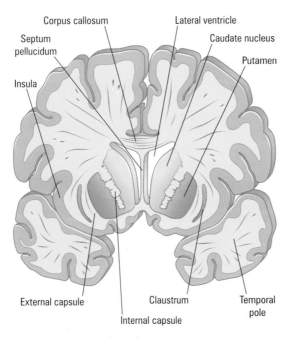

Fig. 16.2 The basal ganglia.

The *anterior cingulate–subcortical circuit* also projects to the important ventral striatum area, on to the globus pallidus and substantia nigra, and then to the dorsomedial nucleus of the thalamus. This nucleus has reciprocal connections with the anterior cingulate.

Disorders of subcortical function

The degenerative diseases Parkinson's disease and Huntington's disease exemplify primarily subcortical disorders. Subcortical tissue includes large areas of myelination axons that are affected in demyelinating conditions (see Ch. 20). Subcortical areas may, of course, be destroyed by fairly indiscriminate processes such as trauma (see Ch. 19), infections (see Ch. 26), tumour (see Ch. 30) and vascular disease (see Ch. 43).

NEUROPSYCHIATRIC CONSEQUENCES OF BASAL GANGLIA DISORDERS

The basal ganglia are important mediators of action and form part of a bi-directional frontal–subcortical circuit. Amotivational syndromes (e.g. apathy, akinesia, akinetic mutism) can occur with lesions to linked areas of the anterior cingulate, medial frontal cortex, caudate, pallidum and white matter pathways. The basal ganglia are well known in the genesis of fine motor control, locomotion, speech and cognition. The psychiatric consequences of basal ganglia lesions are also a common theme in neuropsychiatry. For unclear reasons, the basal ganglia are vulnerable to damage from diverse degenerate conditions such as Huntington's disease and Parkinson's disease, metabolic conditions such as Wilson's disease, and diffuse processes such as cerebrovascular disease and heavy metal intoxication. Pure caudate haemorrhage accounts for about 6% of cases of primary intracerebral haemorrhage. Dementia, depression, apathy, aphasia and possibly psychosis and mania have been associated with basal ganglia lesions (Bhatia & Masden 1994). Obsessional behaviour is also seen in some conditions affecting the basal ganglia, particularly when the bilateral caudate, putamen or globus pallidus are involved. Conversely, the primary psychiatric disorders obsessive–compulsive disorder and depressive disorder feature definite basal ganglia pathology in a subgroup of patients. Bilateral basal ganglia calcifi-

Box 16.2 Diseases featuring basal ganglia damage

- Basal ganglia calcification
- Basal ganglia infarction
- Carbon monoxide poisoning
- Cerebral palsy
- CNS infections
- Creutzfeldt–Jakob disease
- Encephalitis lethargica
- Heavy metal poisoning
- Huntington's disease
- Lesch–Nyhan syndrome
- Multiple system atrophy
- Neuroacanthocytosis
- Parkinson's disease
- Progressive supranuclear palsy
- Sydenham's chorea
- Tourette's syndrome
- Wilson's disease

Table 16.2 Cortical versus subcortical syndromes

Parameter	Cortical dementias	Subcortical dementias
Attention	Normal	Poor
Psychomotor speed	Normal	Slow
Memory	Abnormal retention	Abnormal retrieval
Language	Aphasia	Dysarthria and poor fluency
Affect	Indifference	Depression
Executive function	Normal	Poor

cation (*Fahr's syndrome*, see Ch. 23) is also associated with mood disorders, cognitive impairment and rarely, obsessive–compulsive disorder or psychosis.

Gradually, as more patients are studied, specific syndromes of regional basal ganglia damage are emerging. Lesions of the dorsal caudate appear to produce a dysexecutive syndrome characterized by apathy, whereas damage to the ventral caudate is associated with an orbitofrontal-like syndrome, characterized by disinhibition. Caudate haemorrhage alone has been noted to cause delirium or depression, word-finding difficulty and obsessive–compulsive disorder. The same applies to isolated lesions of the putamen or globus pallidus, although these are very rare. Damage to the striatum and putamen may produce a variety of language disorders. The degree of caudate atrophy has been correlated with the severity of secondary depression in Huntington's disease, Parkinson's disease and idiopathic basal ganglia calcification.

The basal ganglia are important in cognition as well as mood. Their role is largely in executive and attentional processes. Cognitive deficits in Huntington's disease are correlated with abnormalities of basal ganglia structure and function, although this could be confounded by the overall severity of the disease process. Several authors have documented a correlation between caudate atrophy on MRI and impaired

memory (Brandt et al 1995). Reduced dopamine receptor density (dopamine-2 receptors more than dopamine-1 receptors) in the corpus striatum shows the same relationship (Lawrence et al 1998).

In summary, the basal ganglia are involved in the genesis of motor function, locomotion, language, mood, motivation and cognition; these functions are disrupted in certain acquired, developmental and degenerative disorders.

REFERENCES AND FURTHER READING

Albert ML, Feldman RG, Willis AL 1974 The sub-cortical dementia of progressive supranuclear palsy. Journal of Neurology, Neurosurgery and Psychiatry 37:121–130

Bhatia KP, Masden CD 1994 the behavioural and motor consequences of focal lesions of the basal ganglia in man. Brain 117:859

Brandt J, Bylsma FW, Aylward EH et al 1995 Impaired source memory in Huntington's disease and its relation to basal ganglia atrophy. Journal of Clinical and Experimental Neuropsychology 17:868–877

Gerstmann J 1930 Zur symptomatology der Hirnläsionene im Übergangsgebiet der unteren Parietal- und ermittleren Occipitalwindung. Nervenartz 3:691–696

Kerr JB 1999 Atlas of functional histology. Mosby, St. Louis

Lawrence AD, Weeks RA, Brooks DJ et al 1998 The relationship between striatal dopamine receptor binding and cognitive performance in Huntington's disease. Brain 121:1343–1355

Core Neuropsychiatric Disorders

This section summarizes the effects of neurological brain diseases on higher function. Published research does not provide a balanced picture, and thus the weight given to each complication does not accurately reflect its frequency or seriousness.

The most common neuropsychiatric disorders in children and adolescents are the effects of head injury, epilepsy, CNS infections, neurodevelopmental disorders and, increasingly, illicit drugs. In mid-life the common conditions are head injury, epilepsy,

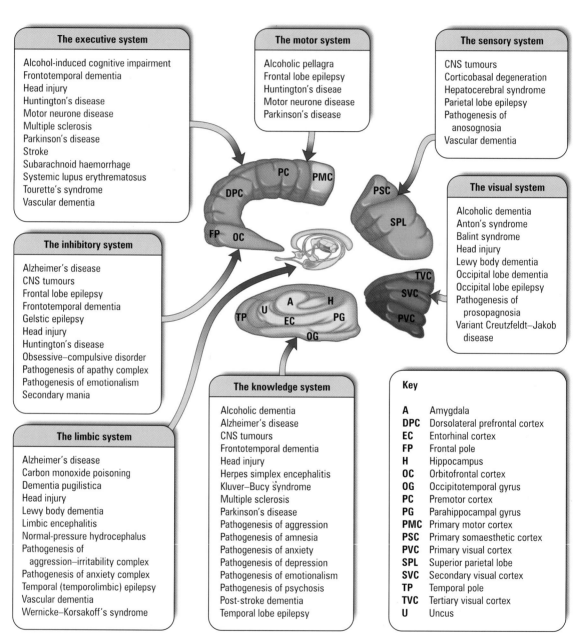

The executive system

Alcohol-induced cognitive impairment
Frontotemporal dementia
Head injury
Huntington's disease
Motor neurone disease
Multiple sclerosis
Parkinson's disease
Stroke
Subarachnoid haemorrhage
Systemic lupus erythematosus
Tourette's syndrome
Vascular dementia

The motor system

Alcoholic pellagra
Frontal lobe epilepsy
Huntington's diseae
Motor neurone disease
Parkinson's disease

The sensory system

CNS tumours
Corticobasal degeneration
Hepatocerebral syndrome
Parietal lobe epilepsy
Pathogenesis of
   anosognosia
Vascular dementia

The visual system

Alcoholic dementia
Anton's syndrome
Balint syndrome
Head injury
Lewy body dementia
Occipital lobe dementia
Occipital lobe epilepsy
Pathogenesis of
   prosopagnosia
Variant Creutzfeldt–Jakob
   disease

The inhibitory system

Alzheimer's disease
CNS tumours
Frontal lobe epilepsy
Frontotemporal dementia
Gelstic epilepsy
Head injury
Huntington's disease
Obsessive–compulsive disorder
Pathogenesis of apathy complex
Pathogenesis of emotionalism
Secondary mania

The knowledge system

Alcoholic dementia
Alzheimer's disease
CNS tumours
Frontotemporal dementia
Head injury
Herpes simplex encephalitis
Kluver–Bucy syndrome
Multiple sclerosis
Parkinson's disease
Pathogenesis of aggression
Pathogenesis of amnesia
Pathogenesis of anxiety
Pathogenesis of depression
Pathogenesis of emotionalism
Pathogenesis of psychosis
Post-stroke dementia
Temporal lobe epilepsy

The limbic system

Alzheimer's disease
Carbon monoxide poisoning
Dementia pugilistica
Head injury
Lewy body dementia
Limbic encephalitis
Normal-pressure hydrocephalus
Pathogenesis of
   aggression–irritability complex
Pathogenesis of anxiety complex
Temporal (temporolimbic) epilepsy
Vascular dementia
Wernicke–Korsakoff's syndrome

Key

A	Amygdala
DPC	Dorsolateral prefrontal cortex
EC	Entorhinal cortex
FP	Frontal pole
H	Hippocampus
OC	Orbitofrontal cortex
OG	Occipitotemporal gyrus
PC	Premotor cortex
PG	Parahippocampal gyrus
PMC	Primary motor cortex
PSC	Primary somaesthetic cortex
PVC	Primary visual cortex
SPL	Superior parietal lobe
SVC	Secondary visual cortex
TP	Temporal pole
TVC	Tertiary visual cortex
U	Uncus

Fig. II.1 Exploded view of the cerebral cortices and their neuropsychiatric significance. Schematic representation of each lobe of the right cerebral hemisphere seen from the medial aspect in a sagittal plane. It illustrates the possible functional significance of each area of the brain in relation to common neuropsychiatric disorders. Where disorders impact upon multiple areas the principal influence is shown. All clinicoanatomical relationships listed are discussed in more detail in the text.

multiple sclerosis, movement disorders, CNS infections and the effects of alcohol, illicit drugs and environmental toxins. In the elderly, the dementias, delirium, cerebrovascular diseases and CNS tumours are important. I have included chapters on infectious diseases of the CNS, autoimmune diseases and substance abuse because of their importance across the life span.

Two points should be borne in mind while reading this section. First, neuropsychiatric features are often presented as clusters or syndromes that aid clinical decision-making. However, the distress and dysfunction caused by individual symptoms and signs should not be forgotten. At the same time, the frequency of a complication greatly depends on whether symptoms or syndromes are rated. The second point is that the majority of information is summarized from original studies. These summary statistics are a crude representation of a complex interplay between disease and patient. Consider head injury. Is the rate of irritability the same in early and late head injury victims, or in closed (blunt) and open (penetrating) head injury, or in men and women?

As further original work is completed we receive increasingly accurate information about particular complications. Nevertheless, at any particular point in time we must acknowledge that the information we have is, at best, a simplification of what is, more often than not, a very complicated picture.

17

Cerebro-vascular Disease

May I be allowed to make a proposition as to the nomenclature. If as we have seen the processes of the primary fatty and atheromatous degeneration are intimately involved in the sclerosing processes, then the name arteriosclerosis is not sufficient to include the entire disease. I therefore would like to recommend for this the expression 'atherosclerose', or, if you prefer, 'sclero-atherosis'. (Felix Jacob Marchand 1846–1928)

BACKGROUND

Vascular diseases are the most common cause of mortality worldwide, accounting for approximately 30% of all deaths. About one-quarter of the population aged above 65 years has evidence of silent brain infarcts. One in four men and nearly one in five women aged 45 years can expect to have a stroke if they live to their 85th year. Prevalence is higher in oriental, hispanic and black populations. There is a close relationship between cerebrovascular disease and psychiatric disorder. Arteriosclerosis was linked with dementia, psychosis and mood disturbance at the turn of the 20th century. It was Kraepelin who defined arteriosclerotic insanity and arteriosclerotic dementia in 1883 (Kraepelin 1883). At that time syphilitic general paresis was the most common psychiatric presentation and tended to swamp other aetiological processes. Vascular risk factors are

Box 17.1 Possible risk factors for vascular cognitive impairment

Unmodifiable
Apolipoprotein Eε4 and genetic factors
Lower educational level
Male sex
Old age
Previous stroke

Modifiable
High cholesterol level
Hypertension
Smoking

Diseases
Diabetes mellitus
Lyme disease
Neurosyphilis (endarteritis)
Epilepsy
Stroke and transient ischaemic attack
Vasculitis

Cardiovascular
Atrial fibrillation and other arrhythmias
Previous coronary artery bypass grafts
Endocarditis
Ischaemic heart disease
Ventricular septal defect

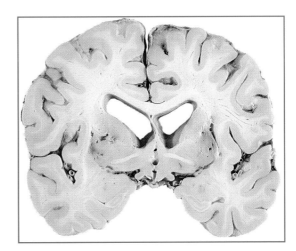

Fig. 17.1 Lacunar infarcts are seen as small slit-shaped cavities (S), a few millimetres in size, in the basal ganglia. From Stevens & Lowe (2000).

themselves linked to both depression and cognitive impairment, although the association is a modest one. Cerebrovascular disease may be divided into microvascular disease, macrovascular disease and vasculitis (Fig. 17.2).

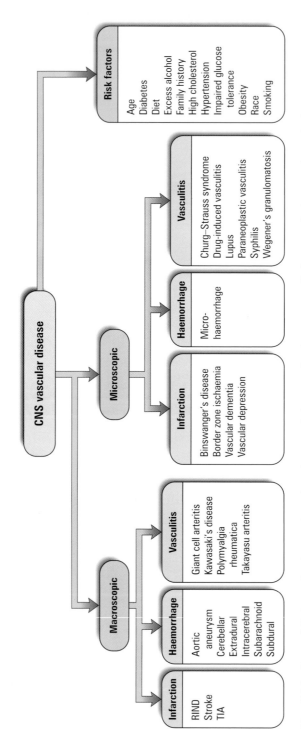

Fig. 17.2 Types of CNS vascular disease. Several conditions, including vascular dementia, usually feature multiple types of vascular lesions. RIND, reversible ischaemic neurological deficit; TIA, transient ischaemic attack.

MICROVASCULAR DISEASE

Binswanger's disease

Encephalitis subcorticalis progressiva, or Binswanger's disease, is a syndrome of dementia associated with white matter damage bilaterally in the periventricular area. On CT there is evidence of low attenuation of the white matter, a finding also seen in 20% of the healthy elderly. Functional neuroimaging demonstrates bilateral frontal lobe hypoperfusion. Post-mortem characteristics are lacunes, subcortical white matter demyelination, état criblé (dilated perivascular 'Virchow–Robin' spaces), ventricular dilatation and astrocytic gliosis, leading to loss of myelin without definite necrosis.

Clinically, there is as a progressive dementia with focal deficits, frontal signs, pseudobulbar palsy, gait disturbance and incontinence (Roman 1996). Affective and psychotic symptoms are also seen. It is probably a variant of vascular dementia, although some patients have an underlying hyperviscosity or hypercoagulabilty diathesis.

Transient ischaemic effects, carotid artery disease and lacunar state

At least 18 studies have examined cognitive function in patients with occlusive carotid artery disease (Bakker et al 2000). The majority of studies have concluded that cognitive deficits were present in patients with and without focal neurological signs and that the degree of deficits varied considerably. If one examines cognition in patients with systemic vascular disease, those with peripheral vascular disease alone have impairments that are barely detectable. People with a history of transient ischaemic attacks tend to have mild deficits and those with a history of stroke have moderate or severe deficits.

Atherosclerotic small vessel brain disease may be undetectable on CT scans. Vascular brain disease is better detected on T2-weighted MRI, in the form of white matter lesions. White matter lesions are conventionally divided into those around the ventricular system (periventricular lesions) and those elsewhere, such as the basal ganglia (deep white matter lesions or *leukoaraiosis*, which is Greek for 'white rarefaction'). Larger lacunal lesions (up to 1.5 cm in diameter) are also seen, especially in subcortical areas (see Fig. 17.1). Lacunae are thought to result from the occlusion of small penetrating lenticulostriate (basilar) and long medullary arterioles. Areas involved include the internal capsule, basal ganglia, thalamus and pons. Patients with these lesions are liable to develop sudden focal cognitive impairments, with later progression toward dementia. Clinically, the syndromes of cognitive impairment associated with cerebrovascular disease may be usefully subdivided into three types: vascular cognitive impairment, vascular dementia and mixed dementia with a vascular component (Fig. 17.3). There is considerable variation in presentation of vascular cognitive impairment and vascular dementia. Vascular cognitive impairment has been compared with the syndrome of mild cognitive impairment, in that there is an approximately 50% risk of developing dementia (predominantly Alzheimer's disease or vascular dementia) in a 5-year follow-up study (Wentzel et al 2001). Mortality is high, at 50% over 5 years of follow-up. Patients may present with cortical or subcortical features, or both. There is typically a history of vascular disease and the presence of vascular risk factors. Neuropsychological testing often reveals regional impairments, reflecting the underlying vascular damage. Vascular dementia itself is discussed in Chapter 43.

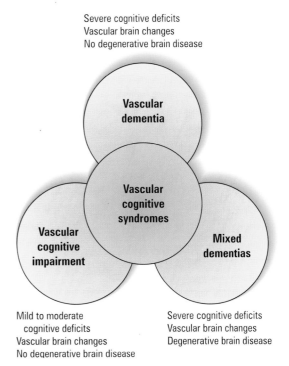

Fig. 17.3 Syndromes of vascular cognitive impairment.

Limited studies have examined non-cognitive neuropsychiatric variables in patients with evidence of small vessel cerebrovascular disease. Only mood disorder has been studied to any extent. The rate of depression is higher than expected in patients with microvascular and macrovascular cerebrovascular disease, whether defined by clinical history of TIAs or stroke, by neuroimaging findings or by carotid artery disease. To what extent depression varies between these subgroups has not been adequately addressed. One provisional study found no significant differences in the severity of depression in 25 TIA patients compared with 25 stroke patients (Rao et al 2001).

Studies of elderly depressed patients have shown that they have significantly more extensive and probably more frequent white matter lesions (O'Brien et al 1996). Such differences are reduced when vascular risk factors are taken into account. White matter lesions in depressed patients have been associated with treatment resistance, cognitive impairment and a lower frequency of family history of affective disorder. With these differences in mind, an independent syndrome of *vascular depression* has been proposed. Depressed patients with vascular brain disease have higher amino acid homocysteine levels (Bell et al 1992). Plasma homo-

cysteine is a marker of cobalamin and folate status and it is also elevated in vascular dementia and, to a lesser extent, in Alzheimer's disease.

MACROVASCULAR DISEASE

Stroke

A stroke is a focal neurological deficit caused by an interruption in blood supply to the brain. Two-thirds of strokes are due to a cerebral infarct, of which two-thirds are thrombotic and one-third are embolic. One-third of strokes are due to haemorrhage, approximately one-half of which are intracerebral and one-half are subarachnoid. Vasculopathies and coagulopathies account for less than 5% of all strokes. Stroke is the second most common cause of death, causing 5 million fatalities per year worldwide. Stroke can occur at any age, but half of all strokes occur in people over 70 years old, making

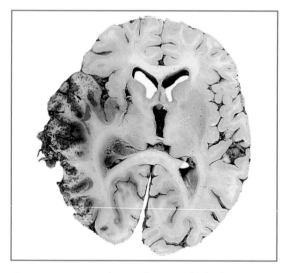

Fig. 17.4 A recent haemorrhagic cerebral infarct. A large infarct, corresponding to the territory of the middle cerebral artery is seen as an area of swollen haemorrhagic brain (I). The haemorrhage was caused by reperfusion after lysis of an occluding thrombus. From Stevens & Lowe (2000).

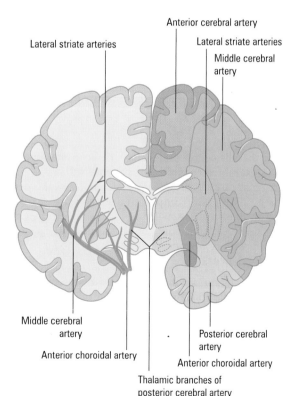

Fig. 17.5 Distribution of perforating branches of the middle cerebral, anterior choroidal and posterior cerebral arteries. From Fitzgerald & Folan-Curran (2001).

Table 17.1 Modified Short Hachinski Scale

	Points
1. Abrupt onset	2
2. History of stroke	1
3. Focal neurological symptoms	2
4. Focal neurological signs	2
5. Low-density areas on CT scanning:	1
– isolated	2
– multiple	3

A score >4 suggests cerebrovascular disease

Box 17.2 Investigations for suspected stroke

- Autoantibodies
- Clotting factors
- CT scan or MRI of the head
- ECG
- Echocardiogram
- Glucose and lipid levels
- Haemoglobin, platelets and white cell count
- Non-invasive neck scan
- Physical and neurological examination
- Plasma viscosity
- Syphilis serology

stroke the most common cause of significant neurological disability in the elderly.

About a third of patients make a full recovery, a third have persistent disability and a third die (mostly within the first month). Death is more common after cerebral haemorrhage. Similarly, alteration in consciousness is much more common in haemorrhagic stroke than in thromboembolic stroke. Various syndromes of stroke have been defined based either on clinical presentation or the vascular territory affected. It is of considerable interest that different lesions can cause recognizable patterns of neuropsychiatric impairment, albeit subject to considerable individual and temporal variation. Common complications of stroke are shown in Fig. 17.6 (Langhorne et al 2000).

Classification of stroke

There are several ways of classifying stroke. Most attempt to follow a clinicoanatomical framework for symptoms and signs (Table 17.2).

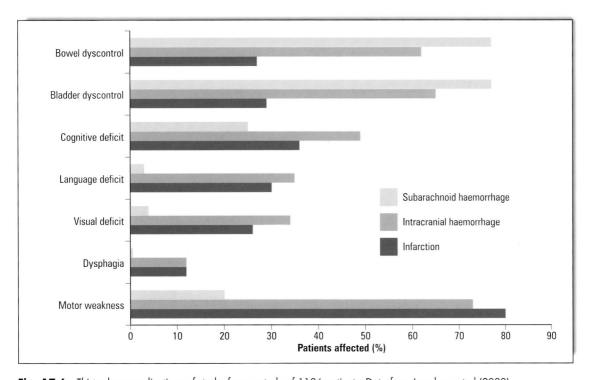

Fig. 17.6 Thirty-day complications of stroke from a study of 1136 patients. Data from Longhorn et al (2000).

Bamford et al (1991) in Oxford formulated a simple system, with four common but overlapping types of stroke, to which haemorrhage has been added. This method of classification can be used as a guide to prognosis. Table 17.3 illustrates the approximate percentages of patients achieving good or bad outcome after stroke, based on initial type of stroke. Note that primary intracerebral haemorrhage was not studied.

NEUROPSYCHIATRIC COMPLICATIONS OF STROKE

Neuropsychiatric presentations after stroke include (from common to rare) the syndromes of cognitive impairment, depression, anxiety, irritability, apathy, emotionalism and mania (Starkstein & Robinson 1994). These presentations co-exist. Neuropsychiatric symptoms such as depression and dementia (both pre-stroke and post-stroke dementia) are independent risk factors for accelerated mortality after stroke.

Post-stroke affective disorder

Depression

Depression after stroke has been studied extensively. The first-year prevalence of new cases of depression (post-stroke depression) is approximately 50% among inpatients and 30–60% in outpatients (Burvill et al 1995, Lowery et al 2002). Approximately half of these cases can be classified as minor depression, which is included in the research section of DSM-IV. Minor depression is characterized by predominantly psychological rather than somatic symptoms of depression, with a severity that shows some correlation with early functional impairment (Paradiso et al 1996). Post-stroke major depression should not be assumed to be a direct consequence of functional disability. It has a similar clinical profile to primary major depressive disorder, with the exception of its higher rate of cognitive impairment, fatigue and anxiety symptoms (Lipsey et al 1986).

Mechanism of post-stroke depression
Much interest has focused on the anatomical localization of post-stroke depression. The most popular theory is that anatomical damage contributes, through local or remote neuronal loss, to depression. In a classic study, Robinson et al (1984), from Baltimore, screened a consecutive series of 184 inpatients with acute stroke, excluding those with severe aphasia or reduced consciousness. In 48 patients who had had their first stroke and who had single vascular lesions visible on CT scan, the severity of post-stroke depression correlated with the proximity of the lesion to the frontal pole of the left hemisphere. However, a recent systematic review of 48 subsequent studies failed to find a consistent

Table 17.2 Clinicoanatomical correlations of stroke

Locations	Vessel involved	Symptoms
Primary intracerebral haemorrhage (PICH) – 10% of strokes	Penetrating lenticulostriate vessels	Headache (35%); vomiting (44%); loss of consciousness; caudate, thalamic, brainstem and cerebellar symptoms
Total anterior circulation infarct (TACI) – 17% of strokes	Middle and anterior cerebral arteries	All three of: higher cognitive dysfunction (dysphasia plus visuospatial deficit), homonymous hemianopia, and motor or sensory deficit
Partial anterior circulation infarct (PACI) – 24% of strokes	Upper or lower division of middle cerebral artery	Higher cognitive dysfunction (dysphasia plus visuospatial deficit (alone)) or two of the three TACI features
Lacunar infarct (LACI) – 25% of strokes	Perforating arteries	Pure motor or sensory symptoms (or sensorimotor stroke) or ataxic hemiparesis; no other features
Posterior circulation infarct (POCI) – 24% of strokes	Vertebrobasilar arteries	Cranial nerve palsy plus contralateral sensorimotor deficit, or bilateral sensorimotor deficit; conjugate eye movement problems; cerebellar dysfunction without ipsilateral long tract signs; isolated homonymous hemianopia

Table 17.3 Stroke outcome based on anatomical area involved

	TACI (%)	PACI (%)	LACI (%)	POCI (%)	Raw numbers
Outcome at 30 days					
Dead	40	5	5	5	56
Dependent	55	40	30	30	214
Independent	5	55	65	65	273
Outcome at 1 year					
Dead	60	15	10	20	124
Dependent	35	30	30	20	150
Independent	5	55	60	60	269

'Dependent' defined as functionally dependent (Rankin grades 3–5)
'Independent' defined as functionally independent (Rankin grades 0–2)
LACI, lacunar infarct; PACI, partial anterior circulation infarct; POCI, posterior circulation infarct; TACI, total anterior circulation infarct

---

Clinical Pointer 17.1

Diagnosing vascular dementia and vascular depression

A vascular contribution to dementia or depression is often overlooked in clinical practice. In an elderly patient with established cardiovascular or peripheral vascular disease, or in those with risk factors of hypertension, smoking or diabetes, the presence of occult cerebrovascular disease should be assumed to be present, until it has been ruled out. A history of unexplained falls or loss of consciousness is suspicious. A physical examination should be repeated in case focal neurological signs, cardiovascular disease or a carotid bruit have been overlooked. In addition, cognitive examination may find evidence of focal cortical or subcortical lesions. First-onset depression or dementia in late life associated with abrupt onset and absence of a family history support the diagnosis. Confirmation with CT or MRI is helpful. Long-term aspirin as well as conventional psychotropic treatment, may be indicated. Psychotropic agents that influence blood pressure should be avoided and patients should be counselled about reversible vascular risk factors.

One problem area, however, is that microinfarcts and lacunar infarcts are each found in about 30% of cases of Alzheimer's disease. Frank haemorrhages are seen in 7% and systematic (cardiovascular) disease in 80%. One possible explanation is that amyloid angiopathy (especially in conjunction with hypertension) leads to spontaneous haemorrhages in the white matter of the frontal or occipital lobes. The pathology of Alzheimer's disease also includes cerebral amyloid angiopathy and microvascular degeneration. A further 30% of the healthy elderly and 60% of patients with Alzheimer's disease show evidence of white matter lesions if these are looked for. Thus, either we are missing many cases of vascular dementia and calling them Alzheimer's disease (which is likely) or Alzheimer's disease is partly a vascular disease (which is also plausible).

Further reading *Chiu E, Kantona CLE, Ames D 2002 Vacular disease and affective disorders. Martin Dunitz, London
Kalaria RN, Skoog I 2000 Vascular factors in Alzheimer's disease. In: O'Brien J, Ames D, Burns A (eds) Dementia, 2nd edn. Arnold, London*

---

association between lesion location and post-stroke depression (see Fig. 70.2) (Carson et al 2000). Overall, we must conclude that there is no single anatomical basis for emotional disorder after stroke and, furthermore, that findings may be explained by functional consequences of aphasia and anosognosia in some cases. In addition, the course of post-stroke mood disorder does not mirror the course of the tissue destruction and recovery, strongly suggesting that the other mechanisms are involved. One possible mechanism is secondary neuroendocrine change. Eight studies involving 336 subjects and using the dexamethasone suppression test to measure hypothalamus–pituitary adrenal axis function have demonstrated a significant link with post-stroke depression, with a mean test sensitivity of 49.6% and a test specificity of 87.2%.

Anxiety

Anxiety is a much overlooked mood disorder in stroke victims. Only a handful of studies have assessed any type of anxiety disorder. As a result, the confidence interval for estimates of the prevalence of anxiety disorder after stroke is very wide. Rates of generalized anxiety disorder of between 1% and 30% at 3 and 6 months post-stroke have been reported. Approximately half of these cases occur in association with depression. A 'ballpark' figure is that around 10% of patients suffer pure generalized anxiety disorder at 6 months post-stroke. In one prospective study, there was very little recovery up to 3 years (Astrom 1996). Agoraphobia also occurs, perhaps half as commonly as generalized anxiety disorder. Data on other types of anxiety disorders is simply insufficient to report.

Other mood problems

Only about 1% of patients suffer mania post-stroke, although approximately 5–10% of patients have transient unstable mood (usually uncontrollable crying), known as *emotionalism*. Mania has been suggested to be more common with right-sided cortical or subcortical damage, but this has yet to be critically examined.

Irritability–aggression after stroke has been studied by three groups. In the first study, anger was present in 21% of those who had sustained an acute thromboembolic stroke (Ghika-Schmid et al 1997). In the second study, aggression was present acutely after stroke in 17% (Aybek et al 2002). In the third study of 145 post-acute patients, inappropriate irritability or anger was reported by 32%, but in only 8% was it totally unprovoked (Kim et al 2002).

At least the same proportion of people suffer apathy early after stroke, half of these in combination with depression. The overlap of apathy, indifference and denial has not been properly studied, although all are common post-stroke (Aybek et al 2002). The course of apathy post-stroke has also not been reported.

The relative risk of suicide is increased after stroke, although this effect is modest in most patients. Men have a six-fold and women a 13-fold increased risk of suicide compared with age-matched controls (Stenager et al 1998). Those at particular risk are patients with stroke in midlife.

Post-stroke cognitive impairment

Post-stroke dementia overlaps with vascular dementia, but the two are not synonymous. Subclinical strokes are thought to be responsible for many cases

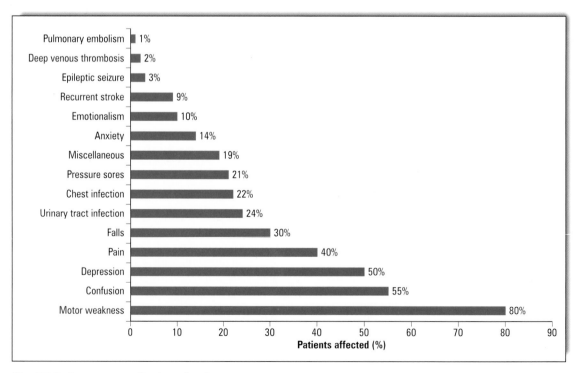

Fig. 17.7 Long-term complications of stroke.

of vascular dementia. Moreover, silent infarcts are five times more prevalent than clinical infarcts in the general population. As many as half of all individuals (depending on risk factors) who experience stroke develop problematic cognitivie deficits. These are unstable, with half again deteriorating to dementia.

Non-dementia cognitive impairment

Two large studies have recently reported rates of post-stroke cognitive impairment of approximately 40–55%. Madureira et al (2001) found that 3 months after stroke, 55% of 220 patients had evidence of cognitive impairment. Of these only 6% had dementia. Thus, nearly 50% had mild to moderate cognitive impairment insufficient for a diagnosis of dementia. Approximately half of these non-dementia cases had predominant memory problems and half had other types of cognitive deficit. In the second study, Patel et al (2001) found that 248 of 645 subjects were cognitively impaired at 3 months after stroke. Predictors of cognitive impairment were:

- age over 75 years (odds ratio 2.5)
- Asian, Caribbean or African ethnicity (odds ratio 1.9–3.4)
- manual socioeconomic class (odds ratio 2.1)
- left hemispheric lesion (odds ratio 1.6)
- visual field defect (odds ratio 2.0)
- urinary incontinence (odds ratio 4.8).

Cognitive impairment was significantly associated with both death and disability at 4 years' follow-up. Neither study accounted for post-stroke delirium, which also causes cognitive dysfunction after stroke.

One group has examined neuroimaging correlates of post-stroke cognitive impairment. Ballard et al (2002) found that impairments in reaction time and working memory on the Cognitive Drug Research Computerized Battery were correlated with severity of white matter hyperintensities in the insular cortex (Ballard et al 2002). It is important to recognize that clinically minor strokes, or even occult strokes, are associated with cognitive deficits that can be evaluated using bedside assessment (e.g. Reverse Digit Span, Trail Making, verbal fluency and Clock Drawing Tests) (Acharya et al 2002).

Delirium

Delirium is well recognized in the acute post-stroke period and may take some weeks to resolve. At least one in four stroke patients suffers delirium.

Delirium can result from a lesion in any critical area and thus is not well localized to any one area. Risk factors for post-stroke delirium include:

- pre-existing cognitive impairment
- extensive stroke
- medical comorbidity
- old age
- polypharmacy.

Dementia

The relative risk of dementia after stroke is five-fold compared with that in age-matched controls. The relative risk is protracted, lasting longer than 4 years, although it is highest in the first 6 months (Tatemichi et al 1994). After excluding approximately 15% of patients, who have prior dementia, the cumulative risk over 3 years is 30% (Hénon et al 2001). There is a strong influence of age, such that the prevalence in those aged under 65 is less than 10%, but in those aged over 85 it may be greater than 50%. Vascular lesions can cause global deficits despite apparently focal brain lesions (see Ch. 43). Risk factors for post-stroke dementia (Hénon et al 2001, Pohjasvaara et al 2000) are:

- atrial fibrillation
- reduced years of education
- older age
- diabetes mellitus
- severity of stroke at admission
- premorbid cognitive impairment
- radiological characteristics, including large infarcts in the dominant superior middle cerebral artery territory, the extent of white matter lesions and medial temporal lobe atrophy.

Thus, both the volume and location of the lesion are important in determining post-stroke dementia. Where the mechanism is neuronal loss, 100 ml is sometimes quoted as the critical amount of infarcted tissue necessary for dementia (Miekle et al 1992). This is undoubtedly an oversimplification.

Box 17.3 Location of vascular dementia syndromes

- Lacunar state – lenticulostriate arteries
- Binswanger's disease – periventricular medullary artery
- Stroke – single intracranial artery
- Thalamic dementia – posterior cerebral or posterior communicating artery
- Watershed ischaemia – carotid artery distribution

Specific focal strokes can cause dementia; examples include the syndromes of *thalamic dementia* (amnesia, amotivational state, drowsiness, ocular palsies and acathexis), *occipital dementia* (amnesia plus delirium and hemianopia) and *angular gyrus syndrome* (Gerstmann's syndrome, visuospatial disorientation and fluent aphasia). Specific infarcts to the caudate and globus pallidus, basal forebrain and hippocampus can also cause severe cognitive impairment. Conversely, vascular lesions can cause focal cognitive syndromes. Examples are hippocampal ischaemia causing a specific deficit in new learning. Of course, other mechanisms can contribute to cognitive impairment, such as pre-existing Alzheimer's disease, stroke-related complications such as hydrocephalus, seizures and adverse drug effects. Depression is another important variable.

We have seen elsewhere that neuropsychiatric complications tend to overlap. Several studies have shown that depression post-stroke is a risk factor for cognitive impairment, and vice versa. In a 12-month prospective study of 106 stroke patients, Kauhanen et al (1999) demonstrated that post-stroke depression was significantly associated with reduced memory, non-verbal problem-solving and attention and psychomotor speed. Conversely, Hénon et al (2001) from the University of Lille found that 56% of patients with post-stroke dementia also had moderate or severe depression over a 3-year period compared with 34% of those stroke patients without dementia. One important finding from this study was that, although most cases of post-stroke dementia were of vascular origin, up to one-third were of the Alzheimer type.

Post-stroke psychosis

Psychosis may take several forms following stroke. The most common types are the transient psychotic symptoms that occur in the context of delirium and more persistent psychotic symptoms in post-stroke dementia. Patients with severe mood disorder, either depression or mania, also experience psychotic episodes after stroke. The overall rate of psychotic symptoms gradually reduces to roughly 10% at 1 year. In elderly patients, occult cerebrovascular disease may cause a diathesis for psychotic forms of depression. Case reports of schizophrenia-like psychosis have been reported after stroke, but such cases are rare. Of note, there may be an association with post-stroke seizures and right-sided lesions in this group. Vivid hallucinations, pseudo-hallucinations and illusions in association with midbrain or occipitotemporal lesions that are complex and feature retained insight are called *peduncular hallucinosis*.

SUBARACHNOID HAEMORRHAGE

There are about 30,000 cases of subarachnoid haemorrhage (SAH) in the USA each year. SAH results

---

Clinical Pointer 17.2

What to do with the tearful stroke patient

First, do not to assume tearfulness after stroke is normal. It may be understandable to be upset after a stroke, but coming to terms with the loss in role, function and relationships may take both time and professional help. Distress and anxiety in the context of these losses can be called an adjustment disorder, but may still require symptomatic treatment despite being temporary. More severe or prolonged low mood should be managed with a combination of antidepressants and support. One of the most important aspects is encouraging the stroke patient to maximize quality of life in spite of the current impairments. In terms of drug choice, SSRIs are safe and effective and hence the usual first-line treatment (see Ch. 47). Relatives often need help too, since they suffer the consequences of the stroke indirectly.

Sudden and unexpected bouts of crying (with or without underlying depression) that are felt to be intense and uncontrollable raise the possibility of pathological crying or emotionalism. However, this should be distinguished from irritability, frustration and anger, which are common complaints in men with enduring acquired disability. The pharmacological treatment of emotionalism is also with antidepressants, usually SSRIs. The response is often better than is seen in post-stroke depression. In all cases, after the patient begins to improve, continue to offer support and antidepressants for at least a year, since this will maximize the chances of improvement in rehabilitation and minimize the chances of relapse.

Further reading   Robinson RG 1998 The clinical neuropsychiatry of stroke. Cambridge University Press, Cambridge

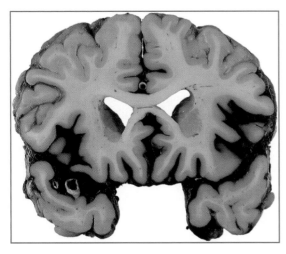

Fig. 17.8 Subarachnoid haemorrhage caused by the rupture of a berry aneurysm just visible in the sylvian fissure. Blood is present in the subarachnoid space. Berry aneurysms are found in 1% of the population. From Stevens & Lowe (2000).

Box 17.4 Hunt and Hess grading system for subarachnoid haemorrhage	
Grade 0	Unruptured
Grade 1	Asymptomatic
Grade 2	Moderate to severe headache, nuchal rigidity, no neurological deficit other than cranial nerve palsy
Grade 3	Drowsiness, mild neurological deficit
Grade 4	Stupor, moderate to severe hemiparesis, possible early decerebrate rigidity, vegetative disturbances
Grade 5	Deep coma, decerebrate rigidity, moribund appearance

After Hunt & Hess (1968)

from the rupture of a latent berry aneurysm and, less commonly, direct head injury or bleeding from arteriovenous malformations. Presenting features are sudden, severe, diffuse headache associated with temporary loss of consciousness, vomiting, nuchal rigidity and focal signs. Diagnosis is usually made on the basis of CT scanning or lumbar puncture (xanthochromia or red cell lysis is seen). About 50% endure permanent disability after SAH, and one of the most common disabilities is cognitive impairment. The prognosis of SAH is poor in many cases. Between 20% and 40% die from the haemorrhage in the first month, and there is about a 20% chance of rebleeding.

NEUROPSYCHIATRIC COMPLICATIONS OF SAH

Mood following SAH

Mood symptoms may be rarer after SAH than after stroke. A shortcoming is that studies of cognition and mood after SAH tend to look at long-term postoperative outcomes and should thus be compared with equivalent long-term outcome studies in stroke. As with stroke, there is limited correlation between functional disability and severity of depression. Nevertheless, this does not imply that a biological mechanism must be present, since depression is multifactorial and the link between function and the development of low mood is certain to be complex. Anxiety is a particular problem after SAH, occurring more freequently than in rehabilitation controls. Further studies are needed to delineate the relationship between locations and extent of bleed after SAH and the effect upon depression, apathy, anxiety and irritability.

Cognition following SAH

Even patients considered to have a relatively good outcome after SAH may suffer from a significant degree of cognitive dysfunction. In one of the few prospective studies in this area, Kreiter et al (2002) measured neuropsychological function in 113 non-traumatic SAH patients at 2 and 12 weeks post-insult. A total of 36% of subjects had global deficits and about half of these had sufficiently severe cognitive impairment to be diagnosed with dementia (personal communication). Within individual domains, deficits in verbal memory and motor functioning were most common. The authors also measured predictors of cognitive impairment (Box 17.5). The demographic variables of age, education, ethnicity and fluency in English imposed a larger effect than disease-related variables. In multivariate analysis, disease-related predictors were complex, but included the type of SAH, the location of the bleed and complications such as cerebral oedema and left-sided infarction. The link with complications was interesting, since 50% of infarcts resulted from procedural complications rather than from the vasospasm itself. Recent operative techniques have reduced the number of postoperative complications, and accordingly the prevalence of affective and cognitive deficits 1 year or more after aneurysm repair appears to be falling.

The special case of the anterior communicating artery aneurysm

The anterior communicating artery (ACoA) connects the two anterior cerebral arteries and is the most common site for berry aneurysms (Fig. 17.9). Berry (or saccular) aneurysms may be inherited or acquired, and are likely to be occult until they rupture. Fusiform aneurysms are more commonly associated with atherosclerosis and are less likely to rupture. Over 80% of aneurysms develop in the anterior portion of the circle of Willis, most commonly at the junction of the ACoA and the anterior cerebral artery, the origin of the anterior cerebral artery, at the origin of the middle cerebral artery or the junction of the posterior communicating artery and the middle cerebral artery. Extensive brain areas may be involved following ACoA rupture, including the orbital frontal lobe, the anterior cingulate gyrus, the basal ganglia and the diencephalon. Thus, the clinical picture is varied, although core features of amnesia, confabulation and personality change are most frequently seen.

Cognitive changes following ACoA rupture are difficult to study, owing to the presence of confounding factors. The typical pattern is one of anterograde

---

Box 17.5 Predictors of cognitive impairment after subarachnoid haemorrhage

Demographic variables
Old age

Disease variables
Hunt and Hess grade (weakly predictive)
Cerebral oedema
Left-sided infarction
Non-posterior subarachnoid haemorrhage
Regional bleed (anterior interhemispheric and sylvian fissures)

Treatment complications
Vasospasm

After Kreiter et al (2002)

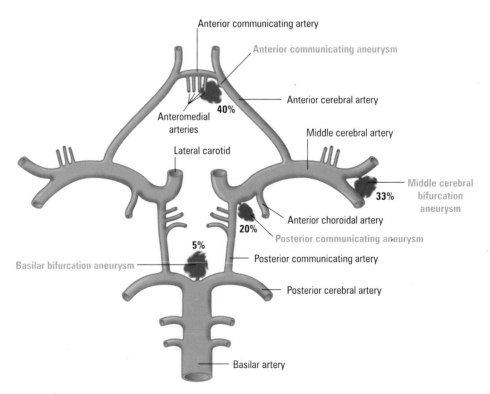

Fig. 17.9 Sites of Berry aneurysms.

amnesia with little retrograde amnesia. Intelligence, attention and visuospatial functions are generally preserved. Executive function is often impaired, and this has been found to predict confabulation, along with involvement of the basal forebrain. Non-cognitive symptoms of ACoA aneurysm have not been widely studied, but include a variety of emotional and behavioural responses, including 'frontal-lobe-type' problems, low mood, anxiety, apathy and irritability.

RARE CEREBROVASCULAR DISORDERS

CADASIL

CADASIL (cerebral autosomal-dominant arteriopathy with subcortical infarcts and leukoencephalopathy) is a rare vascular disorder of midlife caused by mutation in the Notch3 gene on chromosome 19. This results in thickening of the penetrating cerebral small arteries. The clinical features are migraine with aura and stroke with progressive cognitive impairment. Infarcts are as likely to be silent as they are to manifest themselves clinically. Two studies have found that subcortical white matter lesion volume (on structural MRI) and regional cerebral blood volume (on functional MRI) correlate with disability and cognitive impairment (Bruening et al 2001, Dichgans et al 1999).

Hypertensive encephalopathy

Severe and sudden increases or decreases in blood pressure may exceed the capacity for autoregulation. Hypertensive damage may occur gradually if the cause is essential hypertension or renal disease, but more often the presentation is as an emergency in eclampsia or with drug interactions or illicit-drug abuse. The clinical presentation comprises severe headache, nausea and vomiting, epistaxis, dyspnoea and, in severe cases, focal signs, seizures and delirium. Cerebral infarction (and, to a lesser extent, haemorrhage) and acute pulmonary oedema are the end-organ complications of severe hypertension. Cognitive impairment from stroke-like episodes occur, but accumulating damage from long-standing hypertension is more common. Interestingly, modest but persistent hypertension is now recognized as a cause of deteriorating cognitive performance (Knopman et al 2001).

SUMMARY

Stroke is one of the most common causes of neurological and neuropsychiatric disability in those over 60 years of age. Each year in the USA almost half a million patients are discharged from hospital having suffered a stroke. Depression, anxiety, apathy, cognitive impairment and delirium are the most likely impediments to quality of life and rehabilitation success. Although stroke is an excellent model for studying the anatomical and neurochemical basis of psychiatric disorders, no anatomical region is robustly linked with post-stroke mood disorder, and the exact mechanism underlying the neuropsychiatric complications of stroke and other cerebrovascular diseases remains poorly understood.

Occult microvascular disease is increasingly recognized as a common and important cause of dementia, depression, delirium and parkinsonism, yet it is frequently overlooked in clinical practice. The presence of vascular risk factors and a past history of systemic vascular disease should always prompt consideration of this important differential diagnosis. Future developments include more accurate prediction of post-stroke depression, better delineation of the syndrome of post-stroke cognitive impairment and, perhaps most important of all, effective prevention.

REFERENCES AND FURTHER READING

Acharya AB, Edwards DF, White DA et al 2002 How mild is mild stroke? Cognitive impairment in persons with mild stroke. Presented at the American Academy of Neurology 54th Annual Meeting, Denver, 13–20 April

Astrom M 1996 Generalized anxiety disorder in stroke patients. A 3-year longitudinal study. Stroke 27:270–275

Aybek S, Carota A, Berney A et al 2002 Emotional behavior in hyperacute stroke. Presented at the American Academy of Neurology 54th Annual Meeting, Denver, CO, 13–20 April

Bakker FC, Klijn CJM, Jennekens-Schinkel A et al 2000 Cognitive disorders in patients with occlusive disease of the carotid artery: a systematic review of the literature. Journal of Neurology 247:669–676

Ballard C, O'Brien J, Stephens S et al 2002 Cognitive impairments in elderly stroke patients without dementia: profile and MRI correlates. Presented at the American Academy of Neurology 54th Annual Meeting, Denver, 13–20 April

Bamford J, Sandercock P, Dennis M et al 1991 Classification and natural history of clinically identifiable subtypes of cerebral infarction. Lancet 337:1521–1526

Bell IR, Edman JS, Selhub J et al 1992 Plasma homocysteine in vascular-disease and in nonvascular dementia of depressed elderly people. Acta Psychiatrica Scandinavica 86:386–390

Bruening R, Dichgans M, Berchtenbreiter C et al 2001 Cerebral autosomal dominant arteriopathy with subcortical infarcts and leukoencephalopathy: Decrease in regional cerebral blood volume in hyperintense subcortical lesions inversely correlates with disability and cognitive performance. American Journal of Neuroradiology 22:1268–1274

Burvill PW, Johnson GA, Jamrozik KD et al 1995 Prevalence of depression after stroke: the Perth Community Stroke Study. British Journal of Psychiatry 166:320–327

Carson AJ, MacHale S, Allen K et al 2000 Depression after stroke and lesion location: a systematic review. Lancet 356:122–126

Dichgans M, Filippi M, Bruning R et al 1999 Quantitative MRI in CADASIL: correlation with disability and cognitive performance. Neurology 52:1361–1367

Fitzgerald MJT, Folan-Curran J 2001 Clinical neuroanatomy and related neuroscience, 4th edn. Saunders, Philadelphia

Ghika-Schmid F, Ghika J, Vuilleumier O et al 1997 Bihippocampal damage with emotional dysfunctional. Impaired perception of fear. European Journal of Neurology 38:276–283

Hénon H, Durieu I, Guerouaou D et al 2001 Poststroke dementia incidence and relationship to prestroke cognitive decline. Neurology 57:216–1222

Hunt W, Hess R 1968 Surgical risks as related to time of intervention in the repair of intracranial aneurysms. Journal of Neurosurgery 28:14–20

Kauhanen ML, Korpelainen JT, Hiltunen P et al 1999 Poststroke depression correlates with cognitive impairment and neurological deficits. Stroke 30:1875–1880

Kim JS, Choi S, Kwon SU et al 2002 Inability to control anger or aggression after stroke. Neurology 58:1106–1108

Knopman D, Boland LL, Mosley T et al 2001 Cardiovascular risk factors and cognitive decline in middle-aged adults. Neurology 56:42–48

Kraepelin E 1883 Lehrbuch der psychiatrie. 8th edn. Macmillan, London

Kreiter KT, Copeland D, Bernardini GL et al 2002 Predictors of cognitive dysfunction after subarachnoid hemorrhage. Stroke 33:200–208

Langhorne P, Stott DJ, Robertson L et al 2000 Medical complications after stroke: multicenter study. Stroke 31:1223–1229

Lipsey JR, Spencer WC, Rabins PV et al 1986 Phenomenological comparison of post-stroke depression and functional depression. American Journal of Psychiatry 143:527–529

Lowery KJ, Rodgers H, Rowan E et al 2002 Psychiatric morbidity in older stroke survivors. Presented at the American Academy of Neurology 54th Annual Meeting, Denver, CO, 13–20 April

Madureira S, Guerreiro M, Ferro JM 2001 Dementia and cognitive impairment three months after stroke. European Journal of Neurology 8:621–627

Miekle R, Herholz K, Grond M et al 1992 Severity of vascular dementia is related to volume of metabolically impaired tissue. Annals of Neurology 49:909–913

O'Brien JT, Ames D, Schwietzer I 1996 White matter changes in depression and Alzheimer's disease: a review of magnetic resonance imaging studies. International Journal of Geriatric Psychiatry 11:681–694

Paradiso S, Robinson RG, Lamberty G 1996 Validation of the DSM IV construct of minor depression in patients with stroke. Biological Psychiatry Abstracts 39:664

Patel M, Coshall C, Rudd AG et al 2001 Post-stroke cognitive impairment: clinical determinants and its associations with long-term stroke outcomes. Journal of Neurological Science 187(suppl 1):S23

Pohjasvaara T, Mantyla R, Salonen O et al 2000 How complex interactions of ischemic brain infarcts, white matter lesions, and atrophy relate to poststroke dementia. Archives of Neurology 57:1295–1300

Rao R, Jackson S, Howard R 2001 Depression in older people with mild stroke, carotid stenosis and peripheral vascular disease: a comparison with healthy controls. International Journal of Geriatric Psychiatry 16:175–183

Robinson RG, Kubos KG, Starr LB 1984 Mood disorders in stroke patients: importance of location of lesion. Brain 107:81–93

Roman GC 1996 From UBOs to Binswanger's disease. Impact of magnetic resonance imaging on vascular dementia research. Stroke 27:1269–1273

Starkstein SE, Robinson RG 1994 Neuropsychiatric aspects of stroke. In: Coffey CE, Cummings JL (eds) Textbook of geriatric neuropsychiatry, American Psychiatric Press, Washington, DC, p 457–477

Stenager EN, Madsen C, Stenager E et al 1998 Suicide inpatients with stroke: epidemiological study. British Medical Journal 316:1206

Stevens A, Lowe J 2000 Pathology, 2nd edn. Mosby, St. Louis

Tatemichi TK, Paik M, Bagiella E et al 1994 Dementia after stroke is a predictor of long-term survival. Stroke 25:1915–1919

Wentzel C, Rockwood K, MacKnight C et al 2001 Progression of impairment in patients with vascular cognitive impairment without dementia. Neurology 57:714–716

18

Epilepsy

I suppose that in cases of epilepsy and of epileptiform seizures there is a very local discharge-lesion (physiological fulminate) of a few highly unstable cells of one half of the brain. (John Hughlings Jackson 1864)

BACKGROUND

Epilepsy is the tendency to recurrent motor, sensory or behavioural seizures caused by a discrete electrical brain abnormality. The cellular correlate of a seizure is the paroxysmal depolarization shift in which there is greater excitatory than inhibitory activity (Fig. 18.1). About 5% of the population experience a seizure, but only 0.5% have epilepsy. Psychiatric symptoms have been estimated to occur in about 60% of sufferers of refractory epilepsy and are particularly common in those with temporal lobe epilepsy (TLE) and in patients with established brain pathology. Many famous people have suffered from probable TLE, including Julius Caesar, Alexander the Great, Lewis Carroll and Vincent van Gogh.

CLASSIFICATION

The classification of epilepsy is complex. The revised criteria proposed by the International League Against Epilepsy (Box 18.1) are widely cited, but have been criticized for not representing many common presentations in primary care. Alternatives

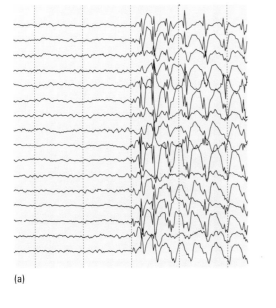

(a)

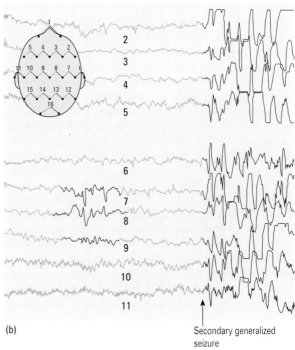

(b)

Secondary generalized seizure

Fig. 18.1   EEG in a patient with epilepsy. From Haslett (1999).

113

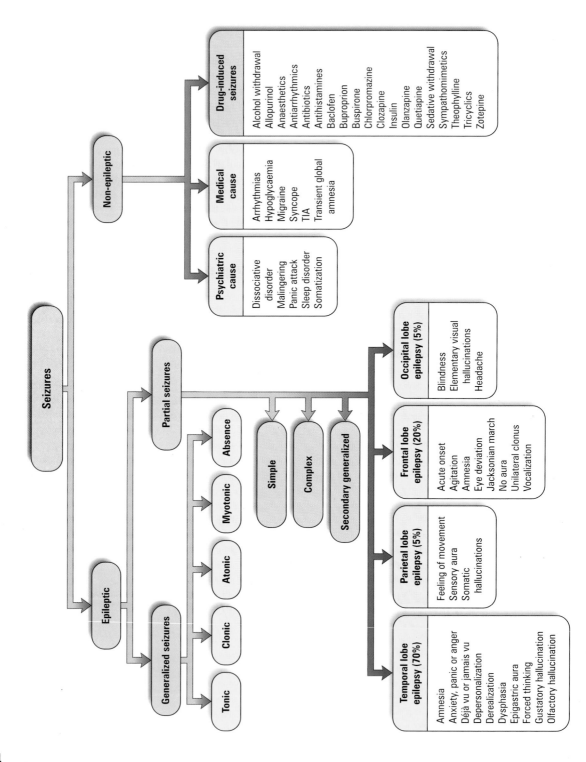

based on clinical signs alone (seizure semiology) have been proposed.

In broad terms, seizures can be divided into three main groups:

- About one-third of patients suffer from a form of epilepsy that cannot be localized to one part of the brain. These generalized epilepsies are usually idiopathic, presumably largely attributable to genetic factors. They include childhood absence seizures, juvenile myoclonic seizures and tonic–clonic seizures.
- At least one-third of patients have an identified focus of seizure activity in the brain from which the epileptic activity begins and then spreads. Clinically these are hailed by a specific symptom described by the conscious patient. This specific symptom is an aura. These localization-related epilepsies include simple partial seizures, in which the seizure is localized, and complex partial seizures in which the depolarization spreads to impair consciousness. A partial seizure may become secondarily generalized if activity spreads to both hemispheres (Fig. 18.3). As this happens quickly, the initial focal nature of the seizure is easily overlooked.
- The remaining one-third of patients have rarer subtypes or undetermined causes of epilepsy. In cases in which a lesion is suspected but not yet found, the term 'cryptogeneic epilepsy' is sometimes used.

The special case of partial seizures

Partial seizures have special significance in neurology and psychiatry. Partial seizures are usually symptomatic of an underlying cerebral lesion. This lesion acts as the pacemaker for the seizures and determines the type of focal symptoms. The presence of a cerebral lesion makes this type of epilepsy

Box 18.1 International classification of epileptic seizures

I. *Partial seizures*
A. Simple partial seizures (consciousness not impaired):
- with motor symptoms
- with somatosensory symptoms (visual, auditory, olfactory)
- with autonomic symptoms (nausea, vomiting, flushing)
- with psychic symptoms

B. Complex partial seizures (consciousness impaired):
- beginning as simple partial seizures
- with impairment of consciousness at onset
- with psychomotor (automatisms)

C. Partial seizures secondarily generalized symptoms

II. *Generalized seizures*
Absence (petit mal) seizures
Myoclonic seizures
Clonic seizures
Tonic seizures
Tonic–clonic seizures (grand mal)
Atonic seizures

III. *Unclassified epileptic seizures*
Usually two clear (unprovoked) seizures are required before diagnosis

Adapted from the Commission on Classification and Terminology of the International League Against Epilepsy (1981)

Fig. 18.2 *(opposite)* Classification of seizure disorders. In 1981, the International League Against Epilepsy (ILAE) revised Gastaut's 1970 proposal in the form of the International Classification of Epileptic Seizures (ICES) (see Box 18.1). Other descriptive methods of classification have been suggested which rely on seizure semiology rather than EEG findings. A taskforce of the ILEA is currently reconsidering its classification system (see http://www.epilepsy.org/ctf). In this figure, an anatomic subdivision of partial seizures and a schema of non-epileptic seizures has been added to the ICES.

less likely to respond to treatment than others. The underlying lesion is easier to identify in some cases (tumours, infiltrations, angiomas and cysts) than others (hamartomas and tissue gliosis).

Partial seizures can be subdivided by anatomy or by pathology. In mesial temporal sclerosis there is extensive neuronal loss and gliosis within all cornu ammonis (CA) fields of the hippocampus (but particularly the CA1 or Sommer sector). This is usually accompanied by atrophy of the ipsilateral entorhinal cortex and amygdala. In a small proportion there is no clear hippocampal lesion, but possible evidence of cortical dysgenesis. This has been called 'paradoxical TLE'. If seizures with a localizable onset are subdivided according to anatomical origin, the most common subtypes are TLE and frontal lobe epilepsy (FLE). However, this distinction is not absolute, since seizures beginning in one region often involve neighbouring regions. In addition, patients with TLE also have a higher rate of damage to extratemporal areas, which could be important in the genesis of neuropsychiatric complications. For these reasons some authors prefer the descriptive term 'temporolimbic epilepsy' to TLE. It is very important to remember that the hippocampus can be both the origin of seizures and the area damaged as a consequence of chronic seizures (Briellmann et al 2002). This would have the effect of creating a feed-forward loop of increasing vulnerability to seizures and may explain the mysterious phenomenon of *kindling*.

CLINICAL FEATURES

The hallmark of the partial seizure is a specific motor, sensory or neuropsychiatric symptom that helps to pinpoint the onset of the seizure to one area of the brain. Because the seizure often spreads to involve other areas, the earliest symptom (usually the aura) is most helpful. In most cases, consciousness is not entirely normal at the outset and the patient is amnesic for the time of the seizure and for a short period either side. This is the *complex partial seizure*. Although preserved consciousness suggests a *simple partial seizure*, it is a presentation easily confused with migraine (if headaches are present) and transient ischaemic attacks (if focal symptoms are present). As a group, extratemporal (and particularly medial frontal) epilepsies are poorly localised using surface EEG recordings. One pointer is the absence of interictal spikes, which suggests extratemporal epilepsy in those with definite seizures. Lesions in specific brain regions may cause identifiable neuropsychiatric symptoms.

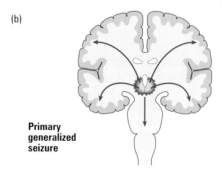

(a)

Partial seizure
± secondary
generalization

(b)

**Primary
generalized
seizure**

Fig. 18.3   (a) Partial seizure with or without secondary generalization. (b) Primary generalized seizure. From Haslett (1999).

Temporal lobe epilepsy

In TLE, both the aura and seizure may consist of simple or complex motor and sensory symptoms,

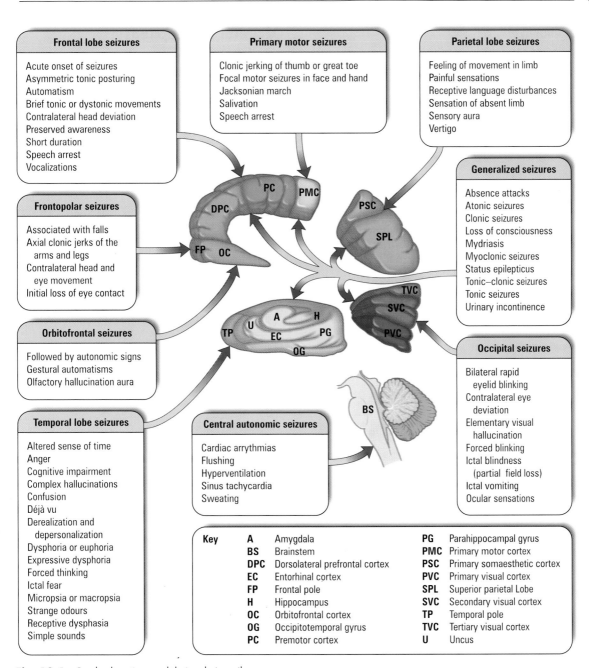

Frontal lobe seizures

Acute onset of seizures
Asymmetric tonic posturing
Automatism
Brief tonic or dystonic movements
Contralateral head deviation
Preserved awareness
Short duration
Speech arrest
Vocalizations

Primary motor seizures

Clonic jerking of thumb or great toe
Focal motor seizures in face and hand
Jacksonian march
Salivation
Speech arrest

Parietal lobe seizures

Feeling of movement in limb
Painful sensations
Receptive language disturbances
Sensation of absent limb
Sensory aura
Vertigo

Frontopolar seizures

Associated with falls
Axial clonic jerks of the
   arms and legs
Contralateral head and
   eye movement
Initial loss of eye contact

Generalized seizures

Absence attacks
Atonic seizures
Clonic seizures
Loss of consciousness
Mydriasis
Myoclonic seizures
Status epilepticus
Tonic–clonic seizures
Tonic seizures
Urinary incontinence

Orbitofrontal seizures

Followed by autonomic signs
Gestural automatisms
Olfactory hallucination aura

Occipital seizures

Bilateral rapid
   eyelid blinking
Contralateral eye
   deviation
Elementary visual
   hallucination
Forced blinking
Ictal blindness
   (partial field loss)
Ictal vomiting
Ocular sensations

Temporal lobe seizures

Altered sense of time
Anger
Cognitive impairment
Complex hallucinations
Confusion
Déjà vu
Derealization and
   depersonalization
Dysphoria or euphoria
Expressive dysphoria
Forced thinking
Ictal fear
Micropsia or macropsia
Strange odours
Receptive dysphasia
Simple sounds

Central autonomic seizures

Cardiac arrythmias
Flushing
Hyperventilation
Sinus tachycardia
Sweating

Key	A	Amygdala	PG	Parahippocampal gyrus
	BS	Brainstem	PMC	Primary motor cortex
	DPC	Dorsolateral prefrontal cortex	PSC	Primary somaesthetic cortex
	EC	Entorhinal cortex	PVC	Primary visual cortex
	FP	Frontal pole	SPL	Superior parietal Lobe
	H	Hippocampus	SVC	Secondary visual cortex
	OC	Orbitofrontal cortex	TP	Temporal pole
	OG	Occipitotemporal gyrus	TVC	Tertiary visual cortex
	PC	Premotor cortex	U	Uncus

Fig. 18.4 Cerebral cortices and their role in epilepsy.

changes in speech, abnormalities of perception, temporary cognitive impairment (confusion), almost any emotion and forced thinking (the neurological equivalent of thought insertion) (Box 18.2). Symptoms of TLE overlap with those generated by the amygdala and the central autonomic network.

The central autonomic network comprises the hypothalamus, midbrain periaqueductal grey matter, pons and medulla. Partial seizures of this network are thought to be responsible for many of the autonomic features of epilepsy, including tachycardia, hyperventilation, sweating and flushing. Discharges in the amygdala have been associated with piloerection and post-ictal nose-wiping.

Frontal lobe epilepsy

In FLE simple partial motor (or jacksonian) seizures identify the origin as the primary motor cortex. Complex motor seizures (e.g. contralateral head deviation) may suggest involvement of the supplemental motor area. Unusual behaviour is often reported in FLE, but this is a difficult symptom to evaluate scientifically. Agitation may be a more specific symptom that has been reported with seizures in orbitofrontal and frontopolar regions. Recently, one group found that epigastric auras (particularly those evolving into oral or gestural automatisms) were much more common in TLE than in FLE (Henkel et al 2002). Other features of FLE include an acute onset of seizures of short duration, characterized by brief tonic or dystonic movements and vocalizations and automatisms. Such seizures have a tendency to occur at night and run in clusters, although post-ictal confusion is less prominent.

Occipital lobe epilepsy

Patients with occipital lobe seizures can experience hallucinations and blindness. These seizures are described as simple patterns in the visual field contralateral to the seizure focus. Not infrequently, occipital lobe seizures spread to involve the temporal or frontal lobe.

Parietal lobe epilepsy

Sensory aura can suggest a parietal lobe seizure, and in some cases this is a painful sensation. Two very interesting parietal lobe symptoms are the feeling that the one limb is moving or is absent. Spread

---

Box 18.2   Neuropsychiatric auras in temporal lobe epilepsy

Cognition
Confusion
Derealization and depersonalization
Altered sense of time
Forced thinking

Memory-like*
Déjà vu
Déjà vecu
Déjà entendu
Jamais vu

Mood
Fear or anxiety
Dysphoria
Euphoria
Anger

Perceptions
Micropsia or macropsia
Hallucinations and illusions

Speech
Expressive dysphasia
Receptive dysphasia

*These are alterations in sense of familiarity, not memory

Box 18.3   Differential diagnosis of epilepsy (non-epileptic causes of seizures)

Cardiovascular disorders
Arrhythmias
Syncope

Neurological disorders
Migraine
Stroke
Tic disorders and tremor
Transient global amnesia
Transient ischaemic attacks

Metabolic disorders
Hypocalcaemia
Hypoglycaemia
Hypomagnesaemia
Hyponatremia (water intoxication)
Hypoxia

Intoxication
Cocaine
D-Amphetamine
Isoniazid
Mercury and lead poisoning
Theophylline

Drug withdrawal
Alcohol withdrawal
Barbiturate withdrawal
Benzodiazepine withdrawal
Cocaine withdrawal

Psychiatric disorders
Narcolepsy, cataplexy
Night terrors
Panic attacks and hyperventilation
Psychogenic seizures
Sleep disorders
Somnambulism

occurs from the superior parietal lobule to the frontal lobe and from the inferior parietal lobule to the temporal lobe.

NEUROPSYCHIATRIC COMPLICATIONS OF EPILEPSY

Psychiatric disorders are common, but by no means invariable, in patients with epilepsy (Table 18.1). Historically, many have overestimated the frequency of psychiatric disorders in people with seizures. The longest follow-up study suggests that the relative risk of psychiatric disorder is approximately four-fold. One common error is to fail to distinguish psychiatric symptoms (which may be linked with seizure frequency) from psychiatric disorders (which tend to be seizure independent). Furthermore, one should specify whether the symptoms are pre-ictal, ictal or post-ictal.

Psychosis in epilepsy

Psychosis in epilepsy principally occurs in three situations:

- shortly after a seizure, often associated with confusion leading to post-ictal psychosis
- between seizures, with no obvious relationship to the seizure frequency (interictal psychosis)
- upon treatment with anticonvulsants (drug-induced psychosis).

The fact that seizure frequency is not closely related to interictal and drug-induced psychoses suggests that distinct mechanisms are at work in each of these situations.

Post-ictal psychosis

Post-ictal epileptic psychosis accounts for approximately 25% of psychotic episodes seen in epilepsy. Post-ictal psychosis and confusion may occur fol-

lowing a cluster of complex partial seizures after a short lucid interval. There is usually evidence of focal discharges on the EEG. Clinically, the psychosis is likely to involve pure delusions or hallucinations (in a non-auditory modality). The patient usually has preserved affect and personality.

Interictal chronic schizophrenia-like psychosis

A non-seizure-related psychosis without confusion occurs between five and 10 times more commonly in patients with seizures than in the general population, (i.e. with a prevalence rate of 5–10%). Mendez et al (1993) compared the rate of interictal schizophrenic disorders in 1600 outpatient patients with epilepsy and 2000 patients with migraine. The rate in migraine sufferers was 1% and in epilepsy sufferers 9%. In children with established TLE, the risk of interictal psychosis over the next 30 years is 10% (Lindsay et al 1979). About two-thirds of such seizures occur in association with TLE and one-quarter in association with extratemporal partial seizures. Less than 10% are due to generalized epilepsy. Recently, it has been suggested that both positive and negative symptoms of schizophrenia occur in epilepsy sufferers. Risk factors for interictal psychosis are proxy markers of TLE (autonomic aura and temporal EEG foci), together with an early age of onset and reduced IQ. The association between left-sided medial temporal lesions and psychosis documented in some studies is not conclusive, and requires a thorough meta-analysis before conclusions can be drawn (see Ch. 76).

Drug-induced psychosis

A paradoxical relationship between seizure activity and psychosis has been commented on by several authors. Brief psychotic episodes have been record-

---

Box 18.4 Conditions conferring a high risk of convulsions

- Acute CNS infection
- Arteriovenous abnormality
- Brain tumour resection
- Haemorrhagic stroke
- Penetrating head injury
- Supratentorial craniotomy

Table 18.1 Approximate frequency of psychiatric disorders in temporal lobe epilepsy

Disorder	Frequency (%)
Major depression	30
Cognitive impairment	20
Anxiety	15
Aggressive behaviour	10
Bipolar affective disorder	8
Psychosis	5
Sexual dysfunction	Unknown
Obsessive–compulsive disorder	Rare

Table 18.2 Phenomenology of interictal psychoses in epilepsy

Psychosis	Frequency (%)
Schizophrenia	40
Schizophreniform	25
Delusional disorder	20
Brief psychosis	11
Schizoaffective disorder	1

Adapted from Kanemoto et al (2001)

ed after treatment of seizure activity (sometimes called *forced normalization*; Landholt (1953) originally reported improvements in EEG activity during psychotic periods). Certain anticonvulsants such as felbamate, vigabatrin and zonisamide have been implicated in causing new psychotic episodes. Psychosis has been noted not only following drug treatment, but also as a consequence of neurosurgery. As neither neurosurgery nor psychosis is common, this combination has not been well studied. From limited data, predictors of post-surgical psychosis include pre-existing brain damage, right temporal lobe operations and ongoing seizures. This suggests that failure to resolve the underlying epilepsy might account for many such cases.

Mood disorder in epilepsy

Depression

Depression and epilepsy have a somewhat curious relationship. There is no doubt that both depression and anxiety occur frequently in epilepsy. In a large survey of TLE patients, Currie et al (1971) documented a 19% point prevalence of anxiety disorder and 11% point prevalence of depressive disorder. Mendez et al (1986) asked the question whether the rate of depression in outpatients with epilepsy was more common than in disabled non-epileptic controls. On self-report measures, 55% of the epileptic group reported depression, compared with 30% of matched controls. In a recent large community survey of 2281 people with epilepsy, 29% reported major depression – about twice the rate found in either diabetes or asthma (Blum et al 2002). There is also evidence that the rate of depression is higher in patients with non-epileptic seizures and that it strongly influences quality of life in patients with epileptic and non-epileptic seizures.

Several studies have also shown that the rate of suicide is about 5% in patients with epilepsy, which is much higher than in the general population. In most patients the symptom of depressed mood is not directly linked with seizure frequency, although both pre-ictal, ictal and post-ictal dysphoria have all been described. It should be of no surprise that depression is less frequent in those with epilepsy in full remission. Temporary dysphoria may occur as a prodrome or aura and typically lasts a few hours, although occasionally it may persist for days. Interictal depression is the most important type of depressive disorder for most patients and is seen in about 20% of sufferers, although the incidence may be as high as 40% in those with intractable seizures and in those with confirmed TLE. The phenomenology of interictal depression is usually similar to primary depression, although atypical features and irritability have been described more frequently than expected. Hermaan & Wyler (1989) found that, in a cohort of 37 patients who had undergone temporal lobe surgery, those in whom interictal depression improved were also those in whom seizures abated. This may suggest that in most patients with depression and TLE it is the disruptive effect of the TLE on their lives that accounts for the depression. It can be argued that a biological effect (specific neuronal discharge) could also account for the remission of depression, but what mechanism would effect depression interictally?

Mechanism of interictal depression

Several studies have found that a higher proportion of TLE patients than patients with other types of epilepsies suffer depression, and in many cases symptoms resolve with successful neurosurgery (Altshuler et al 1999, Lambert & Robertson 1999). One study found that it was mesial temporal sclerosis in particular that was important in the genesis of depression (Quiske et al 2000). Depression may be more common in epilepsies with a left-sided focus and, although the literature is not altogether consistent on this point, this finding has been replicated using PET scanning (Fig. 18.6) (Victoroff et al 1994). Other risk factors are subject to dispute, including the frequency and duration of seizures. Possible associations with depression include stressful life events, poor adjustment to ongoing seizures, a past psychiatric history, hypofrontality on SPECT and low serum folate. One impressive study, available only in abstract form, examined 5-hydroxyindole acetic acid and the dopamine metabolite homovanillic acid in blood, urine and CSF in 85 epilepsy patients, 36 patients with epilepsy and depression, 27 patients with depression alone and 50 controls.

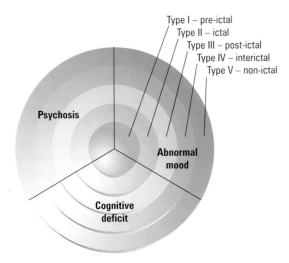

Type I – pre-ictal
Type II – ictal
Type III – post-ictal
Type IV – interictal
Type V – non-ictal

Psychosis

Abnormal mood

Cognitive deficit

Fig. 18.5 Neuropsychiatric semiology in epilepsy. Conceptually, neuropsychiatric symptoms in epilepsy may be considered in terms of the phase in which they begin. Pre-ictal symptoms occur as a prodrome, linked with later seizure onset. Ictal symptoms include aura experiences that represent the first onset of an abnormal brain electrical activity. Post-ictal and interictal symptoms may be affiliated with seizure frequency, but this becomes more difficult to establish the longer the delay between the seizure and symptom. Non-ictal symptoms do not correlate with seizure frequency.

The authors found that levels of 5-hydroxyindole acetic acid were lowest in the depressed patients with epilepsy, although this was only statistically significant in comparison with controls (Maheshwari et al 2001).

Anxiety disorders

Anxiety disorders are common in patients with epilepsy and, as with other neuropsychiatric complications, can either be seizure related or non-seizure related. Panic disorder, in particular, occurs in about one in five people with epilepsy, many times the rate in the general population. Interictal anxiety is non-seizure-related anxiety, in which the sufferer can normally describe the focus of their worries. It may be health-related ('I am fearful of having another fit'), related to disability ('I am anxious about how I am going to cope in the future'), related to leaving the home ('I get anxious every time I go out, in case something happens') or related to social situations ('I cannot meet my friends any more because I always stand out'). Fear of leaving the home is observed in one-fifth of patients (Mittan 1986). These anxieties can be classified as persistent (gen-

eralized anxiety disorder, agoraphobia and social phobia) or episodic (panic disorder).

Seizure-related anxiety is called *ictal fear*. This is a sudden, brief feeling of apprehension at the onset of a seizure that occurs 'out of the blue'. Intensity is on a sliding scale from slight nervousness to complete terror. It is different from the anticipatory anxiety that a seizure is going to occur. The frequency of ictal fear in patients with TLE is 20–40%. Partial seizures are increasingly recognized as a cause of panic attacks, particularly nocturnal panic. Closely related is agitation, which has been linked with FLE.

Mechanism of epilepsy-related anxiety

Intraoperative studies involving electrical stimulation of the brain suggest that the amygdala, more than the hippocampus and parahippocampal gyrus, is involved in eliciting the fear response (see Ch. 71).

Mania

Mania is recognized as a complication of TLE, and estimates put the lifetime risk at 8–20%, at least twice the observed rate in asthma or diabetes (Blum et al 2002). Unfortunately, this presentation has not been described in sufficient detail in the literature for a summary to be provided here.

Cognitive impairment in epilepsy

There can be little doubt that epilepsy is associated with a modest deterioration in cognition in those with previously normal performance, but defining the exact nature of the deficits has proven elusive. One reason for this is that these deficits are multifactorial, involving some factors that are seizure related (site and severity of neuronal damage) and others that are not (developmental effects and adverse medication effects). Patients with subclinical spike and wave recordings are now recognized to suffer cognitive deficits. This can be interpreted in two ways. The first is that subclinical seizures are not really subclinical, since close examination will reveal transient cognitive impairment in 50% of patients at the time of abnormal electrical activity. More contentiously, the second interpretation is that some people will develop persistent cognitive changes even with the mildest forms of seizure disorder. The latter conclusion is supported by the discovery of poor attention, memory and processing speed in relatively stable outpatients with partial epilepsy treated with carbamazepine. This has important implications for complex activities such as driving and work competence (Engelberts et al 2002).

At the other end of the epilepsy spectrum, patients with recurrent refractory seizures certainly suffer cognitive deficits that may persist after successful surgical treatment (see below). From the reverse angle, is it possible that early cognitive impairments are a risk factor for refractory epilepsy? This has been studied at the Kuopio University Hospital, Finland. The development of refractory seizures in 89 consecutive patients was predicted by poor immediate and delayed recall on the List Learning Test done 2 years previously (Aikia et al 1999). As a consolation, some recent evidence shows that the

pre-existing deficits deteriorate very little, if at all, over a 10-year period (Helmstaedter et al 2000).

Mechanisms of cognitive impairment in epilepsy

Various groups are beginning to explore cognitive function in epilepsy in relation to seizure foci and epilepsy subtypes. Duration of illness and frequency of seizures are modestly related to deterioration in cognitive function, but not all deficits neatly correlate with seizure burden. An early age of onset is associated with more severe impairment, particularly in IQ rather than memory alone (but see the discussion of learning disability, below). In TLE, there are impairments in declarative memory, shown as deficits in naming to confrontation, but sparing of attention, concentration and executive functions. Head-to-head comparisons of cognition in TLE versus other types of epilepsy are rare. In one study in children, those with FLE had deficits in planning and impulse control not seen in those with TLE (Hernandez et al 2002). There is also an interaction with depression. Not only do depressed patients perform more poorly than non-depressed patients with TLE on cognitive testing, but also those depressed sufferers with left-sided TLE generally perform

---

Box 18.5 Cognitive impairment in each stage of epilepsy

- Impairments in attention and concentration, which typically occur in the ictal phase
- Impairments in recent anterograde and retrograde memory, which typically occur in the post-ictal phase
- Impairments in calculation and reading, which typically occur in the interictal phase

---

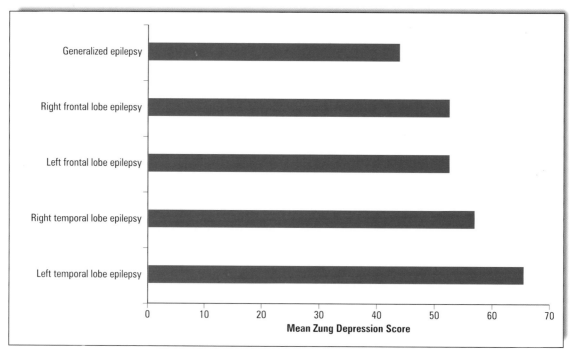

Fig. 18.6 Zung Depression Scores in temporal lobe epilepsy, frontal lobe epilepsy and generalized epilepsy. Data from Piazzini & Canger (2001).

more poorly than depressed patients with right-sided TLE (Paradiso et al 2001). The relationship between medial temporal atrophy and cognitive performance is particularly interesting. Severity of hippocampal atrophy correlates with memory difficulties in TLE, although other limbic sites also may play a role (Lencz et al 1992).

Epilepsy and learning disability

There is a strong overlap between epilepsy and learning disability, because brain pathology acquired early in life causes both seizures and cognitive impairment (see Box 18.6). Fifty per cent of people with a profound learning disability have epilepsy and, conversely, 25% of those with epilepsy have learning disability. Epilepsy occurring in people with learning disability is more difficult to treat, for a number of reasons (see Ch. 48). The presence of one or more pathological foci will continue to generate seizures, but at the same time prove difficult or impossible to manage surgically. Therefore, the likelihood of seizure control depends on the type and extent of seizure-generating pathology more than on the learning disability syndrome (unless the two are related, as in the case of the neurocutaneous syndromes). The odds ratio for mortality is three-fold higher in those with epilepsy than those without, but it is only in cases of profound learning disability that deaths are commonly attributable to seizures in the form of status epilepticus, sudden unexpected death in epilepsy, or seizure-related trauma or drowning (Nashef et al 1995).

Cognitive effects of antiepileptic drugs

There is increased understanding of the effects of antiepileptic drugs (AEDs) on cognition, but research is still in the early stages. Drugs influence cognition positively by reducing seizure frequency. Indeed, most studies support the observation that drug-naive patients with epilepsy perform worse than those treated with AEDs. However, drugs may affect cognition negatively via a direct neurotoxic effect on the brain, or indirectly via sedation, induced low mood, impaired motivation, effect on sleep, effect of drug interactions and effects of drug withdrawal. When examining studies of prescribed drugs and cognition, the following levels of sensitivity may help to understand to magnitude of any drug effect (Box 18.7).

Studies of individual AEDs examine either absolute drug effects, (i.e. the on-drug performance compared with the same patient's off-drug performance

---

Box 18.6 Syndromes featuring learning disability and epilepsy

Perinatal brain injury, cerebral palsy

Prenatal infections

Postnatal infections

Chromosomal disorders:
- Down's syndrome
- fragile X syndrome
- Wolf–Hirschhorn syndrome
- Angelman's syndrome

Childhood autistic disorders

Cortical dysplasia

Neurocutaneous syndromes:
- neurofibromatosis
- tuberous sclerosis
- Sturge–Weber syndrome

Metabolic disorders:
- phenylketonuria
- maple-syrup disease
- homocystinuria
- ornithine deficiencies

Neurodegenerative disorders:
- Unverricht–Lundborg disease
- Batten's disease
- Lafora body disease
- Rett's syndrome

Specific epilepsy syndromes:
- Lennox–Gastaut syndrome
- West's syndrome
- Rasmussen's syndrome
- Landau–Kleffner syndrome

Adapted from Lhatoo & Sander (2001)

Box 18.7 Levels of cognitive disturbance induced by antiepileptic drugs

Level I Does the drug impair cognition in toxic overdose?

Level II Does the drug impair cognition in vulnerable groups (e.g. the elderly, the learning disabled)?

Level III Does the drug impair cognition at high doses, over a long period?

Level IV Does the drug impair cognition in combination with other drugs?

Level V Does the drug impair cognition at normal doses in those who are seizure free?

Level VI Does the drug impair cognition when given acutely to healthy volunteers?

Clinical Pointer 18.2

Making the diagnosis of pseudoseizures (non-epileptic seizures)

Psychogenic pseudoseizures are always high on the list for the neurologist investigating unusual or refractory seizures. The diagnosis of non-epileptic seizures can be difficult, and this is reflected in the observation that most patients who eventually receive this diagnosis have previously been diagnosed with epilepsy (Benbadis et al 1999) and also in the average time to diagnosis of 7 years (Reuber & House 2002). Roughly one in five patients referred to epilepsy clinics are thought to have non-organic seizures. The proportion of patients with epilepsy who also experience non-epileptic seizures is difficult to estimate. Similarly, the proportion of patients with apparent pseudoseizures who develop evidence of epilepsy is uncertain, but may be above 10%.

On close inspection, the term 'pseudoseizures' actually encompasses three separate phenomena. There are seizures not caused by epilepsy but by some other medical condition (such as transient ischaemic attacks and hypoglycaemia). These are more precisely labelled as *symptomatic seizures*. There are seizures in patients who have a somatoform (somatization) disorder, sometimes known as *dissociative pseudoseizures*. There are also people who are labelled as having non-organic seizures, but who have *unusual forms of epilepsy*. One should also add that, very rarely, patients may feign seizures at times of distress (a form of malingering).

Helpful pointers for distinguishing the dissociative pseudoseizures and true epilepsy are that non-epileptic seizures tend to occur in vulnerable people (perhaps with a psychiatric history), who have a tendency to present distress in a physical way, often after a period of social adversity. Women are twice as likely as men to suffer dissociative pseudoseizures, and there is also a link with unemployment. Clinical pointers are contentious, but the following pointers have been suggested. The seizures usually occur in the daytime, with others present, and they are often modifiable by direct command. The patient rarely sustains any injures and has no autonomic or pupillary changes and no significant rise in prolactin. Note that a stress hormone response is seen in about 50% of sufferers of complex partial seizures and less often in those with simple and absence attacks. During the seizure the patient is more likely to maintain body tone and to shout. Motorless swooning, hyperventilation, whole-body shaking and pelvic thrusting are possible indicators of non-epileptic seizures (Jedrzejczak et al 2001). Afterwards the patient tends to be alert and orientated and can recall events clearly. Neuropsychological testing has not proven a reliable method of distinguishing epileptic from non-epileptic seizure disorders. Routine EEGs are rarely useful, because it is unlikely that a patient will have a seizure at the moment an EEG is being recorded. Twenty-four-hour recording with video telemetry is an option in difficult cases. There is an unresolved debate as to whether to use provocative testing to elucidate seizure threshold in the most challenging cases. Follow-up studies show that about half of patients continue to experience seizures 2 years or more after the diagnosis is made. Simple reassurance is rarely effective; rather, the principles of consistency, support and reattribution of symptoms (see Ch. 66) are required.

Further reading Agrawal V, Tatum WO 2001 How many patients with psychogenic non-epileptic seizures also have epilepsy? Neurology 57:915–917
Benbadis SR 1999 How many patients with pseudoseizures receive antiepileptic drugs prior to diagnosis? European Journal of Neurology 41:114–115
Benbadis SR, Ettinger AB, Devinsky O et al 1999 A comprehensive profile of clinical, psychiatric, and psychosocial characteristics of patients with psychogenic nonepileptic seizures. Epilepsia 40:1292–1298
Jedrzejczak J, Grabowska A, Owczarek K et al 2001 The analysis of frequency of morphological events in patients with psychogenic pseudo-epileptic seizures. Journal of the Neurological Sciences 187(suppl 1):S417
Reuber M, House AO 2002 Treating patients with psychogenic non-epileptic seizures. Current Opinion in Neurology 15:207–211

or the performance of drug-naive controls) or relative drug effects (i.e. a comparison of cognitive performance in two groups of patients on different AEDs) (Aldenkamp 2001). In most comparative studies of anticonvulsants, it is the sedative barbiturates and, to a lesser extent, the benzodiazepines that come out worst (see Table 48.1). These drugs have a strong dose-dependent relationship with impaired attention, reaction times and, to some extent, measures of short-term memory and performance IQ. This effect is seen even at therapeutic doses. Patients can also become disinhibited (or, in the case of children, hyperactive) while taking medium doses. Note the comparable effects of alcohol at medium doses. Phenytoin and carbamazepine are both capable of interfering with cognition, although this is often overlooked clinically. There is a clearer dose–response relationship with carbamazepine than with phenytoin. In head-to-head studies impairments due to phenytoin and carbamazepine are not easily distinguishable, provided that patients with toxic levels are accounted for. Sodium valproate is considered to have a modest adverse cognitive profile, with several small studies demonstrating mild effects on psychomotor speed that are not dose related.

Cognitive effects of newer anticonvulsants have been better studied as awareness of this area has grown. Topiramate causes a decline in attention, concentration and verbal fluency, both acutely and chronically, although tolerance may occur. In comparison, gabapentin, lamotrigine and vigabatrin have yet to be shown to have significant adverse cognitive adverse effects. Further work on levetiracetam and oxcarbazepine is required.

Cognitive effects of neurosurgery for epilepsy

In 1972, Falconer at the Maudsley Hospital in London developed the en bloc temporal lobectomy, which entailed removal of the anterior temporal neocortex, the amygdala and the body of the hippocampus. Postoperative neurological deficits such as stroke, dysphasia and hemianopia are rare, but disastrous deficits in new learning can occur if both temporal lobes are removed (as famously described in Brenda Milner's case reports of HM). Just as with AEDs, neurosurgery can cause an improvement as well as a deterioration in memory, depending on the pre-existing cognitive impact of the seizures and the success in reducing seizure burden. In those considered for surgery the benefits are thought to outweigh the risks. The main reason why neurosurgery is considered only when medical management has failed is because of the possible neurological and cognitive adverse effects. Many patients, but not all, who undergo left anterior temporal lobectomy experience a decline in verbal memory. Those who receive right anterior temporal lobectomy suffer visuospatial memory decline, although patients find this less disruptive. Those with mesial temporal sclerosis on MRI do better than those without.

PERSONALITY IN EPILEPSY

It is impossible to assign a certain personality type to people with epilepsy. Nevertheless, having a chronic relapsing and remitting CNS disease will cause adjustment and behavioural difficulties in most previously healthy people. Characteristics that have been ascribed, probably erroneously, to sufferers with epilepsy include viscous or sticky thoughts, religiosity, expressiveness, irritability and hypergraphia. This is sometimes called the *Gastaut–Geschwind syndrome*. Without more scientific evidence it is more important to consider not how patients with epilepsy are different in terms of character, but how they are subject to disadvantage by the attitudes of others. As an example, one recent multicentre study illustrated that over 50% of people with epilepsy felt stigmatized (Baker et al 2000).

SUMMARY

Epilepsy is a syndrome encapsulating several diseases. It is one of the most prevalent neurological disorders, with an estimated 40 million people suffering from epilepsy worldwide. Complex partial seizures, particularly TLE, have special neuropsychiatric significance, notably in relation to anxiety disorders, cognitive impairment and psychosis. Seizure-related ictal fear, dysphoria, confusion and amnesia are very different entities from the non-seizure-related interictal disorders. The EEG is a valuable tool in the differential diagnosis of epilepsy-related disorders, but clinical judgement is equally valuable, particularly in evaluating neuropsychiatric complications. Clinical concern about drug-induced seizures should not stop the appropriate psychotropic treatment of disabling psychiatric complications. Important future developments will include an increased understanding of the mechanisms underlying anxiety, depression and neuropsychological impairments in different types of epilepsy. Minimizing stigma and handicap remain a high priority.

REFERENCES AND FURTHER READING

Aikia M, Kalviainen R, Mervaala E et al 1999 Predictors of seizure outcome in newly diagnosed partial epilepsy: memory performance as a prognostic factor. Epilepsy Research 37:159–167

Aldenkamp AP 2001 Effects of antiepileptic drugs on cognition. Epilepsia 42(suppl 1):46–49

Altshuler L, Rausch R, Delrahim S et al 1999 Temporal lobe epilepsy, temporal lobectomy, and major depression. Journal of Neuropsychiatry and Clinical Neuroscience

11:436–443

Baker GA, Brooks J, Buck D et al 2000 The stigma of epilepsy: a European perspective. Epilepsia 41:98–104

Blum D, Reed M, Metz A 2002 Prevalence of major affective disorders and manic/hypomanic symptoms in persons with epilepsy: a community survey. Presented at the American Academy of Neurology 54th Annual Meeting, Denver, CO, 13–20 April

Briellmann RS, Berkovic SF, Syngeniotis A et al 2002 Seizure-associated hippocampal volume loss: a longitudinal magnetic resonance study of temporal lobe epilepsy. Annals of Neurology 51:641–644

Commission on Classification and Terminology of the International League Against Epilepsy 1981 Proposal for revised clinical and electroencephalographic classification of epileptic seizures. Epilepsia 22:489–501

Currie S, Heathfield KWG, Henson RA et al 1971 Clinical course and prognosis of temporal lobe epilepsy: a survey of 666 patients. Brain 94:173–190

Engelberts NHJ, Klein M, van der Ploeg HM et al 2002 Cognition and health-related quality of life in a well-defined subgroup of patients with partial epilepsy. Journal of Neurology 249:294–299

Gastaut H 1970 Clinical and electroencephalographical classification of seizures. Epilepsia 11:102–113

Haslett C 1999 Davidson's principles and practice of medicine. Churchill Livingstone, Edinburgh

Helmstaedter C, Kurthen M, Lux S et al 2000 Long-term clinical neuropsychological, and psychosocial follow-up in surgically and nonsurgically treated patients with drug-resistant temporal lobe epilepsy. Nervenarzt 71:629–642

Henkel A, Noachtar S, Pfander M et al 2002 The localizing value of the abdominal aura and its evolution: a study in focal epilepsies. Neurology 58:271–276

Hermann BP, Wyler AR 1989 Depression, locus of control, and the effects of epilepsy surgery. Epilepsia 30:332–338

Hernandez MT, Sauerwein HC, Jambaque I et al 2002 Deficits in executive functions and motor coordination in children with frontal lobe epilepsy. Neuropsychologia 40:384–400

Jackson JH 1864 Loss of speech with hemiplegia of the left side, valvular disease, epileptiform seizures affecting the side paralysed. Medical Times Gazette 2:166–167

Kanemoto K, Tsuji T, Kawasaki J et al 2001 Re-examination of interictal psychoses based on DSM IV Psychosis and International Epilepsy Classification. Epilepsia 42:98–103

Lambert MV, Robertson MM 1999 Depression in epilepsy: etiology, phenomenology, and treatment. Epilepsia 40(suppl 10):S21–S47

Landholt H 1953 Serial electroencephalographic investigations during psychotic episodes in epileptic patients and during schizophrenia attacks. In: Lorentz de Haas AM (ed) Lectures on epilepsy. Elsevier, Amsterdam, p 91–133

Lencz T, Mccarthy G, Bronen RA et al 1992 Quantitative magnetic resonance imaging in temporal-lobe epilepsy: a relationship to neuropathology and neuropsychological function. Annals of Neurology 31:629–637

Lhatoo SD, Sander JWAS 2001 The epidemiology of epilepsy and learning disability. Epilepsia 42(suppl 1):6–9

Lindsay J, Ounstead C, Richards P 1979 Long term outcome in children with temporal lobe seizures. III. Psychiatric aspects of childhood and adult life. Developmental Medicine in Child Neurology 21:630–636

Maheshwari PK, Pal T, Hazra DK et al 2001 Epilepsy and depression: their prognostic significance in relation to serotonin and dopamine metabolites. Journal of the Neurological Sciences 187(suppl 1):S413

Mendez MF, Cummings JL, Benson F 1986 Depression in epilepsy: significance and phenomenology. Archives of Neurology 43:766–770

Mendez MF, Grau R, Doss RC et al 1993 Schizophrenia in epilepsy: seizure and psychosis variables. Neurology 43:1073–1077

Mittan RJ 1986 Fear of seizures. In: Whitman S, Hermann BP (eds) Psychopathology in epilepsy: social dimensions. Oxford University Press, New York, p 90–121

Nashef L, Fish DR, Garner S et al 1995 Sudden-death in epilepsy: a study of incidence in a young cohort with epilepsy and learning-difficulty Epilepsia 36:1187–1194

Paradiso S, Hermann BP, Blumer D et al 2001 impact of depressed mood on neuropsychological status in temporal lobe epilepsy. Journal of Neurology and Neurosurgical Psychiatry 70:180–185

Piazzini A, Canger R 2001 Depression and anxiety in patients with epilepsy. Epilepsia 42 (suppl 1):29–31

Quiske A, Helmstaedter C, Lux S et al 2000 Depression in patients with temporal lobe epilepsy is related to mesial temporal sclerosis. Epilepsy Research 39:121–125

Victoroff JL, Benson DF, Grafton ST et al 1994 Depression in complex partial seizures. Archives of Neurology 51:155–163

Zafonte RD, Hammond FM, Mann NR et al 1996 Revised Trauma Score. An additive predictor of disability following traumatic brain injury. American Journal of Physical Medicine and Rehabilitation 75:456–460

19

Head and Brain Injury

Fibres as delicate as those of which the organ of mind is composed are liable to break as a result of violence to the head. (JHP Gama 1835)

BACKGROUND

Head injury (often referred to as traumatic brain injury) is not one single condition but a heterogeneous mix of penetrating, non-penetrating, focal and diffuse injuries of any severity. It is thus not surprising that the neuropsychiatric complications are diverse and, in many respects, poorly described.

In the Epidemiological Catchment Area Study (Silver et al 2001), 8.5% of adults reported a history of head injury with loss of consciousness or confusion. At the other end of the spectrum, 4000 deaths per year in the UK and 50,000 deaths in the USA occur as a result of severe head injury, making head injury the leading cause of death in young people. In the young and middle-aged, road traffic accidents and violent assaults are the most common causes, while in the very old and very young falls are most often to blame. In adults alcohol is a significant contributory factor in 50% of cases, particularly those involving injuries from assaults (Bogner et al 1991). Other important causes are occupational and sports injuries. One frightening statistic is that, in the USA, the number of head injuries from firearms and road traffic accidents are comparable. In terms of disability, because 80% of head injuries are survivable (gunshot being the obvious exception) there is a huge prevalence of head-injury-related disability. The Centers for Disease Control and Prevention in the USA estimates that 5.3 million US citizens are living with disability as a result of a traumatic brain injury.

PATHOGENESIS

The mechanism of tissue damage following head injury is a combination of direct effects and the effects of secondary complications (Box 19.1). The direct effects are both macroscopic (compression and contusion) and microscopic (diffuse axonal injury and cavitation). Certain areas of the brain are vulnerable to traumatic damage, just as certain areas are vulnerable to vascular damage. The anterior surfaces of the frontal and temporal lobes lie close to bony skull prominences and are damaged with sudden deceleration forces (Fig. 19.1). The occipital pole is also vulnerable to impact. Rotational forces produce shearing injury in the white matter of cortical, subcortical and limbic areas. This shearing stretching strain is not as well tolerated as compressive strain.

Significant head injury may fail to produce demonstrable brain injury during life. Microscopic damage to neurones occurs in the majority of severe head

---

Box 19.1 Pathogenesis of head injury

Primary injury
Focal:
- contusion
- haematoma or haemorrhage
- skull fracture (linear or depressed)
- penetrating brain lesion (destructive and/or irritative)
- diffuse axonal injury (localized)

Diffuse:
- hypoxic–ischaemic injury
- diffuse axonal injury (non-localized)

Secondary
Oedema and raised intracranial pressure

Herniation (subfalcine, midline, tentorial, tonsilar)

Extracranial:
- infection (abscess, meningitis)
- fat embolism (from fractures)
- hypovolaemia and hypoxia

Haematoma:
- extradural (middle meningeal arteries)
- subdural (cerebral veins)
- intracerebral (cortical arteries)

---

injuries and a substantial number of mild to moderate cases. This is known as diffuse axonal injury although this is a misnomer because regional (not diffuse) brain areas are affected. Neuroimaging detects perhaps 10% of the burden of diffuse axonal injury that can be seen microscopically at postmortem. Modern techniques such as anti-β-amyloid precursor protein immunocytochemistry reveal accumulation of β-amyloid precursor protein, a subtle marker of reversible neurone injury that represents derangement of fast axonal transport before wallerian axonal degeneration. Diffuse axonal injury results from rapid acceleration or deceleration of the brain and is associated with biologically severe injuries, loss of consciousness and possibly amnesia.

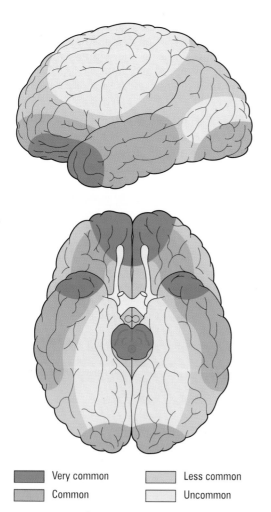

| | Very common | | Less common |
| | Common | | Uncommon |

Fig. 19.1 Sites of contusions. From Stevens & Lowe (2000).

CLASSIFICATION OF HEAD INJURY IN RELATION TO OUTCOME

There is considerable debate about how best to describe head injuries, and in particular what is meant by the concept of 'mild traumatic brain injury.' The aim of classification is to categorize the injury in a way that is most helpful for intervention and prognosis.

When an object penetrates the skull and enters the brain there is little debate that neurological complications will ensue, and therefore the term 'severe traumatic brain injury' is appropriate. In the absence of such prima facia evidence, other methods of separating injury types are required. Neuroimaging techniques (skull X-ray, head CT or MRI) have high sensitivity for demonstrating contusions or haemorrhages that follow moderate or severe open and closed head injuries. However, if used unselectively, CT and plain skull X-ray have diminishing value in milder head injuries because they cannot identify small regional non-haemorrhagic lesions caused by diffuse axonal injury (Haydel et al 2000). Even MRI cannot detect the smallest lesions. For this reason, clinical indicators are used to classify cases in which trauma to the brain cannot be visualized. The two classic methods used are the Glasgow Coma Scale and the length of coma, but both come with caveats (Asikainen et al 1998). First, if there is a delay in presentation a late assessment will be misleading. Secondly, there is a ceiling effect, making these methods relatively insensitive to subtle injuries. Thirdly, a witnessed account may be required (Table 19.1; see also Table 5.1). Fourthly, these methods are better at predicting neurological than neuropsychiatric outcomes. For these reasons, the concept of an altered mental state and, in particular, amnesia in grading mild head injuries has become important (Figs 19.5 and 19.6).

POST-TRAUMATIC AMNESIA

Amnesia caused by head injury is conventionally divided into retrograde amnesia for previously learnt material and anterograde amnesia for newly presented information. Whereas the duration of retrograde amnesia is short, the duration of anterograde amnesia is typically 10 times longer. Russell & Nathan (1946) suggested using the period of antero-

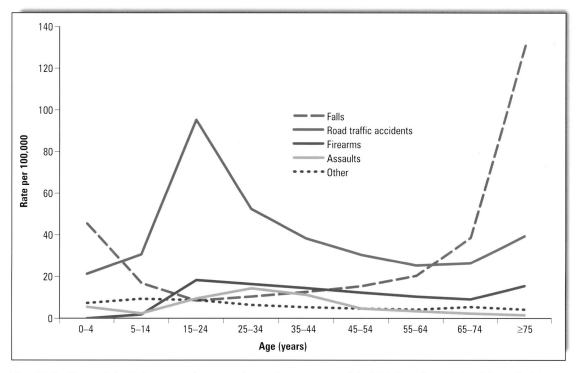

Fig. 19.2 Traumatic brain injury rates by age and cause in seven states of the USA. Data from National Center for Injury Prevention and Control (1999).

Table 19.1 Loss of consciousness on admission and most likely outcome 12 years after head injury				
Length of coma	<7 years*	8–16 years*	17–40 years*	>40 years*
Up to ½ hour	Moderate disability	Good recovery	Good recovery	Good recovery
Up to 6 hours	Moderate disability	Moderate disability	Moderate disability	Severe disability
Up to 24 hours	Moderate disability	Moderate disability	Moderate disability	Moderate disability
Up to 7 days	Severe disability	Moderate disability	Moderate disability	Severe disability
More than 7 days	Severe disability	Moderate disability	Severe disability	Severe disability

*Age at time of injury
Based on data from Asikainen et al (1998)

grade post-traumatic amnesia that follows a closed head injury as a prognostic indicator. This can be assessed retrospectively as the time period from injury to re-commencement of *continuous* episodic memory function. Patients may be tested using bed-side memory tests or measures such as the Galveston Orientation and Amnesia Test (GOAT), the Westmead Post Traumatic Amnesia Scale or the Modified Oxford Post Traumatic Amnesia Scale. All these scales assess orientation as well as memory,

consistent with the observation that disorientation and amnesia are highly correlated during recovery from closed head injury (in the presence of antero-grade amnesia a patient will have great difficulty acquiring awareness of time). The close relationship between amnesia, orientation and attention leads to the logical conclusion that post-traumatic amnesia is simply one measurable facet of post-traumatic delirium (Stuss et al 1999). Against this, there are cases in which post-traumatic confusion resolves but amnesia runs a more protracted course. The opposite pattern has been observed in severe head injuries (Tate et al 2000).

OUTCOME

Morbidity and mortality

Initial recovery from head injury tends to follow a predictable temporal course. As the initial coma recovers, there are fluctuations in orientation, disturbed sleep–wake cycle, overarousal and agitation (i.e. the syndrome of delirium). The course of delirium can be prolonged if secondary complications intervene. Information processing ability improves relatively quickly but this often leaves residual problems with sleep, irritability and memory. Depending on the type of injury, apathy and other anxiety disorders may surface. Predicting these late neuropsychiatric complications is extremely difficult (Fig. 19.10).

Predicting mortality after severe head injury is much more straightforward than predicting longer term functional outcome after mild or moderate injury (Champion et al 1989). Combining the Glasgow Coma Scale score with systolic blood pressure and respiratory rate in the *Revised Trauma Score* strongly predicts mortality (Zafonte et al 1996).

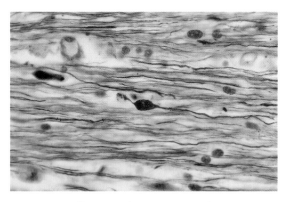

Fig. 19.3   Diffuse axonal injury. From Cooke & Stewart (1995).

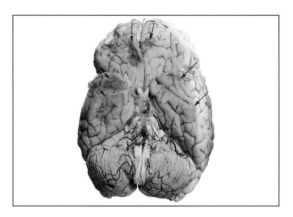

Fig. 19.4   Frontal and temporal contusions after fatal head injury (arrows). From Peter Rochford, Museum Curator, James Vincent Duhig Pathology Museum, University of Queensland.

Box 19.2   Predictors of poor functional outcome after head injury

Demographic factors
Male sex

Markers of injury severity
Glasgow Coma Scale score
Raised intracranial pressure*
Hyperglycaemia*
Length of coma
Length of post-traumatic amnesia
Length of post-traumatic disorientation
Late seizures

Neuroimaging findings
Depressed skull fracture
Haemorrhage*
Contusion
Diffuse axonal injury

Early physical function
Admission functional independence measure (FIM)
Discharge disability rating scale score

Cognitive deficits
Planning and reasoning
Verbal fluency
Verbal memory
Visuospatial ability
Attention, orientation and processing speed

Neuropsychiatric complications
Depression
Poor motivation

Vulnerability factors
Extremes of age
Poor premorbid function
Premorbid unemployment

Treatment
Inadequate medical management
Little ongoing support

*Predictors of mortality

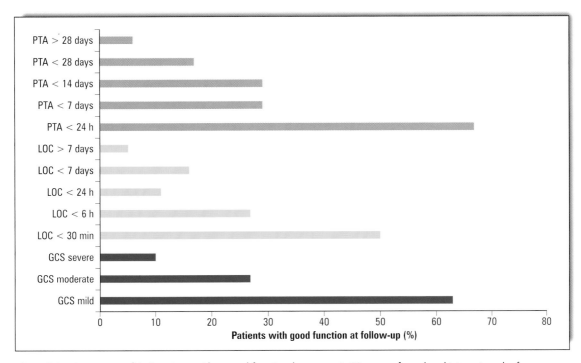

Fig. 19.5 Percentage of 342 patients with a good functional outcome 5–20 years after a head injury. Length of coma (LOC), duration of post-traumatic amnesia (PTA) and initial Glasgow Coma Scale (GCS) score were all predictive. Data from Asikainen et al (1998).

Factors influencing disability include pre-existing vulnerability factors, as well as injury-related variables and immediate complications (Box 19.2). There is good evidence that the predictors of functional recovery (exemplified by return to independent work) are different from the predictors of recovery of social function or the predictors of future independence. For example, within the cognitive domain, memory predicts occupational activity, whereas cognitive speed and judgement predict social competence (Tate & Broe 1999). A large number of studies show that post-traumatic amnesia is an accurate and stable predictor of outcome of closed head injuries that have not involved crushing trauma (see above). The main advantage of using post-traumatic amnesia is its ability to predict outcome for superficially minor injuries. Many other factors modify outcome after head injury long after amnesia and confusion have resolved. For example, patients who score poorly on the Trail Making Test B at 1 month after injury are half as likely to be productive 1 year later as those who perform well (Boake et al 2001).

Post-traumatic epilepsy

A seizure may occur immediately upon impact but this has little prognostic significance. The degree of brain damage predicts the emergence of seizures. Penetrating injuries confer a 30% chance of post-traumatic epilepsy and a 10% chance of status epilepticus. On average, early seizures (often focal motor seizures) occur in 5% of head injury victims. In a further 5%, seizures (often complex partial seizures) occur for up to 1 year. Approximately one-third of people will convert from early to late seizures. Compared with a baseline risk of 0.5% in the population, the relative risk of seizures in a 5-year period following injury is 1.5-fold after mild injury (defined as a loss of consciousness for less than 30 minutes), 3-fold after moderate injury, and nearly 20-fold after severe injury (defined as a loss of consciousness or amnesia for more than 24 hours) (Annegers et al 1998). The occurrence of post-traumatic seizures has an influence on poor outcome, particularly recovery in function. Predictors of late epilepsy include early epilepsy, haematoma,

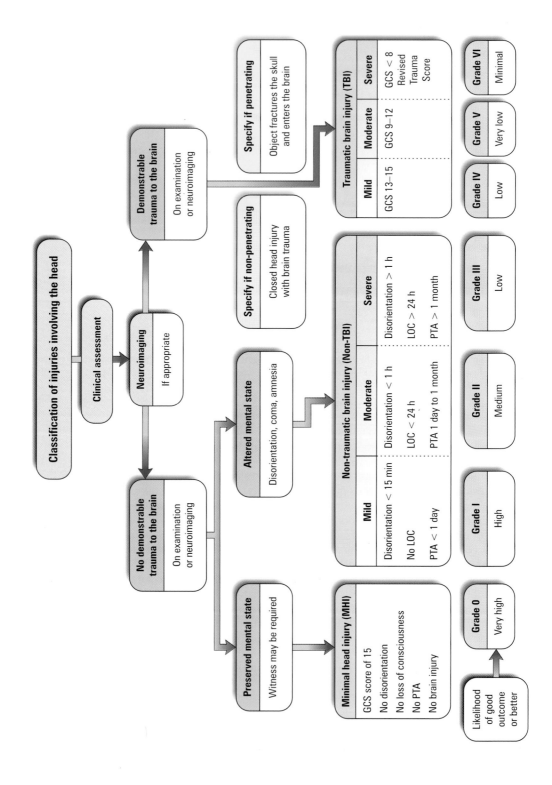

Classification of injuries involving the head

Clinical assessment

Neuroimaging
If appropriate

Demonstrable trauma to the brain
On examination or neuroimaging

No demonstrable trauma to the brain
On examination or neuroimaging

Specify if penetrating
Object fractures the skull and enters the brain

Specify if non-penetrating
Closed head injury with brain trauma

Altered mental state
Disorientation, coma, amnesia

Preserved mental state
Witness may be required

Traumatic brain injury (TBI)

Mild	Moderate	Severe
GCS 13–15	GCS 9–12	GCS < 8 Revised Trauma Score

Non-traumatic brain injury (Non-TBI)

Mild	Moderate	Severe
Disorientation < 15 min	Disorientation < 1 h	Disorientation > 1 h
No LOC	LOC < 24 h	LOC > 24 h
PTA < 1 day	PTA 1 day to 1 month	PTA > 1 month

Minimal head injury (MHI)
GCS score of 15
No disorientation
No loss of consciousness
No PTA
No brain injury

Grade VI	Grade V	Grade IV	Grade III	Grade II	Grade I	Grade 0
Minimal	Very low	Low	Low	Medium	High	Very high

Likelihood of good outcome or better

depressed skull fracture (especially if there is also anterograde amnesia or dural tear or focal signs) and penetrating injury. The merit of prophylactic anticonvulsants has been examined in several prospective series (see Ch. 49).

NEUROPSYCHIATRIC COMPLICATIONS OF HEAD INJURY

Cognitive impairment after head injury

Some form of memory disturbance usually accompanies moderate or severe head injuries. The patient is unlikely to recover memories of the accident and its immediate temporal vicinity if such memories were disrupted at the time of the injury. On the other hand, substantial cognitive deficits occur in less than 5% of head injuries. Reduced attention is common with any type of injury (involving selective, sustained and switching deficits), but is usually transient. A dysexecutive syndrome is not uncommon, and it is often associated with confabulation. Problems in new learning and short-term memory are typical. Verbal deficits are seen after dominant injuries and visuospatial deficits after non-dominant injuries. Expressive dysphasia and word-finding difficulties are also seen. Risk factors are long periods of post-traumatic amnesia, penetrating injuries, head injuries in elderly patients, and lesions to frontal or dominant temporal lobes. Atrophy of the hippocampus is correlated with memory difficulties, although the mechanism is unknown (Bigler et al 1996). In rare cases (such as KC described by Tulving et al (1988)) bilateral hippocampal damage produces a dense anterograde or episodic memory loss. Global cognitive impairment

Fig. 19.6 (opposite) Classification of head injuries. Injuries to the head are difficult to classify satisfactorily. Neuroimaging (MRI where available) is probably valuable in all cases except minimal head injury. However, no single factor perfectly predicts outcome. Predictors of mortality are not synonymous with predictors of morbidity. Head injuries involving clear trauma to the brain have high a mortality rate that can be predicted by an admission Glasgow Coma Scale score or Revised Trauma Score (see text). The residual disability after closed head injuries but may be better assessed by any of early disorientation, loss of consciousness or post-traumatic amnesia. The predictors of emotional and behavioural complications are not well studied.

after repeated head injury may occur despite the individual insults being relatively minor (see below).

Mood disorder after head injury

Depression occurs in approximately one-quarter of patients 1 month after injury, but in many cases it resolves by 6 months (Jorge et al 1993). About half this number of patients develop depression later in the course of recovery. Similar rates are seen in studies of paediatric head injury. One good-quality study examined the lifetime rate of depression in World War II veterans who suffered closed head injury. Veterans had a 50% increased lifetime risk of depression (i.e. 18.5%) (Holsinger et al 2002).

It is sometimes forgotten that mood disorder in the context of spinal cord injury is also associated with both acute-onset and delayed-onset depression. Depression is often overlooked in clinical practice, but it is vital because it will dominate progress in rehabilitation. Fundamental psychological symptoms of depression are no different in head injury from those in primary depression, although the focus is typically on what the patient has lost, what they are not able to do and why from the patient's perspective things will never be the same again. Multiple somatic symptoms can be used as a marker of severity in depression, although it has been reported that certain symptoms, such as loss of libido, poor concentration and sleep disturbance, commonly result from head injury itself, and therefore in isolation are not discriminating. Federoff et al (1992) compared depressed and non-depressed patients with acute closed head injury ($n = 66$). Patients who were depressed showed more functional impairment and more alcohol and illicit drug abuse, but no greater cognitive impairment than their non-depressed counterparts. In contrast, other studies have linked depression with neuropsychological impairment after head injury. Depression has many complications, including aggravated disability, aggression and suicide. Suicide accounts for 10% of head injury deaths.

Mania is a recognized but relatively unusual complication of head injury that tends to occur early and may or may not predispose to bipolar disorder. In post-head-injury mania, patients tend to be more irritable and aggressive than their primary mania counterparts. Hypomania is probably more common in the later phases, often in combination with depression (bipolar affective disorder, type II). Patients with head injury appear to be at particular risk of rapid cycling (i.e. four or more episodes per year).

Pure irritability and comorbid irritability and anger are extremely important neuropsychiatric complications of head injury. Men are both more prone to anger and more likely to suffer head injury. There is often deep resentment at the injury, frustration at slow progress and sometimes there is self-blame, particularly if alcohol was involved. The anger is often irrational and commonly sparked by arguments in the family home. One recent study found that almost 20% suffered acute-onset irritability and 15% suffered delayed-onset irritability after closed head injury, although relatives rated temper problems in over half of head injury patients (Kim et al 1999). Acute-onset irritability is associated with a higher frequency of left cortical lesions, and delayed onset irritability is linked with poor function. Anger outbursts can be broadly subdivided into those generated by frustration or abnormal mood and those generated by disinhibition. Each requires a specific form of management.

Emotionalism has been reported by McGrath (2000) in up to 40% of patients with severe head injury, although only half of these patients reported crying spells as distressing. In this study of 82 patients, the independent variables that predicted crying behaviour were female sex and focal damage to the right cerebral hemisphere.

Apathy is one of the most serious and yet most common neuropsychiatric complications of head injury. After studying 83 outpatients with closed head injury, Kant et al (1998) concluded that apathy occurred in some form in an astonishing 71% of patients. In the majority of cases (60% of the 71%) apathy co-existed with depression. This finding has been replicated and refined, and it now appears to be the behavioural and emotional aspects of apathy that overlap with depression more than the cognitive aspects of apathy (Andersson & Bergedalen 2002). Furthermore, the cognitive components of apathy are often closely affiliated with deficits in memory, executive function and processing speed after severe head injury. Apathy is a very destructive

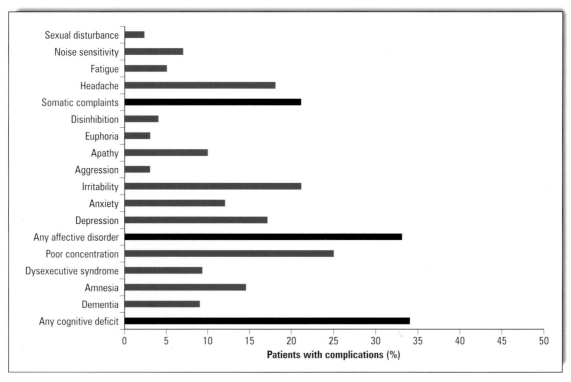

Fig. 19.7 Neuropsychiatric complications 1–5 years after penetrating head injury. Data from Lishman (1968).

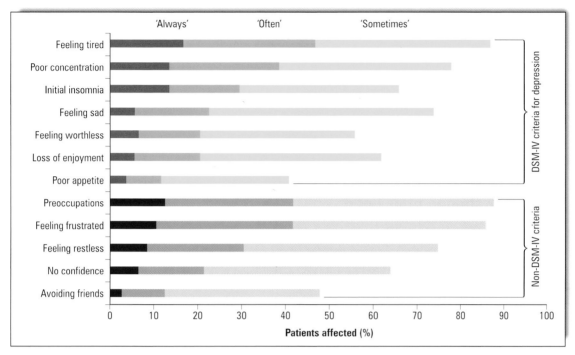

Fig. 19.8 Depressive symptoms in head injury. This study gives a very clear illustration of the difference between depressive symptoms and a depression syndrome following a brain insult. Using a low threshold for eliciting troublesome symptoms it can be seen that at least 70% of people endorse several problem areas. The stricter threshold required by DSM-IV for major depression reduces the rate to about 20%. Not all complaints associated with depression are captured in the DSM-IV criteria. Data from Kreutzer et al (2001).

complication because it leads to social isolation, dysphoria, low self-esteem, loss of support, poor compliance and a reduced quality of life.

Anxiety disorders are less common, and consequently are frequently overlooked. Panic disorder has been reported in 10% of patients in the first year after head injury. Post-traumatic stress disorder (PTSD) occurs in about 10–20% of severe head injuries, but PTSD is actually less likely if there is dense amnesia for the trauma. Up to half of those with PTSD may also suffer from depression and other anxiety disorders. As with depression, PTSD interferes with function and rehabilitation progress. Risk factors for onset and outcome of PTSD have been studies (Freedman et al 1999). Adequacy of social support and comorbid depression are the most important prognostic factors found to date. Obsessive–compulsive disorder (OCD) is sometimes classified as a form of anxiety disorder, and is a recognized but relatively rare consequence of head injury. OCD may occur after mild injury, but is more likely after significant brain injury with involvement of the frontal cortices or subcortical structures such as the caudate nucleus.

Psychotic disorder after head injury

Psychosis occurring after head injury is not common but it should not be overlooked for several reasons. Psychosis early after a substantial impact is most probably a symptom of delirium and hence a predictor of poor outcome if untreated. Early psychosis is also associated with agitation, which is disruptive for all concerned. The phenomenology includes suspiciousness, persecutory delusions and illusions or visual hallucinations. Unsurprisingly, memory problems are a prominent associated feature. Persistent psychotic symptoms without disorientation are rare. Isolated hallucinations, particularly olfactory and haptic (sensory) hallucinations, can be a reflection of undiagnosed post-traumatic epilepsy. The misidentification syndrome *reduplicative paramnesia*, in which the patient believes something has been duplicated and exists as a double, has been linked with early head injury and also with epilepsy. Schizophrenia-like psychosis developing late after head injury appears to be two to three times more common than in the general population. Risk factors for psychosis after head injury are not well known, but may include previous neurological disorder in childhood, previous psychiatric disorder and seizures. Several case series implicate the left temporal lobe as central to the development of psychosis after head injury in the absence of clouding of consciousness.

Personality change after head injury

Personality change after head injury is a major concern for relatives. Studies have shown that the majority of patients who suffer severe brain injury experience significant difficulty regaining complex social and behavioural skills. Approximately 30% of patients reach criteria for personality change (avoidant, impulsive and paranoid being most common). A further 20% develop maladaptive personal-

ity traits short of major distress or dysfunction. Personality change is often linked with cognitive impairment.

Changes are varied, but what relatives usually describe is that 'the patient is not the same person as before'. This encompasses irritability or aggression; labile, depressed or anxious moods; withdrawal and poor motivation; reduced insight and judgement; and, less commonly, obsessional or antisocial traits. In some patients, but by no means all, there is an anatomical basis for the change in personality. When assessing a patient with disinhibition and poor judgement, ask: 'is there an orbitofrontal lesion?' When assessing a patient with a syndrome of poor motivation ask: 'has a mesial frontal (anterior cingulate) injury occurred or perhaps a lesion to the hypothalamus, medial subthalamic nuclei or basal ganglia?' Unfortunately for sufferers and their families, changes in personality and social functioning are among the most persistent complications of head injury, although they may show slow improvements up to 2 years after the injury (Hoofien et al 2001).

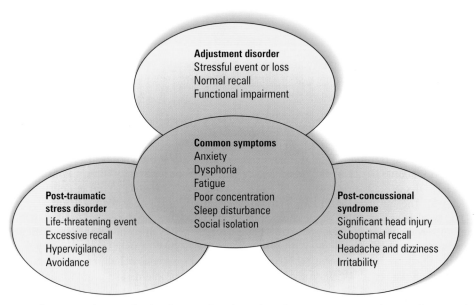

Fig. 19.9 Overlapping syndromes after head injury. The relationship of post-concussion syndrome, adjustment disorder and post-traumatic stress disorder after head injury is more complex than it first appears. Many symptoms are shared between these overlapping presentations. Although the majority of people suffer unpleasant symptoms early after head injury, a minority continue to experience such symptoms to a disabling degree. The specificity of individual symptoms (as suggested by various diagnostic schedules) has not yet been properly tested. However, Trahan et al (2001) in Texas found that depression was an important confounder in this already complex relationship.

Clinical Pointer 19.1

Minimal brain dysfunction in children and minimal brain injury in adults

Adults who experience a mild head injury with a short period of loss of consciousness and no immediate CT or skull X-ray evidence of damage are often labelled as having mild or minimal brain injury. It is now recognized that apparently minor head injuries (including those with no loss of consciousness) can still result in cognitive complaints and adjustment disorder or a post-concussion syndrome. Thus, defining severity of head injury using loss of consciousness or the Glasgow Coma Scale is more successful after moderate or severe injuries than minimal or mild injuries. One reason for this difficulty in classification is that patients may not accurately recall the severity of the impact or the duration of unconsciousness. Attempts to find better predictors of prognosis after mild head injury have not been particularly successful. For example, although there are changes on MRI or SPECT demonstrable after mild head injuries, there appears to be little correlation with neuropsychiatric sequelae. Until such clinical or radiological markers are available, it is reasonable to classify closed head injuries without disorientation or loss of consciousness as minimal brain injury, yet to monitor for possible neuropsychiatric complications (in primary care) if the impact to the head was substantial.

This should not be confused with the syndrome of minimal brain dysfunction, in which perinatal trauma causes neurological soft signs but no localizing signs. Epidemiologically, a history of this kind of damage is found more often than expected in children with learning disability, cerebral palsy, attention deficit hyperactivity disorder, conduct disorder and possibly autism. Of course, such brain injuries are at one end of a spectrum. Clear perinatal brain injuries (50% of which are due to hypoxic–ischaemic encephalopathy or prematurity) with radiological evidence of focal lesions, hydrocephaly, intraventricular haemorrhage or white matter lesions cause (in approximate decreasing order of frequency) cerebral palsy, epilepsy, learning disability, strabism, microcephaly, visual impairment, and hyperkinesis or attention deficit hyperactivity disorder. Understandably, the term minimal brain dysfunction has fallen from use as the consequences of such early insults are often far from minimal.

Further reading   *Hofman PAM, Stapert SZ, van Kroonenburgh MJPG et al 2001 MR imaging, single-photon emission CT, and neurocognitive performance after mild traumatic brain injury. American Journal of Neuroradiology 22:441–449*
Garaizar C, Prats-Vinas JM 1998 Perinatal and late intrauterine brain lesions at the neuropediatric clinic. Revista de Neurologia 26:934–950
Rantakallio P, Vonwendt L, Koivu M 1987 Prognosis of perinatal brain damage: a prospective study of a one year birth cohort of 12000 children. Early Human Development 15:75–84

OTHER HEAD-INJURY-RELATED CONDITIONS

Persistent vegetative state

Originally described in 1972, the persistent vegetative state is a chronic condition in which a person is awake (or, more correctly, has a preserved sleep–wake cycle) but not consciously aware (Jennett & Plum 1972). The cause is usually severe head injury or severe hypoxia. In contrast to brain death, the diagnosis can be difficult, because consciousness is not easily measured. There are important legal and ethical questions; not least, is it ethically correct to withdraw treatment? In every case in which the High Court has been consulted, it was decided that there was no benefit from continued treatment and hence permission (but not a directive) to stop treatment was given.

A study of 650 severe closed head injury patients in the USA found that 14% were discharged in a persistent vegetative state. Of 84 vegetative patients, 40% regained consciousness by 6 months post-trauma, with an additional 11% regaining consciousness by 1 year, and another 6% regaining consciousness by 3 years. The chances of recovery are better after traumatic rather than non-traumatic causes. Thus, if a patient does not regain consciousness by 1 year, the prognosis is poor but not hopeless. Where the chances of recovery are small, the term 'permanent vegetative state' is sometimes preferred.

Dementia pugilistica

Dementia pugilistica or 'boxing encephalopathy' results from repeated non-penetrating trauma to the head. It occurs in mild forms in about 20% of boxers. Symptoms are those of cognitive impairment, overvalued ideas, morbid jealousy and coarsening of personality. Signs include ataxia, dysarthria, pyramidal and extrapyramidal features. The pathology is characterized by cerebral atrophy, ventricular enlargement, lesions to the septum pellucidum and neurofibrillary tangles (not senile plaques or Lewy bodies). There is neuronal loss to the hippocampal gyrus, substantia nigra and amygdala. The syndrome is considered irreversible.

Post-concussion syndrome

This is a cluster of psychological and somatic symptoms that occurs after mild, moderate and severe head injury, beginning in the first few days or weeks. The exact boundaries of the post-concussion syndrome have not been delineated. The syndrome appears to overlap with post-traumatic stress disorder and post-traumatic mood or adjustment disorder (Fig. 19.9) (King et al 1999).

The proportion of patients who experience several characteristic symptoms is estimated at between 25% and 50% at 3 months (but definitions, and hence estimates vary). The symptoms usually resolve spontaneously, but in an important subgroup of 10–20% of patients the symptoms are persistent for months or years. Risk factors for the post-concussion syndrome have been described in detail by Lishman (1988) (Box 19.3). In many ways the features are similar to those of an adjustment disorder, and indeed there are usually fears about loss of independence and role. Symptoms can be quite disabling, with many patients feeling unable able to work or socialize normally. All the symptoms of adjustment disorder occur, although it is noteworthy that headache, fatigue, dizziness and insomnia are more common after head injury than in simple adjustment disorder, being present in over half of patients. Psychological complaints are sensitivity to noise, irritability, mood swings, depression and anxiety.

Only 3% have focal neurological findings on physical examination. Patients also complain of mild cognitive changes (including reduced concentration

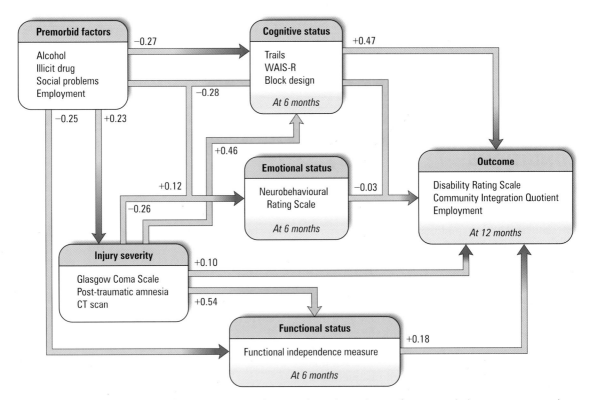

Fig. 19.10 Contributions to head injury outcome. Pathway analysis of contributions from premorbid, injury severity, and recovery variables in 107 patients who had severe head injury up to 1 year previously. A composite outcome measure was most strongly related to cognitive function, premorbid factors and injury severity. Surprisingly, functional status and emotional stability at 6 months did not significantly determine outcome, although the authors noted that emotional problems in their sample were effectively treated. Adapted from Novak et al (2001).

Clinical Pointer 19.2

The effect of head injury on family and carers

An understanding gained from the study of the effect of head injury on carers can be applied to many neuropsychiatric conditions. Two-thirds of marriages in which one partner has sustained a head injury end in divorce within 2 years of the injury. The burden on family members can be separated into general effects of living with an acquired debilitating disorder and the specific effects of head injury. People who acquire a severe disability in mid-life often cope less well than those who acquire comparable disabilities in childhood. Patients with an acute severe illness adopt a sick role in which they are reliant upon carers, asking, for example, 'Can you do this for me today?' Patients with chronic illness must make the transition towards asking 'what can I do for myself' and focusing on what they can do rather than what they cannot. Carers are often angry and resentful towards their loved one for failing to improve rapidly; anger and resentment may also be felt towards medical staff. This resentment is difficult to express to someone who continues to be unwell. Carers may also neglect to look after their own physical and mental health, and perhaps adopt a parenting role with their loved one.

Patients with head injury are typically frustrated as they attempt to regain former skills. This is often expressed as irritability directed towards carers. They may also have deficits in communication skills that cause friction between themselves and carers. Change in personality is a major complaint of carers. However, that is a simple description of a complex problem. Enduring differences in empathy, judgement and warmth are huge problems in spousal relationships. Inappropriateness, depression and indifference are more closely related to family functioning and carer stress level than injury severity (Groom et al 1998).

Further reading Perlesz A, Kinsella G, Crowe S 1999 Impact of traumatic brain injury on the family: a critical review. Rehabilitation Psychology 44:6–35
Groom KN, Shaw TG, O'Connor ME et al 1998 Neurobehavioral symptoms and family functioning in traumatically brain-injured adults. Archives of Clinical Neuropsychology 13:695–711

and attention, and recent memory complaints), and there has been some work investigating whether these cognitive findings might predict the development of the full syndrome. Structural investigations are usually fruitless, with changes on CT seen in only 5% and changes on MRI in 10% following mild closed head injury. However, this does not rule out a subtle contribution of neuronal damage to the syndrome. Indeed, some authors believe that delayed brainstem evoked potentials or SPECT abnormalities can be found in up to half of sufferers with per-sistent symptoms (Kant et al 1997). One line of research worth examining in more detail is the contribution of post-traumatic damage to the vestibulo-cochlear system and central control mechanisms. Disorders of balance increase with increasing severity of head injury, but are difficult to predict accurately (Greenwald et al 2001). Patients are often described as suffering from simple dizziness when they actually have post-traumatic vestibular disease (Mallinson & Longridge 1998). In a provocative report, Guerts et al (1999) demonstrated increased postural instability in those with the post-concussional syndrome, hinting that a combination of neurological and psychological factors underpin this poorly understood condition.

Box 19.3 Suggested risk factors for the post-concussion syndrome

Pre-traumatic
Age
Psychiatric history
Personality factors
Alcohol

Traumatic
Markers of tissue damage
Circumstances of injury

Post-traumatic
Residual impairments
Post-traumatic epilepsy
Compensation factors

SUMMARY

Head injury is one of the most common causes of neuropsychiatric disorder in young people. Each year about half a million people in the UK and 2 million people in the USA suffer a head injury of suffi-cient severity to require hospital attention. Twenty per cent of these require admission and 1% require a neurosurgical opinion. Eighty per cent of cases are mild, 10% are moderate and 10% are severe, based on an initial Glasgow Coma Score. Patients without coma or demonstrable brain injury are still at risk of significant neuropsychiatric sequelae. Assessment using the duration of post-traumatic amnesia (with or without disorientation) along with simple cognitive tests help predict outcome.

Unfortunately, alcohol has a lot to answer for, since it is both the cause of many head injuries and a negative influence on recovery. Although amnesia is widely discussed in the context of head injury, problems with irritability, attention, low mood, adjustment disorder (post-concussion syndrome), post-traumatic stress disorder and the frontal lobe syndromes are also very problematic and often lead to what is crudely described as personality change. Predictors of neurological recovery are not the same as the predictors of functional outcome or predictors of psychological adjustment. Appropriate support and rehabilitation are essential to recovery. It is to be hoped that developments in head injury research will include improved detection and treatment of irritability, apathy and cognitive impairment.

REFERENCES AND FURTHER READING

Andersson S, Bergedalen AM 2002 Cognitive correlates of apathy in traumatic brain injury. Neuropsychiatry, Neuropsychology and Behavioral Neurology 15:184–191

Annegers JF, Hauser WA, Coan SP et al 1998 A population-based study of seizures after traumatic brain injuries. New England Journal of Medicine 338:20–24

Asikainen I, Kaste M, Sarna S 1998 Predicting late outcome for patients with traumatic brain injury referred to a rehabilitation programme: a study of 508 Finnish patients 5 years or more after injury. Brain Injury 12:95–107

Bigler ED, Johnson SC, Anderson CV et al 1996 Traumatic brain injury and memory: the role of hippocampal atrophy. Neuropsychology 10:333–342

Boake C, Millis SR, High WM et al 2001 Using early neuropsychological testing to predict long-term productivity outcome from traumatic brain injury. Archives of Physical and Medical Rehabilitation 82:761–768

Bogner JA, Corrigan JD, Mysiw J et al 1991 A comparison of substance abuse and violence in the prediction of long-term rehabilitation outcomes after traumatic brain injury. Archives of Physical and Medical Rehabilitation 82:571–577

Champion HR, Sacco WJ, Copes WS et al 1989 A revision of the trauma score. Journal of Trauma 29:623–629

Cooke RA, Stewart B 1995 Color atlas of anatomical pathology, 2nd edn. Churchill Livingstone, Edinburgh

Crepeau F, Scherzer P 1993 Predictors and indicators of work status after traumatic brain injury: a meta-analysis. Neuropsychological Rehabilitation 3:5–35

Federoff JP, Starkstein SE, Forrester AW et al 1992 Depression in patients with acute traumatic brain injury. American Journal of Psychiatry 149:918–923

Freedman SA, Brandes D, Peri T et al 1999 Predictors of chronic post-traumatic stress disorder. A prospective study. British Journal of Psychiatry 174:353–359

Gama JHP 1835 Traite des plaies de tete et de l'encephalite. In: Strich SJ (ed) Shearing of nerve fibres as a cause of brain damage due to head injury: a pathological study of twenty cases. Lancet 2:443–448

Geurts ACH, Knoop JA, van Limbeek J 1999 Is postural control associated with mental functioning in the persistent postconcussion syndrome? Archives of Physical and Medical Rehabilitation 80:144–149

Greenwald BD, Cifu DX, Marwitz JH et al 2001 Factors associated with balance deficits on admission to rehabilitation after traumatic brain injury: a multicenter analysis. Journal of Head Trauma Rehabilitation 16:238–252

Haydel MJ, Preston CA, Mills TJ et al 2000 Indications for computed tomography in patients with minor head injury. New England Journal of Medicine 343:100–105

Holsinger T, Steffens DC, Phillips C et al 2002 Head injury in early adulthood and the lifetime risk of depression. Archives of General Psychiatry 59:17–22

Hoofien D, Gilboa A, Vakil E et al 2001 Traumatic brain injury (TBI) 10–20 years later: a comprehensive outcome study of psychiatric symptomatology, cognitive abilities and psychosocial functioning. Brain Injury 15:189–209

Jennett B, Plum F 1972 Persistent vegetative state after brain damage. A syndrome in search of a name. Lancet i:734–737

Jorge RE, Robinson RG, Arndt SV et al 1993 Depression following traumatic brain injury: a 1 year longitudinal study. Journal of Affective Disorders 27:233–243

Kant R, SmithSeemiller L, Isaac G et al 1997 Tc-HMPAO SPECT in persistent postconcussion syndrome after mild head injury: comparison with MRI/CT. Brain Injury 11:115–124

Kant R, Duffy JD, Pivovarnik A 1998 Prevalence of apathy following head injury. Brain Injury 12:87–92

Kim SH, Manes F, Kosier T et al 1999 Irritability following traumatic brain injury. Journal of Nervous and Mental Disorders 187:327–335

King NS, Crawford S, Wenden FJ et al 1999 Early prediction of persisting post-concussion symptoms following mild and moderate head injuries. British Journal of Clinical Psychology 38:15–25

Kreutzer JS, Seel RT, Gourley E 2001 The prevalence and symptom rates of depression after traumatic brain injury: a comprehensive examination. Brain Injury 15:563–576

Lishman WA 1968 Brain damage in relation to psychiatric disability after head injury. British Journal of Psychiatry 114:373–410

Lishman WA 1988 Physiogenesis and psychogenesis in the post-concussional syndrome. British Journal of Psychiatry 153:460–469

Maes M, Delmeire L, Mylle J et al 2001 Risk and preventive factors of post-traumatic stress disorder (PTSD): alcohol consumption and intoxication prior to a traumatic event diminishes the relative risk to develop PTSD in response to that trauma. Journal of Affective Disorders 63:113–121

Mallinson AI, Longridge NS 1998 Specific vocalized complaints in whiplash and minor head injury patients. American Journal of Otology 19:809–813

McGrath J 2000 A study of emotionalism in patients undergoing rehabilitation following severe acquired brain injury. Behavioural Neurology 12:201–207

National Center for Injury Prevention and Control 1999 Traumatic brain injury in the United States. A report to Congress. Centers for Disease Prevention, Atlanta, GA

Novak TA, Bush BA, Meythaler JM et al 2001 Outcome after traumatic brain injury: pathway analysis of contributions from premorbid, injury severity and recovery variables. Archives of Physical Medicine and Rehabilitation 82:300–305

Pelegrin-Valero C, Fernandez-Guinea S, Tirapu-Ustarroz J et al 2001 Differential diagnosis of postconcussional syndrome. Revista de Neurologia 32:867–884

Report of the Quality Standards Subcommittee, American Academy of Neurology 1997 Practice parameter: the management of concussion in sports. Neurology 48:581–585

Russell WR, Nathan PW 1946 Traumatic amnesia. Brain 69:280–300

Silver JM, Kramer R, Greenwald S et al 2001 The association between head injuries and psychiatric disorders: findings from the New Haven NIMH Epidemiological Catchment Area Study. Brain Injury 15:935–945

Stevens A, Lowe J 2000 Pathology. Mosby, St. Louis

Stuss DT, Binns MA, Carruth FG et al 1999 The acute period of recovery from traumatic brain injury: posttraumatic amnesia or posttraumatic confusional state? Journal of Neurosurgery 90:635–643

Tate RL, Broe GA 1999 Psychosocial adjustment after traumatic brain injury: what are the important variables? Psychology and Medicine 29:713–725

Tate RL, Pfaff A, Jurjevic L 2000 Resolution of disorientation and amnesia during post-traumatic amnesia. Journal of Neurological and Neurosurgical Psychiatry 68:178–185

Trahan DE, Ross CE, Trahan SL 2001 Relationships among postconcussional-type symptoms, depression, and anxiety in neurologically normal young adults and victims of mild brain injury. Archives of Clinical Neuropsychology 16:435–445

Tulving E, Schacter DL, McLachlan DR et al 1988 Priming of semantic autobiographical knowledge: a case study of retrograde amnesia. Brain and Cognition 8:3–20

Voe PE, Battistin L, Birbamer G et al 2002 EFNS guideline on mild traumatic brain injury: report of an EFNS task force. European Journal of Neurology 9:207–219

Zafonte RD, Hammond FM, Mann NR et al 1996 Revised trauma score: an additive predictor of disability following traumatic brain injury? American Journal of Physical and Medical Rehabilitation 75:456–460

20

Multiple Sclerosis

The trembling ... does not show itself except on the occasion of intentional movements ... Nystagmus is a symptom of great diagnostic importance ... There are cases in which the nystagmus is wanting so long as the look remains vague, without precise direction; but manifests itself suddenly, in a manner more or less marked so soon as the patients are requested to fix their attention on an object. A symptom more frequent still than nystagmus ... is a peculiar difficulty in articulation ... The speech is slow, drawling, and now and again almost unintelligible.
(Jean Martin Charcot 1880)

BACKGROUND

Multiple sclerosis (MS) is hugely important because it is the most common cause of chronic neurological disability in young adults, estimated to affect over 1 million people worldwide and 80,000 in the UK. Within 15 years of diagnosis 50% of patients will be unable to work or walk independently. Integrity of the lipid sheath that covers many neurones is vital for higher brain function. MS destroys this myelin coat. MS is the perfect example of a neurological disease that causes psychiatric symptoms, something that was recognized from the earliest descriptions. The French neurologist Charcot listed three prominent psychological symptoms: mental depression, stupid indifference and foolish laughter. MS afflicts sufferers in early to midlife at a mean age of 30 years with frightening symptoms that include problems with coordination, balance, walking, motor and sensory disturbance, optic neuritis and sexual and bladder dysfunction. Lhermitte's symptom (an electric-shock-like sensation when flexing the neck) and

Uhtoff's symptom (heat-induced disability) are often cited as relatively specific features of MS. Plaques of demyelination cause symptoms disseminated in time and space. Sites most commonly affected include the optic nerves, brainstem, cerebellum and spinal cord. Patients usually recover from these attacks, only to suffer a subsequent relapsing and remitting course. After some years, the residual disability tends to accumulate and the exacerbations become less pronounced. This is the secondary progressive phase of MS.

The 1983 criteria for MS have recently been updated and simplified (McDonald et al 2001). A single episode, even when supported by MRI-proven white matter lesions (hyperintensities on T2-weighted scans), is insufficient for a diagnosis, although over 80% of patients presenting in this way will develop MS within 10 years. Diagnosis of 'clinically definite MS' requires a clinical relapse (i.e. a second attack) along with specific MRI data, or two relapses and no MRI data. CSF oligoclonal bands, visual evoked potentials and spinal cord MRI are useful if an MRI scan of the brain shows no identifying features and also in patients with progressive MS.

Progressive MS is characterized pathologically by tissue destruction (axonal loss), and this is revealed on MRI as hypodense lesions on T1-weighted scans and, when severe, by gross atrophy. There is much interest in the ability of MRI to highlight preclinical lesions and to help predict the disease course. Neuroimaging developments, such as enhancement with the heavy metal gadolinium, do help detect early lesions (or, more accurately, associated disturbance of the blood–brain barrier), but these findings are not as strongly predictive of future decline as white matter lesions in patients with characteristic initial symptoms.

Table 20.1 Laboratory findings in multiple sclerosis

	Approximate frequency (%)
CSF	
Oligoclonal bands	90
High immunoglobulin levels	80
High lymphocyte levels	33
Evoked potentials	
Visual	90
Sensory	80
Brainstem	33
Neuroimaging	
High signal	90
CT changes	33

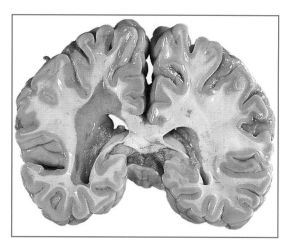

Fig. 20.1 Multiple sclerosis: a large plaque is seen adjacent to the lateral ventricle. From Stevens & Lowe (2000).

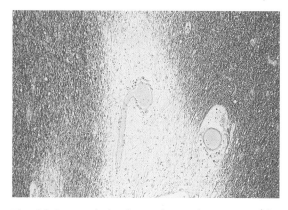

Fig. 20.2 A multiple sclerosis chronic plaque consists of a sharply defined area of myelin loss (which appears pale in this preparation) containing fibrillary astrocytes. From Underwood (2000).

NEUROPSYCHIATRIC COMPLICATIONS OF MULTIPLE SCLEROSIS

Psychiatric symptoms are varied. They include cognitive impairment, mood disorder (depression, emotionalism and euphoria) and psychosis. Treatment with steroids can easily cause or exacerbate psychiatric complaints. In contrast with several other neurological conditions, it is unusual for patients to present with psychiatric complications, although these often develop later (Skegg et al 1988). Stress is sometimes mentioned as a cause of both physical and mental symptoms of MS. This is almost certainly true, but it is also true of many conditions (see Clinical Pointer 81.1).

Mood disorder in multiple sclerosis

Depressive disorder

Over the course of the illness, depression appears to occur more commonly than in most other medical illnesses, with a prevalence of around 50%. Even in community samples, on cross-sectional assessment about 40% of people with MS have significant depressive symptoms and 20% are depressed, by DSM-IV criteria (Chwastiak et al 2002). Hypomania, mania and mixed affective states occur in about 10% of patients, a rate which is at least two-fold higher than in healthy individuals. Symptoms of euphoria and disinhibition are much more common than the syndromes of mania or hypomania, but these concepts are often confused. Emotional lability or pseudobulbar affect is well recognized (and was described in Charcot's original reports). Studies in selected groups of patients suggest that depression in MS is more common than depression in rheumatoid arthritis, motor neurone disease, muscular dystrophy and spinal cord injury. It has been found that patients with both predominantly spinal cord injury and predominantly brain injury suffer depression frequently, but in the latter the depression is usually more severe.

Certain depressive symptoms are probably more common in the context of MS. For example, many patients have difficulty coming to terms with their illness (possible adjustment disorder) and display significant anger and worry about the future. Core symptoms of cognitive impairment and fatigue occur more commonly than in primary depression. Fatigue in MS is contributed to by the direct effects of MS itself and by depression in approximately equal measure (Randolph et al 2000). Fatigue can be an episodic or persistent complaint in about one-third of MS patients. Most evidence also suggests that the fatigue is central rather than peripheral in origin (Comi et al 2001). However, it is less severe and has a different mechanism than the fatigue reported by patients with chronic fatigue syndrome (Taillefer et al 2002).

Mechanism of depression in MS

In a cross-sectional study of 76 outpatients with MS, Voss et al (2002) examined disability, fatigue and psychosocial factors in relation to self-reported depressive symptoms. Physical disability and fatigue were indirectly associated with depression via their effects on recreational functioning. Disability also influenced work and social function, but these functions were not linked with depressed mood. Fatigue was also an independent risk factor for depression over and above the effect on handicap.

Correlates of depression in MS have also been examined using MRI. Several authors have reported that the association between depression and severity of physical symptoms is very weak. Similarly, the association of lesion load on MRI and depression is not a robust one, and is certainly a lot weaker than the association of lesion load and cognitive impairment. Clinical experience and the results of one study suggest that there is a stronger association between lesion load and high mood than there is between lesion load and low mood (Diaz-Olavarrieta et al 1999). There is an overlap between impaired cognition and depression in MS (particularly in patients with maladaptive coping strategies), although this has been infrequently studied. Several authors have asked whether any specific regions of the brain are liable to cause depression when affected by MS. The jury is still out on this and we await larger studies but, provisionally, dominant hemisphere involvement, particularly in the temporal lobe may have particular importance (Berg et al 2000).

Apathy

Apathy has not been well studied in MS, despite being a major problem. Apathy is less common than depression or anxiety, but is probably more common than euphoria or disinhibition (see Fig. 20.3). It is likely that apathy in MS has a contribution from both biological factors and psychological factors, but more work needs to be done.

Anxiety disorders

Anxiety symptoms in MS are under-researched, despite their impact on quality of life (Stenager et al 1994). Anxiety shows an intercorrelation with depression and cognition in MS patients. Approximately the same percentage of sufferers have significant anxiety as depression, as determined by cross-sectional assessment (Hakim et al 2000). Two recent studies have assessed the clinicoanatomical basis of anxiety in MS using MRI, but no association was found(Diaz-Olavarrieta et al 1999, Zorzon et al 2001).

Suicide

Suicide rates in MS have now been observed in relatively large samples so that meaningful conclusions can be drawn. In a Danish cohort of 5525 patients, the completed suicide rate was twice the mean rate of the adjusted population and was higher in those with an onset of MS before 40 years of age (Stenager et al 1992). A Canadian study followed 3126 patients for up to 16 years and found a suicide rate of 7.5 times the age-adjusted population rate, although adjustments were not made for sex distribution, and therefore this figure may be an overestimate (Sadovnik et al 1991).

Psychosis in multiple sclerosis

Psychosis is most often seen in MS in response to prolonged steroid treatment and as an affective psychosis. However, a schizophrenia-like psychosis can occur, particularly when there is extensive temporal lobe involvement. Ron & Logsdail (1989) examined 116 patients with and without psychosis and found a relationship between delusions or thought disorder and demyelination in temporal–parietal regions. This should not be thought of as an exclusive relationship, since lesions in the frontal lobes, basal ganglia and limbic areas have also been linked with psychosis in MS. There are probably several different types of psychosis in MS (compare with psychosis in Parkinson's disease; see Ch. 21). In patients with severe cognitive impairment, delirium and dementia are major risk factors for psychosis. In young people a schizophreniform psychosis may

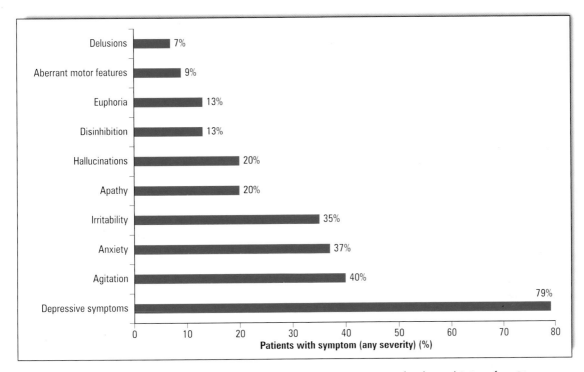

Fig. 20.3 Neuropsychiatric features of multiple sclerosis (cognition was not measured in this study). Data from Diaz-Olavarrieta et al (1999).

occur, with preserved cognition and insight. In these cases, patients may be perplexed at sudden odd hallucinations and beliefs that may have an unreal quality.

Cognitive impairment in multiple sclerosis

Cognitive impairment is increasingly recognized as affecting up to half of all MS sufferers, and it can dramatically worsen quality of life. Deficits appear early in the course of disease, and indeed are often present before the full diagnosis is made, when only symptoms of optic neuritis have presented. Fortunately, in most cases progression of these deficits is slow, probably paralleling the extent of irreversible brain lesions. An Italian 10-year follow-up study of 45 patients with MS revealed that the percentage of patients unimpaired early in the course of disease (mean duration 2 years) was 74%, but this had fallen to 44% by 10 years (Fig. 20.4) (Amato et al 2001). In this study, more aggressive disease, increasing age and increasing degree of physical disability predicted cognitive decline.

The classical neuropsychological picture is widely stated as subcortical, with white matter demyelination causing a slowing of information processing and attention performance (independently of motor speed) and leaving the cortical functions of language and praxis pretty much intact (Zakzanic 2000). On closer inspection there are considerable individual differences that are rarely discussed in neuropsychological studies. Recent work shows that patients with MS often have difficulty with verbal fluency, comprehension, reading and naming – not what one would expect in a classical subcortical dementia. Executive functions and memory show frequent and early deterioration in MS which, using the old favourite rule of thirds, neatly packages into one-third with minimal deficits, one-third with moderate deficits and one-third with severe deficits. Studies have attempted to elucidate whether deficits in acquisition or retrieval predominate and whether visual or verbal material is most affected (Gaudino et al 2001). No pattern is totally convincing, although studies to date do suggest that many patients with MS have impaired verbal abilities that are greater than their impairments in visual learning abilities and recall, which are in turn greater

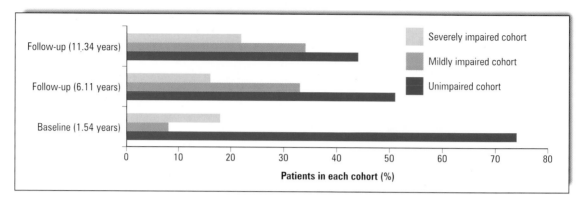

Fig. 20.4   Cognitive decline in multiple sclerosis over 10 years. Data from Amato et al (2001).

than their recognition impairments, (i.e. a retrieval-based memory deficit). (Remember that recognition is said to be preserved in the subcortical dementias.) However, this is neither a consistent nor a specific finding.

Patients with progressive disease have more severe cognitive impairments than those with relapsing–remitting forms, and this appears to hold true after controlling for degree of physical disability. In addition, on meta-analysis there is a trend for patients with chronic progressive MS to have more frontal executive deficits than patients with relapsing–remitting MS, who suffer more memory deficits (Zakzanic 2000). This is almost certainly a reflection of the severity of brain involvement. Cognitive deficits tend to be slowly progressive, although longer follow-up studies are needed to characterize this more precisely. In early relapsing–remitting MS, about one-third of those with cognitive impairment at baseline would be expected to deteriorate over a period of 2 years. This is accompanied by an 8% loss of brain parenchymal volume (Zivadinov et al 2001b).

Dementia can certainly occur with severe MS, but it is thankfully uncommon, developing in perhaps 5% of patients. Future work will have to take better account of the stage of the disease and the nature and distribution of the lesions.

Clinicoanatomical relationships

Cognitive dysfunction is weakly associated with disease duration and physical disability, but is more strongly affiliated with lesion load. The strength of this association is dependent on the method used to assess lesion load, with modern methods such as

volume quantification, and magnetization transfer imaging being the most successful (Zivadinov et al 2001a). Areas of particular significance include the frontal lobes, periventricular areas, corpus callosum and medial temporal lobes (Pozzilli et al 1993). As frontal–subcortical links are strong, a picture of executive dysfunction may be seen without evidence of frank frontal lobe involvement. If visible lesions explain only a modest degree of the variance in cognitive dysfunction, an important question is, what explains the remaining variance? It is likely that microscopic damage, invisible on current tests, adds up to a greater cumulative burden than expected. Up to 80% axonal loss is now recognized in 'normal-appearing white matter'. Whole brain volume may be a crude marker of diffuse loss of axons and appears to correlate with cognitive deterioration and disability in MS over time (Kalker et al 2001, Zivadinov et al 2001b).

SUMMARY

Multiple sclerosis is a devastating disease of young people that gradually worsens with time. Many factors, including problems adjusting to loss, changes in lifestyle and level of support, influence the development of neuropsychiatric complications. Disturbances in mood and cognition are definitely affected by active (and probably inactive) brain lesions and often vary in severity as a result. The magnitude of the neuropsychiatric complications is not tightly correlated with the extent of demyelination visible on MRI and is probably a reflection of the underlying burden of invisible microscopic damage. Studies that have attempted to characterize a set of cognitive impairments have, so far, taken insufficient account of the possibility that cognition varies according to the stage of disease. Sufferers and families who are told what complications to expect are more likely to present early for help and handle such complications more competently. There is a great need for better neuropsychiatric studies concerning the less recognized complications of apathy, anxiety and irritability.

REFERENCES AND FURTHER READING

Amato MP, Ponziani G, Stracusa G et al 2001 Cognitive dysfunction in early-onset multiple sclerosis. Archives of Neurology 58:1602–1606

Berg D, Supprian T, Thomae J et al 2000 Lesion pattern in patients with multiple sclerosis and depression. Multiple Sclerosis 6:156–162

Charcot JM 1880 Clinical lectures on diseases of the nervous system. In: Talbott JH (ed) A biographical history of medicine, p 825–826

Chwastiak L, Ehde DM, Gibbons LE et al 2002 Depressive symptoms and severity of illness in multiple sclerosis: epidemiologic study of a large community sample. American Journal of Psychiatry 159:1862–1868

Comi G, Leocani L, Rossi P et al 2001 Physiopathology and treatment of fatigue in multiple sclerosis. Journal of Neurology 248:174–179

Diaz-Olavarrieta C, Cummings JL, Velazquez J et al 1999 Neuropsychiatric manifestations of multiple sclerosis. Journal of Neuropsychiatry and Clinical Neurosciences 11:51–57

Gaudino EA, Chiaravalotti ND, DeLuca J et al 2001 A comparison of memory performance in relapsing–remitting primary progressive and secondary progressive multiple sclerosis. Neuropsychiatry, Neuropsychology, Behavior and Neurology 14:32–44

Hakim EA, Bakheit AMO, Bryant TN et al 2000 The social impact of multiple sclerosis: a study of 305 patients and their relatives. Disability and Rehabilitation 22:288–293

Kalker NF, Bergers E, Castelijn JA et al 2001 Optimizing the association between disability and biological markers in MS. Neurology 57:1253–1258

McDonald WI, Compston A, Edan G et al 2001 Recommended diagnostic criteria for multiple sclerosis: guidelines from the International Panel on the Diagnosis of Multiple Sclerosis. Annals of Neurology 50:121–127

Pozzilli C, Gasperini C, Anzini A et al 1993 Anatomical and functional correlates of cognitive deficits in multiple sclerosis. Journal of Neurological Science 115:S66

Randolph JJ, Arnett PA, Higginson CI et al 2000 Neurovegetative symptoms in multiple sclerosis: relationship to depressed mood, fatigue and physical disability. Archives of Clinical Neuropsychology 15:387–398

Ron MA, Logsdail SJ 1989 Psychiatric morbidity in multiple sclerosis: a clinical and MRI study. Psychology and Medicine 19:887–895

Sadovnik AD, Eisen K, Ebers GC et al 1991 Cause of death in patients attending multiple sclerosis clinics. Neurology 41:1193–1196

Skegg K, Corwin PA, Skegg DGC 1988 How often is multiple sclerosis mistaken for a psychiatric disorder? Psychology and Medicine 18:733–736

Stenager EN, Stenager E, Koch-Henrikson N et al 1992 Suicide and multiple sclerosis: an epidemiological investigation. Journal of Neurology and Neurosurgical Psychiatry 55:542–545

Stenager E, Knudsen L, Jensen K 1994 Multiple sclerosis: correlation of anxiety, physical impairment and cognitive dysfunction. Italian Journal of Neurological Sciences 15:97–101

Stevens A, Lowe J 2000 Pathology, 2nd edn. Mosby, St. Louis

Taillefer SS, Kirmayer LJ, Robbins JM et al 2002 Psychological correlates of functional status in chronic fatigue syndrome. Journal of Psychosomatic research 53:1097–1106

Underwood JCE 2000 General and systematic pathology. Churchill Livingstone, Edinburgh

Voss WD, Arnett PA, Higginson CI et al 2002 Contributing factors to depressed mood in multiple sclerosis. Archives of Clinical Neuropsychology 17:103–115

Zakzanic KK 2000 Distinctive neurocognitive profiles in multiple sclerosis subtypes. Archives of Clinical Neuropsychology 15:115–136

Zivadinov R, De Masi R, Nasuelli D et al 2001a MRI techniques and cognitive impairment in the early phase of relapsing–remitting multiple sclerosis. Neuroradiology 43:272–278

Zivadinov R, Sepcic J, Nasuelli D et al 2001b A longitudinal study of brain atrophy and cognitive disturbances in the early phase of relapsing–remitting multiple sclerosis. Journal of Neurology and Neurosurgical Psychiatry 70:773–780

Zorzon M, de Masi R, Nasuelli D et al 2001 Depression and anxiety in multiple sclerosis. A clinical and MRI study in 95 subjects. Journal of Neurology 248:416–421

21

Parkinson's Disease

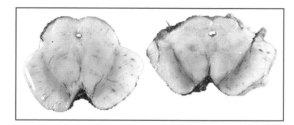

Fig. 21.1 Loss of neuromelanin pigmentation in Parkinson's disease substantia nigra. From Professor Edward C Klatt, Florida State University, College of Medicine.

The patient can [rarely] form any recollection of the precise period of its commencement. The first symptoms perceived are, a slight sense of weakness, with a proneness to trembling in some particular part; sometimes in the head, but most commonly in one of the hands and arms ... The propensity to lean forward becomes invincible ... As the debility increases and the influence of the will over the muscles fades away, the tremulous agitation becomes more vehement. (James Parkinson 1817)

BACKGROUND

Idiopathic Parkinson's disease is the most common movement disorder and the second most common neurodegenerative disorder, with a prevalence of 1%, rising to 3.5% in those aged over 85 years. The average age of onset is 60 years. It is characterized by a triad of tremor, rigidity and bradykinesia. Other common clinical symptoms include a festinant gait, micrographia and a mask-like facies. Nigrostriatal dopaminergic neurones are dramatically (but not exclusively) affected. Other neurotransmitters are reduced in Parkinson's disease, including serotonin and noradrenaline (norepinephrine). These reductions could be important in the pathogenesis of neuropsychiatric sequelae. The three headline psychiatric complications seen in Parkinson's disease are depression, psychosis and cognitive impairment.

Idiopathic Parkinson's disease is distinguishable pathologically from other degenerative parkinsonian syndromes such as progressive supranuclear palsy and multiple system atrophy. Acquired parkinsonism is a common complication of antipsychotic

drugs and a well-recognized complication of vascular disease and encephalitis (see Box 2.3). With so many competing causes and no diagnostic test, an accurate clinical diagnosis of Parkinson's disease can be challenging (Table 21.1 and Clinical Pointer 21.1; see Clinical Pointer 42.1). It has been estimated that false-positive diagnoses occur in 50% of cases in general practice and 25% of cases in secondary care. The most common causes of misdiagnosis are essential tremor, Alzheimer's disease and vascular parkinsonism.

PATHOGENESIS

Dopamine originating in the pars compacta of the substantia nigra innervates the cerebral motor cortex. This occurs via an indirect pathway mediated via D2 receptors and a direct pathway mediated via

Table 21.1 Causes of parkinsonism presenting to neurologists

Disorder	% of presentation
Parkinson's disease	77.7
Parkinsonism plus	12.2
Progressive supranuclear palsy	7.5
Shy–Drager syndrome	1.7
Olivopontocerebellar atrophy	1.1
Corticobasal degeneration	0.9
Striatonigral degeneration	0.4
Alzheimer's disease plus parkinsonism	0.4
Motor neurone disease	0.1
Secondary parkinsonism	8.2
Hereditary parkinsonism	0.6
Unknown	1.3

Data from Baylor College of Medicine, Parkinson's Disease Center and Movement Disorders Clinic (*n* = 2052)

D1 receptors. In Parkinson's disease, loss of inhibitory input to the striatum of the basal ganglia, via both pathways, allows activation of the subthalamic nucleus, which is usually held relatively inactive. This discharges inhibitory GABA signals onto the critical ventral nucleus of the thalamus, which normally reinforces motor signals of the supplementary motor area (see Fig. 51.2).

Pathology

Degeneration of central dopaminergic systems in the basal ganglia is the hallmark of Parkinson's disease, but extranigral pathology is invariably present. Braak & Braak (2003) have recently described the development of the pathology of Parkinson's disease through six stages (Fig. 21.2). Clinical symptoms manifest themselves years after the onset of pathology, when a critical threshold of about 70% neuronal loss has occurred. Using PET, abnormalities in the dopaminergic system can be demonstrated in one-third of relatives at risk of Parkinson's disease. About one-quarter of patients diagnosed by neurologists with Parkinson's disease actually have other diagnoses at post-mortem, including progressive supranuclear palsy, multiple system atrophy, Alzheimer's disease and vascular basal ganglia dis-

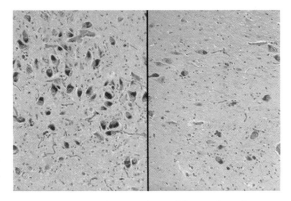

Fig. 21.2 Lesions begin in the medulla, involving the nuclei of the ninth and tenth cranial nerves and anterior olfactory nucleus (stage I). Brainstem involvement progresses with atrophy of the nucleus ceruleus and caudal raphe nuclei of the pons (stage II). In stage III, degeneration affects the substantia nigra. Cortical involvement ensues, with the medial temporal transentorhinal region (mesocortex) in stage IV and then the high-order parietal and prefrontal association cortices in stage V. Finally, the first-order sensory and motor fields succumb (stage VI) (Braak et al 2003). From Professor Edward C Klatt, Florida State University, College of Medicine.

ease. In unselected cases the pathology of Parkinson's disease is not straightforward. Roughly one-third of patients have evidence of Alzheimer's disease at post-mortem (due in part to an elevated rate of Alzheimer's disease pathology in Parkinson's disease and due in part to diagnostic error). About 10% have evidence of distributed Lewy bodies. Lewy bodies are also found in substantia nigra and locus ceruleus (see Ch. 42).

Aetiology

The aetiology of idiopathic Parkinson's disease has been one of medicine's greatest mysteries, but the puzzle may be close to being solved. Clues as to what causes basal ganglia damage come from rare mutations in the α-synuclein gene on chromosome 4, a mutation affecting the ubiquitin pathway and mutations in the parkin gene on chromosome 6. Of major importance, in idiopathic cases, a defect of complex I (and also complex II/III) of the mitochondrial respiratory chain has been quite consistently described. This could mean that the cause is a mutation in mitochondrial DNA, and it opens up a range of new therapies such as supplementation with coenzyme Q_{10}.

OUTCOME

As with many neurological diseases, Parkinson's disease is incurable. There is an increased mortality rate (relative risk is about two-fold), which appears to be slightly higher in men than women. The mean duration of disease at time of death is approximately 10 years, although this is strongly influenced by the age at which people are diagnosed.

NEUROPSYCHIATRIC COMPLICATIONS OF PARKINSON'S DISEASE

Mood disorder in Parkinson's disease

Depression

There is a higher than expected prevalence of depression in Parkinson's disease when compared to similarly disabled patients with osteoarthritis or diabetes. In a sample of over 1000 patients, 50% had depression of mild severity or greater (The Global Parkinson's Disease Survey 2002). About 20% have moderate or severe depression (DSM-IV major depressive disorder) and 30% have mild symptoms of depression. Despite this, results from various studies show that less than 10% of patients are offered antidepressants. One explanation might be that somatic symptoms of depression are confused with the physical symptoms of Parkinson's disease. Thus, psychomotor retardation, early morning wakening and anergia may not carry the usual diagnostic weight for severe depression when occurring in Parkinson's disease (see Table 70.2) (Starkstein et al 1990). Nevertheless, the presence of multiple psychological and somatic features should alert the clinician to likely depression.

Some authors have suggested there are differences in the organic mood syndrome of Parkinson's disease compared with primary depression (Allain et al 2000). They quote less frequent thoughts of guilt and self-harm in the depression of Parkinson's disease. In reality, one cannot reliably distinguish a primary and organic depressive syndrome on the basis of cross-sectional clinical features. However, there are likely to be subtle differences due to the effects of contamination with pre-existing physical symptoms. In addition, patients with an acquired depression in middle to late life are less likely to have a family history of depression and are less likely to blame themselves for their depression. Mood may vary rapidly in some patients (sometimes with 'off' motor symptoms linked with low mood).

A follow-up study of 485 patients indicated that the rate of suicide is lower than in primary depression (see Ch. 78). Outcome of depression in Parkinson's disease has been studied and serves as a template for the outcome of other cases of depression in neurological disease (see Fig. 21.3).

Mechanisms of mood disorder in Parkinson's disease

Depression is more common in late stages of the disease, but it can also herald the onset of neurological symptoms early in the disease. Severe and akinetic forms of Parkinson's disease are risk factors for more severe depression. Other correlates of depression include cognitive impairment and functional limitation (particularly patient-rated disability and handicap), but there is only moderate correlation with neurological motor signs (Schrag et al 2001). One new line of investigation is whether Parkinson's with predominantly right-sided symptoms (or a right-sided onset) predisposes to depression. Given the historical interest in monoamine

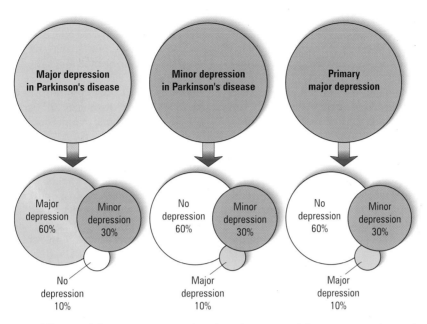

Fig. 21.3 One-year follow-up of depression in PD. By describing the severity of depression according to the DSM descriptions of 'major' and 'minor', it is possible to track what happens to the typical sufferer over time. A patient diagnosed with major depression at initial assessment is likely to remain unwell at 1-year follow-up. A patient diagnosed with minor depression at baseline has a good chance of remission by 1 year. This may be different to the situation in primary depression, where the course of major depression resembles the course of minor depression of PD. After Starkstein et al (1992).

theories of depression, a dopaminergic hypothesis of depression in Parkinson's disease is attractive. Unfortunately, in the real world it has received little support, as there is no appreciable correlation between depression and levels of CSF dopamine metabolites. That said, one group has reported that depressed patients with Parkinson's disease have dysfunction of dopamine projections from the midbrain to the anterior cingulate and of noradrenergic projections from the locus ceruleus to the thalamus compared with non-depressed patients with Parkinson's disease; this report is based on a small PET study (Remy et al 2002).

Conceivably, the factors that influence depression could vary with the stage of illness. For example, one group found that depression correlated with disability, but only in late stages of the disease. This is likely to be a two-way relationship, in that depression adversely affects function and poor function predisposes to depression. Parkinson's disease is an interesting neuropsychiatric model to use to study the biological basis of depression. Various associations have been found on neuroendocrine, neuroimaging and neuropsychological examination. However, distinct differences in comparison with

primary depression have rarely been seen. One hypothesis under active investigation is that brainstem midline raphe nuclei are preferentially affected in depression of Parkinson's disease, although this could be an epiphenomenon of depression (Berg et al 1999). Antiparkinsonian medication (particularly levodopa) can contribute to depression (see Ch. 51).

Anxiety

Anxiety symptoms may actually be more common than symptoms of depression in Parkinson's disease. Indeed, both generalized and episodic anxiety symptoms are more common in Parkinson's disease than in the general population and also more common than in controls with medical disease. Research in this area is in its infancy. The point prevalence of anxiety disorders is 40% in Parkinson's disease, if examined closely. The most common type appears to be panic disorder, often beginning in the early stages of Parkinson's disease. In most reports, generalized anxiety is about half as common, although Schiffer et al (1988) found that 75% of patients had generalized anxiety disorder at some point in the disease. Agoraphobia and social phobia are also seen more commonly than in the general population (Stein et al 1990). Certain somatic symptoms of Parkinson's disease, particularly autonomic symptoms (e.g. flushing, palpitations, dizziness and urinary frequency) can be mistaken for anxiety symptoms in Parkinson's disease. As with depressive symptoms, anxiety symptoms can occur before the onset of the first motor symptoms, but since this does not occur consistently it is difficult to know if this observation has any more than chance significance. In more than two-thirds of cases, anxiety disorders co-occur with depression, and there is some evidence that anxiety disorders are more common in depressed patients with Parkinson's disease than depressed patients with multiple sclerosis, which raises a question about the pathophysiology of anxiety. In some reports, anxiety levels are higher in the 'off' state than in the 'on' state, but this could have a number of explanations, including normal fears about disability and prognosis and the effects of medication. The mechanisms involved in the genesis of anxiety remain speculative (see Ch. 71).

Apathy and emotional liability

Apathy is a major problem in one-third to one-half of patients with Parkinson's disease. The majority have both depression and apathy, but about 10% of patients with Parkinson's disease suffer 'pure apathy' (Isella et al 2002). Patients with apathy perform worse on neuropsychological testing, but such patients are not necessarily those with more severe motor symptoms. It is tempting to ascribe diminished motivation to dopamine reductions in frontal–anterior cingulate–subcortical circuits, given the role of dopamine in motivation and reward, but the direct evidence for this mechanism is not strong.

At the opposite end of the emotional spectrum, emotional lability is seen in about 10% of patients with Parkinson's disease, and clinically it is almost always overlooked. It is typified by sudden, little-provoked, intense crying episodes that are brief but frequent. About two-thirds of cases occur with co-existent depression and one-third of cases are of pure 'pathological crying'.

Psychosis in Parkinson's disease

The relative risk of psychosis is very high in Parkinson's disease compared with aged-matched controls. The prevalence is somewhere between 15%

and 25%, depending on the definition used and the population studied. The prevalence in Parkinson's sufferers with dementia may be as high as 40%, which is more common than the hallucinations of Alzheimer's disease. The difficult question to answer is, why is it so common? Examination of the epidemiology of psychosis in Parkinson's disease reveals that psychotic symptoms are more accurately divided into three major types (Fig. 21.4). The most common symptoms are fleeting illusions and, typically, visual hallucinations associated with good insight (in 10–20% of patients). A small proportion of these symptoms are drug induced. These resemble the Charles Bonnet syndrome. The other types are characterized by more severe delusions and hallucinations with variable insight, and occur in 5–10% of patients (Aarsland et al 1999). These resemble the organic psychosis seen in Alzheimer's disease (Diederich et al 2000). Rarely, other psychotic syndromes occur, such as schizophreniform psychosis and affective psychosis. An important clue to the underlying mechanism is that visual hallucinations are much more common than auditory hallucinations or delusions. Typically, the hallucinations are non-threatening, in contrast to delusions which, when they do occur, are often persecutory in nature.

Mechanism of psychosis in Parkinson's disease

One eloquent explanation for the high rate of visual hallucinations is that patients with Parkinson's disease have subtle visual abnormalities, including poor colour perception and visual contrast sensitivity, which are thought to result from retinal dopamine deficiency. This loss in acuity predisposes patients to low-grade visual hallucinations (Rodnitzky 1998). Other possible mechanisms of hallucinations in Parkinson's disease include changes in the sleep–wake cycle and medication effects. The mechanisms underlying psychosis are probably different in the different types of psychotic presentations discussed above. In Parkinson's dementia, psychosis could be related to pathology in the limbic system and temporal cortex (Harding et al 2002).

The role of dopaminergic medication is no doubt important in some patients, but is widely misunderstood and misrepresented by the term 'levodopa psychosis'. Under controlled conditions, dopaminergic stimulation using intravenous levodopa causes dyskinesias much more commonly than hallucinations. Psychosis has been reported following treatment with bromocriptine, ropinirole, selegiline, pergolide, lisuride and cabergoline. That said, many clinical

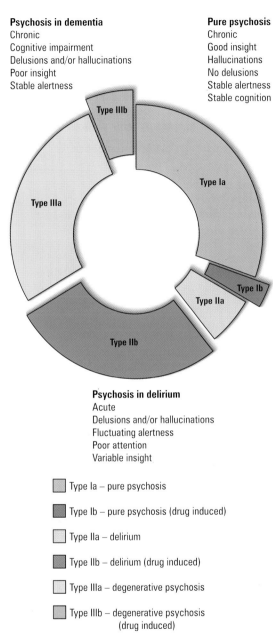

Psychosis in dementia
Chronic
Cognitive impairment
Delusions and/or hallucinations
Poor insight
Stable alertness

Pure psychosis
Chronic
Good insight
Hallucinations
No delusions
Stable alertness
Stable cognition

Psychosis in delirium
Acute
Delusions and/or hallucinations
Fluctuating alertness
Poor attention
Variable insight

Type Ia – pure psychosis

Type Ib – pure psychosis (drug induced)

Type IIa – delirium

Type IIb – delirium (drug induced)

Type IIIa – degenerative psychosis

Type IIIb – degenerative psychosis
(drug induced)

Fig. 21.4 Proposed classification of psychosis in PD. Schematic representation of the types of psychosis that are commonly seen in PD. It is an oversimplification to consider psychotic symptoms to represent one type of pathology in complex diseases. In patients with brain disease psychosis is commonly a symptom of delirium (type II) or dementia (type III). Interesting, there appear to be specific reasons why patients with Parkinson's disease may suffer pure visual hallucinations (see text for details).

studies confirm that medication variables have a weak relationship with persistent psychotic symptoms in Parkinson's disease. This may suggest that in cases where there is an association it is often due to an idiosyncratic effect. The vital point is that true drug-induced psychosis must be distinguished from drug-induced delirium, which *is* a common complication of treatment with levodopa, bromocriptine, selegiline, pergolide, amantadine and anticholinergic agents. Indeed, if one examines closely the data of well-conducted studies, the reported rate of antiparkinsonian drug-induced delirium is approximately 10% – and this frequency would account for one-third of all psychosis in Parkinson's disease.

As with the treatment of depression, treatment of psychosis is difficult because of the exacerbation of symptoms with conventional antipsychotic agents, and therefore atypical antipsychotic agents are often preferred (see Ch. 51).

Cognitive impairment in Parkinson's disease

The majority of patients with Parkinson's disease have some degree of neuropsychological impairment. Common problem areas include executive performance, which is more severely affected than visuospatial function, which in turn is more severely affected than memory and language. Often there is also reduced attentional ability. One study found that specific deficits were associated with specific clinical presentations. Rigidity was associated with impaired verbal fluency and visuospatial performance, whereas tremor was associated with impaired auditory verbal learning, visual memory and reaction time. Bradykinesia was associated with more widespread cognitive impairment (Reid et al 1989).

Dementia is increasingly recognized as a complication in about 1 in 10 cases cross-sectionally or 1 in 3 cases longitudinally (Brown & Marsden 1984, The Global Parkinson's Disease Survey 2002). Some authors report higher rates (of up to 80% (Aarsland et al 2003)). In the elderly, Parkinson's dementia is more common, with about 70% of those over the age of 80 years suffering dementia. Patients who develop dementia in Parkinson's disease almost always have a late age of disease onset. Of interest, poor performance on verbal fluency tasks, but not motor deficits, has been found by two groups to predict onset of Parkinson's dementia (Jacobs et al 1995, Mahieux et al 1998). It is not yet clear whether executive deficits, and in some cases visuospatial deficits (such as the picture completion subtest of the Weschler Adult Intelligence Scale (WAIS)), can be used clinically to predict which patients with Parkinson's disease will develop dementia. Parkinson's disease characteristically causes subcortical neuropsychological changes, including slowed thought tempo (or bradyphrenia) and poor recent memory. Other clinical characteristics include a high rate of visuospatial problems, visuomotor impairments and visual hallucinations.

Alzheimer-type pathology is seen up to five times more often in Parkinson's disease patients than in age-matched controls, but this does not appear to be the predominant cause of Parkinson's dementia. In fact, no single pathological process (including nigrostriatal cell loss, concomitant Alzheimer's disease or vascular disease) has been consistently found to explain this dementia, although correlations with regional cerebral hypoperfusion, locus ceruleus neuronal loss and hippocampal atrophy have been the subject of considerable interest. One recent candidate mechanism producing Parkinson's dementia is cholinergic depletion in the nucleus basalis of Meynert. Another candidate mechanism – cortical Lewy bodies – has been revisited using α-synuclein immunostaining, rather than the comparatively crude haematoxylin and eosin stain. Emerging work forwards the exciting hypothesis that Lewy bodies are a principal explanatory variable in Parkinson's dementia, and hence there is even

more convergence of Lewy body dementia and Parkinson's disease (see Clinical Pointer 42.1) (Hurtig et al 2000). It is probable that the dementia syndrome of Parkinson's disease is multifactorial and compounded by several other distinct pathological processes. In some cases, treatment of primary Parkinson's disease results in a partial improvement in cognition but, in general, Parkinson's patients with dementia are less responsive to treatment than Parkinson's patients without dementia.

Risk factors for Parkinson's dementia are:

- old age or old age of onset
- long disease duration
- severe neurological symptoms (especially postural instability and gait problems)
- severe physical disability
- family history of dementia
- depression
- akinetic rather than tremor-dominant disease
- hallucinations at onset of disease.

Some studies have implied that Parkinson's disease patients who subsequently develop dementia have a specific neuropsychological profile early in the course of the disorder. On closer inspection the differences are usually quantitative rather than qualitative. There is almost certainly an interaction between cognition and depression in Parkinson's disease. Depression alone will cause subtle (and not so subtle) cognitive deficits, and an important question is whether there is an additive effect in

Table 21.2 Profile of neuropsychological impairments in parkinsonian syndromes, Alzheimer's disease, frontotemporal dementia and depression

Cognitive test	Depression	Parkinson's disease	Progressive supranuclear palsy	Multiple system atrophy	Alzheimer's disease	Fronto-temporal dementia
Spatial recognition (working memory)	Impaired	– (mild)	Impaired	Impaired	Impaired	Impaired
Delayed matching to sample (short-term memory)	Impaired (in proportion to difficulty)	Impaired	Impaired	–	Impaired	–
Planning	Impaired	–	–	Impaired	–	Impaired
Thinking time	–	Impaired	Impaired	–	?	–
Movement time	Impaired	Impaired (elderly)	Impaired (severe)	Impaired	–	–
Attention set shifting	–	Impaired	Impaired	Impaired	–	Impaired

Adapted from Elliot et al (1996) and Robbins et al (1994)

Parkinson's disease. Norman et al (2002) found that memory (but not attentional or executive) deficits in Parkinson's disease were largely explained by depression and comparable to those seen in primary depression. Another study found more severe deficits in depressed patients with Parkinson's disease than a comparable group with Alzheimer's disease (Tröster et al 1995).

It is important to remember that delirium is more common in patients with underlying cognitive impairment, the elderly, those with medical illness, those on CNS drugs and those taking polypharmacy. Elderly Parkinson's disease patients fulfil all these criteria. Particular care must be taken, therefore, when starting and stopping antiparkinsonian and psychotropic medication.

PERSONALITY IN PARKINSON'S DISEASE

Patients with Parkinson's disease have been described as industrious, stoical and inflexible, speculatively all attributes of low novelty seeking that links with dopamine deficiency (see Ch. 77). In the largest study, recently completed at the University of Lubeck, Germany, Jacobs et al (2001) found no difference in novelty seeking but higher harm avoidance in 122 Parkinson's disease patients compared with 122 controls. However, on closer analysis it appeared to be higher rates of depression that explained the difference. This emphasizes the need for studies in clinically matched control groups before conclusions can be drawn, and also teaches a valuable lesson about the influence of episodic symptoms on cross-sectional assessments of personality.

UNUSUAL PARKINSONIAN SYNDROMES

Progressive supranuclear palsy

Progressive supranuclear palsy (PSP), or Steele–Richardson–Olszewski syndrome, is a hypokinetic basal ganglia condition featuring bradykinesia. It is less common than Parkinson's disease. Whereas Parkinson's disease usually begins with a unilateral tremor and, later, postural instability, PSP features early postural instability and then symmetrical bradykinesia and vertical gaze palsy. Pathologically,

Table 21.3 Perceptual abnormalities in Parkinson's disease

Perceptual abnormality	% of patients
Illusions (total)	25
Illusions (isolated)	15
Visual hallucinations (total)	22
Visual hallucinations (isolated)	10
Auditory hallucinations (total)	10
Auditory hallucinations (isolated)	2
Abnormal perceptions (any)	40

PSP shows greater involvement of the related basal ganglia nuclei (the putamen, caudate and globus pallidus) and possible greater frontal involvement than Parkinson's disease. Microscopically, there are globose neurofibrillary tangles, granulovacuolar degeneration, neuronal loss and gliosis in the substantia nigra, globus pallidus and subthalamic nucleus. Other areas are more variably affected. Electron microscopy of the neurofibrillary tangles shows straight filaments in addition to the paired helical filaments of Alzheimer's disease. The electrophoretic profile of aggregated tau proteins demonstrates a characteristic tau doublet in PSP (initially in the subcortex and later in the neocortex), rather than the triplet of Alzheimer's disease. Compared with Parkinson's disease, the nigrostriatal loss is greater in PSP, whereas the mesolimbic loss is less. The caudate and putamen are affected to approximately the same degree. On neuroimaging, there is atrophy of the internal globus pallidus.

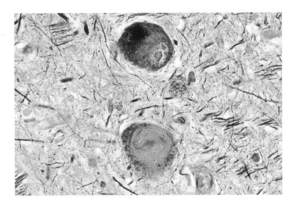

Fig. 21.5 Progressive supranuclear palsy with globose tangles in neurones of the brainstem. Bielschowky silver stain. From Professor Edward C Klatt, Florida State University, College of Medicine.

There is evidence to suggest that apathy, agitation and disinhibition are more severely affected in PSP than Parkinson's disease, whereas dysphoria, anxiety, delusions and hallucinations may be more frequent in Parkinson's disease and Lewy body dementia (see Fig. 21.6) (Aarsland et al 2001). Depression or dysphoria is probably less common in PSP than in Parkinson's disease, especially in severe Hoehn and Yahr stages. Solitary delusions are very rare. There is also the risk of pseudobulbar palsy (presenting with emotionalism) in patients with upper motor neurone lesions involving cranial nerve nuclei. Neuropsychologically, patients with PSP have executive deficits, impaired verbal fluency, and reductions in attention and long-term memory. The rate of cognitive decline may be rapid in some cases of PSP, but in most cases it is gradual. Abnormali-ties of cortical function (apraxia, aphasia and agnosia) are usually absent. Ultimately, the prog-nosis of PSP is worse than that of idiopathic Parkinson's disease.

Multiple system atrophy

Multiple system atrophy (MSA) is a severe degenerative disorder featuring variable degrees of pyramidal and extrapyramidal signs (the essential feature of striatonigral degeneration or MSA type P), autonomic failure (sometimes referred to as Shy–Drager syndrome) and cerebellar ataxia (the essential fea-

---

Box 21.1 Criteria for progressive supranuclear palsy

All of:
- onset over 40 years
- progressive course
- supranuclear palsy
- bradykinesia

Three of:
- dysarthria
- dysphagia
- extended neck posture
- minimal tremor
- greater axial than limb rigidity
- pyramidal signs
- early gait disturbance or frequent falls

Without:
- early or progressive cerebellar signs
- unexplained polyneuropathy
- dysautonomia (except isolated postural hypotension)

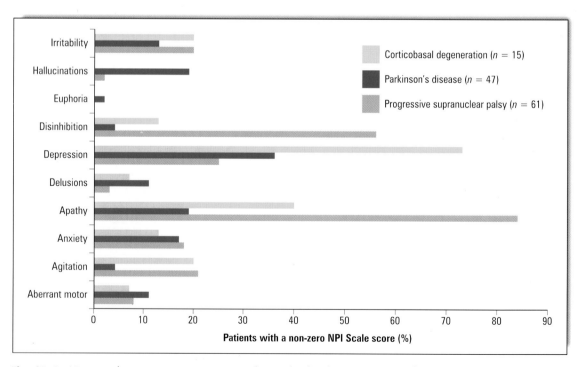

Fig. 21.6 Neuropsychiatric symptoms in PD, PSP and corticobasilar degeneration. Data from Aarsland et al (2001) and Litvan et al (1998).

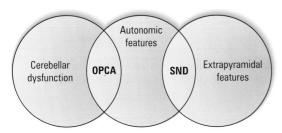

OPCA, olivopontocerebellar atrophy (MSA type C), 20% of cases
SND, striatonigral degeneration (MSA type P), 80% of cases

Fig. 21.7 Revised classification of multiple system atrophy.

ture of olivopontocerebellar atrophy or MSA type C) (Gilman et al 1999). Although the disorder is idiopathic, there is some evidence to call MSA an α-synucleinopathy akin to Parkinson's disease and Lewy body dementia. Although Lewy body pathology is not present, filamentous glial cytoplasmic inclusions, immunostaining positive for α-synuclein, are the pathological hallmark of MSA. These are found in areas known to be affected in the disease – but, unlike in Lewy body dementia, it is glial cells rather than neurones that are affected (in the substantia nigra, putamen and caudate).

Patients with MSA have frontal lobe deficits in cognitive function, broadly similar to those with Parkinson's disease. The rate of dementia probably varies according to the type of inheritance and is less common in sporadic cases (30%) than familial cases (60%). Depression has been recorded as both common and rare in MSA, and the conclusion must await better studies. Response to antiparkinsonian medication is often limited, and prognosis is worse than in idiopathic Parkinson's disease.

Encephalitis lethargica

Encephalitis lethargica is a viral encephalitis, noted for the 1918–1920 epidemic. The acute phase was typical of an encephalitis with stupor, agitation and pyramidal and extrapyramidal signs. The majority of survivors developed postencephalitic parkinsonism, often accompanied by depression, obsessive–compulsive disorder and impulsivity.

Corticobasal degeneration

In 1968, Rebeiz et al first reported three patients with parkinsonism in the absence of tremor – a syndrome now known as corticobasal degeneration, a rare but conceptually important syndrome that has features of both cortical and subcortical disease. It accounts for roughly 1% of patients who present to neurologists with parkinsonism and usually it presents with an asymmetric akinetic–rigid syndrome. The picture is one of posterior cortical dysfunction and subcorticofrontal dysfunction. Proposed diagnostic criteria are alien limb phenomena (spontaneous hand movements outside the patient's control), cortical sensory signs, focal limb dystonia, action tremor and myoclonus. Focal reflex myoclonus is thought to be a distinctive feature of this condition, occurring either spontaneously or in response to stimuli. There is usually cognitive impairment early in the condition, but dementia may develop later and is often mild in severity. Neuropsychiatric features include depression irritability and agitation, possibly more frequently than patients with PSP, but less apathy, anxiety, disinhibition and delusions.

Pathological examination shows neuronal loss and gliosis and swollen ballooned neurones (staining for tau protein and α-B-crystallin but not ubiquitin) in all cortical layers, especially in superior frontal and parietal gyri. The tau abnormality in corticobasal degeneration is similar to that in PSP, with a characteristic tau doublet involving the 4R tau isoform. There is extensive loss of myelinated axons in the white matter. Scattered neuronal inclusions similar to Pick bodies may be seen. Neuronal loss and gliosis are also observed in the nuclei of the basal ganglia and substantia nigra. Lewy bodies are absent. Cognitive impairment is milder than in Alzheimer's disease, but dementia still occurs late in the disease in about half of cases. Corticobasal degeneration presents with more pronounced visuospatial deficits than does Parkinson's disease, which is suggestive of parietal involvement. It has been hypothesized that the French composer Maurice Ravel (1875–1937) suffered from corticobasal degeneration.

SUMMARY

Parkinson's disease is a progressive neurodegenerative disease, observed in 1% of the adult population and affecting approximately 1 million people in the USA alone. It features one of the highest rates of depression, apathy and hallucinations seen in any neurological disease. The explanation may lie in the early damage to critical parts of the basal ganglia or the importance of associated subcorticofrontal involvement. Considerable progress has been made in describing changes in higher function in Parkinson's disease. Increasingly, the role of delirium and drug-induced delirium are being recognized. The neuropsychiatric complications have more than one type of common presentation (major and minor depression, mild and severe cognitive impairment, hallucinations with and without loss of insight), underlining the importance of not oversimplifying what is a complex condition. Psychotic symptoms in young people may be very different to psychotic symptoms seen in older patients. More research needs to be done towards understanding the pathogenesis and treatment of these complications.

REFERENCES AND FURTHER READING

Aarsland D, Larsen JP, Cummings JL et al 1999 Prevalence and clinical correlates of psychotic symptoms in Parkinson's disease. Archives of Neurology 56:595–601

Aarsland D, Litvan I, Larsen JP 2001 Neuropsychiatric symptoms of patients with progressive supranuclear palsy and Parkinson's disease. Journal of Neuropsychiatry and Clinical Neuroscience 3:42–49

Aarsland D, Andersen K, Larsen JP et al 2003 Prevalence and characteristics of dementia in Parkinson's disease. An 8-year prospective study. Archives of Neurology 60:387–392

Allain H, Schuck S, Mauduit N 2000 Depression in Parkinson's disease. British Medical Journal 320:1287–1288

Baylor College of Medicine, Parkinson's Disease Center and Movement Disorders Clinic. Available: http://www.parkinsons-information-exchange-network-online.com/archive/091.html

Berg D, Supprian T, Hofmann E et al 1999 Depression in Parkinson's disease: brainstem midline alteration on transcranial sonography and magnetic resonance imaging. Journal of Neurology 246:1186–1193

Braak H, Tredici KD, Rüb U et al 2003 Staging of brain pathology related to sporadic Parkinson's disease. Neurobiology of Aging 24:197–211

Brown RG, Marsden CD 1984 How common is dementia in Parkinson's disease? Lancet ii:1262–1265

Diederich NJ, Pieri V, Goetz CG 2000 Visual hallucinations in patients with PD and the Charles–Bonnet syndrome: a phenomenological and pathogenetic confrontation. Fortschritte der Neurologie Psychiatrie 68:129–136

Elliot R, Sahakian BJ, McKay AP et al 1996 Neuropsychological impairments in unipolar depression: the influence of perceived failure on subsequent performance. Psychology and Medicine 26:975–989

Fenelon G, Mahieux F, Huon R et al 2000 Hallucinations in Parkinson's disease: prevalence, phenomenology and risk factors. Brain 123:733–745

Friedman JH, Factor SA 2000 Atypical antipsychotics in the treatment of drug-induced psychosis in Parkinson's disease. Movement Disorders 15:201–211

Gilman S, Low PA, Quinn N et al 1999 Consensus statement on the diagnosis of multiple system atrophy. Journal of Neurological Science 163:94–98

Harding AJ, Broe GA, Halliday GM 2002 Visual hallucinations in Lewy body disease relate to Lewy bodies in the temporal lobe. Brain 125:391–403

Hauw JJ, Daniel SE, Dickson D et al 1994 Preliminary NINDS neuropathologic criteria of Steele–Richardson–Olszewski syndrome (progressive supranuclear palsy). Neurology 44:2015–2019

Hurtig HI, Trojanowski JQ, Galvin J et al 2000 Alpha-synuclein cortical Lewy bodies correlate with dementia in Parkinson's disease. Neurology 54:1916–1921

Isella V, Melzi P, Grimaldi M et al 2002 Clinical, neuropsychological and morphometric correlates of apathy in Parkinson's disease. Movement Disorders 17:366–371

Jacobs DM, Marder K, Cote LJ et al 1995 Neuropsychological characteristics of preclinical dementia in Parkinson's disease. Neurology 45:1691–1696

Jacobs H, Heberlein I, Vieregge A et al 2001 Personality traits in young patients with Parkinson's disease. Acta Neurologica Scandinavica 103:82–87

Litvan I, Cummings JL, Mega M 1998 Neuropsychiatric features of corticobasal degeneration. Journal of Neurology and Neurosurgical Psychiatry 65:717–721

Mahieux F, Fenelon G, Flahault A et al 1998 Neuropsycho-logical prediction of dementia in Parkinson's disease. Journal of Neurology and Neurosurgical Psychiatry 64:178–183

Norman S, Troster AI, Fields JA et al 2002 Effects of depression and Parkinson's disease on cognitive functioning. Journal of Neuropsychiatry 14:31–36

Parkinson J 1817 Essay on the shaking palsy. London

Rebeiz JJ, Kolodny EH, Richardson EP 1968 Corticodentatonigral degeneration with neuronal achromasia. Archives of Neurology 18:20

Reid WG, Broe GA, Hely MA et al 1989 The neuropsychology of de novo patients with idiopathic Parkinson's disease: the effects of age of onset. International Journal of Neuroscience 48:205–217

Remy P, Doder M, Lees AJ 2002 Depression in Parkinson's disease is associated with impaired catecholamine terminal function in the midbrain, thalamus and anterior cingulate cortex. Presented at the American Academy of Neurology 54th Annual Meeting, Denver, CO, 13–20 April

Robbins TW, James M, Owen AM et al 1994 Cognitive deficits in progressive supranuclear palsy, Parkinson's disease, and multiple system atrophy in tests sensitive to frontal lobe dysfunction. Journal of Neurology and Neurosurgical Psychiatry 57:79–88

Rodnitzky RL 1998 Visual dysfunction in Parkinson's disease. Clinical Neuroscience 5:102–106

Schiffer RB, Kurian R, Rubin A et al 1988 Evidence for atypical depression in Parkinson's disease. American Journal of Psychiatry 145:1020–1022

Schrag A, Jahanshahi M, Quinn NP 2001 What contributes to depression in Parkinson's disease? Psychology and Medicine 31:655–673

Starkstein SE, Preziosi TJ, Berthier ML et al 1990 Specificity of affective and autonomic symptoms of depression in Parkinson's disease. Journal of Neurology and Neurosurgical Psychiatry 53:869–873

Starkstein SE, Mayberg HS, Preziosi TJ et al 1992 A prospective longitudinal study of depression, cognitive decline, and physical impairments in patients with Parkinson' disease. Journal of Neurology and Neurosurgical Psychiatry 55:377–382

Stein M B, Heuser IJ, Juncos JL et al 1990 Anxiety disorders in patients with Parkinson's disease. American Journal of Psychiatry 147:217–220

The Global Parkinson's Disease Survey (GPDS) Steering Committee 2002 Factors impacting on quality of life in Parkinson's disease: results from an international survey. Movement Disorders 17:60–76

Tröster AI, Paolo AM, Lyons KE et al 1995 The influence of depression on cognition in Parkinson's disease: a pattern of impairment distinguishable from Alzheimer's disease. Neurology 45:672–676

22

Huntington's Disease

The hereditary chorea ... is confined to ... a few families, and has been transmitted to them, an heirloom from generations ... back in the dim past ... It is attended generally by all the symptoms of common chorea, only in an aggravated degree, hardly ever manifesting itself until adult or middle life, and then coming on gradually but surely ... until the hapless sufferer is but a quivering wreck of his former self. (George Sumner Huntington 1872)

BACKGROUND

Huntington's disease is a disease that affects neurological, psychological and behavioural integrity in the majority of sufferers. It was first described by George Huntington on 15 February 1872, at the Meigs and Mason Academy of Medicine meeting at Middleport, Ohio, USA. It is a rare disorder, with a prevalence of 6 per 100 000, and it affects both sexes equally. Chorea is the most common manifestation of basal ganglia involvement, but almost any other symptom of basal ganglia disease is possible. About half of all patients present with neurological features that include fidgeting and slow saccadic eye movements. Over time, dysarthria, dysphagia, ataxia, dystonia, rigidity and epilepsy develop.

The condition has an established genetic basis, namely an abnormality on the short arm of chromosome 4, causing an expansion of the polyglutamine tract (polyQ) in the amino-group terminal region of the protein huntingtin, which is inherited as an autosomal-dominant trait with complete penetrance. In other words, everyone carrying the gene eventually develops the condition. Paternal trans-

mission tends to increase the number of trinucleotide repeats on the first exon of the huntingtin gene and hence reduces the age of onset in the next generation (a phenomenon called *anticipation*). The disease is a progressive disorder in which symptoms gradually worsen over 10–20 years. One in 20 cases develops before the age of 20 years. In most cases of this juvenile-onset form the disease is inherited from an affected father, because CAG-repeat instability is greater in spermatogenesis than oogenesis. The clinical picture is also different, being characterized by an akinetic–rigid syndrome with more severe intellectual decline, seizures and myoclonus. This is known as the *Westphal variant*. Neuropsychiatric complications are usually most evident in the early and middle stages but, unlike Alzheimer's disease, insight is often retained even in the late stages, increasing the risk of depression and suicide.

The core clinical feature of Huntington's disease is an abnormality of involuntary movement (Clinical Pointer 22.1). In addition, very young patients or very old patients often experience myoclonus or seizures. Most patients also have impairments in everyday voluntary movement, such as clumsiness, abnormal gait and abnormal eye tracking. These symptoms may be more disabling than the chorea itself. A rating scale has been developed to rate the severity of Huntington's disease by motor function, cognitive function, behavioural abnormalities and functional capacity (Huntington Study Group 1996).

PATHOGENESIS

There appears to be selective loss of the GABA neurones that project from the pallidum (striatum) to the lateral or external globus pallidus. This pathway usually inhibits the GABA neurones acting on the subthalamic nucleus. Without the first set of GABA neurones, the subthalamic nucleus becomes relatively inactive and in turn overactivates the lateral nucleus of the thalamus and the motor cortex (see Fig. 52.1).

Pathology

Caudate atrophy is caused by neuronal loss of the GABAergic neurones that innervate the globus pallidus and substantia nigra. There is neuronal loss and gliosis in the frontal cortex, basal ganglia, substantia nigra, locus ceruleus, hippocampus and

Recognizing the chorea of Huntington's disease

Fully developed chorea consists of excessive spontaneous movements that are irregularly timed, generally non-repetitive (at one location), randomly distributed and medium to abrupt in speed. The chorea is usually first apparent in the face and the upper extremities, but generally progresses to involve all the extremities, the trunk and the muscles of articulation and deglutition. The chorea is exacerbated during action of the involved body part (e.g. walking) and is suppressible to only a modest extent by patient effort. The inability to maintain voluntary contraction, called *motor impersistence*, is seen during manual grip or tongue protrusion and is a characteristic feature of chorea. It results in dropping objects and clumsiness. Gait disturbances, eye movement abnormalities, dysarthria and dysphagia are virtually universal in the fully developed syndrome. Patients are often not fully aware of the abnormal movements. In contrast to Sydenham's chorea, the movements of Huntington's disease tend to be more jerky and less flowing, at least in the early stages. EMG bursts of asynchronous activity of 10–30 ms and 50–100 ms (shorter than in Sydenham's chorea) are seen in antagonist muscles.

hypothalamus. The majority of patients show at least 30% atrophy of the cerebral cortex, white matter and thalamus.

Within affected brain regions certain neurones degenerate more than others. Huntington's disease preferentially affects projection neurones. In the striatum, medium spiny GABA neurones are preferentially lost and in the cortex large pyramidal neurones in the deeper cortical layers V and VI degenerate. The severity of neuropathological change can be rated on the Vonsattel scale (Vonsattel et al 1985).

Aetiology

The huntingtin gene is on the short arm of chromosome 4 (4p16.3), leading to an expansion of trinucleotide repeats (CAG) from 11–30 to 36–121 repeats. There is a very strong correlation between number of trinucleotide repeats and the degree of atrophy in the caudate and putamen. The pattern of

neuronal loss is very similar to that caused by to toxins that act by excessive glutamate activation and by inhibiting mitochondrial oxidative phosphorylation, possibly indicating glutamate-induced neurotoxicity as the pathogenetic mechanism in Huntington's disease.

Investigations

Laboratory studies useful in cases of movement disorders are given in Table 4.1. The EEG shows a flattened trace (<25 mV), but it is the DNA test that is diagnostic. Subtle preclinical changes in functional,

Box 22.1   Causes of chorea
Neurological disorders Basal ganglia stroke Benign hereditary chorea Cerebral palsy Huntington's disease Neuroacanthocytosis Senile chorea Sydenham's chorea Wilson's disease
Iatrogenic (drug induced) Dopamine agonists Lithium toxicity Oral contraceptives
Systemic disorders AIDS Chorea gravidarum Heavy metal poisoning Paraneoplastic syndromes Polycythaemia Systemic lupus erythematosus Thyrotoxicosis

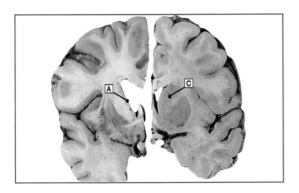

Fig. 22.1 Two coronal brain slices. On the right is a healthy brain with a normal caudate (C); on the left is a brain of a patient with Huntington's disease with an atrophic caudate (A). From Stevens & Lowe (2000).

more than structural, imaging of the basal ganglia have been demonstrated (see Ch. 4). Carriers may also have mild deficits on neuropsychological testing.

OUTCOME

No disease-modifying treatment is available, although symptomatic treatment is offered. Presymptomatic genetic testing is available and should be considered carefully (Clinical Pointer 22.3). The prognosis is relatively poor, and death typically occurs 15 years or so after the disease becomes manifest.

NEUROPSYCHIATRIC COMPLICATIONS OF HUNTINGTON'S DISEASE

Many neuropsychiatric symptoms in Huntington's disease appear to be more frequent than in other dementias and other basal ganglia disorders. Patients currently hospitalized with established Huntington's disease almost universally have neuropsychiatric complications. Outpatients and those with early disease also have a high frequency of psychiatric symptoms, although these are usually less severe and may even go unreported by patients. The severity of cognitive dysfunction and the degree of apathy shows a significant correlation (adjusted for age) with both the duration of disease and the num-

---

Clinical Pointer 22.2

Differential diagnosis of patients presenting with unusual body movements

Sustained and painful contortions of the neck, spine, eyes or tongue that begin rapidly after a first antipsychotic prescription should be recognized as a dystonia and treated with a rapid-acting benzodiazepine. If recurrent, a diagnosis of chronic dystonia may be appropriate. Rare causes of chronic dystonia include Huntington's disease, Wilson's disease, kernicterus, hypoxic brain damage and Parkinson's disease. Inherited dystonia presenting in the first decade of life accompanied by parkinsonism may show responsiveness to levodopa. This is the dopa-responsive dystonia (Segawa disease) caused by a autosomal-dominant mutation in the guanosine triphosphate cyclohydrolase I gene on 14q 22.1. Carpopeadal spasm should be distinguished from drug-induced dystonia by observing for hyperventilation (or by checking blood gases) and ruling out hypocalcaemia.

Athetoid movements are slow, almost rhythmic (snake-like) movements. Choreiform movements are usually briefer, jerky involuntary actions. Hemiballismus is an extreme type of chorea in which an extremity is violently flung out to one side of the body.

Tardive dyskinesia is a very important type of choreoathetoid involuntary movement that is associated with prolonged dopamine receptor blockade (usually due to typical antipsychotic agents) and is essentially irreversible. The movements seen in tardive dyskinesia most commonly affect the lips, face and trunk. Slower movements in the same distribution are sometimes labelled as 'tardive dystonia'.

Rapid and recurrent vocal or motor outbursts, which are often partially suppressed by the patient, are tics. Tics result from Tourette's syndrome, but are also as seen as part of a spectrum in obsessive–compulsive disorder, attention-deficit hyperactivity disorder and Asperger's syndrome.

Fixed movements or postures are usually associated with catatonia in schizophrenia, but bizarre overactivity featuring agitation, mannerisms (apparently purposeful), preservation and echolalia are grouped together under the term 'catatonic excitement'.

Paroxysmal movement disorders are unusual and present a diagnostic challenge. In paroxysmal kinesigenic dyskinesia episodes of choreiform movements are provoked by sudden voluntary movement or startle. In contrast, in those with paroxysmal non-kinesigenic dyskinesia, dystonic attacks occur spontaneously or are triggered by alcohol, caffeine, stress or fatigue. Other types of paroxysmal dyskinesias include episodes precipitated by prolonged exertion (paroxysmal exercise-induced dyskinesia) or sleep (paroxysmal hypnogenic dyskinesia). These conditions bear marked similarities to the channelopathies that cause periodic paralysis following rest.

Further reading   Joseph AB, Young RR 1999 Movement disorders in neurology and neuropsychiatry. Blackwell, Boston
Lees AJ 2002 Odd and unusual movement disorders. Journal of Neurology, Neurosurgery and Psychiatry 72(suppl I) :i17–i21

Clinical Pointer 22.3

Genetic testing for Huntington's disease

It is almost impossible to predict the reaction of an individual who has been told not only that they have a progressively fatal disease but also that no good treatment is available. This is sometimes called the *tiresias complex* (Wexler 1992). Diagnosis on the basis of genetics carries implications for future health, relationships, offspring, occupation and insurance, to name just a few areas. Patients should give informed consent (i.e. they should understand the risks and benefits of genetic testing and the impact it may have on their life). Furthermore, patients will need to know the technical details about the testing process and the clinical significance of results. Although there is no upper age limit for the development of Huntington's disease, an older individual is less likely to develop the disease and also less likely to develop a severe form of the disease.

The Practice Committee Genetics Testing Task Force of the American Academy of Neurology makes the following recommendation:

Before ordering a genetic test for a major neurological disorder, neurologists should ordinarily establish that a patient or lawful surrogate is capable of comprehending relevant disclosures and capable of exercising informed choice. If these conditions exist, the neurologist or collaborating genetic counsellor should disclose why the test is recommended, the predictive weight of the test, the potentially adverse consequences of a positive test (e.g. extreme emotional distress, stigmatization, loss of health insurance or employment), the benefits of enhanced knowledge about genotype (whether the test is positive or negative), and any negative consequences of not testing (e.g. transmission of a detectable disease-associated genotype to offspring).

Important aspects to discuss include the following.

- the purpose of the test
- potential test outcomes
- risks of genetic testing
- benefits of genetic testing
- alternatives to genetic testing for assessing risk status
- confidentiality
- post-testing surveillance and disease-treatment options.

Further reading   Broadstock M, Michie S, Marteau T 2000 Psychological consequences of predictive genetic testing: a systematic review. *European Journal of Human Genetics* 8:731–738
Wexler NS 1992 The tiresias complex – Huntington's disease as a paradigm of testing for late-onset disorders. *FASEB Journal* 6:2820–2825

---

ber of CAG repeats (Craufurd et al 2001). No such relationship has been documented for depression or anxiety (Berrios et al 2001). Up to 50% of people with moderate Huntington's disease (and a greater proportion of those with more severe disease) experience a pervasive change in mood or behaviour which is essentially a change in personality. These cases are difficult to classify and can include disinhibited, apathetic, irritable and paranoid subtypes.

One of these largest and most valuable studies is from the multicentre Huntington Study Group. A total of 2095 patients with a diagnosis of definitive Huntington's disease and almost 700 with presymptomatic Huntington's have been examined prospectively (Paulsen & Robinson 2001). The results show high rates of psychiatric symptoms in both the presymptomatic and the symptomatic phase. They

also show that neuropsychiatric complications influence functional outcome (Marder et al 2000).

Mood disorder in Huntington's disease

Depression in Huntington's disease

The Huntington study group found that 58% of the 2095 patients with definitive Huntington's disease felt that they had depression. The rate of depression was equally high in those with soft signs of Huntington's disease only, and it was also present in 45% of asymptomatic carriers (Paulsen & Robinson 2001). To some extent this very high rate of depression reflects the method of mood assessment in this study. Other reports have found that the point prevalence of depression is about 30–40%

and that depression may precede chorea in about half of cases. Depression is also common in people who do not know they are at risk, implying that the cause of depression is not simply explained by living with the fear of diagnosis. Roughly 40% of patients have a family history of depression, compared with half this number in patients with Alzheimer's disease. Patients with a late onset of disease may be more at risk of developing depression, but this requires confirmation.

In the early stages of Huntington's disease the phenomenology of depression is very similar to that in conventional depression. As the disease progresses the behavioural picture of Huntington's disease becomes increasingly dominant. Patients are often withdrawn, have poverty of speech or mutism, insomnia, loss of drive and psychomotor retardation. Valuable pointers include tearfulness, guilt, suicidal thoughts and overvalued beliefs or delusions. The diagnosis of depression can be difficult, and therefore a trial of antidepressant medication is indicated if diagnostic doubt persists.

The risk of suicide is high in Huntington's disease. Farrer (1986) analysed the cause of death in 452 patients with Huntington's disease using the National Huntington's Disease Register. Six per cent died from suicide. Even though the capture rate was likely to be higher in this study than comparable population surveys, the rate was comparable to that seen in primary affective disorders. Clearly, depression is a major risk factor for suicide in Huntington's disease, but the burden of living with inevitable decline is also very hard. In an impressive postal survey, Almqvist et al (1999) found that 1% of 4527 patients undergoing screening for Huntington's disease had attempted suicide or been admitted for psychiatric treatment. All those who committed suicide had signs of Huntington's disease, whereas almost 50% of those attempting suicide or requiring admission were asymptomatic. Risk factors associated with these poor outcomes included a history of psychiatric problems and unemployment.

Mechanism of mood disorder in Huntington's disease

Studies of the biological correlates of depression in Huntington's disease have been slow in coming to fruition, because Huntington's disease is much less common than Parkinson's disease, multiple sclerosis or Alzheimer's disease. In fact, only one study of

Table 22.1 Frequency of neuropsychiatric problems in Huntington's disease

Neuropsychiatric problem	Patients affected* (%)
Apathy cluster	
Loss of energy	88
Poor quality of work	76
Lack of initiative	76
Lack of perseverance	66
Blunting of affect	66
Poor self-care	64
Irritability–aggression cluster	
Self-centred, demanding	64
Inflexibility, uncooperative	52
Irritability	44
Verbal outbursts	40
Threatening behaviour	22
Jealousy	1
Anxiety–depression cluster	
Anxiety	37
Depressed mood	33
Early wakening	32
Depressive cognitions	20
Suicidal ideation	8
Obsessions	5
Somatic–behavioural cluster	
Loss of libido	62
Physically tense	61
Disturbed temperature regulation	44
Drowsy during the day	43
Bolting food	43
Increased appetite	37
Initial insomnia	37
Pathological preoccupations	24
Sexual disinhibition	6
Somatization	6
Psychosis cluster	
Delusions	3
Auditory hallucinations	3
Tactile hallucinations	.2
Other hallucinations	0

*Proportion of 134 outpatients with Huntington's disease reporting symptoms in the previous 4 weeks, confirmed by a family member

Adapted from Craufurd et al (2001)

note was identified. Kurlan et al (1988) looked at CSF levels of 5-hydroxyindole acetic acid and corticotrophin-releasing hormone in 56 unmedicated patients early in the course of their illness. Patients with depression did not differ from those without depression on these measures. Of passing

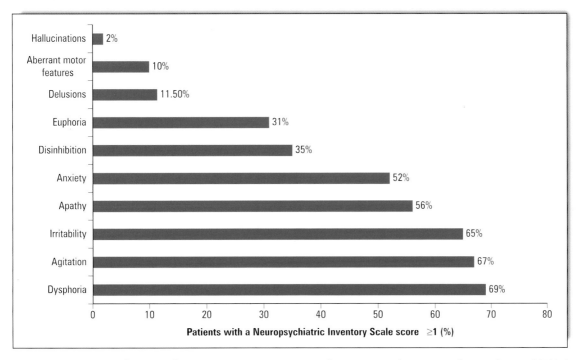

Fig. 22.2 Frequency of neuropsychiatric symptoms in 52 patients with Huntington's disease. Data from Paulsen et al (2001).

interest, there was a correlation between the severity of depression and CSF levels of corticotrophin-releasing hormone (see Table 81.1).

Anxiety

Anxiety is most likely to co-occur with irritability, depression or psychomotor agitation. In other words, anxiety can be a symptom of depression, a symptom of hostility or a solitary symptom. Some have reported that anxiety is the most common prodromal symptom. No studies have compared the rate of anxiety symptoms with that in other medically ill patients, so it is not known how much more common these symptoms are in patients with Huntington's disease. Case series in Huntington's disease suggest that these symptoms occur in about two-thirds of patients (Paulsen et al 2001). Clinical experience suggests that pure anxiety disorders and obsessive–compulsive disorder are probably more common in Huntington's disease than in medically ill controls.

Irritability–aggression

Irritability, when combined with disinhibition, leads to aggression. As in other conditions, verbal outbursts are at least twice as common as threatening behaviour (Craufurd et al 2001). Burns et al (1990) compared the rate of irritability and apathy in 26 patients with Huntington's disease with that of 31 patients with Alzheimer's disease. Irritability was present in almost 60% in both groups, while aggression was more common in Huntington's disease (59%) than Alzheimer's disease (32%). In the largest study of irritability and disruptive behaviour, over 2500 patients were rated using the Unified Huntington Disease Rating Scale. Irritability was present in 45% of subjects and disruptive behaviour in 29% of subjects to a mild or greater degree (Table 22.2).

The likelihood of aggression in Huntington's disease increases as the condition worsens. In milder cases, irritability is precipitated by stress, but in more severe cases irritability and agitation increasingly intrudes spontaneously into daily living. Patients may have poor recollection of irritability (unlike their spouses).

Apathy

Apathy can be a major problem for patients with Huntington's disease. The rate of apathy appears comparable to that in Alzheimer's disease. It is not yet clear how apathy and depression overlap in Huntington's disease. Preliminary work suggests that pure apathy without depression is more common in Huntington's disease than in Alzheimer's disease or after head injury. Patients with apathy usually do not have somatic features of depression, unless the somatic features are caused by Huntington's disease. (Somatic complaints are common in Huntington's disease. Sleep disturbance progresses with severity of the disease. Abnormal movements usually diminish partially during sleep. Loss of libido also occurs, as does, less commonly, increased sexual interest.) To make matters worse, apathy can increase with disease severity and at the same time insight may be lost. It is not unusual for patients with Huntington's disease to deny or refuse to accept their illness. This makes the process of engaging the patient with treatment more difficult.

Some authors have suggested that there is an association between hypokinetic movement disorders (e.g. Parkinson's disease) and apathy and between hyperkinetic movement disorders (e.g. Huntington's disease) and agitation. This may hold true in the early stages of each disease but in the late stages apathy is more severe and frequent than agitation in Huntington's disease. Speculatively, the proposed relationship might have a clinicoanatomical basis

Table 22.2 Irritability–aggression in 2562 patients with Huntington's disease

	Patients affected (%)
Irritability rating	
Not present	39
Slight	15
Mild	23
Moderate	18
Severe	4
Disruptive behaviour	
Not present	58
Slight	10
Mild	13
Moderate	12
Severe	4

After Marshall et al (2001)

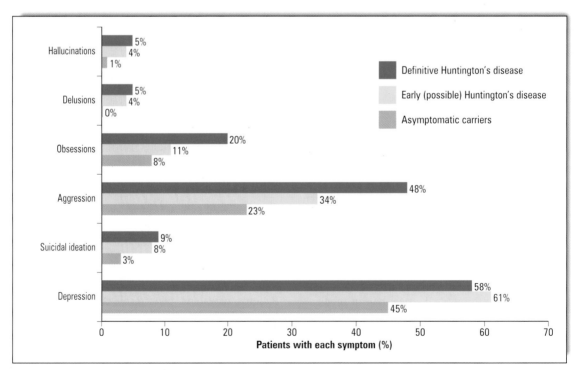

Fig. 22.3 Psychiatric symptoms in Huntington's disease, by stage of disease. From Paulsen & Robinson (2001).

Table 22.3 Degenerative diseases caused by polyglutamine trinucleotide repeat

Disease	Gene	Gene product	Dementia	Pyramidal signs	Extrapyramidal signs	Peripheral neuropathy	Central neuropathy	Retinopathy	Ophthalmoplegia	Ataxia
Huntington's disease	4p16.3 (autosomal dominant)	Huntingtin	✓	✓	✓					
Dentatorubral–pallidoluysian atrophy	12p13 (autosomal dominant)	Atrophin-1	✓	✓	✓					
Spinobulbar muscular atrophy	Xq13-q21 (X-linked recessive)	Androgen receptor							✓	
Spinocerebellar ataxia type 1	6p23 (autosomal dominant)	Ataxin-1	✓	✓	✓	✓	✓		✓	✓
Spinocerebellar ataxia type 2	12q24.1 (autosomal dominant)	Ataxin-2	✓	✓	✓	✓	✓	✓	✓	✓
Spinocerebellar ataxia type 3 (Machado–Joseph disease)	14q32.1 (autosomal dominant)	Ataxin-3	✓	✓	✓	✓	✓		✓	✓
Spinocerebellar ataxia type 6	19q13 (autosomal dominant)	CANA1A								✓
Spinocerebellar ataxia type 7	3p12-13 (autosomal dominant)	Ataxin-7	✓					✓		✓

Adapted from Zoghbi & Orr (2000)

with cingulate disruption in the former and orbitofrontal–dorsolateral dysfunction in the latter.

Cognitive impairment in Huntington's disease

Changes in executive function and memory function are thought to be the hallmarks of cognitive disturbance in Huntington's disease. Neuropsychological impairments are often noticeable at least 2 years before the clinical development of the condition in at-risk carriers. Deficits are progressive. Impairments in executive function involve problems with planning, abstraction, sequencing, organization and judgement. Using the Tower of London Test, Huntington's disease patients have slower initial and subsequent thinking times and poor planning, proportional to the severity of their disease.

Deficits in memory include problems with encoding, storage and retrieval (especially on effortful tasks), although it may be retrieval that is more affected than recognition (at least for verbal material). A higher than expected rate of intrusion errors (perseverations) occur. Some work suggests that memory and verbal fluency are improved by the use of contextual retrieval cues to a greater degree in Huntington's disease than in Alzheimer's disease. Recent and remote memories are similarly affected.

Box 22.2 Summary of cognitive deficits in
Huntington's disease

- Executive dysfunction
- Deficits in memory
- Retrieval (especially in effortful tasks)
- Subcortical deficits

Deficits in declarative memory are relatively mild, but procedural memory is severely affected compared with the case in Alzheimer's disease. Visuospatial and language changes are generally minor and generally occur late in the course of disease. Specific deficits in motor learning (particularly movement sequences) may be a feature of Huntington's disease; they are presumably related to basal ganglia damage. Gradual longitudinal decline occurs in attention and executive functions, more so than in memory, but possible predictors of decline (e.g. reaction time and depression) have not been successfully demonstrated.

The point prevalence of dementia in definite Huntington's disease is somewhere between 30% and 50%, depending on the sample and instrument used (Peavy et al 2002). The dementia of Huntington's disease is often described as a subcortical dementia, based on observations of psychomotor slowing, and reduced selective and sustained attention. This hypothesis has gained credence from neuroimaging investigations showing a correlation between cognitive performance and caudate size on MRI, frontal lobe volume on MRI and dopamine receptor density in the corpus striatum. That said, there are also important similarities with cortical dementias on neuropsychological testing.

Most, but not all, studies have found that the severity of cognitive impairment is determined by the number of CAG repeats. Over the course of time, deficits in fluency, recall and attention may deteriorate more quickly than executive deficits.

Psychosis in Huntington's disease

There is considerable difficulty in studying the co-existence of two uncommon syndromes. Psychosis is certainly observed in Huntington's disease, but it is usually in the context of dementia, delirium, depression and drug-induced states. The Huntington Study Group found that the rate of delusions and hallucinations was not elevated in asymptomatic carriers, but that the rate in definitive

Huntington's disease was about 5%. Both delusions and hallucinations tend to increase in frequency as the disease progresses.

There is no compelling evidence that schizophrenia occurs more commonly in Huntington's disease sufferers or probands, once the contaminating conditions have been accounted for. In the absence of significant cognitive impairment the presence of delusions or hallucinations should raise the question of underlying mood disorder and, quite possibly, delirium.

RARE DISEASES CHARACTERIZED BY CHOREA

Abetalipoproteinaemia

Abetalipoproteinaemia is an autosomal-recessive condition. Vitamin E deficiency results in a progressive spinocerebellar syndrome associated with peripheral neuropathy and retinitis pigmentosa.

Dentatorubral–pallidoluysian atrophy

Dentatorubral–pallidoluysian atrophy is a rare autosomal-dominant neurodegenerative disease characterized by neuronal degeneration in the dentate nucleus, globus pallidus, thalamus, striatum and subthalamic nuclei. The disorder is more common in Japan. The clinical features are various combinations of ataxia, choreoathetosis, myoclonus, epilepsy and dementia. Rarely, parkinsonism or psychosis develops. Age of onset is also variable. It is caused by a specific unstable trinucleotide repeat expansion in a gene on the short arm of chromosome 12 coding for the protein atrophin-1 (Clinical Pointer 22.4).

Neuroacanthocytosis

Neuroacanthocytosis is a disorder named after the appearance of acanthocytosis on more than 10% of the blood film, but the cause of the disorder is unknown (although a genetic basis is postulated). Acanthocytosis is said to result from ultrastructural abnormalities of the erythrocyte. In fact, two other hereditary neurological conditions are associated with it. The disorder is probably familial. Pathologically there is atrophy of the caudate and putamen and, to a lesser extent, the globus pallidus.

Chorea is characteristic, but dysarthria, tics, absent tendon reflexes, dystonia, orofaciolingual dyskinesia and parkinsonism are also recognized. Dementia, personality change and self-mutilation (self-harm) are the main neuropsychiatric complications. In the few patients reported to have undergone cognitive testing, most have cognitive abnormalities. Fifty per cent have memory impairment without high-level language deficits associated with frontal lobe executive skills and psychiatric morbidity (Kartsounis & Hardie 1996).

Spinocerebellar ataxias

The spinocerebellar ataxias are trinucleotide repeat (polyQ) disorders characterized by ataxia and, in some cases, a late-onset form of dementia. Eight types have been proposed, although types SCA4, SCA5 and SCA10 have yet to be adequately characterized. Variable features include chorea, parkinsonism, ophthalmoplegia, pyramidal signs and retinopathy.

SUMMARY

Huntington's disease is a degenerative movement disorder inherited as an autosomal-dominant disorder, caused by glutamate-enhancing triple repeats (polyQ). It is unusual in that its clear genetic basis allows preclinical genetic testing, but this in itself carries implications for asymptomatic carriers. It is a progressive condition for which there is no disease-modifying treatment. It has significant neuropsychiatric complications, including high rates of dementia, apathy and depression. The fact that psychiatric problems appear to be elevated in asymptomatic carriers reminds us of the burden of living with the fear of a disorder that is destined to develop, as well as raising the question of early preclinical biological effects. There is some correlation between the CAG repeat length and both the pathological findings and cognitive impairment, but there is no clear correlation with other psychiatric symptoms. This autosomal-dominant disorder takes a heavy toll on families with an affected relative.

REFERENCES AND FURTHER READING

Almqvist EW, Bloch M, Brinkman R et al 1999 A worldwide assessment of the frequency of suicide, suicide attempts, or psychiatric hospitalization after predictive testing for Huntington disease. American Journal of Human Genetics 64:1293–1304

Berrios GE, Wagle AC, Markova IS et al 2001 Psychiatric symptoms and CAG repeats in neurologically asymptomatic Huntington's disease gene carriers. Psychiatry Research 102:217–225

Burns A, Folstein S, Brandt J et al 1990 Clinical assessment of irritability, aggression, and apathy in Huntington and Alzheimer disease. Journal of Nervous and Mental Disorders 178:20–26

Craufurd D, Thompson JC, Snowden JS 2001 Behavioral changes in Huntington's disease. Neuropsychiatry,

Neuropsychology and Behavioural Neurology 14:219–226

Farrer LA 1986 Suicide and attempted suicide in Huntington's disease: implications for preclinical testing of persons at risk. American Journal of Medical Genetics 24:305–311

Haslett C 1999 Davidson's principles and practice of medicine. Churchill Livingstone, Edinburgh

Huntington G 1872 On chorea. Medical and Surgical Reports 26:317–321

Huntington Study Group 1996 Unified Huntington's disease rating scale: reliability and consistency. Movement Disorders 11:136–142

Kartsounis LD, Hardie RJ 1996 The pattern of cognitive impairments in neuroacanthocytosis – a frontosubcortical dementia. Archives of Neurology 53:77–80

Kurlan R, Caine E, Rubin A et al 1988 Cerebrospinal fluid correlates of depression in Huntington's disease. Archives of Neurology 45:881–883

Marder K, Zhao H, Myers RH et al 2000 Rate of functional decline in Huntington's disease. Neurology 54:452–458

Marshall FJ, Marder K, Taylor S et al 2001 The frequency and severity of disruptive behavior and irritability in Huntington's disease. Movement Disorders 16(suppl 1):143

Paulsen JS, Robinson RG 2001 Huntington's disease. In: Hodges JR (ed) Early-onset dementia: a multidisciplinary approach. Oxford University Press, Oxford, p 338–366

Paulsen JS, Ready RE, Hamilton JM et al 2001 Neuropsychiatric aspects of Huntington's disease. Journal of Neurology, Neurosurgery and Psychiatry 71:310–314

Peavy GM, Salmon DP, Hamilton JM et al 2002 A comparison of dementia prevalence in Huntington's disease as assessed by clinical impression and established criteria. Presented at the American Academy of Neurology 54th Annual Meeting, Denver, CO, April 13–20. Available [abstract only]: http://www.abstracts-on-line.com/abstracts/aan

Stevens A, Lowe J 2000 Pathology, 2nd edn. Harcourt, St. Louis

Vonsattel JP, Myers RH, Stevens TJ et al 1985 Neuropathological classification of Huntington's disease. Journal of Neuropathology and Experimental Neurology 44:559–577

Zoghbi HY, Orr HT 2000 Glutamine repeats and neurodegeneration. Annual Reviews of Neuroscience 23:217–247

23

Wilson's Disease

Progressive lenticular degeneration is a disease of the motor nervous system, occurring in young people and very often familial. It is not congenital or hereditary ... The neurological symptoms constitute a syndrome of the corpus striatum ... Although cirrhosis of the liver is constantly found in this affection, and is an essential feature of it, there are no signs of liver disease during life ... The morbid agent is probably of the nature of a toxin ... It is probable that the toxin is associated with the hepatic cirrhosis. (Samuel Alexander Kinnier Wilson 1912)

BACKGROUND

Wilson's disease, also known as *hepatolenticular degeneration*, is an autosomal-recessive condition characterized by an error in copper metabolism, causing prominent damage to the liver and brain. It is a rare disorder, occurring in approximately 1 in every 40 000 births. Onset is in early or mid-life, but rarely before the age of 6 years. Approximately 20–40% of patients complain of psychiatric symptoms (but typically less than half of these present to psychiatrists). The most common presentation is with hepatic dysfunction. There is an average 8-year latency until neurological manifestations are apparent. Early symptoms are tremor and dysarthria. A variety of abnormal movements can occur. A classic, but nevertheless unusual, early feature is a wing-beating tremor, in which the arms beat up and down at the shoulders. Other abnormal movements include dystonia, chorea, parkinsonism, cerebellar signs or dysarthria.

PATHOGENESIS

There is impaired transport of copper from the liver to the biliary system. Copper is involved in various neurotransmitter systems. The pathogenesis is thought to be absence or dysfunction of a copper transporting P-type ATPase causing faulty biliary excretion of copper. In 1993, the abnormal ATP7B gene was located on chromosome 13q14. An abnormal ATP7A gene causes X-linked Menkes' disease, a copper malabsorption disease of childhood.

Pathology

Neuronal loss and astrocytosis is caused by direct pericapillary copper deposition and secondary damage. Secondary damage is reflected in gliosis, spongy necrosis and demyelination. Areas affected include the basal ganglia (especially the putamen, but also the caudate and the globus pallidus), frontal cortex, brainstem and cerebellum (Fig. 23.1). Copper deposition also occurs in the liver, skin, heart, kidney and eye.

Investigations

A variety of abnormalities are found (Clinical Pointer 23.1), including impaired liver function tests, haemolytic anaemia, the Kayser–Fleischer ring in Descemet's membrane, low ceruloplasmin levels and high levels of urinary copper.

OUTCOME

Management

In 1956, Walshe first treated patients with penicillamine, a chelating agent that increases urinary copper excretion. Other less toxic agents, such as tetrathiomolybdate, are now used. Zinc is a copper-depleting agent that is recommended during pregnancy because D-penicillamine is teratogenic.

Liver transplantation is an option for patients with liver failure, and possibly for patients with neurological and psychiatric disease without liver insufficiency.

Dietary advice is required, but the merits of a low copper diet is controversial (see Ch. 54).

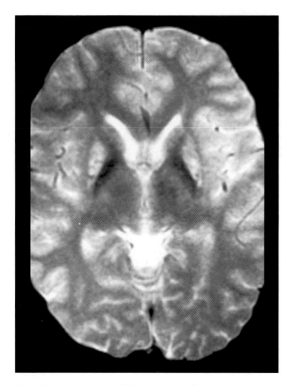

Fig. 23.1 MRI scan of the brain in Wilson's disease. From James G Smirniotopoulos, Uniformed Services University.

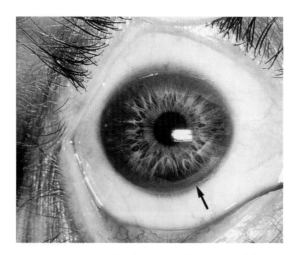

Fig. 23.2 Kayser–Fleischer rings at the junction of the cornea and sclera are associated with neurological rather than hepatic Wilson's disease. From Haslett (1999).

Prognosis

To a great extent the prognosis depends on how far the disease has progressed when treatment is instituted. If the condition is recognized and treated, survival is possible for 20 years or more. Improvement usually begins 5–6 months after therapy is started and continues for about 24 months. Without treatment, death can occur within 6 months of the onset of neurological symptoms.

NEUROPSYCHIATRIC COMPLICATIONS OF WILSON'S DISEASE

Wilson noted that eight of the 12 patients he described had psychiatric symptoms, including euphoria, hypersexuality, hallucinations and catatonia. The most common psychiatric problems are cognitive impairment, mood disorder and irritability. Symptoms vary between patients and between families.

One of the most commonly observed changes, in up to half of sufferers of Wilson's disease, is the irritability symptom complex, consisting of various degrees of frustration, irritability and aggression. At the same time there is often impulsivity and disinhibition. Of interest, there may be an association between irritability and/or disinhibition and brainstem or basal ganglia lesions. When persistent, these changes are considered to be a form of personality change. Personality change has been record-

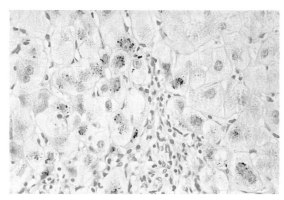

Fig. 23.3 Liver biopsy stained for copper (dark granules), showing excessive copper in periportal liver cells. From Underwood (2000).

Clinical Pointer 23.1

How to diagnose Wilson's disease

Wilson's disease can mimic a number of other movement disorders and cognitive disorders. The onset can be at any age, because a threshold for damage to the CNS is gradually achieved. The presenting complaint may be simplified as hepatitis-like symptoms in one-third of patients, movement disorder in one-third and psychiatric symptoms in one-third. In the early stages, cognitive symptoms are relatively mild, although they gradually become more severe until a dementia ensues. Clinical observation may reveal a combination of abnormal movements, including dystonia, chorea and tremor. Deposits of brown, green or gold pigment at the corneal margin should be visible with the naked eye, or after slit-lamp examination. Ninety per cent of patients have low ceruloplasmin levels (<20 mg/dl), accompanied by high unbound serum copper and high urinary copper excretion (>100 μg in 24 hours). Ten per cent have neither Kayser–Fleischer rings nor low caeruloplasmin concentrations. A high urinary copper level distinguishes Wilson's disease from the rare syndromes of hereditary ceruloplasmin deficiency and Menkes' syndrome. Occasionally, Kayser–Fleischer rings and copper accumulation are seen in the obstructive liver diseases such as primary biliary cirrhosis. If doubt remains, a liver biopsy should show increased copper deposition (> 200 μg/g) and MRI may show increased signal intensity in the basal ganglia and thalamus. DNA marker analysis can also be used.

Further reading *Richards RJ, Hammitt JK, Tsevat J 1996 Finding the optimal multiple-test strategy using a method analogous to logistic regression: the diagnosis of hepatolenticular degeneration (Wilson's disease). Medical Decision Making 16:367–375*

ed in two-thirds of patients who have reached the symptomatic neurological stage of Wilson's disease.

Cognitive impairment accumulates with time parallelling the extent of cerebral lesions (if untreated). No characteristic set of cognitive deficits has been described, but these often encompass mild and diffuse deficits in visuospatial perception, new learning, abstract reasoning and constructional ability. Reduced attention and slowed speed of cognitive processing are particularly common. Reduced motor speed may contaminate cognitive testing. Cognitive problems can be influenced by liver failure or seizures. Many disturbances in mood have been described, but their characteristics have not been adequately studied. Although an insidious dementia is recognized, milder neuropsychological deficits are much more common.

Depression is more likely to occur than anxiety and is found in about one-quarter of patients. It was found in a cross-sectional study that depression was associated with cognitive impairment, parkinsonism and ventricular enlargement (Oder et al 1993). Bipolar illness, pure mania and emotionalism are occasionally seen.

Psychosis occurs in about 5% of patients, with a variety of features including delusions, hallucinations and schneiderian first-rank symptoms. There is no reason to suspect that schizophrenia is more common in Wilson's disease than in the general population.

Box 23.1 Neuropsychiatric manifestations of Wilson's disease

Neurological
Autonomic dysfunction
Cerebellar involvement
Chorea
Dysarthria
Dystonia
Oculomotor palsies
Parkinsonism
Poor handwriting
Seizures
Tics
Tremor

Psychiatric
Anxiety disorders
Depression and dysphoria
Disinhibition
Emotionalism
Hyperactivity (attention deficit hyperactivity disorder) in children
Irritability and aggression
Mania and hypomania
Personality change
Progressive cognitive impairment
Psychosis

Predictors of psychiatric complications include:

- disease severity (measured by the presence of dysarthria or global neurological impairment)
- problems within the family

- long periods of hospitalization
- young age at disease onset.

OTHER RARE DEPOSITION DISEASES

Fahr's syndrome

Fahr's syndrome is characterized by abnormal calcification of the basal ganglia and related areas. CT scanning reveals calcification in the globus pallidus, which often extends into the putamen and caudate. The cerebellum and cerebral cortex are less commonly involved. Basal ganglia calcification is more often bilateral than unilateral, and is only of clear significance when it is symptomatic. The disorder may be idiopathic or associated with systemic disorders such as hypercalcaemia.

Approximately half of patients develop neurological complications, which include parkinsonism, chorea, dysarthria, dystonia and seizures. An overlapping 50% of patients develop psychiatric complications, most notably depression, cognitive impairment and obsessive–compulsive disorder. Most patients suffer some degree of progressive cognitive impairment, although in one-third dementia with a frontal, temporal, subcortical or mixed pattern is recognized. In most cases the cognitive decline is very slow.

On post-mortem examination the calcification is usually clearly visible. In those with dementia there is neuronal loss in the frontotemporal cortex and the nucleus basalis of Meynert. There may be neocortical neurofibrillary tangles, but no senile plaques.

Hallervorden–Spatz disease

Hallervorden–Spatz disease (or Martha Alma disease) is a very rare condition characterized by excess deposition of iron in the basal ganglia, especially the globus pallidus and substantia nigra. Peculiarly, extracerebral iron is unaffected. The disease is inherited as an autosomal-recessive condition, with onset usually before the age of 20 years. There are pyramidal and extrapyramidal signs, abnormal postures, optic atrophy, nystagmus and a gradually progressive dementia. MRI may reveal hypodense regions in the basal ganglia. Pathological analysis reveals brown discolouration of the affected areas, which stain sea-blue with Perls' iron stain.

SUMMARY

Wilson's disease is a rare multisystem movement disorder caused by an inborn error in copper metabolism, which predominantly affects the basal ganglia. Disinhibition, irritability and depression are the most common neuropsychiatric features. Cognitive impairment and dementia also occur, but are not well characterized. Early recognition and treatment is essential in order to alter the course of the disease.

REFERENCES AND FURTHER READING

Haslett C 1999 Davidson's principles and practice of medicine. Churchill Livingstone, Edinburgh

Oder W, Prayer L, Grimm G et al 1993 Wilson's disease: evidence of subgroups derived from clinical findings and brain lesions. Neurology 431:120–124

Underwood JCE 2000 General and systematic pathology. Churchill Livingstone, Edinburgh

Walshe JM 1956 Penicillamine: a new oral therapy for Wilson's disease. American Journal of Medicine 21:487–495

Wilson SAK 1912 Progressive lenticular degeneration: a familial nervous disease associated with cirrhosis of the liver. Brain 134:295–509

24

Tourette's Syndrome

This illness is hereditary; it is characterized by motor inco-ordination in the form of abrupt muscular jerks that are often severe enough to make the patient jump; ... the incoordination may be accompanied by articulated or inarticulated sounds. When articulated, the words are often repetitions of words which the patient may have just heard ... Among the expressions which the patient may repeatedly utter, some may have the special character of being obscene (coprolalia); ... the physical and mental health of these patients is otherwise basically normal. The condition seems incurable and life long, with onset in childhood. (George Gilles de la Tourette 1884)

BACKGROUND

Tourette's syndrome is a syndrome of motor and phonic tics. The first recorded case was that of the Marquise de Dampierre, originally described by Itard in 1825 and then by Tourette in 1884. Several famous people are thought to have suffered from Tourette's syndrome, including Samuel Johnson (1709–1784) and professional basketball player Mahmoud Abdul-Rauf. It is not considered a dementing disorder. It begins in early life, certainly before 21 years of age, and is three times more common in boys than girls. The prevalence is about 0.1%. As anticipated, the prevalence is higher in selected populations with established attentional problems, impulsivity or those with special educational needs.

CLINICAL FEATURES

The clinical features are variable. Most patients suffer an urge or sensory experience that precedes the tic. This is known as the *premonitory feeling* or *sensory tic*. Many also have an urge to reveal socially inappropriate actions or comments. Classically, tics are subdivided into:

- simple motor tics – blinking, grimacing, shrugging and, occasionally, dystonic tics
- complex motor tics – touching, hopping, throwing, bending, gesturing, hitting and biting
- simple vocal tics – snorting, hissing, coughing, throat-clearing and barking
- complex vocal tics – echolalia (repetition of others' phrases), palilalia (repetition of one's own words and phrases) and obscenities (coprolalia).

Other associated features include obsessions and compulsions, aggression (unlike simple obsessive–compulsive disorder), bipolar spectrum disorder, attention-deficit hyperactivity disorder (or pure hyperactivity), oppositional defiant disorder or conduct disorder, and substance abuse. There is also an association with self-injurious behaviour (as opposed to attempted suicide), which resembles that found in those with severe learning disabilities.

PATHOGENESIS

The mechanism of the disease is not established.

Pathology

Caudate atrophy is found in some cases. Frontal supplementary motor area activation on functional imaging or subcortical grey lesions on structural imaging are recorded in cases of secondary tics (such as in encephalitis, head injury, stroke and drug-induced tics) (Singer 1997). Childhood tics can be caused by the PANDAS syndrome (paediatric autoimmune neuropsychiatric disorders associated with streptococcal infections; see Ch. 28).

Investigations

On EEG some tics are not preceded by the pre-movement potential (*Bereitschafts*) that immediately antedates volitional movements, including the action of mimicking the tic movement.

Aetiology

The aetiology is unknown, but several clues exist. A genetic influence is shown by the monozygous concordance of 70% and dizygous concordance of 25%. An autosomal-dominant inheritance via chromosome 4, 8 or 18 (with variable penetrance) has been suggested. In some mothers, first-trimester illness and perinatal illness may predispose to more severe tics in their offspring.

OUTCOME

Management

Usually a package of care is required, with education, support and pharmacological management to minimize tics and maximize quality of life.

Prognosis

Occasional remissions occur, but the disorder is persistent in two-thirds of cases. In one-third of cases, the disorder resolves by late adolescence. Even in those with chronic forms of the disorder, gradual long-term improvement can be expected if the condition is treated.

NEUROPSYCHIATRIC COMPLICATIONS OF TOURETTE'S SYNDROME

Systematic studies of psychiatric features of Tourette's syndrome are gradually beginning to appear. Most notably, Kulisevsky et al (2001) applied the Neuropsychiatric Inventory to 26 patients with Tourette's syndrome, 29 patients with Huntington's disease and 34 with progressive supranuclear palsy. There was no difference between the groups in the total Neuropsychiatric Inventory scores. However, patients with hyperkinetic disorders (Huntington's disease and Tourette's syndrome) exhibited significantly more agitation, irritability, anxiety, euphoria and hyperkinesia, whereas patients with hypokinetic disorders (progressive supranuclear palsy) exhibited more apathy (Fig. 24.1). Patients with Tourette's syndrome had greater anxiety symptoms than did patients with Huntington's disease or progressive supranuclear palsy. Interestingly, the severity of tics was associated with the degree of anxiety and irritability.

Box 24.1 Classification of tics

Primary
Tourette's syndrome
Transient tic disorder of childhood
Adult onset tic disorder

Secondary
Degenerative:
- neuroanthocytosis
- progressive supranuclear palsy

Developmental:
- pervasive developmental disorder
- childhood encephalopathy

Drug induced:
- antipsychotic agents
- stimulants

Hereditary:
- Down's syndrome
- fragile X syndrome
- Huntington's disease

Infections and autoimmune causes:
- Sydenham's chorea
- encephalitis
- Creutzfeldt–Jakob disease
- rubella

Psychiatric causes:
- somatoform disorder (pseudo-tic)
- anxiety disorder (pseudo-tic)
- obsessive–compulsive disorder (tic or pseudo-tic)*

Toxic causes:
- carbon monoxide poisoning
- hypoglycaemia

*Obsessions and tics may occur together as symptoms. Abnormal movements in primary obsessive–compulsive disorder can be mistaken for tics

---

Cognition in Tourette's syndrome

The extent and nature of cognitive deficits in Tourette's syndrome are not well studied. The majority of deficits appear to be subtle dysexecutive problems, perhaps due to developmental delay or an overlap with attention-deficit hyperactivity disorder. A substantial proportion have more severe deficits in several domains, including severe executive dysfunction, visuospatial skills and memory. One study found that predictors of cognitive dysfunction were an early onset of tics, the presence of complex motor tics and behavioural disturbances, but not obsessive–compulsive disorder or use of neuroleptics

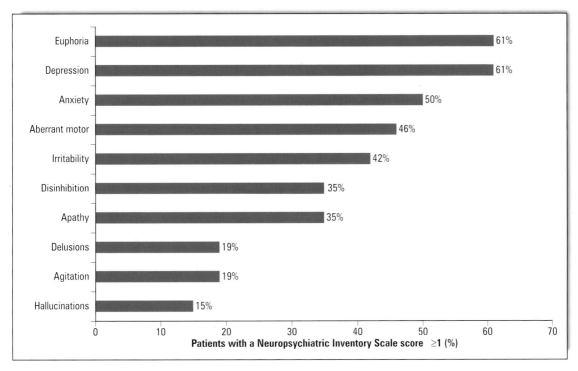

Fig. 24.1 Neuropsychiatric features of Tourette's syndrome. Data from Kulisevsky et al (2001).

Clinical Pointer 24.1

The differential diagnosis of tics

Tics usually have a purposeful and repetitive quality that distinguishes them from choreoathetoid movements and myoclonus. The phenomenology of tics should be distinguished from mannerisms, akathisia, anxiety and stereotypies. Occasionally, patients with unusual postural compulsions give a history of similar movements, although these are associated with obsessional thoughts. Tics presenting for the first time in adult life are less likely to be due to Tourette's syndrome. Indeed, Tourette's syndrome peaks at 10 years of age and may resolve by 18 years. Tourette's syndrome is suggested by tics that persist for more than 1 year accompanied by abnormal vocalizations. Tardive dyskinesia following chronic dopamine blockade is one differential diagnosis. Drug-induced tardive tics occur with dopamine-stimulating drugs and, rarely, with anticonvulsants. Other rare causes of secondary tics include Huntington's disease, Sydenham's chorea, encephalitis, tuberous sclerosis, Wilson's disease and childhood developmental disorders.

Further reading   Joseph AB, Young RR 1999 Movement disorders in neurology and neuropsychiatry. Blackwell, Boston

---

(Levin et al 2001). A second study found that attention-deficit hyperactivity disorder, obsessive–compulsive disorder, specific learning disability and tic severity all influenced separate domains of executive function (Lichter et al 2002). Impairments in attention and working memory were related to attention-deficit hyperactivity disorder, impairments in set-shifting were related to obsessive–compulsive disorder, and impairments in letter word fluency correlated with tic severity.

Mood disorder in Tourette's syndrome

Depression in Tourette's syndrome has not been directly compared with depression in other chronic childhood disorders. Thus, while depression is common in Tourette's syndrome, it is not necessarily more common than expected given developmental and social hardships. Anxiety disorders may actually be more common than depression.

Typically, worries focus on illness, tics, daily function and sleep. The rates of generalized anxiety disorder, panic disorder and phobias all appear to be elevated in Tourette's syndrome. High rates of anxiety are correlated with high rates of depression, agitation and irritability. In studies to date, the risk of generalized anxiety disorder in Tourette's probands is not elevated, suggesting genetic independence of these conditions.

OTHER MOVEMENT DISORDERS

Essential tremor

Essential tremor is one of the most common movement disorders, with a prevalence of 0.5–5%. Although it is often mild, it is usually persistent. Essential tremor is characterized by a peripheral postural tremor of the upper limbs, and sometimes other parts of the body. The physiological basis of the tremor is thought to be different in essential, cerebellar, parkinsonian and psychogenic tremors – involving oscillations due to either neuronal pacemaker activity, disturbed feedback loops or abnormal reflexes. The anatomical origin of essential tremor is unknown, although an involvement of the cerebellum and inferior olivary nucleus seems likely.

Traditionally, essential tremor is viewed as an entirely peripheral disorder, but recent evidence challenges this assumption. Preliminary cognitive testing has revealed subtle deficits in executive function and memory, not dissimilar to patients with Parkinson's disease (Gasparini et al 2001). In addition, mood abnormalities are greater than in control populations, with higher rates of depression, disinhibition and, in some cases, blunted affect (Lombardi et al 2001). The degree to which this reflects

neurobiological changes in the brain is totally unknown.

SUMMARY

Tourette's syndrome is a syndrome of simple and complex motor and vocal tics of unknown aetiology. Tics, obsessions and compulsions, hyperactivity and aggression are the common neuropsychiatric complications. The pathology appears to reside in the basal ganglia. The disorder probably has a genetic basis, but this has yet to be identified.

REFERENCES AND FURTHER READING

Gasparini M, Bonifati V, Fabrizio E et al 2001 Frontal lobe dysfunction in essential tremor: a preliminary study. Journal of Neurology 248:399–402

Gilles de la Tourette G 1884 Study of a neurologic condition characterized by motor incoordination accompanied by echolalia and coprolalia (jumping, latah, myriachit). Archives of Neurology 8:68–74

Kulisevsky J, Litvan I, Berthier ML et al 2001 Neuropsychiatric assessment of Gilles de la Tourette patients: comparative study with other hyperkinetic and hypokinetic movement disorders. Movement Disorders 16:1098–1104

Levin OS, Moscovczeva GM, Glozman GM 2001 Cognitive disturbances in patients with Tourette's syndrome. Journal of Neurological Science 187(suppl 1):S309

Lichter DG, Jackson LA, Bisker SM 2002 Discrete influences on executive function in Tourette syndrome. Presented at the American Academy of Neurology 54th Annual Meeting, Denver, CO, 13–20 April. Available: http://www.abstracts-on-line.com/abstracts/aan/

Lombardi WJ, Woolston DJ, Roberts JW et al 2001 Cognitive deficits in patients with essential tremor. Neurology 57:785–790

Singer HS 1997 Neurobiology of Tourette syndrome. Neurologic Clinics of North America 15:357–379

25

Creutzfeldt–Jakob Disease

We are dealing with a disease process ... characterized by the following features: ... unknown cause ... relapsing course with remissions ... cortical symptoms referable to the motor and sensory centers ... mental symptoms of the type of intellectual defect with predominance of psycho-motor manifestations ... course ... a noninflammatory focal disintegration at the neural tissue of the cerebral cortex ... a noninflammatory diffuse cell disease with cell outfall throughout almost the entire gray substance.
(Hans Gerhard Creutzfeldt 1920)

BACKGROUND

There has been a huge resurgence of interest in Creutzfeldt–Jakob disease following the discovery of a new and distinctive form of the disease. The infectious agent in new variant Creutzfeldt–Jakob disease has identical characteristics to the bovine spongiform encephalopathy agent, raising the distinct possibility of transmission of bovine spongiform encephalopathy or 'mad cow disease' to humans. Although bovine spongiform encephalopathy is relatively common in the UK, variant Creutzfeldt–Jakob disease remains a very rare disease, with only about 100 neuropathologically confirmed cases ever having been reported worldwide. However, there is still great concern because these diseases can have an extremely long incubation period, and thus the majority of cases may not have had time to manifest themselves.

Creutzfeldt–Jakob disease is a prion disease, a prion being a proteinaceous infective particle that is extremely resistant to degradation. Prion protein is an essential membrane protein, normally coded for by chromosome 20. When a transmissible form is inoculated, a transformation occurs into a non-degradable isoform. Prion diseases include scrapie, kuru, bovine spongiform encephalopathy, Gerstmann–Straussler syndrome, fatal familial insomnia and Creutzfeldt–Jakob disease (Box 25.1). They all cause an subacute spongiform enceph-alopathy of the brain, a condition characterized by microscopic cysts or vacuoles in the grey matter (Fig. 25.1).

Ninety per cent of cases of Creutzfeldt–Jakob disease are spontaneous mutations (i.e. sporadic Creutzfeldt–Jakob disease). The remainder of cases are either iatrogenic or familial in nature.

CLINICAL AND NEUROPSYCHIATRIC FEATURES OF CREUTZFELDT–JAKOB DISEASE

Sporadic Creutzfeldt–Jakob disease

Rarely, there is a prodromal illness, but more often sporadic Creutzfeldt–Jakob disease presents as a dementia associated with myoclonus or cerebellar symptoms. If prodromal symptoms occur there may be ill-defined confusion, disorientation and forgetfulness. As the disease progresses a picture of multifocal cortical and subcortical dementia may emerge. Myoclonus occurs in 80% of patients. Additional features are pyramidal and extrapyramidal signs, choreoathetoid movements, dysarthria and visual disturbances. Akinetic mutism and cortical blindness can occur (*Heidenhain's syndrome*).

Box 25.1 The prion diseases

Human prion diseases
Creutzfeldt–Jakob disease
Fatal familial insomnia
Fatal sporadic insomnia
Gertmann–Sträussler–Scheinker disease
Kuru

Animal prion diseases
Bovine spongiform encephalopathy
Chronic wasting disease of deer
Exotic ungulate encephalopathy
Feline spongiform encephalopathy
Scrapie (in sheep)

Neuropsychiatric features are very variable. Cognitive impairment is the most characteristic feature, although delirium is an important complication. Apathy, depression, emotional lability, anxiety and aggressive behaviour are common.

Familial Creutzfeldt–Jakob disease

Many mutations of the prion protein gene on chromosome 20 can produce a classical form of Creutzfeldt–Jakob disease. Mutations on codons 200 and 178 are the most common. The condition has incomplete penetrance, and many carriers live to old age.

Iatrogenic Creutzfeldt–Jakob disease

About 300 cases of Creutzfeldt–Jakob disease have been caused by the administration of contaminated growth hormone or contamination during neurosurgical procedures. These errors are now much less likely, but the possible long incubation period of up to 30 years remains a cause for concern. The clinical presentation is similar or identical to that of sporadic Creutzfeldt–Jakob disease.

New variant Creutzfeldt–Jakob disease

In late 1995, two cases of sporadic Creutzfeldt–Jakob disease were reported in two UK teenagers. Subsequent cases have largely been confined to the

UK. Unlike classical Creutzfeldt–Jakob disease, this disease primarily affects young adults (mean age 26 years) and features prodromal psychiatric symptoms. Sixty-five per cent present with prodromal or initial psychiatric features, such as dysphoria, anxiety, panic attacks, apathy, withdrawal and aggression, whereas 15% present with neurological symptoms (particularly cognitive problems, gait disturbance and sensory symptoms). Later features include disorientation, hallucinations, confabulation and abnormal movements. A progressive cerebellar syndrome with myoclonus often develops within months, producing ataxia and progressive dementia, which may culminate in akinetic mutism. Notably, no particular symptom or sign is characteristic of variant Creutzfeldt–Jakob disease (Spencer et al 2002).

PATHOGENESIS

Pathology

Microscopic features are more striking than the macroscopic appearance. Histologically, there is spongiform change accompanied by neuronal loss, gliosis and deposition of abnormal prion protein. In variant Creutzfeldt–Jakob disease there are amyloid plaques surrounded by spongiform vacuoles in the cerebral and cerebellar cortex. These are unique 'florid' kuru-like plaques. The occipital cortex and thalamus may also be severely affected in variant Creutzfeldt–Jakob disease.

Aetiology

Normal brain prion protein changes into an insoluble form, which accumulates as amyloid and results in cell death and spongiform change. The exact mechanism by which abnormal forms of prion protein are neurotoxic is incompletely understood at this time.

Investigations

The following changes may aid diagnosis:

- CT shows atrophy in the cortex and cerebellum.
- EEG shows periodic (triphasic) complexes (0.5-second slow waves) in classical, sporadic Creutzfeldt–Jakob disease, but only non-specific slow wave activity in variant Creutzfeldt–Jakob

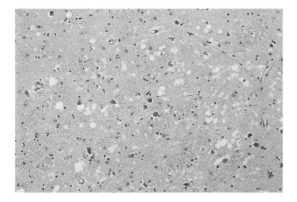

Fig. 25.1 Brain biopsy from a patient with Creutzfeldt–Jakob disease, showing numerous grey matter vacuoles with gliosis and neuronal loss. From Underwood (2000).

disease. The sensitivity and specificity of EEG changes is approximately 70%.

- CSF proteins (14-3-3 protein, neurone-specific enolase, S-100b and tau protein) are elevated.
- In variant Creutzfeldt–Jakob disease, characteristic prion protein can be detected on tonsilar biopsy.
- MRI shows a hyperintense signal in the basal ganglia in sporadic Creutzfeldt–Jakob disease and an increased thalamic signal intensity in variant Creutzfeldt–Jakob disease.

OUTCOME

Prognosis

The prognosis of classical Creutzfeldt–Jakob disease is very grave, with most cases proving fatal within months. A small handful survive for 2 years or more. In variant Creutzfeldt–Jakob disease the prognosis is still grave, but the average duration of illness is 14 months, compared with 4 months in classical Creutzfeldt–Jakob disease.

SUMMARY

Creutzfeldt–Jakob disease is a rare human prion disease that is rapidly fatal. In the new variant form, which is thought to be transmitted from bovine spongiform encephalopathy, there is a neuropsychiatric prodrome in the majority of patients. There is a very long latent period, shared by the spongiform disorders, and this raises uncomfortable questions about the true prevalence. There is also the concern that the disease could be transmitted via blood transfusion. Use of cadaveric growth hormone and dura mater graft have caused over 250 cases of iatrogenic classical Creutzfeldt–Jakob disease, often after an extended incubation period. Myoclonus and cognitive impairment are the most recognized features, but no neuropsychiatric symptom or sign is pathognomonic. An EEG is the most useful diagnostic test, although tissue biopsy may be required. Even with early diagnosis, the prognosis is very poor.

REFERENCES AND FURTHER READING

Creutzfeldt HG 1920 Uber eine eigenartige herdformige erkrankung des zentralnervensystems. Zeitschrift fur Gesamte Neurol Psychiatrie 57:1–18

Spencer MD, Knight RSG, Will RG 2002 First hundred cases of variant Creutzfeldt–Jakob disease: retrospective case note review of early psychiatric and neurological features. BMJ 324:1479–1482

Underwood SAK 2000 General and systematic pathology. Churchill Livingstone, Edinburgh

26

HIV and AIDS

We recently treated several young, previously healthy, homosexual men for multiple episodes of Pneumocystis carinii pneumonia, extensive mucosal candidiasis, and severe viral infections. The clinical manifestations and studies of cellular immune function ... indicated a ... severe acquired T-cell defect ... This syndrome represents a potentially transmissible immune deficiency.
(Michael Gottlieb 1981)

BACKGROUND

Acquired immune deficiency syndrome (AIDS) is a systemic immune deficiency caused by the retrovirus human immunodeficiency virus type 1 (HIV-1). AIDS was first reported in 1981, although it was not initially recognized as a new syndrome. The infective agent was identified in 1984 as a human retrovirus. HIV invades lymphoid tissue and the CNS early in the course of infection. As the virus replicates, the host loses the capacity to fight off the infection. Immunocompromise also predisposes to a variety of secondary infections of the CNS (Table 26.1). There are estimated to be 1 million patients in the USA and 33 million worldwide (Fig. 26.1). In the UK, 90% of AIDS occurs in men, although there

Table 26.1 Presenting complaints in AIDS

Complaint	Patients presenting (%)
Pneumocystis carinii pneumonia	40
Kaposi's sarcoma	15
Oesophageal candidiasis	15
Neuropsychiatric complications	10
Lymphoma	5

are geographical variations. In both men and women one-quarter of cases are due to intravenous drug injection. In women, the remainder of cases are due to heterosexual contact, whereas in men the majority are due to homosexual contact.

CLINICAL FEATURES

A few weeks after infection there is wide dissemination of the virus, coinciding with a flu-like illness. The host produces antibodies that fight the infection (seroconversion), but invariably these are not completely successful. A dynamic balance between viral replication and viral destruction is usually achieved quickly and maintained for several years. This is reflected in the number of viral particles per cubic millimetre of blood. Lymphoid tissue and the CNS act as reservoirs for the virus. In this prolonged asymptomatic stage, infected individuals may unknowingly spread the disease. Eventually the virus overcomes the body's capacity for defence and viral titres rapidly rise in association with falling $CD4^+$ cell counts. (Approximately 30% of those with HIV infection suffer a decline of $CD4^+$ cell counts to below $200/\mu l$ every 5 years.) At this stage, AIDS is diagnosed and neoplastic and neurological manifestations ensue (Fig. 26.3).

PATHOGENESIS

Pathology

CNS pathology in HIV can be complex, but includes HIV encephalopathy (AIDS dementia), aseptic meningitis and vacuolar myelopathy, cere-

---

Box 26.1 Causes of susceptibility to secondary infections

- AIDS
- Alcoholism
- Diabetes mellitus
- Glucocorticoid therapy
- Malignancy (particularly of the lymphoreticular system)
- Pregnancy
- Sarcoidosis
- T-cell diseases (Di George's syndrome and Nezelof's syndrome)
- Vasculitis (e.g. systemic lupus erythematosus)

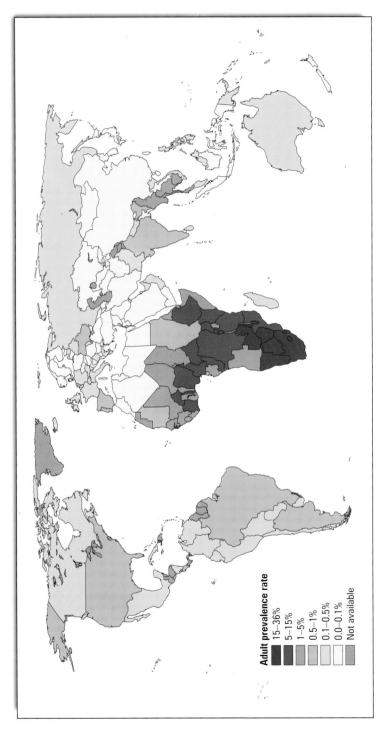

Fig. 26.1 Worldwide prevalence of AIDS in adults in 2000. Ninety per cent of people with HIV/AIDS live in developing countries and are not aware of their diagnosis. In sub-Saharan Africa the adult prevalence is 9%, and 50% of these are women. Although epidemics are growing in many countries, prevention has been shown to be successful in Uganda.

Adult prevalence rate

15–36%
5–15%
1–5%
0.5–1%
0.1–0.5%
0.0–0.1%
Not available

brovascular infarction or haemorrhage, and secondary effects of CNS tumours and infections. HIV aseptic meningitis or encephalitis is characterized by foci of microglia, macrophages and multinucleated giant cells. Vacuolar myelopathy refers to intramyelinic or periaxonal vacuoles, present in the terminal phases and associated with weakness and sphincter disturbance.

Investigations

Diagnosis of HIV infection is usually made from ELISA or Western blot antibody detection. These tests only give a positive result about 2 months after initial infection. Markers of CNS involvement include ventricular enlargement, cortical atrophy, subcortical white matter lesions and an abnormal CSF. It has been reported that perfusion deficits are seen in two-thirds of asymptomatic patients.

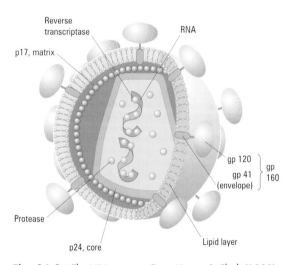

Fig. 26.2 The HIV structure. From Kumar & Clark (1998).

OUTCOME

Management

The management of HIV-infected patients is becoming increasingly sophisticated. There is also prevention and screening to consider. Beyond symptomatic management, antiretroviral treatment is briefly reviewed in Chapter 58.

Prognosis

It is universally acknowledged that prognosis is poor. Death often occurs within a year of developing dementia, although there is considerable individual variability. Constant therapeutic developments are improving the prognosis.

Table 26.2 Characteristics of 2864 patients with HIV in the USA

Characteristic	Proportion of patients (%)
Male	77.4
White	49.2
African-American	32.8
Hispanic	14.8
Heterosexual	40.4
Homosexual	47.4
Bisexual	5.4
Sexually abstinent	6.8
CDC asymptomatic	7.6
CDC symptomatic	33.6
CDC AIDS	58.8
Any psychiatric disorder	47.9
Illicit drug use	50.1
Drug dependence	12.5
Alcohol use	53.4

CDC, Centers for Disease Control and Prevention
Adapted from Bing et al (2001)

Clinical Pointer 26.1

Recognizing AIDS-induced cerebral lesions

AIDS causes a wide variety of lesions that can have an impact on the CNS. Metabolic encephalopathy, cerebrovascular accidents, malignancies and opportunistic infections are the most common causes. Ominous new symptoms in patients with established HIV infection include headaches, pyrexia, weakness, disturbed vision, partial seizures or any sign of localized CNS disease. *Toxoplasma gondii* causes cerebral toxoplasmosis, the most common infection. CT scanning reveals multiple ring-shaped lesions. Syphilis and tuberculosis are serious infections in immunosuppressed patients; they usually present with meningitis. Primary cerebral lymphoma presents like toxoplasmosis, but with solitary rather than multiple lesions. Infection with the JC virus causes progressive multifocal leukoencephalopathy, presenting in a similar fashion to multiple sclerosis. See also Chapter 29.

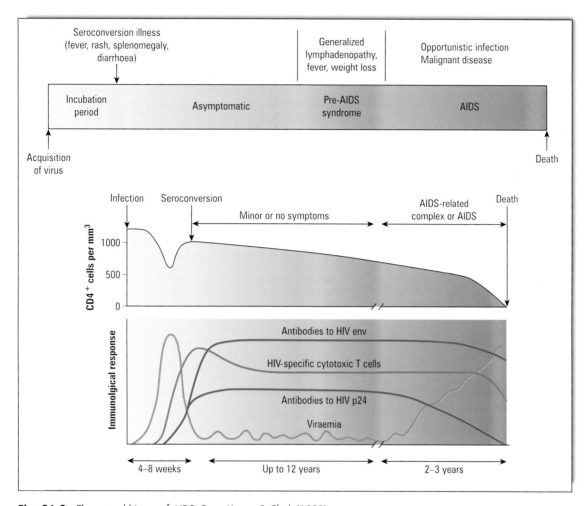

Fig. 26.3 The natural history of AIDS. From Kumar & Clark (1998).

NEUROPSYCHIATRIC COMPLICATIONS OF HIV AND AIDS

Given sufficient time, HIV will invade the CNS in most cases. HIV is capable of crossing the blood–brain barrier early in the course of disease via infected monocytes. Once in the CNS the virus infects macrophages and microglia rather than neurones themselves. At autopsy, around 75% of cases have neuropathological findings and one-third have multiple CNS lesions. The most severe complication is AIDS dementia, which is now one of the most common causes of dementia in young men.

Much valuable information about the psychiatric complications of HIV comes from the large Health Costs and Services Utilization Cohort, a nationally representative sample of HIV-infected adults receiving outpatient medical care in the USA (Bing et al 2001). In this sample, multiple regression analyses showed that the likelihood of screening positive for a psychiatric disorder was greater in those under 35 years old, in people of white ethnic groups, in those who lived alone, in those who were unemployed and in those who were disabled.

Cognitive impairment in HIV

Cognitive impairment can occur in early stages of HIV infection and tends to fluctuate with time. Among those with mild or even asymptomatic neuropsychological impairment, about half will remain stable over the first 5 years of follow-up. In those treated with antiretroviral therapy, approximately half of patients with baseline deficits will show substantial improvements over 3 years (Tozzi et al 2001). In patients who have progressed to AIDS, delirium and AIDS dementia are also important causes of cognitive impairment.

Mild cognitive impairment

Mild impairment is much more common than severe cognitive deficits. Indeed, subtle neuropsychological changes are seen in one-quarter to one-third of HIV-positive people under 40 years old who are otherwise asymptomatic (Fig. 26.4) (Starace et al 1998). In people with AIDS aged over 50 years the proportion with some degree of cognitive impairment may reach 90%. This category is sometimes referred to using the cumbersome term 'minor cognitive–motor disorder'. DSM-IV has no established place for this condition, but proposes research criteria. Mild cognitive deficits are not insignificant, because they are associated with social difficulties, problems with driving, reduced compliance with medication, and unemployment (Grant 2002). These deficits also have a negative influence on survival.

Most patients with mild cognitive impairment develop problems with attention, information processing speed, retaining new information and, to a lesser extent, verbal fluency. These are the same type of deficits seen in many people with more severe types of HIV-related cognitive impairment.

HIV-related delirium

Delirium is seen in about 10% of patients who are HIV-positive and in 25–50% of hospitalized patients with AIDS. Delirium may be the most common single neuropsychiatric complication in AIDS sufferers. As with all types of delirium, delirium in HIV is associated with poor outcome, including longer hospital stays, increased need for long-term care at discharge and higher mortality rates (Uldall et al 2000). In one study, only one-third of patients who recovered from AIDS delirium had full recovery of cognitive function (Fernandez et al 1989).

The presentations of delirium and organic psychosis overlap in patients with HIV (Fig. 26.5). Delusions and hallucinations are features of both conditions. Approximately half of all cases of new-onset psychosis in HIV infection have underlying cerebral disease, most commonly cerebral oppor-

---

> **Box 26.2 Causes of delirium in HIV and AIDS**
>
> Cerebral opportunistic infections:
> - Aspergillus
> - Candida albicans
> - Coccidioides immitis
> - Cryptococcus neoformans
> - cytomegalovirus
> - herpes simplex virus
> - Mycobacterium tuberculosis
> - Toxoplasma gondii
> - Treponema pallidum
>
> Metabolic encephalopathy
>
> Cerebrovascular accidents
>
> Malignancies:
> - Kaposi's sarcoma
> - CNS lymphoma
>
> Drug-induced:
> - illicit drugs and alcohol
> - prescribed drugs
>
> Primary CNS HIV infection
>
> AIDS dementia
>
> HIV-related systemic illness

---

tunistic infections or metabolic encephalopathy (Alciati et al 2001). The majority of such cases present with features of delirium. The syndrome of delirium may manifest without evidence of organic pathology, although this is rare. For this reason all HIV-infected patients with new-onset psychosis, fluctuating attention or cognition and out-of-character agitation should be fully investigated for cerebral involvement.

AIDS dementia

This increasingly common dementia occurs in 7% or more of patients who are HIV-positive and 25% of patients with late-stage AIDS. From the database of the Centers for Disease Control and Prevention in the USA, which contains data on 144,184 people with AIDS, those diagnosed before the age of 14 years and those diagnosed after the age of 60 years had a 10–15% probability of having AIDS dementia as their initial presentation (Hinkin et al 2001).

Brain and CSF levels of HIV-1 RNA correlate with the severity of the dementia. However, another 25% of patients who die from AIDS have evidence of encephalitis at post-mortem, most commonly due to cytomegalovirus (recognized by comorbid retinitis, colitis and disturbed adrenal function). The pathology responsible does not appear to be one single process, but a combination of neuronal loss, diffuse white matter vacuolar lesions and small-vessel vascular disease. Microscopically one finds reduced density of dendritic spines and foci of inflammatory multinucleated giant cells in the hippocampi and cerebral cortex. There are also reduced *N*-acetylaspartate concentrations. Macroscopically there is ventricular enlargement and cortical atrophy. HIV can invade any brain region, although the greatest concentration of the virus tends to be in subcortical grey structures, such as the basal ganglia. Thus, AIDS dementia is most commonly described as a subcortical dementia, but this may be misleading since diverse neuropsychological complications can occur as a result of diverse pathological processes.

Early neuropsychiatric features of HIV dementia include changes in behaviour, mood and cognition. Patients may present with parkinsonian features. Notable behavioural problems are social withdrawal and reduced function both at work and at home. Psychiatric problems are those of apathy, blunted affect and depression. Cognitively, patients complain of forgetfulness, bradyphrenia and poor concentration, although insight is usually preserved. Neuropsychological tests typically reveal abnormalities in spontaneity, motor speed and visual memory. Language function is usually relatively preserved. These findings are accompanied by neurological signs of poor coordination, loss of balance, tremor and, in some cases, inaccurate eye tracking. In the advanced stages of disease, hyperreflexia, dysdiodokokinesia (rapid alternating movements), ocular pursuit abnormalities, myoclonus and frontal

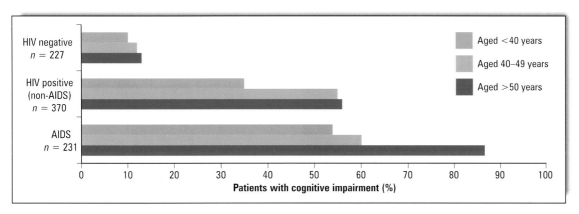

Fig. 26.4 Cognitive impairment in 976 patients with HIV infection and AIDS. Data from Hardy et al (1999).

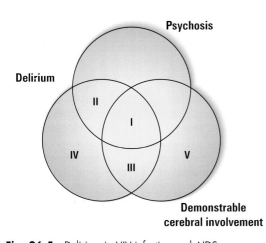

Explanation

Psychotic symptoms in patients with neurological disease should always raise the suspicion of delirium. Delirium may be present in the following ways:

I – delirium with psychotic features and clear cerebral involvement
II – delirium without demonstrable cause
III – delirium without psychotic features
IV – delirium without psychotic features or demonstrable cause
V – asymptomatic cerebral predisposition to delirium

Fig. 26.5 Delirium in HIV infection and AIDS.

release signs develop. Gradually, there is a global deterioration in cognitive function, with incontinence, seizures or myoclonus and, eventually, progression to mutism.

Mechanisms of dementia in HIV and AIDS

It is reasonable to postulate a direct relationship between the area of the brain affected by HIV and the type and severity of the cognitive deficit. Proving this hypothesis is a challenge because it is difficult to map accurately the affected brain regions during life. General markers of the severity of HIV infection tend to show a weak correlation with cognitive deficits. CSF viral load is a better marker than plasma viral load, but a poor marker nevertheless. Low levels of haemoglobin and elevated levels of CSF B2 microglobulin have been suggested to be risk factors for dementia in very provisional work. Intravenous drug abusers, particularly those using methamphetamine, may be at particular risk of developing cognitive impairment.

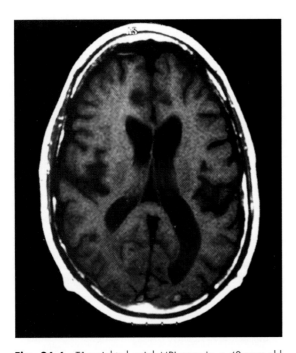

Fig. 26.6 T1-weighted axial MRI scan in a 43-year-old man with AIDS dementia. This patient with advanced AIDS presented with a gradual decline in motivation and marked impairment in multiple cognitive areas. The scan shows no focal lesions, but there is ventricular dilatation and sulcal predominance. From James M Powers, Deparment of Neurology, University of Rochester School of Medicine and Dentistry.

One interesting line of research concerns the effect of HIV infection on the basal ganglia. HIV selectively targets the basal ganglia, resulting in major loss of dopaminergic neurones. Patients with AIDS dementia often present with parkinsonian features and are sensitive to antidopaminergic medication. One study found that low concentrations of a dopamine metabolite, homovanillic acid, in the CSF correlated with neuropsychological impairments in AIDS dementia (Di Rocco et al 2000). Other indicators of cognitive dysfunction have been found on post-mortem analysis, for example reductions in dendritic spine density in the frontal lobes.

Mood disorder in HIV infection and AIDS

Adjustment disorder

When diagnosed with an irreversible disease of poor prognosis, patients are forced to face the implications for themselves and their loved ones. Adjustment is more difficult when the disorder is widely feared and misconceived by the public. Where worries interfere with normal function for several weeks or more, the diagnosis of adjustment disorder is made. Adjustment disorders are therefore common, being typified by shock, distress and protest, and later by gradual resolution. It is usual to specify anxious, depressed or mixed subtypes.

Depression

Depression in HIV infection is a dynamic process that is heavily influenced by cultural variables. The rates of depression in the following groups are of interest to those studying the neuropsychiatric aspects of HIV infection: healthy controls with HIV-related risk factors alone, asymptomatic HIV-positive individuals, symptomatic HIV-positive individuals and patients with AIDS.

A recent meta-analysis has helped to document the rates of depression in these groups. Using two meta-analytic techniques, Ciesla & Roberts (2001) examined 10 studies involving over 2500 depressed patients with HIV. A total of 9.4% of HIV-positive people had major depression, compared with 5.2% of those who were HIV-negative. Furthermore, 4% of HIV-positive individuals had dysthymia, compared with 2% of those who were HIV-negative. The drawback of this meta-analysis was that the HIV-positive group included both symptomatic and asymptomatic individuals and the HIV-negative group included high-risk and low-risk controls. If one compares the rates of depression in presymptomatic HIV-seropositive people, symptomatic HIV-positive people and high-risk groups, there are subtle differences (Table 26.3). The rate of depression (at least in Western cultures) in symptomatic sufferers is of the order of 20% (Maj 1997). Note that this figure may not be robust because the condition continually evolves and thus studying a comparable cohort is difficult. At least one study has found that major depression, in patients who have progressed to AIDS, may affect as many as two-thirds of sufferers (Hinkin et al 2001). Symptoms of depression in HIV infection feature high rates of fatigue and insomnia. In early stages of HIV infection these somatic symptoms are more valid indicators of depression than underlying HIV activity measured by CD4$^+$ cell counts (Perkins et al 1995). Comorbidity in depressed patients with HIV infection is frequently present. A useful rule of thumb is that one-third of depressed patients have alcohol problems, one-third have medical problems and one-third have depression alone (Fig. 26.7).

The relative risk of suicide is greatly elevated in HIV-infected people compared with that of an age-matched healthy population, but it may not be appreciably increased relative to high-risk HIV-negative groups. Risk factors for depression and suicide in HIV infection are:

- previous psychiatric history
- accidental inoculation
- lack of social support or confiding relationship, loss of friends and exposure to stigma
- loss of job, role, status or finances
- severe, rapidly progressive, disabling or overt disease
- experience of HIV-related bereavements.

Mania

Bipolar affective disorders are beginning to be examined in seropositive patients, with one suggestion being that high rates of soft bipolar disorders (i.e. bipolar disorders not reaching the full criteria for mania or hypomania) exist premorbidly. Bipolar affective disorders are more common in patients with AIDS than in those with non-AIDS HIV infection, and true mania tends to develop late in the disease. Case series suggest that the majority of cases of new-onset mania in HIV-seropositive individuals are cases of secondary mania. Thus mania is suggestive of CNS disease and should prompt further investigations to rule out a treatable brain lesion.

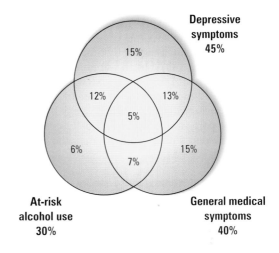

Explanation

Self-reported complications of HIV infection in 768 subjects (mean age 49 years) treated with HAART. Includes 115 patients with CD4$^+$ counts below 200 cells/mm^3. The majority of those with general medical complaints had either depression or excessive alcohol use. The rate of problematic drinking was not significantly elevated in HIV sufferers who were neither depressed nor experiencing medical comorbidity.

Fig. 26.7 Comorbidity in HIV-infected patients with depressive symptoms. Data from Kilbourne et al (2001).

Table 26.3 Rates (%) of major depression and cognitive impairment across a spectrum of HIV-related disorders

	Healthy control	High-risk group (IV drug users)	Asymptomatic HIV-positive	Symptomatic HIV-positive	HIV-positive IV drug users
Depression	5	5–10	10	11–20	20
Cognitive impairment	2.5	8			23

IV, intravenous

Apathy

Apathy is seen in HIV-positive patients with approximately the same frequency as depression. In fact, apathy has been associated with depression and cognitive impairment in HIV. Conceivably the predictors of apathy may vary according to the stage of the disease. In all stages one would anticipate that depression is the main predictive factor but in the later stages, particularly in patients approaching AIDS dementia, cognition is likely to show increasing inverse correlation with apathy.

Anxiety

There have been relatively few studies of anxiety disorders in HIV-positive individuals. In a modest sample of 113 HIV-positive men, one study found a low 12-month prevalence rate of generalized anxiety disorder of 2.4% but a higher lifetime prevalence of 15% (Drew et al 1997). In the same study, adjustment disorder with anxious mood was very common, with a 12-month prevalence rate of 23%. Risk factors for anxiety disorder were a psychiatric history, low support from partner and a 'low sense of mastery'. Other studies suggest that the rate of panic disorder is about 5% and not greatly elevated. However, these studies have not examined anxiety over an extended period. Post-traumatic stress disorder can develop in response to various life-threatening traumatic events during the course of infection with HIV.

Mechanism of HIV-related mood disorders

Of developing interest is whether depression affects immune parameters in HIV infection and, furthermore, whether depression affects mortality. To date, studies do not show any relationship between antidepressant therapy or antidepressant response and severity of immunosuppression. In the large-scale HIV Epidemiologic Research Study (Ickovics et al 2001), an association between depression and mortality was seen (see Clinical Pointer 58.1).

Psychosis in HIV infection and AIDS

There is a slightly higher than expected prevalence of schizophrenia-like psychosis in patients with HIV infection, of about 6% (Walkup et al 1999).

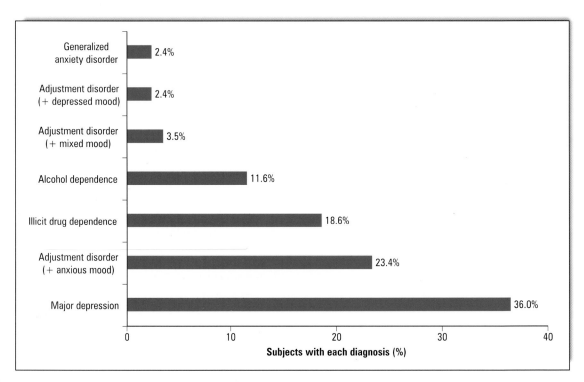

Fig. 26.8 One-year prevalence of various psychiatric diagnoses in HIV-positive men. Data from Drew et al (1997).

Clinical Pointer 26.2

Distinguishing bereavement and depression in people with HIV infection

HIV dramatically increases the exposure of young people to the effects of losing a loved one through death. In many cases, it is not clear whether a presentation with dysphoria and distress is due to normal grief, a complicated bereavement reaction or a depressive disorder. The core feature of grief is a yearning or pining after the deceased. It is important to remember that every depressive symptom can occur in the context of normal grief. This is probably because bereavement and depression are closely related conditions that overlap considerably. Bereavement itself is the single most common life event that causes depression. Nevertheless, certain symptoms are good indicators that depression is present and requires treatment. These include pessimism about the future, low self-esteem, guilt (unrelated to the deceased) and recurrent suicidal thoughts. Furthermore, the presence of severe distress or dysfunction may be reasonably considered enough to begin treatment with antidepressants. The majority of such patients will benefit, although a minority will require a reduction of dose to help them express what they consider to be normal emotional responses. A short course of antidepressants (of up to 3 months) may suffice.

Further reading Prigerson HG, Bierhals AJ, Kasl SV et al 1996 Complicated grief as a disorder distinct from bereavement-related depression and anxiety: a replication study. *American Journal of Psychiatry* 153:1484–1486

Psychosis is also a recognized complication of direct HIV-related CNS disease and is seen in at least 15% of patients with AIDS dementia. Medical complications in the late stages of AIDS and concurrent illicit drug use are confounding factors in the relationship between HIV infection and psychosis. Patients who develop first-onset psychosis after the diagnosis of AIDS appear to have a higher than expected mortality rate. Most psychotic disorders are thus of organic origin (whether or not the cause is identified) rather than a primary schizophreniform illness. Many psychotic disorders have an affective flavour, particularly manic presentations. Interestingly, these may respond better to treatment than the schizophreniform psychoses.

prisingly, have difficulty coming to terms with a much-feared diagnosis. There can be no doubt that HIV-positive intravenous drug users and symptomatic HIV-positive patients have increased rates of depression and cognitive impairment. The direct and indirect effects of HIV infection on the brain should not be underestimated when assessing problems in cognition, mood or psychosis, even though this impact cannot easily be measured during life. Given sufficient time the virus almost invariably invades the CNS. Most sufferers will at some point have signs of cognitive impairment, although only a minority will go on to develop AIDS dementia. A new onset of psychotic or manic symptoms in a person with HIV infection is a clear indication for investigation of direct CNS involvement.

SUMMARY

Infection with HIV devastates cell-mediated immunity, enabling opportunistic infections and cancer to invade the CNS. Although AIDS has not reached the epidemic proportions in the Western world that some had predicted, it has become one of the most common causes of cognitive impairment in young people. Furthermore, a rapidly increasing rate in the developing world (particularly in women and children) along with limited resources means that, worldwide, the impact is severe. An estimated 1% of adults worldwide are infected with HIV. HIV infection is frequently associated with chaotic lifestyles that make studying the association of HIV infection and neuropsychiatric complications difficult. Asymptomatic people with HIV infection have increased rates of adjustment disorder and, unsur-

REFERENCES AND FURTHER READING

Alciati A, Fusi A, Monforte AD et al 2001 New-onset delusions and hallucinations in patients infected with HIV. Journal of Psychiatry and Neuroscience 26:229–234

Bing EG, Burnam MA, Longshore D et al 2001 Psychiatric disorders and drug use among human immunodeficiency virus infected adults in the United States. Archives of General Psychiatry 58:721–728

Ciesla JA, Roberts JE 2001 Meta-analysis of the relationship between HIV infection and risk for depressive disorders. American Journal of Psychiatry 158:725–730

Di Rocco A, Bottiglieri T, Dorfman D et al 2000 Decreased homovanillic acid in cerebrospinal fluid correlates with impaired neuropsychologic function in HIV-1-infected patients. Clinics in Neuropharmacology 23:190–194

Drew MA, Becker JT, Sanchez J et al 1997 Prevalence and predictors of depressive, anxiety and substance use disorders in HIV-infected and uninfected men: a longitudinal evaluation. Psychology in Medicine 27:395–409

Fernandez F, Levy JK, Mansell PWA 1989 Management of delirium in terminally ill AIDS patients. International Journal of Psychiatry in Medicine 19:165–172

Gottlieb MS, Schroff R, Schanker HM et al 1981 *Pneumocystis carinii* pneumonia and mucosal candidiasis in previously healthy homosexual men: evidence of a new acquired cellular immunodeficiency. New England Journal of Medicine 1305:1425–1431

Grant I 2002 The neurocognitive complications of HIV infection. In: Ramachandran VS (ed) Encyclopedia of the human brain. Academic Press, San Diego

Hardy ?? 1999 Poster presented at Fourth Annual Research Conference on Aging. University of California, Los Angeles

Hinkin CH, Castellon SA, Atkinson JH et al 2001 Neuropsychiatric aspects of HIV infection among older adults. Journal of Clinical Epidemiology 54:s44–s52

Ickovics JR, Hamburger ME, Vlahov D et al 2001 Mortality, CD4 cell count decline, and depressive symptoms among HIV-seropositive women: longitudinal analysis from the HIV epidemiology research study. JAMA 285:1466–1474

Kilbourne AM, Justice AC, Rabeneck L 2001 General medical and psychiatric comorbidity among HIV-infected veterans in the post-HAART era. Journal of Clinical Epidemiology 54:S22–S28

Kumar P, Clark M 1998 Clinical medicine, 4th edn. Churchill Livingstone, Edinburgh

Maj M 1997 Depression and AIDS. In: Robertson MM, Katona CLE (eds) Depression and physical illness. Wiley, New York, p 186–207

Perkins DO, Stern RA, Golden RN et al 1995 Somatic symptoms and HIV infection: relationship to depressive symptoms and indicators of HIV disease. American Journal of Psychiatry 155:1776–1781

Starace F, Baldassarre C, Biancolilli V et al 1998 Early neuropsychological impairment in HIV-seropositive intravenous drug users: evidence from the Italian Multicentre Neuropsychological HIV Study. Acta Psychiatrica Scandinavica 97:132–138

Tozzi V, Balestra T, Galgani S et al 2001 Changes in neurocognitive performance in a cohort of patients treated with HAART for 3 years. Journal of Acquired Immune Deficiency Syndrome 28:19–27

Uldall KK, Harris VL, Lalonde B 2000 Outcomes associated with delirium in acutely hospitalized acquired immune deficiency syndrome patients. Comprehensive Psychiatry 41:88–91

Walkup J, Crystal S, Sambamoorthi U 1999 Schizophrenia and major affective disorder among Medicaid recipients with HIV/AIDS in New Jersey. American Journal of Public Health 89:1101–1103

27

Neurosyphilis

My clinical observations have led me to the following classification of the symptoms of syphilis ... Primary symptom (accident primitif), chancre from the direct action of the virus which it produces, and by means of which it propagates itself ... Secondary symptoms, or symptoms of general infection ... Tertiary symptoms, (accidents tertiares) occurring at indefinite periods, but generally long after the cessation of the primary affection. (Phillippe Ricord 1838)

BACKGROUND

Syphilis is a systemic infection caused by *Treponema pallidum*, a spirochaete, discovered by Schaudinn

Table 27.1 Symptoms of neurosyphilis

Symptom	Patients affected (%)
Hyporeflexia	50
Sensory impairment	48
Pupillary changes	43
Cranial neuropathy	36
Personality change	33
Ataxia	28
Romberg's sign	24
Stroke	23
Ophthalmic symptoms	17
Urinary symptoms	17
Charcot joint	10
Lightning pains	10
Headache	10
Dizziness	10
Hearing loss	10
Seizures	7
Optic atrophy	7

Adapted from Sotero de Menezes & Knudsen (2001)

and Hoffman while working in Hamburg in 1905. It is a sexually transmitted disease which, after an incubation period of weeks or months, causes a chancre and lymphadenopathy (primary syphilis). If untreated, secondary syphilis, characterized by malaise, rash and ulcers, and later tertiary syphilis, featuring visceral involvement with granulomas called gummas, ensue. Aggressive disease progresses into the CNS and the cardiovascular system. Meningovascular syphilis is now the most common neuropsychiatric complication and can occur at any stage of the infection. Before antibiotics, general paralysis of the insane was the most common cause of dementia worldwide. AIDS has caused a recent resurgence in syphilis.

CLINICAL AND NEUROPSYCHIATRIC FEATURES

The CNS is invaded in 30–40% of infected individuals but only 5% develop symptoms.

Quaternary syphilis

Quarternary syphilis (also known as aggressive tertiary syphilis) involves the CNS, most notably with meningovascular complications, tabes dorsalis and general paralysis of the insane. In neurosyphilis,

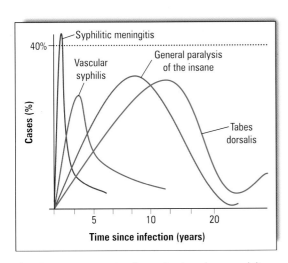

Fig. 27.1 Time course of complications due to syphilis. Data from Simon (1985).

193

there is normally an asymptomatic stage without symptoms but with abnormal CSF findings.

Meningovascular syphilis

Meningovascular syphilis presents 2–10 years after the primary infection. An acute presentation with meningitis or stroke is typical following the inflammation of large vessels. Occasionally, small vessel disease causes an insidious dementia.

General paralysis of the insane

General paralysis of the insane is probably a consequence of chronic meningitis. Disturbance in cognition and mood progressing towards dementia is the typical presentation. Frontal lobe atrophy is common and hence judgement and motivation are often impaired. The onset is often insidious, with subtle changes in personality, motivation and irritability noted by family and friends. Historically, elevated mood was frequently described, but this is now seen in less than 10% of modern cases. Other presentations (as described by Lishman) are simple dementia, depression and mixed presentations with tabes dorsalis. Associated neurological features are seizures (in 50%), dysarthria, the Argyll–Robertson pupil, atrophy of facial muscles and a coarse tremor. Symptoms can wax and wane with time and can be exacerbated by stress. Microscopically, *Treponema pallidum* invades the brain directly, causing enlarged microglia and perivascular infiltrates, especially in the ventricular walls. Macroscopically, the cortex is atrophied with thickened dura (Fig. 27.3).

Tabes dorsalis

In tabes dorsalis there is degeneration and demyelination of the ascending posterior column. This pro-

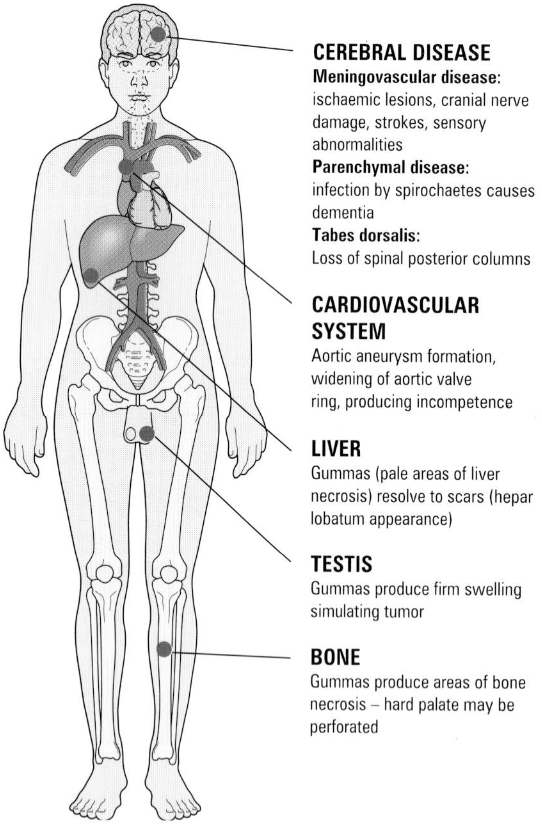

CEREBRAL DISEASE
Meningovascular disease:
ischaemic lesions, cranial nerve damage, strokes, sensory abnormalities
Parenchymal disease:
infection by spirochaetes causes dementia
Tabes dorsalis:
Loss of spinal posterior columns

CARDIOVASCULAR SYSTEM
Aortic aneurysm formation, widening of aortic valve ring, producing incompetence

LIVER
Gummas (pale areas of liver necrosis) resolve to scars (hepar lobatum appearance)

TESTIS
Gummas produce firm swelling simulating tumor

BONE
Gummas produce areas of bone necrosis – hard palate may be perforated

Fig. 27.2 Systemic effects of syphilis. From Stevens & Lowe (2000).

> **Box 27.1 Infections that produce neuropsychiatric disease**
>
> *Bacterial infections*
> Tuberculosis (*Mycobacterium tuberculosis*)
> Whipple's disease (*Tropheryma whippelii*)
> Syphilis (*Treponema pallidum*)
> Lyme disease (*Borrelia burgdorferi*)
>
> *Fungal infections*
> Candida (*Candida albicans*)
> Cryptococcosis (*Cryptococcus neoformans*)
> Coccidioidomycosis (*Coccidioides immitis*)
> Histoplasmosis (*Histoplasma capsulatum*)
>
> *Viral infections*
> Herpes simplex encephalitis type I
> Progressive multifocal leukoencephalopathy (JC virus (papovavirus))
> Subacute sclerosing panencephalitis (measles virus)
> AIDS dementia (HIV)
>
> *Prion diseases*
> Creutzfeldt–Jakob disease
> Fatal familial insomnia
> Kuru
>
> *Parasites*
> Malaria (*Plasmodium* spp.)
> Cysticercosis (*Taenia solium*)
> Toxoplasmosis (*Toxoplasma gondii*)
> Rocky Mountain spotted fever (*Rickettsia rickettsii*)

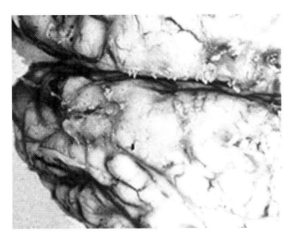

Fig. 27.3 Meningovascular syphilis showing thickening of the meninges on the dorsum of the brain. From Professor G Baumbach, Online Virtual Hospital, University of Iowa.

duces a gradual onset of lightning pain and paraesthesiae in the legs, with loss of proprioception. Other features include incontinence, loss of sexual function, Charcot joints and trophic ulcers (mal perforans). As no spirochaetes have been found in the posterior columns the cause is unclear.

PATHOGENESIS

Pathology

The pathology may be best characterized as an endarteritis obliterans, although direct parenchymal invasion of the brain occurs without arteritis in general paralysis of the insane. Iron pigment in the microglia may be a specific pathological sign.

Investigations

Treponema pallidum can be demonstrated directly using dark-field microscopy. Serological tests are usually employed as follows:

- a venereal disease laboratory test (VDRL) becomes positive within a month of infection, but is negative in treated and latent cases
- the serum fluorescent treponemal antibody (FTA) test looks for IgM and is very sensitive, remaining positive for life

- the *Treponema pallidum* haemagglutination assay is also sensitive in secondary and latent cases
- CSF antibodies (CSF VDRL) can be used to augment the clinical diagnosis of neurosyphilis.

OUTCOME

Prognosis

If neurosyphilis is untreated, the prognosis is poor, with death usually 3–5 years after diagnosis. Treatment can be remarkably effective. In late cases or cases associated with HIV, treatment is more challenging.

SUMMARY

Syphilis has been a source of social stigma for centuries. The term 'syphilis' came from a poem written in 1530 by the Italian poet Hiero Fracastor. The introduction of penicillin in the 1940s led to a dramatic decrease in frequency, but there has been a recent resurgence of the disease, largely accounted for by socioeconomic adversity and HIV. Now about 40,000 cases of syphilis are recorded in the USA each year, 1000 of which are congenital. In the immunocompromised, syphilis can run a more aggressive course. The main pathological processes in neurosyphilis are chronic meningeal inflammation and cerebrovascular disease. Once antibodies have been produced syphilis serology is normally an accurate diagnostic test, although a lumbar puncture may be required to demonstrate CNS involvement. Early intervention is particularly effective.

REFERENCES AND FURTHER READING

Ricord P 1838 Traité pratique des maladies vénériennes. De Just Rouvier and E Le Bouvier, Paris
Simon RP 1985 Neurosyphilis. Archives of Neurology 42:606–613
Sotero de Menezes M, Knudsen RP 2001 Neurosyphilis. eMedicine Journal 2(9). Available: http://www.emedicine.com/NEURO/topic684.htm
Stevens A, Lowe J 2000 Pathology, 2nd edn. Mosby, St. Louis

28

Sydenham's Chorea

This is a kind of convulsion, which attacks boys and girls from the tenth year to the time of puberty. It first shows itself by limping or unsteadiness in one of the legs, which the patient drags. The hand cannot be steady for a moment. It passes from one position to another by a convulsive movement, however, much the patient may strive to the contrary.

Before he can raise a cup to his lips, he makes as many gesticulations as a mountebank; since he does not move in a straight line, but has his hand drawn aside by spasms, until by some good fortune he brings it at last to his mouth. He then gulps it off at once, so suddenly and so greedily as if he were trying to amuse the lookers-on.
(Thomas Sydenham 1686)

BACKGROUND

Sydenham's chorea occurs as an autoimmune complication of rheumatic fever. The proportion of people with acute rheumatic fever who develop chorea has been estimated at 25%. Worldwide, rheumatic heart disease is the most common cardiovascular disease in young adults, affecting at least 12 million people. It is twice as common in girls as boys. It follows within 6 months of infection with β-haemolytic group A *Streptococcus* and is thought to result from cross-reactivity of streptococcal antibodies to neuronal cytoplasmic antigens in caudate and subthalamic nuclei. It is also known as St. Vitus' dance, a name that gives away the main complication (i.e. chorea). There is sometimes a mixed picture of agi-

tation, psychosis and delirium, known as *maniacal chorea*. An acute attack is almost always accompanied by psychiatric symptoms such as irritability, impulsivity, obsessions and compulsions, and tics.

PATHOGENESIS

Aetiology

Streptococcal infection is thought to cause small vessel autoimmune disease (i.e. vasculitis). In addition, encephalitis without vasculitis has been documented.

Investigations

Rheumatic fever titres may be negative. The appearance on MRI may be abnormal, especially in the region of the basal ganglia. Caudate volumes are smaller in those with long-standing obsessive–compulsive disorder, but larger in acute PANDAS syndrome. Sufferers may have a higher percentage of B cells that react with the monoclonal antibody D8/17, a marker for rheumatic fever. This may also be a marker for childhood PANDAS syndrome.

OUTCOME

Management

Immediate and prophylactic treatment for rheumatic fever is essential. Case series show that chorea itself can be managed with sodium valproate, carbamazepine or haloperidol.

Prognosis

The course of the disorder is often self-limiting, with many cases spontaneously resolving within 2 years, although exacerbations of chorea occur with recurrence of rheumatic fever.

NEUROPSYCHIATRIC COMPLICATIONS OF SYDENHAM'S CHOREA

Patients can experience several types of movement disorder. The most common of these is chorea, in a

The presence of two major criteria, or of one major and two minor criteria, indicates a high probability of acute rheumatic fever, if supported by evidence of preceding group A streptococcal infection.

Major criteria
Myocarditis
Polyarthritis
Chorea
Erythema marginatum
Subcutaneous nodules

Minor criteria
Laboratory:
● acute phase reactants
● prolonged PR interval

Clinical:
● arthralgia
● fever
● previous rheumatic fever or rheumatic heart disease

After the American Heart Association (1965)

generalized pattern often associated with dysarthria and weakness. Rarely, seizures, cranial neuropathies and encephalopathy occur. Psychiatric features are those of emotional lability, memory problems, agitation, obsessive–compulsive disorder and poor concentration. Rarely, there is psychosis or delirium develops. In a recent study of 22 children with Sydenham's chorea, 20 with rheumatic fever and 20 healthy children, obsessive–compulsive symptoms were more frequent in both the Sydenham's chorea group and the rheumatic fever group than in the comparison group (Mercadante et al 2000). The Sydenham's chorea group had a higher frequency of major depressive disorder, tic disorders and attention-deficit hyperactivity disorder (ADHD) than both the comparison and rheumatic fever groups. ADHD symptoms were associated with a higher risk of developing Sydenham's chorea.

THE SPECIAL CASE OF PANDAS SYNDROME

PANDAS is an acronym of *paediatric autoimmune neuropsychiatric disorders associated with streptococcal infections.* Children who have had rheumatic fever are also vulnerable to developing a tic disorder (Tourette's syndrome) or obsessive–compulsive disorder. PANDAS syndrome may account for 10% of childhood obsessive–compulsive disorder. As with chorea, symptoms most often begin about 2 months after a streptococcal infection. It can be difficult to differentiate this condition from primary obsessive–compulsive disorder or classical Tourette's syndrome. One distinguishing feature is that children have complete remissions of symptoms between episodes in PANDAS. In addition, the presence of accompanying neurological signs soft signs, or choreiform movements suggests streptococcal involvement. Other psychiatric features include hyperactivity, oppositional behaviour, emotional lability, exaggerated separation anxiety and cognitive deficits. These symptoms qualify for a comorbid diagnosis of attention deficit hyperactivity syndrome, depression or anxiety disorder in 40% of those affected.

The condition is thought to have an autoimmune basis similar or identical to that proposed in Sydenham's chorea. However, families of PANDAS patients have higher than anticipated rates of tics and obsessive–compulsive disorder: in one study, 39% of probands had at least one first-degree relative with a history of tics and 26% had at least one first-degree relative with obsessive–compulsive disorder (Lougee et al 2000). The contribution of streptococcal-related autoimmune disease to adults with obsessive–compulsive disorder and/or tics is not known (Eisen et al 2001).

Ideal treatment is prevention with a full course of antibiotics at the time of the initial infection. If penicillin or cephalosporins are given early enough, neuropsychiatric symptoms can be reversed. More chronic complications tend to be refractory to treatment. Although in these cases the use of intravenous immunoglobulin or therapeutic plasma

● The presence of obsessive–compulsive disorder and/or tic disorder
● Prepubertal onset of symptoms
● Sudden onset or episodic course
● Temporal association with streptococcal infections
● Associated neurological abnormalities

exchange has been suggested, it has not yet been tested scientifically.

SUMMARY

Sydenham's chorea is a movement disorder occurring after approximately 20% of cases of acute rheumatic fever. It is a condition with a peak incidence at 8 years and is more common in girls. Chorea, dysarthria and weakness are the most common features. Sydenham's chorea is often a self-limiting condition, usually spontaneously resolving within 2 years. Children who have had rheumatic fever are also vulnerable to developing a tic disorder or obsessive–compulsive disorder – a condition known by the acronym PANDAS.

REFERENCES AND FURTHER READING

American Heart Association 1965 Jones' criteria (revised) for guidance in the diagnosis of rheumatic fever. Circulation 32:664–668

Eisen JL, Leonard HL, Swedo SE et al 2001 The use of antibody D8/17 to identify B cells in adults with obsessive–compulsive disorder. Psychiatry Research 104:221–225

Lougee L, Perlmutter SJ, Nicolson R et al 2000 Psychiatric disorders in first-degree relatives of children with pediatric autoimmune neuropsychiatric disorders associated with streptococcal infections (PANDAS). Journal of the American Academy of Child Psychiatry 39:1120–1126

Mercadante MT, Busatto CF, Lombroso PJ et al 2000 The psychiatric symptoms of rheumatic fever. American Journal of Psychiatry 157:2036–2038

Sydenham T 1686 Schedula monitoria de novae febris ingressu. Londini, Keyyilby, p 25–28

29

Viral Encephalitis

BACKGROUND

The term 'encephalitis' refers to infection of the brain parenchyma, whereas 'meningitis' refers to infection of the meninges. In viral encephalitis,

---

Box 29.1 Causes of viral meningitis

- Rabies virus: >99% of cases are fatal
- Herpes simplex viruses: >70% of cases are fatal (if untreated)
- Arboviruses: 1–50% of cases are fatal*
- Lymphocytic choriomeningitis virus: common mild encephalitis; rare deaths
- Mumps virus: common mild encephalitis; rare deaths[†]
- Cytomegalovirus: occasional encephalitis with infectious mononucleosis
- Epstein–Barr virus: occasional encephalitis with infectious mononucleosis[†]
- Adenoviruses: rare cases of serious encephalitis in children
- HIV: rare acute encephalitis at the time of primary infection
- Human herpes virus: mild encephalitis in children
- Coxsackie viruses and echoviruses: rare fatal encephalitis in neonates

*California encephalitis is fatal in <1% of children, western encephalitis in 10% of infants, St. Louis encephalitis in 20% of elderly people and eastern encephalitis in 50% of people of all ages

[†]Some fatal cases have the pathology of postinfectious encephalomyelitis; some viruses may cause acute encephalitis and acute disseminated encephalomyelitis

Adapted from Johnson (2001)

---

there is always some involvement of brain and meningeal tissue, so the disease is a really a form of meningoencephalitis. Viral infections may be acute, chronic or latent. Postinfectious encephalomyelitis is an acute, demyelinating disease of the brain and spinal cord that typically occurs a few days or weeks after a respiratory tract infection or after a vaccination, possibly as an autoimmune response. Viruses may account for about 5% of cases of dementia, with the most common single cause being AIDS dementia. Mild viral encephalitis may go virtually unnoticed, with symptoms of mild headache and fatigue, but possible later sequelae. Consistent with this, studies of patients with psychiatric symptoms and fatigue have found higher than expected levels of viral antibodies, a condition originally named *limbic encephalitis* (Glaser & Pincus 1969). The term 'limbic encephalitis' is now usually reserved for a specific paraneoplastic syndrome.

The majority of cases of aseptic meningitis in the western world are caused by enteroviruses. The main cause in the developing world are arboviruses and, needless to say, fatality is much higher (Table 29.1).

SHARED CLINICAL FEATURES

Although there are some common features, the signs and symptoms of viral meningoencephalitis depend on the interaction between the organism and the host. Typically, there is a sudden frontal headache, accompanied by an undulating fever (up to 40°C) with or without a skin rash. Non-specific symptoms of malaise, drowsiness, sore throat, myalgia, bone pain, nausea and vomiting are common. In addition, there may be photophobia, tinnitus, vertigo, paraesthesia and nuchal rigidity. On investigation, the leukocyte count is normal. The CSF appears normal (<500 leukocytes/mm^3), and in the CSF glucose is normal but protein is elevated. Diagnosis usually requires isolation of the virus.

Herpes simplex virus

Of the two types of herpes simplex virus, type 1 accounts for more than 95% of cases, with type 2 being responsible for diffuse encephalitis in newborns of mothers infected with genital herpes. Although most of the population has been infected with herpes simplex virus type 1 at some point, the

Table 29.1   Neuropsychiatric effects of CNS viral infections

Infection (disorder)	Main features and neuropsychiatric symptoms	Investigations	Associated pathological features
Arbovirus (*meningitis*)	These are either mosquito borne (e.g. St. Louis encephalitis, La Crosse virus) or tick borne (e.g. Colorado tick fever) Acute headache and meningeal signs, delirium, tremor, rarely psychosis without delirium	Increased signal on T2-weighted MRI CSF pleocytosis, CSF glucose normal	Eastern equine encephalitis is concentrated in the cortex, Western equine encephalitis in the basal nuclei, and St. Louis encephalitis in the substantia nigra, thalamus, pons, cerebellum, cortex, bulb, and anterior horn cells
Cytomegalovirus (*encephalitis*)	Headache, fever, weakness, delirium, withdrawal	Petechial haemorrhage, neuronal loss (ventricular enlargement), micronecrosis Increased signal on T2-weighted MRI	Myelitis, radiculopathy. At post-mortem, microglial nodules (containing virus around cytomegalic cells). Ependymitis
Epstein–Barr virus (*infectious mononucleosis*)	Prodrome of headache and fatigue followed by lymphadenopathy and pharyngitis. Delirium, meningitis and convulsions in a minority	Monospot test PCR CSF test for DNA	CSF has a lymphocytic pleocytosis, an elevated protein concentration and a normal glucose concentration
Herpes simplex virus (*acute encephalitis*)	Gradual onset of headache, fever, delirium. Focal neurological signs. Amnesia, rarely dementia, Klüver–Bucy syndrome	Increased signal on T2-weighted MRI CSF for HSV DNA (2–10 days)*	Neurotoxic effects noted at post-mortem; limbic tissue necrosis
HIV-1 (*HIV encephalitis*)	Apathy, depression, social withdrawal; later, hyperreflexia, dysdiodokinesia, myoclonus, frontal release signs	Ventricular enlargement, cortical atrophy, subcortical white matter lesions	Indirect invasions of macrophages and microglia, associated aseptic meningitis, vacuolar myelopathy
Influenza A virus (*encephalitis lethargica*)	Headache, delirium, sleep disturbance, oculomotor pareses, oculogyric crises, catatonia, parkinsonism	Antibody test	Secondary infections
Mumps (paramyxovirus) (*acute encephalitis*)	Childhood onset of fever, malaise and myalgia with bilateral parotiditis. Meningitis in 15%	CFS lymphocytosis Increased protein	Perivascular infiltrate, focal perivascular demyelination
Papovavirus and JC virus (*progressive multifocal leukoencephalopathy*)	Hemiplegia, hemianopia, delirium or dementia often leading to death. Occurs in immunosuppressed patients	CSF normal Reduced signal on T1-weighted (non-enhancing) MRI	Destruction of oligodendrocytes leads to inclusion bodies and demyelination in subcortical white matter

contd

Table 29.1 *Contd*

Infection (disorder)	Main features and neuropsychiatric symptoms	Investigations	Associated pathological features
Rabies (rhabdovirus) (*rabies encephalitis*)	Rapid and fatal encephalitis. Acutely (furious phase) causes severe anxiety, agitation, irritability, hydrophobia and seizures. Chronically (paralytic phase) apathy, tachycardia, delirium, generalized flaccid paralysis and, ultimately, death	Isolation of the virus from saliva	Neurotoxic, neuronal eosinophilic cytoplasmic inclusions bodies (Negri bodies)
Measles (*subacute sclerosing panencephalitis*)	Subacute lethargy and delirium, myoclonus, seizures (measles encephalitis). Insidious dementia with later focal signs and seizures progressing to stupor. In adults can present with psychosis	Cortical atrophy on MRI; increased intensity on T2-weighted images EEG rhythmic slow waves	Inclusion bodies in neuroglia with gliosis
Varicella-zoster virus (*chickenpox*)	Rarely, transverse myelitis, cerebellar ataxia, meningitis or encephalitis	Infarcts, haemorrhages or white matter lesions on MRI	Hemorrhagic infarctions secondary to a vasculopathy; deep white matter lesions from mixed ischaemic and/or demyelinative change

*Very high accuracy has been reported in CSF samples taken 2–10 days after onset of symptoms, but accuracy decreases thereafter.

virus is reactivated in a tiny handful of people, with devastating results. Why these individuals succumb to this severe form of the infection is unclear, as they have mounted an early immune response and the virus is the same strain as in those who are unaffected. It is possible that an abnormal immune response causing immune-mediated cell death (as well as direct viral neurotoxicity) is involved.

Herpes simplex encephalitis presents with a severe form of encephalitis, characterized by fever, headache, focal neurological signs, autonomic dysfunction, nuchal rigidity and often delirium and seizures. For unknown reasons, the medial temporal lobes are preferentially affected, with haemorrhagic necrosis observable at autopsy (Fig. 29.1). This could explain the observation that 50% of cases have personality change at the time of diagnosis. Neighbouring orbitofrontal areas are likely to suffer damage.

Histology may reveal eosinophilic Cowdry type A inclusion bodies (Fig. 29.3). CSF shows elevated protein and pleocytosis with red blood cells and normal glucose (low glucose is seen in bacterial menin-

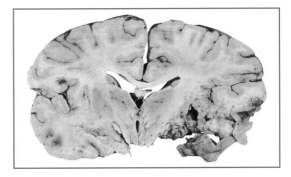

Fig. 29.1 Post-mortem specimen with herpes simplex encephalitis. There is marked necrosis of the right temporal lobe, and petechial haemorrhages and early necrosis in the left temporal lobe. From Cooke & Stewart (1995).

gitis). Historically an EEG has been one of the most useful tests, demonstrating slow waves and periodic spikes in 2-second bursts in over 80% of cases. CT scans are usually unremarkable in the early stages, but on MRI there is increased signal intensity on T2-weighted images of the medial temporal lobe.

Where diagnosis is in doubt, a brain biopsy is purported to be accurate and safe. However, this has been superseded by the polymerase chain reaction analysis of CSF, which detects viral DNA within 24 hours of CNS infection.

Clinically, a dense anterograde amnesia is typical, with variable retrograde amnesia that resembles Korsakoff's syndrome. There may be further cognitive deficits that warrant a diagnosis of dementia or, in some cases, Klüver–Bucy syndrome. Hallucinations and seizures also occur. Mortality can be as high as 70% in those who are comatose and aged above 30 years. Residual neurological deficits are common. Treatment with acyclovir improves outcome, but only if there is little delay in starting treatment.

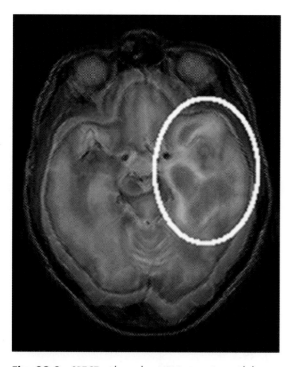

Fig. 29.2 SPECT with overlay MRI in a patient with herpes simplex encephalitis. The patient was alert and oriented but unable to name objects properly. Dysarthria, occasional word substitution and neologisms were noted. Neurological examination was normal. A CT scan showed a low-attenuation lesion involving the medial and posterior aspect of the left temporal lobe and the inferior basal ganglia. SPECT shows an accumulation of radiotracer in the left medial, inferior and superior temporal lobe. From Dr PK Chandak, Department of Radiology, Brigham and Women's Hospital, Harvard Medical School.

Influenza A encephalitis

Influenza A is the cause of *encephalitis lethargica*, the main outbreak of which occurred from 1917 to 1928. The acute syndrome was characterized by headache, fever, reversed sleep rhythm and delirium. In those that survived, about half gradually developed postencephalitic parkinsonism, accompanied by dystonia (particularly oculogyric crises) and sometimes obsessive–compulsive disorder. Pathologically, there was perivascular inflammation in the basal ganglia in the early stages followed by neuronal loss, gliosis and neurofibrillary tangles in the basal ganglia, limbic system and cerebral cortex.

Arbovirus encephalitis

Arboviruses are arthropod-borne viruses that use mosquitoes or ticks as vectors. They typically cause a meningoencephalitis with an acute onset of headache, fever, photophobia, neck stiffness, lethargy and delirium. Severity is very variable and post-infection sequelae can include seizures and dementia.

Rabies

Rabies is a serious disease of the CNS that is transmitted by a bite from a dog, fox, rodent or bat. The World Health Organization attributes more than 30 000 deaths a year to rabies, which is likely to be a

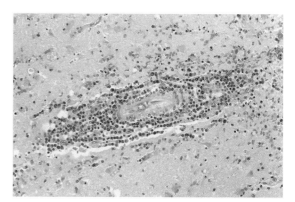

Fig. 29.3 Herpes simplex pathology. In the acute stages, microscopic examination reveals vascular destruction with infiltrates of neutrophils and lymphocytes, followed by haemorrhages. In the later stages, glial proliferation becomes the prominent feature. Cowdry type-A intranuclear inclusions are seen. These are collections of virus, which quickly cause the death of infected cells. From Underwood (2000).

serious underestimate. Of these deaths, 98% occur in the developing world. The further the bite is away from the CNS, the lower the chance of transmission of the virus. Once introduced through the skin or mucous membrane, the virus begins replicating in the striated muscles at the wound site. Migration to the nervous system is via the nearest sensory or motor neurone in the spinal cord. In this incubation period of 1 week or more, immunization will reduce the chances of developing rabies. Once it has infiltrated the nervous system the virus will irreversibly replicate undetected, until the late stages. The incubation period is followed by a short prodromal stage.

Prodromal symptoms are non-specific and include fever, malaise, headache, anorexia, nausea, sore throat (the beginnings of hydrophobia), photophobia and musculoskeletal pain. Some have described local paraesthesiae at the inoculation site due to irritation in the dorsal root ganglion. Two-thirds of patients then develop the more aggressive encephalitic (furious) subtype, and the remainder a paralytic (dumb) subtype. It is possible that localization in the midbrain and medulla is associated with the furious subtype and localization in the spinal cord is associated with the paralytic subtype.

In the furious subtype, patients experience severe overarousal (anxiety, agitation and irritability), inspiratory spasms (aerophobia and hydrophobia), autonomic dysfunction (excessive salivation, lacrimation and perspiration) and fluctuating consciousness. In the paralytic subtype there are cranial nerve signs (weakness of facial muscles, diplopia, asymmetrical pupils and absent corneal reflexes) and systemic symptoms (tachycardia, urinary retention and hyperpyrexia), with or without inspiratory spasms. Generalized flaccid paralysis ensues, followed by coma and death.

After the virus has infected the brain it spreads to all brain regions, and can continue to spread throughout the body, via efferent neural pathways, to the salivary glands, nasal cavities, tears, skin, adrenal glands, pancreas, kidney, heart muscle, hair follicles and cornea. The virus evades and then suppresses the T-cell and natural killer cell immune responses, which are then manifested too late and too weakly to be effective. Research has suggested that death from rabies is not a result of structural damage caused by the virus, but rather a result of a functional change in the neurones. Thus, the neuropathology is relatively mild, with grey matter microglial activation. The pathognomonic histopathological feature was described by Negri in 1905. These *Negri bodies* are cytoplasmic inclusions in infected neurones (Fig. 29.4). The rabies RNA most likely competes with host RNA, impairing neural functions. One of the determining factors of the virulence of rabies is the glycoprotein that makes up the viral membrane.

Investigations may show peripheral leukocytosis, as well as elevated protein and white cells in the CSF. Rapid deterioration is usually associated with hyperintensities of the brainstem, thalamus and temporal lobes on T2-weighted MRI. This pattern may distinguish rabies from other viral infections, such as enterovirus 71, Japanese encephalitis virus, herpes simplex virus, adenovirus and varicella-zoster virus. The diagnosis can be confirmed by detection of the antigen or virus from saliva or CSF. One area of future interest may be the influence of rabies on the hypothalamus–pituitary–adrenal axis and the clinical association with anxiety and immune suppression (Hemachudha & Phuapradit 1997). Vaccination of those at high risk is very safe and highly effective, but is not widely done in developing countries.

Subacute sclerosing panencephalitis

Dawson (1933) described a chronic encephalitis with intranuclear inclusion bodies, which was later recognized as a complication of measles and called subacute sclerosing panencephalitis (SSPE). SSPE is a disease of young people, and occurs more often

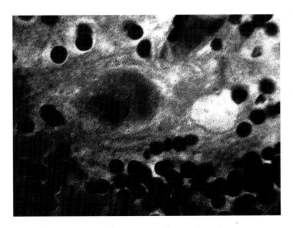

Fig. 29.4 A Negri body in a rabies-infected neurone. From Professor G Baumbach, Online Virtual Hospital, University of Iowa.

in males. It is caused by a reactivation of latent infection with the paramyxovirus. The pathology is characterized by microglial activation in white and grey matter, perivascular inflammation and patchy demyelination. Cortical atrophy and ventricular dilatation may occur. Clinically there is a gradual dementia with myoclonus, and chorea and seizures in later stages. The hallmark is the severe, repetitive myoclonic jerks, generally symmetrical, involving especially the axial musculature and occurring every 5–10 seconds.

Psychosis and catatonic presentations have been described. MRI shows widespread T2 hyperintensities, and CSF may reveal increased protein, oligoclonal bands and the measles antibody. An EEG may be diagnostic, with slow periodic complexes (in 10-second bursts) and 'burst-suppression' pattern. Death most often occurs within 1 year. As the practice of measles vaccination is now widespread, SSPE is extremely rare.

Progressive multifocal leukoencephalopathy

As with SSPE, progressive multifocal leukoencephalopathy (PML) is caused by a reactivation of the ubiquitous JC virus (papovavirus), most often in association with the immunosuppression of AIDS. PML is a serious condition in patients with AIDS, and may account for as many as 5% of all AIDS-related deaths. The pathogenesis of PML is demyelination as a result of direct toxicity to infected oligo-

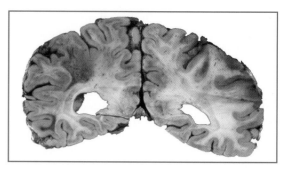

Fig. 29.6 Patchy demyelination in progressive multifocal leukoencephalopathy. The demyelination in this case is widespread, but is particularly prominent in the left hemisphere. Note also the brownish discolouration in some areas of white matter on the left. These areas probably represent advanced destruction of white matter, with residual haemorrhage. From Professor G Baumbach, Online Virtual Hospital, University of Iowa.

dendrocytes. There are then focal signs, including hemiplegia, aphasia or hemianopia. Dementia and delirium are also common complications. MRI shows non-enhancing decreased signal intensity on T1-weighted scans and increased signal in the white matter tracts, particularly in a occipitoparietal distribution. In 10% of cases the lesions are infratentorial. Usually there is no mass effect. Mortality is similar to that in SSPE.

SUMMARY

A number of viruses may penetrate the CNS, with devastating consequences. The sequelae vary enormously, depending on the host and viral factors. Lyssaviruses account for at least 50 000 deaths per year worldwide as rabies, which is endemic in every continent. Rabies is transmitted to humans through close contact with saliva from infected animals. Once the disease invades the CNS it is invariably fatal. In the acute stage, signs of hyperactivity (furious rabies) or paralysis (dumb rabies) predominate. Reactivation of prior infection with the herpes simplex type 1 virus causes haemorrhagic necrosis of the temporal lobes and neighbouring areas. Some survivors are left with a dense and persistent anterograde amnesia. Infections with influenza A caused the 1917–1928 encephalitis lethargica outbreak. Once the virus has adapted to the CNS it appears to have a predilection for the substantia nigra, cerebellum and hippocampus, producing parkinsonism.

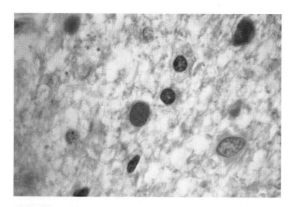

Fig. 29.5 Prominent gliosis in progressive multifocal leukoencephalopathy. There are a number of bizarre giant reactive astrocytes, together with eosinophilic nuclear inclusions in oligodendrocytes. From Professor G Baumbach, Online Virtual Hospital, University of Iowa.

The treatment of this syndrome with levodopa was popularized in the book (Sachs 1983) and film (1990) *Awakenings*.

REFERENCES AND FURTHER READING

American Heart Association 1965 Jones criteria (revised) for guidance in the diagnosis of rheumatic fever. Circulation 32:664–668

Cooke RA, Stewart B 1995 Color atlas of anatomical pathology, 2nd edn. Churchill Livingstone, Edinburgh

Dawson Jr JR 1933 Cellular inclusions in cerebral lesions of lethargic encephalitis. American Journal of Pathology 9:7–16

Glaser GH, Pincus JH 1969 Limbic encephalitis. Journal of Nervous and Mental Disorders 149:59–67

Hemachudha T, Phuapradit P 1997 Rabies. Current Opinions in Neurology 10:260–267

Johnson RT 2001 Viral infections of the nervous system. Presented at the XVII World Congress of Neurology, 17–26 June, London. Available: http://www.wfneurology.org/win/doc/pdf/johnson.pdf

Negri A 1905 Contributo allo studio dell'eziologia della rabia. Bollettino della Societa Medico-chirurgica, Pavia, No. 321

Sachs O 1973 Awakenings. Duckworth, London

Underwood JCE 2000 General and systematic pathology. Churchill Livingstone, Edinburgh

30

CNS Tumours

BACKGROUND

Intracranial tumours comprise 10% of all primary neoplasms. The annual incidence in the UK is about 5 per 100 000 of the population. In the USA there are about 20 000 new CNS tumours diagnosed per year, and 150 000 metastases. Neuropsychiatric symptoms are probably the commonest first indication of CNS malignancies.

The pathology of CNS tumours in complex. Metastases, gliomas and meningiomas are the most common types (Table 30.1). Malignant tumours are much more common than benign tumours. In children, 70% of intracranial neoplasms are infratentorial, whereas in adults 70% are supratentorial. Gliomas include astrocytomas, glioblastomas, oligodendromas and ependymomas. Astrocytomas often involve the subcortical white matter and are classified into low grades (I and II) and high grades (III and IV) (glioblastoma multiforme). Cerebral gliomas are twice as common in males as in females and the frequency increases with age. Medulloblastoma, cerebellar astrocytoma and pineal tumours occur mainly in childhood. Metastases are common from lung, breast, skin, adrenal glands and gastrointestinal tract. Conversely, peripheral metastases from CNS tumours are rare. Widespread dissemination through the brain and spinal cord is seen in cases of medulloblastoma, ependymoma and pineal germinoma (Fig. 30.1).

The cause of CNS tumours is unknown, although certain diseases predispose to CNS tumours, including von Recklinghausen's disease (optic and hypothalamic glioma, schwannomas of the cranial nerves), tuberose sclerosis (periventricular gliomas) and von Hippel–Lindau disease (cerebellar haeman-gioblastoma). Transplant patients and patients with AIDS have an increased risk of intracranial primary lymphoreticular neoplasms.

CLINICAL FEATURES

Clinical features are usually those of direct effects on neighbouring tissue and indirect mass effects. Direct effects include seizures, hemiparesis, dysphasia and visual symptoms. Early consequences of raised intracranial pressure are headache and vomiting and, later, drowsiness. Infratentorial tumours tend to obstruct CSF exiting from the fourth ventricle, leading to hydrocephalus. The site of the tumour is important in the genesis of neuropsychiatric symptoms (Fig. 30.2). In a group of 89 outpatients undergoing chemotherapy for various CNS tumours, Wellisch et al (2002) found that 60% had

Table 30.1 Frequency of various CNS tumours

Tumour	Frequency (%)
Metastases	40
Gliomas	25
Meningioma	10
Pituitary adenoma	5
Acoustic neuroma	5
(Neurinoma) Medulloblastoma	3
Craniopharyngioma	2
Haemangioma	2
Epidermoid cyst	1
Sarcoma	1
Other (chordoma, germinoma, teratoma, pinealoma, neurofibroma)	6

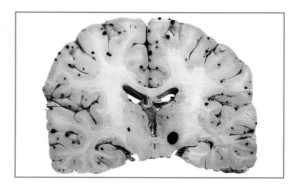

Fig. 30.1 Post-mortem specimen containing widespread metastases. From Peter Rochford, Museum Curator, James Vincent Duhig Pathology Museum, University of Queensland.

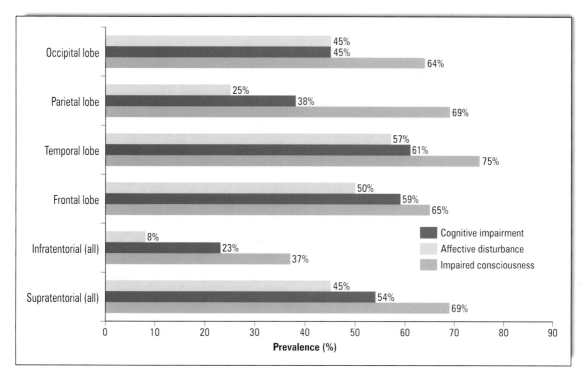

Fig. 30.2 Prevalence of neuropsychiatric complications in 530 patients with cerebral tumours. Data from Lishman (1998).

psychomotor slowing, 55% had attention difficulties and 40% had immediate memory problems. Primary gliomas in adults involve the frontal lobe in 40% of cases, the temporal lobe in 40%, the parietal lobe in 20% and the occipital lobe in 10%. There is often joint involvement of neighbouring areas.

In advanced stages, expansion within the limited confines of the skull leads to herniation below the falx cerebri, at the tentorium cerebelli or at the foramen magnum (Fig. 30.3). Paraneoplastic syndromes involving the brain, neuromuscular junctions and peripheral nervous system are not due to these mechanisms (see below). Ninety per cent of patients die within 2 years of diagnosis.

NEUROPSYCHIATRIC COMPLICATIONS OF CNS TUMOURS

The precise nature and pathogenesis of the psychiatric consequences of brain tumours are not well described. Furthermore, the waters are considerably muddied by the non-specific effects of living with a

terminal illness, secondary neurological impairments, secondary seizure disorder, the presence of cytotoxic medication or radiation, and the systemic effects of terminal illness. As a rule of thumb, the type of tumour has less influence on neuropsychiatric complications than does either the tumour size or the tumour site. Nevertheless, Lishman (1998) quotes a study by Busch showing that roughly one-third of patients with astrocytomas, compared with two-thirds with glioblastomas, had mental symptoms. Multiple tumours (most likely in the form of metastases) greatly increase the likelihood of psychiatric symptoms. One recent small survey of adult brain tumour survivors reported that 90% had some kind of morbidity (Whitton et al 1997). Several small studies have compared the disability and rehabilitation progress of such patients with those with stroke, head injury and spinal cord injury. The degree of disability was very similar.

Cognitive symptoms

Cognitive symptoms are among the most common complaints of patients with frontal lobe and other cortical tumours. Cognitive impairment shows a high correlation with both carer and patient stress (Farace & Shaffrey, 2001). Younger patients diagnosed with CNS germ-cell tumours are at increased risk of psychosocial and physical problems, as well as neuropsychological deficits. Long-term follow-up of such patients reveals that, although only 10% or so are severely disabled, about 50% will suffer permanent cognitive deficits of some type. In adults with brain tumours who are undergoing rehabilita-

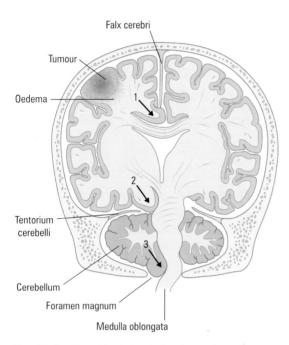

Falx cerebri

Tumour

Oedema

1

2

Tentorium cerebelli

3

Cerebellum

Foramen magnum

Medulla oblongata

Fig. 30.3 Sites of brain herniation. Increasing volume within the rigid confines of the skull can cause several herniation syndromes. In the subfalcine herniation (1), expansion with one cerebral hemisphere displaces part of the cingulate gyrus between the falx cerebri and the corpus callosum. This can cause compression of the anterior cerebral artery. In the transtentorial (uncal) herniation, expansion of a large supratentorial tumour forces part of the medial temporal lobe (parahippocampal gyrus) through the tentorial hiatus (2). Complications include an ipsilateral third cranial nerve lesion, compression of the midbrain, aqueduct of Sylvius, posterior cerebral artery and contralateral cerebral peduncle (the latter producing the false localizing Kernohan notch phenomenon). Occasionally, the midbrain is forced downwards into the rostral aspect of the pons, a phenomenon known as the central diencephalic herniation. In the cerebellar herniation (3), the cerebellar tonsils herniate through the foramen magnum, causing life-threatening compression of the brainstem.

tion, cognitive problems are very common. Mukand et al (2001) studied 51 consecutive patients. The most common deficits were impaired cognition (80%), followed by weakness (78%), visuoperceptual deficit (53%), sensory loss (38%) and bowel and bladder dysfunction (37%). Less common problems were cranial nerve palsy, dysarthria, dysphagia, aphasia, ataxia and diplopia. Seventy-five per cent of patients had three or more concurrent neurological deficits. In the large series quoted by Lishman (1998), cognitive complaints were present in approximately 50% of those with supratentorial tumours, especially those with involvement of the temporal and frontal lobes (see Fig. 30.2).

Psychotic symptoms

Psychotic symptoms are not common among patients with brain tumours, but they are seen in up to 50% of hospice patients receiving terminal care. Hypnagogic or hypnopompic hallucinations are the most common type. In most cases, this is a reflection of the high rate of delirium in these patients. The rate of delirium varies enormously, from about 25% in stable inpatients to 85% in terminally ill patients. In patients with relatively stable CNS tumours, psychosis is more likely with temporal and limbic involvement, particularly as a result of seizures, which occur in about one-third of patients. The phenomenology is sometimes reported as a schizophreniform (or schizophrenia-like) psychosis, but detailed case reports suggest that this is an oversimplification. Psychotic symptoms in patients with temporal lobe tumours are diverse and include hallucinations in all sensory modalities, and derealization with associated confusion or cognitive impairment. Disintegration of affect, function and personality without focal neurological symptoms or signs is very unlikely in the case of a CNS tumour. Although the rates of organic brain disorder appear to be elevated in patients meeting the criteria for schizophrenia, it is not clear whether this applies specifically to CNS tumours. For these reasons, patients with recognized CNS tumours that are causing psychotic symptoms should not be labelled as having schizophrenia.

Mood symptoms

Mackworth et al (1992) found that 50% of outpatients with primary brain tumours endorsed depressive symptoms, although this was unrelated to the

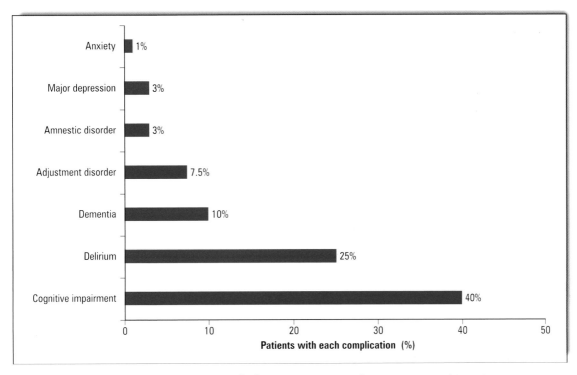

Fig. 30.4 Neuropsychiatric symptoms in terminally ill cancer patients. Data from Minagawa et al (1996).

Clinical Pointer 30.1

The influence of psychological factors on the onset and course of cancer

The influence of psychological factors on cancer has been a hot topic of debate for years. In order to examine this area critically, one has to specify the type of psychological influence (e.g. depression, dysphoria, denial) and the type of cancer (stage and site). At least 40 original prospective studies including over 4000 patients have examined whether psychological outlook (e.g. denial, avoidance, fighting spirit, stoicism) influence the outcome of cancer in terms of mortality or recurrence. A further 12 studies have looked at this question using non-prospective methods. Although the majority of studies in early cancer have found an effect, results in more malignant forms are less consistent. One interesting finding to emerge recently is that the relationship may be unidirectional, in that a high degree of helplessness and hopelessness negatively influences prognosis, while an optimistic outlook may be insignificant (Watson et al 1999). This adds weight to the argument that demanding that patients have a bright outlook or fighting spirit after a diagnosis of cancer is inappropriate. Yet it should equally be remembered that helping patients to plan for the future, understand their prognosis realistically and function maximally will enhance their quality of life.

There is weaker evidence that stress or personality influences the onset of cancer. Several studies are conflicting and the methodology of many studies examining life events in relation to a severe illness is questionable.

Further reading *Butow PN, Hiller JE, Price MA et al 2000 Epidemiological evidence for a relationship between life events, coping style, and personality factors in the development of breast cancer. Journal of Psychosomatic Research 49:169–181*
Porzsolt F, Leonhardt-Huober H, Stephens R 2001 Systematic review of the relationship between quality of life and survival in cancer patients. Breast 10(suppl 3):171–181
Watson M, Haviland JS, Greer S et al 1999 Influence of psychological response on survival in breast cancer: a population-based cohort study. Lancet 354:1331–1336

patients' functioning. In a better study using the Hospital Anxiety and Depression Scale, Grant et al (1994) found depression in 20% and anxiety in 28% of 50 patients with confirmed intracranial glioma. Predictors of depression were problems in limb function, memory problems, language difficulties and handicap. Irle et al (1994) compared the psychopathology of 141 patients following surgery for CNS tumours with that of 29 patients who had undergone surgery for a slipped disk and 18 normal control subjects. Patients with lesions of the ventral frontal cortex and lesions of the temporoparietal cortex reported more postoperative anxiety and depression, irritability and anger, and fatigue than did patients with other lesions and the controls.

Interestingly, lesions in the frontal or parietal association cortex and the paralimbic areas were responsible for the negative mood states. Lesion laterality did not influence the mood states. All groups reported an improvement in mood following surgical treatment. Other case series have reported an effect of laterality, specifically an association between dominant frontal tumours and depression and between non-dominant lesions and mania. These studies have been subject to a narrative review, but not a meta-analysis (Braun et al 1999). In the study by Keschner et al (1938) quoted by Lishman (1998), disturbances of affect were present in 54% of those with supratentorial tumours and 8% of those with infratentorial tumours. Many other diverse changes in mood are possible, including apathy, irritability, anger and emotionalism.

The special case of paraneoplastic syndromes affecting the limbic system

Paraneoplastic syndromes are believed to be immunologically mediated responses that occur when the tumour antigen is similar to a neuronal antigen. Rarely this can result in specific damage to the temporal lobes. This syndrome was brought together by Corsellis et al (1968) under the term *paraneoplastic limbic encephalitis*. Pathological changes are noted in the hippocampus, cingulate gyrus, amygdala, insula and temporal lobe. A large series was recently reviewed by Gultekin et al (2000). Cognitive impairments were the most common presentation, seen in 90% of patients, although seizures were also common (50%), as were miscellaneous psychiatric symptoms (40%) (Fig. 30.6). In this series neuropsychiatric symptoms preceded cancer in 60% of cases. Investigation using MRI, EEG and serology is usually definitive; in this series, 60% of patients had MRI signal hyperintensities in the limbic system and 60% had paraneoplastic antineuronal antibodies.

SUMMARY

Intracranial tumours are a relatively uncommon form of cancer, but are important because they often present with disturbances of higher function. The frontal and temporal lobes are the areas most commonly affected. The type of tumour has less influence on neuropsychiatric complications than does the site or size of the tumour. Almost any neuropsychiatric symptom can result from destruction or irritation of neurones. Symptoms and signs usually follow the clinicoanatomical rules of regional cerebral function (see Chs 12–16), although multiple domains may be involved.

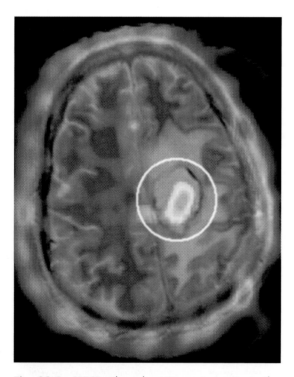

Fig. 30.5 SPECT with overlay MRI scan in a patient with a frontoparietal glioblastoma multiforme. From Dr PK Chandak, Department of Radiology, Brigham and Women's Hospital, Harvard Medical School.

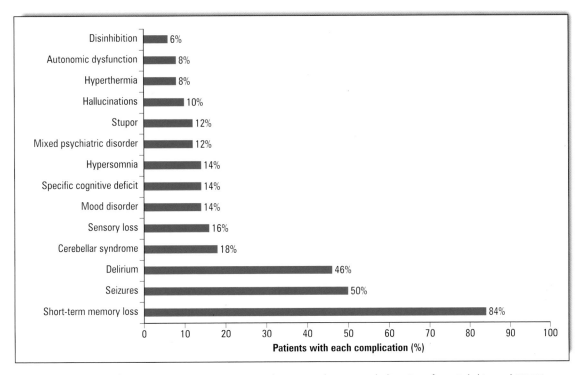

Fig. 30.6 Neuropsychiatric symptoms in 50 patients with paraneoplastic encephalitis. Data from Gultekin et al (2000).

REFERENCES AND FURTHER READING

American Heart Association 1965 Jones criteria (revised) for guidance in the diagnosis of rheumatic fever. Circulation 32:664–668

Braun CMJ, Larocque C, Daigneault S et al 1999 Mania, pseudomania, depression, and pseudodepression resulting from focal unilateral cortical lesions. Neuropsychiatry Neuropsychology and Behavioral Neurology 12:35–51

Corsellis JAN, Goldberg GJ, Norton AR 1968 'Limbic encephalitis' and its associations with carcinoma. Brain 91:481–496

Farace E, Shaffrey ME 2001 Relationship of neurocognitive impairment to quality of life in malignant brain tumour patients. Journal of Neuropsychiatry 13:151

Grant R, Slattery J, Gregor A, Whittle IR 1994 Recording neurological impairment in clinical trials of glioma. Journal of Neuro-oncology 19:37–49

Gultekin SH, Rosenfeld MR, Voltz R et al 2000 Paraneoplastic limbic encephalitis: neurological symptoms, immunological findings and tumour association in 50 patients. Brain 123:1481–1494

Irle E, Peper M, Wowra B et al 1994 Mood changes after surgery for tumors of the cerebral cortex. Archives of Neurology 51:164–174

Lishman WA 1998 Organic psychiatry. The psychological consequences on cerebral disorder. Blackwell, Oxford, p 218–236

Mackworth N, Fobair P, Prados MD 1992 Quality-of-life self-reports from 200 brain-tumor patients – comparisons with Karnofsky performance scores. Journal of Neuro-oncology 14:243–253

Minigawa H, Uchitomi Y, Yamawaki S et al 1996 Psychiatric morbidity in terminally ill cancer patients. Cancer 78:1131–1137

Mukand JA, Blackinton DD, Crincoli MG et al 2001 Incidence of neurologic deficits and rehabilitation of patients with brain tumors. American Journal of Physical Medicine and Rehabilitation 80:346–350

Wellisch DK, Kaleita TA, Freeman D et al 2002 Predicting major depression in brain tumors. Psychooncology 11:230–238

Whitton AC, Rhydderch H, Furlong W et al 1997 Self-reported comprehensive health status of adult brain tumor patients using the health utilities index. Cancer 80:258–265

31

Hydrocephalus

The heads of children sometimes grow enormously large, the sutures give way, and the membranes of the brain are pushed up with the water within, and make a soft tumour rising above the edges of the sutures ... They daily become more and more stupid, with a pulse not above seventy-two. (William Heberden 1802)

BACKGROUND

The CSF has important protective and restorative functions that can be disrupted when the normal balance of CSF production and CSF reabsorption becomes dysregulated. Hydrocephalus refers to an enlargement of part of the ventricular system caused by disrupted CSF dynamics (Fig. 31.1).

In the classical non-communicating variety of hydrocephalus, there is a blockage between the ventricular system and the subarachnoid space, which produces non-communication. Common causes are haemorrhage, meningitis, tumour and head injury.

In the communicating variety of hydrocephalus, there is a build up of pressure caused by an abnormality downstream (e.g. in the arachnoid granulations).

It is probably more useful to divide hydrocephalus into early-onset (developmental) and late-onset (normal-pressure) types. It can also be divided into acute and chronic forms.

CLASSICAL HYDROCEPHALUS

Hydrocephalus that presents acutely as a medical emergency typically causes severe headache and reduced consciousness. Where hydrocephalus builds up gradually it is more likely to feature upper motor neurone signs, papilloedema and features of the hydrocephalus triad:

- slowly progressive gait disorder – related to either ataxia or frontal lobe involvement
- progressive cognitive impairment
- incontinence or urinary urgency from disinhibition of bladder contractility.

By no means all patients have all three features. Indeed hydrocephalus, particularly normal-pressure hydrocephalus, is frequently misdiagnosed. One group found that only 20% of cases referred for suspected normal-pressure hydrocephalus in fact had this condition (Fig. 31.2) (Bech-Azeddinea et al 2001).

NORMAL-PRESSURE HYDROCEPHALUS

Normal-pressure hydrocephalus is a rare but potentially reversible cause of dementia, accounting for less than 0.5% of cases. The majority of cases of normal-pressure hydrocephalus are idiopathic. Abnormalities of CSF dynamics are thought to be the cause, as demonstrated on intracranial pressure monitoring by high CSF outflow pressure and/or waves of elevated pressure (B waves). Compensation to chronic mildly elevated CSF pressure makes measurement difficult. Occasionally, subarachnoid

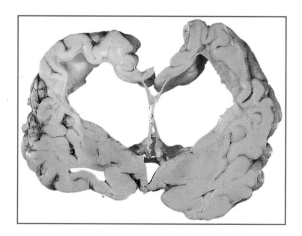

Fig. 31.1 Hydrocephalus. The lateral ventricles, including the temporal horns, are dilated. In this case the cause was obstruction of CSF flow through the cerebral aqueduct. From Stevens & Lowe (2000).

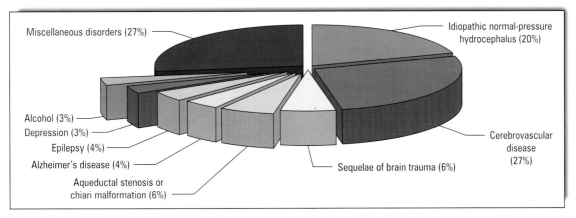

Fig. 31.2 Final diagnosis in 71 cases with suspected normal-pressure hydrocephalus. Data from Bech-Azeddinea et al (2001).

haemorrhage, meningitis, tumour or head trauma can cause an outflow obstruction, but without high intracranial pressure. Classically, normal-pressure hydrocephalus is said to present with the hydrocephalus triad (see above), but without good evidence of raised pressure in the CSF. In practice, the clinical picture is more variable. In the early stages there may be no identifiable signs. As periventricular corticospinal tracts are disrupted, gait becomes unstable, with shuffling steps. Similarly, urinary symptoms begin with urgency and gradually progress to incontinence. Radiological features include periventricular hyperintensities and deep white matter hyperintensities. It is of some interest that periventricular lesions around the frontal horns tend to improve after shunting and that extensive lesions are negatively correlated with improvement in cognitive symptoms as well as with gait disturbance and incontinence (Krauss et al 1996).

Cognitive deterioration

Cognitive deterioration is gradual, with cortical and subcortical features. Short-term memory is usually intact, but there are early executive deficits. For example, deficits in set shifting, verbal fluency and planning have been documented. The nature of the cognitive impairment appears to overlap with that seen in other types of hydrocephalus. Among patients awaiting shunting, about 50% have cognitive impairment in the mild to moderate dementia range. A smaller subgroup have more severe global cognitive impairment.

Predictors of cognitive impairment are not well known, with very limited success having been de-

rived from MRI and functional imaging studies in this regard. That said, the severity of cognitive decline has been correlated with the degree of depression and the extent of hippocampal atrophy (Boksay et al 2000, Savolainen et al 2000). Future studies will elucidate how important white matter lesions are.

Non-cognitive symptoms

Non-cognitive symptoms commonly include irritability, aggression and depression. Movement disorders such as bradykinesia, tremor, hypertonia and hyperkinetic movements occur in up to three-quarters of cases. Other neuropsychiatric complications of chronic hydrocephalus include reduced motivation of varying severity and, occasionally, akinetic mutism. One interesting complication is hypersomnia, which occurs in as many as 40% of sufferers. The neuropsychiatric complications most likely to improve with shunting include somnolence and cognitive impairment (more so than mood disorder and motivation). There are, of course, important functional sequelae to these problems, including the inability to wash, ambulate, cook or dress. Again, these factors would be expected to improve with successful shunting.

PATHOGENESIS

Animal studies suggest that in the initial stages impaired CSF flow and increased intraventricular CSF pressure results in increasing ventricular enlargement. Later the disequilibrium between ven-

Box 31.1 Risk factors for poor prognosis after hydrocephalus shunting

- Incorrect diagnosis
- Long-standing dementia
- Congenital hydrocephalus
- Presence of aphasia
- No improvement after lumbar drainage
- Extensive cortical atrophy
- Extensive periventricular white matter lesions
- Reduced cerebral blood flow in posterior areas
- Occurrence of B waves during 50% or more of the time during continuous monitoring of intracranial pressure
- Resistance to CSF outflow during a continuous lumbar CSF infusion test

tricular and convexity CSF pressures disappears, although episodes of slightly elevated intraventricular CSF pressure may remain (seen as B waves, seen on pressure recording). Clinical symptoms may be due to deteriorating periventricular blood flow (i.e. misery perfusion).

A lumbar puncture is often used to withdraw CSF and to monitor for clinical improvement, but this may be more effective when performed gradually over days rather than as a one-off procedure. Neuroimaging shows proportionately greater ventricular enlargement than cerebral atrophy (Clinical Pointer 31.1). CSF pressure dynamics studies suggest flow abnormalities in the cerebral aqueduct.

OUTCOME

CSF shunting is currently the treatment of choice despite a high rate of complications, which include haematoma and sepsis. Roughly half of all patients will benefit from a CSF shunt, although this is more accurately stated as: two-thirds of patients with a clear acquired cause of hydrocephalus will improve, compared with only one-third of those in whom the cause is unknown. This applies to both cognitive and non-cognitive symptoms, but gait usually shows more improvement than does cognition. Iddon et al (1999) demonstrated significant improvement in cognitive function (pre-shunt mean Mini-Mental State Examination score, 12.5; post-shunt Mean Mini-Mental State Examination score, 27) in a small group of patients with severe idiopathic normal-pressure hydrocephalus. Some groups have used measurement of resistance to CSF outflow or rate of B waves to predict outcome (Box 31.1).

SUMMARY

Hydrocephalus is an enlargement of part of the ventricular system due to a problem with CSF circulation. Broadly, hydrocephalus may be acquired developmentally or in later life. The condition most commonly encountered in adults is normal-pressure hydrocephalus. The cause is unknown, but the me-

Clinical Pointer 31.1

Distinguishing chronic hydrocephalus from hydrocephalus ex vacuo

An enlarged CSF space may be due to primary hydrocephalus or compensation for gross atrophy of cerebral tissue. The latter is sometimes referred to as 'ex vacuo' (i.e from a vacuum). Patients presenting with chronic hydrocephalus without headache, or evidence of papilloedema or gait abnormalities may be difficult to diagnose. Although neuroimaging reveals ventricular enlargement, this is also a feature of the primary dementias. However, in the case of hydrocephalus the degree of ventricular enlargement is disproportionate to the degree of cortical atrophy. Furthermore, the hippocampus is more likely to be affected in Alzheimer's disease than in hydrocephalus, although this is not a useful test on a case-by-case basis. In hydrocephalus there may be greater cognitive deficits in frontal executive function and less in the memory domain than is normally seen in Alzheimer's disease. A diagnostic lumbar puncture will immediately reveal the cause in the case of communicating and non-communicating hydrocephalus but not in normal-pressure hydrocephalus. In these cases, observation for therapeutic benefit may be required.

Further reading Iddon JL, Pickard JD, Cross JJL et al 1999 Specific patterns of cognitive impairment in patients with idiopathic normal pressure hydrocephalus and Alzheimer's disease: a pilot study. Journal of Neurology, Neurosurgery and Psychiatry 67:723–731

Savolainen S, Laakso MP, Paljarvi L et al 2000 MR imaging of the hippocampus in normal pressure hydrocephalus: correlations with cortical Alzheimer's disease confirmed by pathologic analysis. American Journal of Neuroradiology 21:409–414

chanism appears to involve slight elevation of CSF pressure over a long period, which is difficult to measure. Diagnosis using the classical triad of dementia, incontinence and corticospinal weakness cannot be used reliably. Indeed, mild cognitive impairment, movement disorders and sleep–wake disorder are much more common.

REFERENCES AND FURTHER READING

Bech-Azeddinea R, Waldemarb G, Knudsen GM et al 2001 Idiopathic normal-pressure hydrocephalus: evaluation and findings in a multidisciplinary memory clinic. European Journal of Neurology 8:601–611

Boksay I, Graves W, Golomb J et al 2000 Cognitive and behavioural aspects of normal-pressure hydrocephalus (NPH). International Psychogeriatric Association Annual Meeting, April

Heberden W 1802 Commentaries on the history and cure of diseases. T Payne, London

Iddon JL, Pickard JD, Cross JJL et al 1999 Specific patterns of cognitive impairment in patients with idiopathic normal pressure hydrocephalus and Alzheimer's disease: a pilot study. Journal of Neurology, Neurosurgery and Psychiatry 67:723–731

Krauss JK, Droste DW, Vach W et al 1996 Cerebrospinal fluid shunting in idiopathic normal-pressure hydrocephalus of the elderly: effect of periventricular and deep white matter lesions. Neurosurgery 39:292–299

Savolainen S, Laakso MP, Paljarvi L et al 2000 MR imaging of the hippocampus in normal pressure hydrocephalus: correlations with cortical Alzheimer's disease confirmed by pathologic analysis. American Journal of Neuroradiology 21:409–414

Stevens A, Lowe J 2000 Pathology, 2nd edn. Harcourt, St. Louis

Vanneste JAL 2000 Diagnosis and management of normal-pressure hydrocephalus. Journal of Neurology 247:5–14

32

Motor Neurone Disease (Amyotrophic Lateral Sclerosis)

Six months or a year after onset, the symptoms have all appeared and are generally becoming more marked. Death occurs in 2 or 3 years on average, as a result of bulbar symptoms. (Jean-Martin Charcot 1874)

BACKGROUND

Motor neurone disease (MND) is a disease that affects the entire motor system, from the cortex to the peripheral nerves. Patients may present with upper motor neurone signs alone (referred to as *primary lateral sclerosis*) or bulbar signs alone (*progressive bulbar palsy*), but at least 80% have both upper and lower motor neurone signs (*amyotrophic lateral sclerosis* (ALS)). Destruction frequently extends to the interneurones of the prefrontal cortex. Well-known sufferers have included David Niven, Dimitri Shostakovich and Lou Gehrig.

The clinical presentation begins with a gradual onset of weakness in mid-life to late life (mean age of onset 55 years). The condition progresses relentlessly, and both the quality and the length of life are

dramatically affected in MND. The European ALS Health Profile Study examined the quality of life in 451 patients and 415 carers, and found that 96.4% of patients and 50% of carers scored below the mean for physical well-being, and that 63.2% of patients and 72% of carers scored below the mean for mental well-being. Death usually occurs after 2–5 years. This harsh prognosis makes the issue of telling patients and families about the diagnosis particularly difficult (see Clinical Pointer I.1).

PATHOGENESIS

Aetiology

Although the cause of MND is unknown, in 10% of cases the condition is inherited and in about 30% of these an autosomal-dominant factor appears to be responsible. More than one gene may be involved, including the gene coding for the enzyme superoxide dismutase (SOD_1) on chromosome 21 (at 21q22.1) and the ALS2 gene on chromosome 2 (at 2q33). One suggested mechanism for cell death is glutamate-induced excitotoxicity. Two-thirds of patients have a partial loss of the astroglial glutamate transporter (excitatory amino acid transporter 2) in the motor cortex and spinal cord, which causes elevated extracellular glutamate levels (Cleveland & Rothstein 2001). Unusual endemic forms of the disaese (ALS–parkinsonism–dementia complex and lathyrism) may involve the AMPA subclass of glutamate receptors.

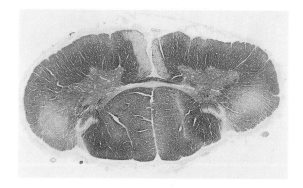

Fig. 32.1 The crossed and uncrossed corticospinal tracts in the cervical spinal cord show pallor resulting from loss of axons in MND. Luxol fast blue-cresyl violet. From Stevens & Lowe (2000).

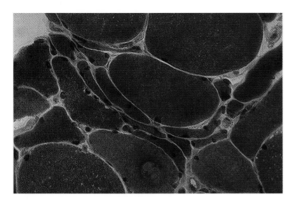

Fig. 32.2 Muscle biopsy using trichrome stain. In MND there are often numerous small regions of grouped angular atrophic muscle fibres. Large muscle fibres may show hypertrophy. From Professor Edward C Klatt, Florida State University, College of Medicine.

Pathology

Grossly, there is atrophy of the motor cortex, corticospinal tracts, anterior temporal lobe, anterior cingulate and corpus callosum. Changes in the subcortical white matter, amygdala, hippocampus and thalamus have also been reported. The major histological change is microvacuolation of the cerebral cortex, with atrophy of the bulbar neurones (especially the hypoglossal nucleus), substantia nigra and anterior horn cells of the spinal cord. Ubiquitinated inclusion bodies and cell loss occurs in large pyramidal cortical neurones of layers II and III and in surviving cranial nerve nuclei and anterior horn cells. There is fibrillary astrocytosis in the subcortical white matter. On T2-weighted MRI scans, signal abnormalities at the level of the motor cortex and the corticospinal tract are a potentially useful marker of MND pathology.

NEUROPSYCHIATRIC COMPLICATIONS OF MOTOR NEURONE DISEASE

Bulbar and pseudobulbar palsy

Loss of the low motor neurones innervating cranial nuclei (bulbar palsy) is the presenting feature in 25% of cases.

Loss of upper motor neurones that connect with cranial nerve nuclei can result in sudden pathological crying and, less often, pathological laughing. This has been called *pseudobulbar palsy* and is demonstrated by dysphagia and a brisk jaw jerk. It is caused by a bilateral disconnection of cortical inhibition from subcortical motor programmes. Voluntary facial movements are lost, but emotional expression is preserved. Speech is usually affected in both bulbar and pseudobulbar palsy. Speech has low volume and is accompanied by dysarthria. Palilalia may feature. There is some evidence that patients with bulbar and pseudobulbar involvement have more severe cognitive deficits than other patients, although with this could simply be because their survival is longer (and hence more complications develop).

Cognition in motor neurone disease

Significant neuropsychological impairment is present in approximately one-third of all sufferers of classical MND. Verbal fluency (part of executive function) appears to be affected more than memory which is, in turn, more affected than visuospatial function. There appears to be a correlation with underlying disease markers such as event-related potentials, the presence of pseudobulbar palsy and failure to suppress antisaccadic eye movements.

Dementia occurs in 5–10% of sufferers, largely as a frontal lobe dementia (see Ch. 41). As it is rare, the characteristics of this dementia are not well described. Provisionally, the features appear to be similar to those of frontotemporal dementia, with impairment of insight, judgement and empathy, and disinhibition. Familial cases are more at risk. Diagnosis is suggested by a rapidly progressing dementia, with frontal features combined with anterior horn signs. Although most often related to the severity of the underlying disease, a frontal lobe dementia can precede the illness by up to 2 years. Authors have begun to investigate whether it is possible to distinguish classical MND from MND with frontotemporal dementia. Provisional work suggests that, on PET functional imaging, comparable frontal and lateral temporal hypometabolism is seen in both conditions, but with greater impairment of

---

Box 31.1 Pseudobulbar syndrome

- Dysarthria
- Dysphagia
- Emotionalism
- Facial paresis
- Upper motor neurone signs

medial temporal lobe activity in MND with frontotemporal dementia (Garraux et al 1999).

Mood in motor neurone disease

Depression and anxiety have not been adequately studied in MND. One group compared the levels of depression in MND with those in multiple sclerosis and found comparable rates (Tedman et al 1997). A second study found a low rate of depression, both in patients and in carers, despite high levels of disability (Rabkin et al 2000). Estimates put the rate of depression at 10–25% and anxiety at 10–20%, but these figures may be inaccurate. It is certainly not the case that everyone who develops this devastating disease becomes depressed, which is in itself a useful lesson for other severe neuropsychiatric disorders.

Psychosis in motor neurone disease

Psychosis most often occurs in the context of dementia or delirium in patients with MND. There is nothing to suggest that the phenomenology of this form of psychosis is unique. That said, there have been reports of a familial association of MND and schizophrenia.

Sleep in motor neurone disease

Sleep problems are very common in MND because of nocturnal hypoxia, myoclonus and periodic leg movements. In addition, the effects of anxiety and depression take their toll on sleep quality and quantity. Sleep apnoea can be monitored by nocturnal pulse oximetry, which measures average blood oxygenation through the night.

SUMMARY

MND is a devastating disease of motor neurones, presenting with weakness, atrophy and spasticity. Although rare, the risk increases with age and the disease is estimated to be responsible for 1 in every 800 deaths. The condition is usually sporadic, but remarkable insights have been gained from the rare familial types. SOD_1 mutations cause an adult-onset variant and ALS2 mutations cause a slowly progressive early-onset variant. The condition only rarely causes dementia, and hence insight can be painfully preserved even in late stages. Surprisingly, rates of mood disorder do not appear to be greatly elevated. Other neuropsychiatric features of this condition require further study.

REFERENCES AND FURTHER READING

Charcot JM 1874 De la sclérose latérale amyotrophique. Progrès en Médecine 2:325, 341, 453

Cleveland DW, Rothstein JD 2001 From Charcot to Lou Gehrig: deciphering selective motor neuron death in ALS. Nature Reviews of Neuroscience 2:806–819

Garraux G, Salmon E, Degueldre C et al 1999 Medial temporal lobe metabolic impairment in dementia associated with motor neuron disease. Journal of the Neurological Sciences 168:145–150

Rabkin JG, Wagner GJ, Del Bene M 2000 Resilience and distress among amyotrophic lateral sclerosis patients and caregivers. Psychosomatic Medicine 62:271–279

Stevens A, Lowe J 2000 Pathology, 2nd edn. Harcourt, St. Louis

Tedman BM, Young CA, Williams IR 1997 Assessment of depression in patients with motor neuron disease and other neurologically disabling illness. Journal of the Neurological Sciences 152(suppl 1):S75–S79

33

Systemic Lupus Erythematosus

BACKGROUND

Systemic lupus erythematosus (SLE) is a connective tissue disease that affects small blood vessels, with a high likelihood of CNS involvement and neuropsychiatric symptoms. This disease affects mainly young adult women. Clinical features include fatigue, arthralgia, a butterfly rash, Raynaud's phenomenon, photosensitivity and multisystem endorgan disease.

There is considerable overlap between CNS lupus (cerebral SLE) and the neuropsychiatric complications of SLE (see Fig. 33.2). CNS lupus is diagnosed clinically in 40% of all SLE sufferers during life and 75% of patients who consent to post-mortem. The core clinical features of CNS lupus are seizures, stroke, peripheral and central nerve involvement and, in some definitions, cognitive impairment. Movement disorders, especially tremor, but also chorea, athetosis or ballism, are rare complications. Abnormal-ities on neuroimaging or CSF analysis support this diagnosis.

Neuropsychiatric symptoms are even more common (Fig. 33.1), since they can occur without demonstrable CNS involvement. The genesis is likely to involve several different factors and is probably caused by CNS vasculitis in the minority of cases. Although it is important to consider the direct

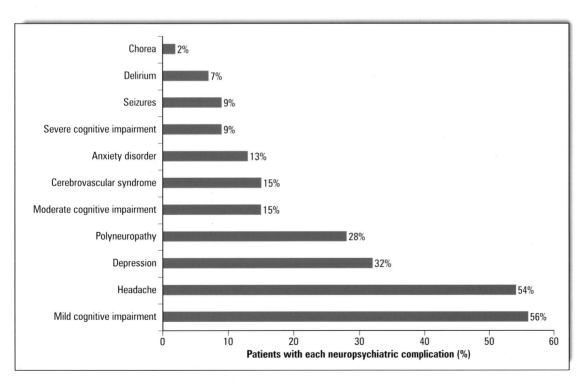

Fig. 33.1 Cross-sectional prevalence of neuropsychiatric complications in 46 patients with SLE. Data from Ainiala et al (2001).

effects of infarcts and haemorrhages, these show a stronger correlation with seizures and stroke than with psychiatric symptoms. There are also indirect effects. For example, patients with SLE are more vulnerable to infections because of immunosuppressant treatment. Some research suggests that diffuse abnormalities in CNS lupus can be attributed to autoantibodies that interact directly with neurones, including the anticardiopin antibodies (antiphospholipid antibodies), antiribosomal pro-

tein antibodies and antineutrophil cytoplasmic antibody (ANCA); ANCA is highly suggestive of Wegener's granulomatosis but is present in 20% of lupus cases. Attempts have been made to distinguish cerebral lupus from systemic lupus on the basis of such diagnostic tests (West et al 1995).

PATHOGENESIS

The pathology may be summarized as:

- systemic small vessel disease
- immune complex-mediated inflammation
- direct cross-reactivity with neurones

INVESTIGATIONS

Autoantibody markers (double-stranded DNA autoantibodies) are usually employed. Possible immunological markers of neuropsychiatric complications (which may simply reflect disease severity) include:

- anticardiolipin (ACA) antibodies
- antiglial fibrillary acidic protein serum antibodies
- antiganglioside immunoglobulin M (IgM) and IgG antibodies
- persistently raised anticardiolipin antibody levels.

OUTCOME

Management

Management involves immunosuppression and symptomatic treatment. One study found no association of neuropsychiatric complications with glucocorticoid treatment (Zanardi et al 2001).

Prognosis

The 5-year survival rate is now higher than 90%, but it is reduced in patients with CNS involvement.

NEUROPSYCHIATRIC COMPLICATIONS OF SLE

The neuropsychiatric complications of SLE are characteristically varied and unpredictable. Some fea-

Neurological lupus

Aseptic meningitis	Delirium/encephalopathy
Ataxia	Guillain–Barré syndrome
Autonomic disorder	Headache
Cerebrovascular disease	Myelitis
Chorea	Peripheral neuropathy
Cranial nerve palsy	Seizures

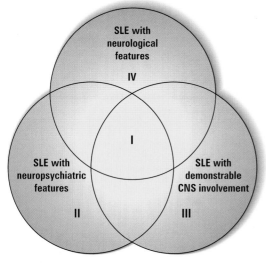

Neuropsychiatric lupus

Anxiety disorder	
Cognitive deficit	
Delirium/encephalopathy	
Depression	
Mania	
Psychosis	

CNS lupus

Adverse drug effects
Emboli
Immune complexes
Secondary infections
Thrombosis
Vasculitis

Fig. 33.2 CNS involvement in SLE. There is significant overlap between psychotic symptoms and neurological symptoms of SLE when the CNS in involved (I). Certain features, including delirium, psychosis and cognitive impairment, rarely occur without CNS involvement (II). However, SLE can manifest with peripheral symptoms alone (IV) and a small proportion of cases with clear CNS involvement do not develop neuropsychiatric symptoms (III).

tures, such as delirium and psychosis, tend to peak with disease relapses and then quickly disappear with remissions. Presumably these are related to small vascular and inflammatory changes. Other features, such as mood and some aspects of cognition (see below), tend to run their own course.

Cognitive impairment in SLE

Cognitive impairment is present in more than half of cases in which cerebral SLE has been established, but it is poorly characterized. About one-quarter of patients with no evidence of CNS disease also have cognitive deficits (Loukkola et al 2001, Monastero et al 2001). Those with cerebral SLE may have more problems with complex attention and psychomotor speed than those without CNS disease but with cognitive impairment nevertheless (Loukkola et al 2001).

Mild cognitive impairment is much more common than moderate cognitive impairment and dementia. Comparative studies have reported cognitive deficits in two-thirds of patients with SLE compared with 20% of those with rheumatoid arthritis. Memory problems, executive impairments, attention deficits and visuospatial deficits have been described, although Hanley et al (1993) found no excess of verbal or visual memory deficits in patients with SLE

Box 33.1 Neuropsychiatric complications of SLE

- Acute confusional state
- Acute inflammatory demyelinating polyradiculo-neuropathy (Guillain–Barré syndrome)
- Anxiety disorder
- Aseptic meningitis
- Autonomic disorder
- Cerebrovascular disease
- Cognitive dysfunction
- Cranial neuropathy
- Demyelinating syndrome
- Headache
- Mononeuropathy (single or multiplex)
- Movement disorder (chorea)
- Myasthenia gravis
- Myelopathy
- Plexopathy
- Polyneuropathy
- Psychosis
- Seizures

---

compared with those with rheumatoid arthritis. Studies have not found a significant relationship between clinical variables (duration or severity of disease, or treatment) and cognitive performance, although samples have been limited. There does, however, appear to be an intercorrelation with depression (Monastero et al 2001). There is some evidence that impaired immediate (working) memory and concentration is associated with temporary disease flare-ups, whereas delayed memory and executive dysfunction is a more permanent maker of underlying disease.

Mood disorder in SLE

Depression and anxiety are common in SLE, although there are wide differences in the estimates of frequency in the few published reports. Predictors of depression onset or prognosis in SLE have not been studied. There is a higher rate of loss of sexual interest, fatigue, pain and insomnia in secondary depression of SLE than in primary depression. In those small studies that have directly compared the rates of depression in SLE and rheumatoid arthritis, no appreciable differences have been found.

Psychosis in SLE

Delirium with psychotic features is a transient but often florid presentation of active disease, seen in about 20% of patients with advanced SLE. This may be related to the underlying acute or subacute encephalopathy that is recognized in SLE.

Psychotic episodes in clear consciousness occur more frequently in SLE than in disabled patients with rheumatoid arthritis. There is a closer correlation between demonstrable brain lesions and cognitive and psychotic episodes than with depression or anxiety.

OTHER VASCULITIC DISEASES INVOLVING THE CNS

Vasculitis of the CNS can occur in primary systemic vasculitides (Table 33.1) or secondary to infections, connective tissue diseases and prescribed drugs. The common feature is intramural inflammation and necrosis of the walls of blood vessels, leading to infarction. Although involvement of the CNS is quite common in vasculitis disease, this usually

Table 33.1 Spectrum of vasculitides

Primary vasculitides	Systemic vasculitis	Frequency of CNS vasculitis (%)	Neuropsychiatric complications
Churg–Strauss syndrome	✓	25	✗
Giant cell (temporal) arteritis	✓✓	30	✓
Kawasaki's disease	✓	10	✗
Polyarteritis nodosa	✓✓	40	✓✓
Primary angiitis of the CNS	✗	100	✓✓
Takayasu arteritis	✓✓	30	✓
Wegener's granulomatosis	✓✓	30	✓✓

occurs in association with systemic vasculitis; solitary vasculitis of the CNS is rare. A proposed classification divides CNS vasculitis into a severe form (primary angiitis of the CNS) and a less severe form (benign angiopathy of the CNS). Clinical presentations vary. Headaches, focal symptoms and signs, seizures and cranial nerve lesions may easily be mistaken for multiple sclerosis or a space-occupying lesion. Psychiatric features are also varied, with most data extrapolated from SLE. These include delirium (encephalopathy), varying degrees of cognitive impairment, organic psychosis and depression. Disease-modifying treatment often involves glucocorticoids or cyclophosphamide.

Behçet's disease

Behçet disease is a multisystem, vascular inflammatory disease probably with an autoimmune basis. In 1937, the Turkish dermatologist Hulusi Behçet described the syndrome, which consists of recurrent oral or genital ulcerations, skin lesions and eye lesions together with a positive pathergy test. Neuro-Behçet syndrome is a recognized syndrome related to large vessel venous sinus thrombosis or small vessel vasculitis. Clinical features include headache, stroke, dementia, meningitis, seizures and abnormal movements. MRI shows white matter lesions in the brainstem and occasionally of the diencephalon and periventricular area.

Polyarteritis nodosa

Polyarteritis nodosa is a systemic vasculitis of small and medium-sized vessels. Most organs can be affected. Pathologically, there is vasculitis, thrombosis and aneurysmal dilatations. Clinical features of CNS involvement are delirium, dementia, headaches, seizures and stroke-like episodes.

SUMMARY

SLE is a systemic autoimmune disease of young people, with diverse dermatological, renal, cardiovascular and haematological complications. The CNS is affected in the majority of sufferers with long-standing disease, although neuropsychiatric complications can present in patients with no evidence of CNS involvement. The pathogenesis of cerebral lupus is subject to intense research. Immune complexes and vasculitis may have a role to play in the genesis of some neuropsychiatric symptoms (such as seizures or stroke), but it is also possible that cross-reactivity of anti-DNA antibodies (e.g. antibodies directed at the N-methyl-D-aspartate receptor) are involved. Cognitive impairment, delirium and psychosis are the neuropsychiatric complications that are most closely affiliated with demonstrable brain involvement. Future developments in the recognition and management of autoimmune disease will certainly improve the management of this fascinating disorder.

REFERENCES AND FURTHER READING

Ainiala H, Loukkola J, Peltola J et al 2001 The prevalence of neuropsychiatric syndromes in systemic lupus erythematosus. Neurology 57:496–500

American College of Rheumatology 1999 Nomenclature and case definitions for neuropsychiatric lupus syndromes. Arthritis and Rheumatism 42:599–608

Behçet H 1937 Uber residivierende, aphtose, durch ein virus verursachte Geschwure am Mund, am Auge und an den Genitalien. Dermatologische Wochenschrift 105:1152–1157

Hanly JG, Walsh NM, Fisk JD et al 1993 Cognitive impairment and autoantibodies in systemic lupus erythematosus. British Journal of Rheumatology 32:291–296

Loukkola J, Laine M, Ainiala H et al 2001 Cognitive impairment in SLE: a population-based neuropsychological study. Journal of the Neurological Sciences 187(suppl 1):S110

Monastero R, Bettini P, Del Zotto E et al 2001 Prevalence and pattern of cognitive impairment in systemic lupus erythematosus patients with and without overt neuropsychiatric manifestations. Journal of the Neurological Sciences 184:33–39

Stevens A, Lowe J 2000 Pathology, 2nd edn. Harcourt, St. Louis

West SG, Emlen W, Wener MH et al 1995 Neuropsychiatric lupus-erythematosus – a 10-year prospective study on the value of diagnostic tests. American Journal of Medicine 99:153–163

Zanardi VA, Magna LA, Costallat LTL 2001 Cerebral atrophy related to corticotherapy in systemic lupus erythematosus (SLE). Clinical Rheumatology 20:245–250

34

Sleep Disorders

It may ... come to pass that someday the person who drives or goes to work while sleepy will be viewed as being as reprehensible, dangerous, or even criminally negligent as the person who drives or goes to work while drunk. If so, perhaps the rest of us can all sleep a little bit more soundly. (Stanley Coren 1996)

BACKGROUND

Some sources report that, in general practice, half of patients harbour a sleep complaint. Insomnia is the most common sleep problem, affecting over one-third of people during the course of a typical year. Between 10% and 20% of people report persistent severe insomnia, and about half this number report hypersomnia. Women, the unemployed, those living alone after divorce or separation and the elderly are more likely to suffer insomnia. Insomnia can occur in several forms:

- changes in pattern of falling asleep, or *initial insomnia*
- waking frequently during the night, or *middle insomnia*
- waking too early, or *early morning waking*
- unrefreshing sleep and daytime tiredness, or *somnolence.*

Insomnia is often not reported until a poor sleep pattern is well established. People often try self-help strategies such as over-the-counter medications and alcohol before seeking help. Insomnia is not an innocent problem, as is often assumed, but is an important symptom of many psychiatric and medical disorders. Insomnia and excessive daytime sleepiness are closely linked. Secondary tiredness is associated with accidents at work and particularly while driving. In one survey 20% of long-distance lorry drivers admitted to dozing off at the wheel at least twice (Hakkanen & Summala 2000). Sleep deprivation from whatever cause is linked with poor concentration and fatigue, and it can progress to disorientation and hallucinations when prolonged. Some disorders of sleep are associated with increased mortality rates.

The assessment of sleep problems is discussed in Clinical Pointer 61.1.

SLEEP DISORDERS OF RELEVANCE TO NEUROPSYCHIATRY

Narcolepsy

Narcolepsy is a fascinating disorder that was described in a case series of 14 patients in 1880 by Gelineau. Narcolepsy is an uncommon chronic sleep disorder with a prevalence of 0.025%. It consists of excessive and powerful daytime sleepiness, with sudden sleep attacks and up to three other features. Only 10% of sufferers have all four features, which are:

- excessive and powerful daytime sleepiness, in 100% of patients (by definition)
- episodes of sudden falling associated with emotion (cataplexy), in 60%
- hypnagogic hallucinations, in 30%
- sleep paralysis, in 20%.

Narcoleptic attacks are described as an irresistible urge to sleep, and this sleep is characterized by an early REM period, usually with dreams, from which the person wakes easily. In cataplexy, subjects lose voluntary muscle tone and fall to the floor, paralysed but conscious. This may be precipitated by a strong emotion. Similarly, in sleep paralysis the subject is unable to move upon waking or falling asleep for up to a minute. *Hypnagogic hallucinations* are dream-like, typically visual images; *hypnopompic hallucinations* are similar experiences on waking. Other psychiatric disorders are common in narcoleptic patients, including schizophreniform psychosis, depression and generalized anxiety disorder.

Box 34.1 Classification of sleep disorders

Dyssomnias (inherent sleep problems)
Intrinsic sleep disorders:
- idiopathic (primary) insomnia (at least 1 month of poor sleep)
- psychophysiological insomnia (prolonged insomnia due to anxiety about sleep)
- idiopathic (primary) hypersomnia (at least 1 month of excessive sleep or somnolence)
- narcolepsy (a syndrome of sudden, uncontrollable sleepiness)
- sleep apnoea (sleep disruption due to breathing disturbance, most commonly obstructive)

Extrinsic sleep disorders

Circadian rhythm disorder (e.g. due to jet lag or shift work)

Other sleep syndromes (e.g. nocturnal myoclonus, restless leg syndrome, Kleine–Levin syndrome)

Parasomnias (disorders that intrude into sleep)
Arousal disorders:
- sleep terror disorder (occurs during deep non-REM sleep, usually in the early night)
- sleepwalking (somnambulism)

REM parasomnias:
- nightmare disorder (nightmares occur during REM sleep, at any time of night)
- REM sleep behaviour disorder

Miscellaneous syndromes (e.g. enuresis, bruxism)

Sleep disorders due to medical conditions

Table 34.1 Secondary sleep disorders

Associated condition	Insomnia	Hypersomnia
Psychiatric causes		
Unipolar depression	✓	✓
Mania	✓	✗
Delirium	✓	✗
Schizophrenia	✓	✗
Anxiety disorders	✓	✗
Post-traumatic stress disorder	✓	✗
Bereavement related	✓	✓
Brief reactive psychosis	✓	✗
Persistent delusional disorder	✓	✗
Alcohol abuse	✓	✗
Illicit drug use	✓	✓
Anorexia nervosa	✓	✗
Psychophysiological insomnia	✓	✗
Neurological causes		
Headaches	✓	✗
Backaches	✓	✗
Sleep-related epilepsy	✓	✗
Parkinson's disease	✓	✓
Any dementia	✓	✓
Fatal familial epilepsy	✓	✗
Brain tumour	✓	✓
Stroke	✓	✓
Epilepsy	✓	✓
Myotonic dystrophy	✓	✓
Encephalitis lethargica	✗	✗
Head injury	✓	✓
Medical causes		
Any respiratory disease	✓	✗
Most cardiovascular diseases	✓	✗
Hyperthyroidism	✓	✗
Cushing's disease	✓	✗
Any pain syndrome	✓	✗
Rheumatological diseases	✓	✗
Orthopaedic problems	✓	✗
Sleeping sickness	✗	✓
Medication-related	✓	✓

Mechanism of narcolepsy

The cause of narcolepsy has been a mystery since its description. In part, this has been due to our inadequate understanding of the mechanisms underlying normal sleep. It is known that narcolepsy can be both familial and sporadic and that there is an association with the human leukocyte antigen (HLA) DR2 (or, more accurately, DQB1*0602). It is also known that narcolepsy can follow tumours and infarcts that damage the hypothalamus and nearby structures. The link between these could be the newly discovered hormone hypocretin (De Lecea et al 1998). Hypocretin stimulates appetite and sleep. Knock-out mice that do not express this hormone have narcoleptic features. Now provisional data suggests that CSF and hypothalamic hypocretin concentrations (but not plasma concentrations) are low in the majority of narcoleptic patients (Thannickal et al 2000). Thus, it is hypothesized that autoimmune destruction of hypocretin-producing cells in the perifornical area of the posterior and lateral hypothalamus, direct lesions to that area, or genetic abnormalities of the preprohypocretin gene may result in narcolepsy.

REM sleep behaviour disorder

If the normal state of atonia is lost during REM sleep then dreams may be enacted, with dramatic and occasionally violent consequences. These coincide with periods of REM sleep, in that they begin within the first 90 minutes of sleep and can occur four or more times during the night. The subject is unaware of his or her condition at the time, but can usually recall the dream on waking. It is difficult to arouse the patient from sleep during the incident, but on waking there is no prolonged confusion or amnesia. The disorder is more common in old age. Of interest to clinicians, this disorder appears to occur much more frequently in patients with Lewy body dementia and Parkinson's disease than in age-matched controls or indeed than in patients with Alzheimer's disease (Boeve et al 2001). The mechanism may involve degeneration of the locus ceruleus and substantia nigra interneurones that usually modulate cholinergic neurones in the pedunculopontine nucleus. The treatment of choice is the long-acting benzodiazepine clonazepam.

SLEEP DISORDERS IN NEUROLOGICAL DISEASE

Acquired brain injury

Brain injury through head injury causes a range of sleep difficulties, including reduced REM sleep in the acute stages and sleep apnoea thereafter. About half of patients with head injury continue to experience sleep problems 2 years after the accident. Of note, sleep problems after head injury are common after mild as well as severe injuries. Rarely, damage to the thalamus may result in pathological hypersomnia in stroke patients.

Dementia

Alzheimer's disease and other dementias regularly disrupt sleep and lead to wandering and behavioural disturbance during the night (sometimes referred to as *sundowning*) and increased napping during the day (day–night reversal is described in one-third of patients). Patients have reduced deep sleep, fragmented sleep and increased sleep apnoea, which may be linked with degeneration of neurones in the suprachiasmatic nucleus, pons, medulla and brainstem. Reduced REM sleep occurs, and this is not seen in 'normal ageing'. Slowing of the EEG is well recognized in Alzheimer's disease, but the same slowing also occurs during sleep and, if anything, is even clearer. This may be due to loss of cholinergic neurones in the nucleus basalis of Meynert. In any case, both waking and sleep EEG slowing has been investigated as a potential diagnostic marker of Alzheimer's disease.

Epilepsy

About 50% of patients with epilepsy experience seizures during sleep. A minority of seizures occur exclusively during the night and may be diagnosed as nocturnal panic attacks, nocturnal paroxysmal dystonia or REM sleep behaviour disorder. Certain forms of epilepsy tend to occur at night (e.g. Rolandic epilepsy of childhood, Lennox–Gastaut syndrome, mesial frontal seizures). Interictal discharges are seen more commonly during sleep, with the greatest activation occurring during non-REM sleep. Sleep deprivation facilitates both epileptiform abnormalities and seizures.

The presence of epilepsy also adversely affects sleep, with patients demonstrating increased latency and fragmented sleep.

Parkinson's disease

As many as 80% of patients with Parkinson's disease complain of sleeping disorders, including disturbance of the circadian rhythm. Hypokinesia and dystonia may be responsible in some cases, although depression and dementia can also be contributory factors. Unlike fatigue, sleep abnormal-

---

Box 34.2 Neurological manifestation of hypothalamic disease

Temperature regulation
Hyperthermia
Hypothermia

Food and water intake
Hyperphagia
Anorexia
Polydipsia
Hypodipsia

Sleep
Hypersomnia
Sleep rhythm disruption
Coma

Autonomic nervous system
Cardiac arrhythmias
Hyperventilation
Sweating

ities tend to progress with disease severity. Dopaminergic drugs (e.g. pramipexole, ropinirole, pergolide) are associated with somnolence and sedation at low doses, although the effect is a modest one. At high doses they can precipitate nightmares and nocturnal hallucinations. REM sleep intrusions in the day and REM sleep behaviour disorder has been linked with hallucinations in small studies in Parkinson's disease.

Patients with Parkinson's disease are prone to the restless leg syndrome and periodic limb movement disorder (Table 34.2). In restless leg syndrome, there is an irresistible desire to move the legs when at rest, which is relieved by movement. In periodic limb movement disorder, there are regular limb movements during sleep. The two conditions overlap and have been linked with a number of neuropsychiatric disorders.

Progressive supranuclear palsy

Progressive supranuclear palsy causes impaired sleep as a result of a variety of physical complaints. There is some evidence that it can specifically affect voluntary control of breathing, but with preserved automatic control of breathing. Interestingly, patients with rare brainstem infarctions can have the reverse problem, with only voluntary breathing during the night, a condition called 'Ondine's curse'.

Tourette's syndrome and Huntington's disease

Tourette's syndrome features nocturnal tics in many patients, causing secondary sleep problems. Tics can occur in any stage of sleep. In contrast, most patients with Huntington's disease have some suppression of chorea during the night, although movements may not be completely absent. When movements do occur it is most often during transient awakenings or in stage 1 of sleep (Fish et al 1991).

Stroke

Patients who have had a stroke can suffer considerable distress related to broken sleep. Particularly common is obstructive sleep apnoea. Sleep apnoea is a predictor of poor prognosis after stroke. Sandberg et al (2001) found that 59% fulfilled the

Table 34.2 Sleep-related movement disorder in neuropsychiatry

	Restless leg syndrome	Periodic limb movement disorder
ADHD	✓	✓
Akathisia	✗	✓
Epilepsy	✗	✓
Huntington's disease	✗	✓
Motor neurone disease	✓	✓
Multiple sclerosis	✓	✓
Myelopathy	✓	✓
Parkinson's disease	✓	✓
Peripheral neuropathy	✓	✓
Polio	✓	✗
PTSD	✗	✓
Radiculopathy	✓	✓
Stiff-man syndrome	✗	✓
Tourette's syndrome	✓	✗

ADHD, attention-deficit hyperactivity disorder; PTSD, post-traumatic stress disorder

criteria for sleep apnoea. Multivariate analysis showed that obesity, low ADL scores, ischaemic heart disease, and depressed mood were independently associated with sleep apnoea. Furthermore, low ADL scores, apnoea-related hypoxaemia, body mass index ≤27 and impaired vision were independently associated with delirium. The presence of sleep apnoea was not associated with any specific type of stroke or with any particular location of the brain lesion.

Fatal familial insomnia

Fatal familial insomnia is a rare prion disorder, inherited as an autosomal-dominant disease. In the initial stages there is insomnia, dysautonomia, sphincter disorder, diplopia with myoclonus and, in men, impotence. In middle stages of the illness there is worsening of the sleep disturbance, dysarthria and dysphagia, and weakness. As the disease progresses there is ablation of non-REM sleep, with only brief periods of REM sleep. The disease preferentially destroys the anteroventral and dorsomedial thalamic nuclei, causing deteriorating attention and memory performance in most cases. After an average of 12 months there is progression to death. Genetically, the disease is closely related to Creutzfeldt–Jakob disease, in that both feature a mutation on the prion protein gene. (In familial

Creutzfeldt–Jakob disease, a D178N mutation occurs whereby valine is encoded at position 129. In fatal familial insomnia, methionine is encoded on the mutated allele.)

Kleine–Levin syndrome

Kleine–Levin syndrome is an episodic illness that was originally described as occurring more commonly in young men. The disorder is characterized by episodes of excessive daytime sleepiness that lasts for days or weeks and then remit, for weeks or months, only to return. Episodes begin with a prodrome of lethargy, sleepiness and headache. There is hyperphagia and disinhibition–aggression–irritability or hypersexuality. In between episodes patients have little memory for the events. Episodes are likely to recur, but with decreasing frequency, and they eventually subside altogether. In women the syndrome is easily confused with the more common menstrual-related periodic hypersomnia. Occasionally EEG disturbances are seen, but these do not appear to be characteristic. A form of encephalitis may be the answer. This disorder is quite different from the two childhood-onset genetic diseases of Prader–Willi syndrome and Laurence–Moon–Biedl syndrome.

Prader–Willi syndrome

Prader–Willi syndrome is a syndrome of hyperphagia, hypogonadism and learning disability caused by a functional deletion on chromosome 15 (15q11-q13). Individuals have higher than expected rates of depression, anxiety, irritability and compulsions. Dysfunction of various hypothalamic systems may cause abnormal luteinizing hormone releasing hormone, lack of growth hormone releasing hormone

or oxytocin, daytime hypersomnolence and insatiable hunger (Swaab 1997).

Laurence–Moon–Biedl syndrome

Laurence–Moon–Biedl syndrome features learning disability, obesity, polydactyly and retinitis pigmentosa. There may be an association with psychosis, but the neuropsychiatric features require further examination.

PATHOGENESIS OF SLEEP DISORDERS

Sleep is an extremely primitive biological drive, but its function is remains a mystery. In order to understand the pathogenesis of sleep disorders it is reasonable to mention the physiology of normal sleep. No one anatomical area is responsible for sleep, but rather different parts of the brain are involved in different ways. There seems to be a balance between sleep-promoting GABAergic and galaninergic neurones in the ventral preoptic hypothalamus and wake-promoting hypocretin neurones in the lateral hypothalamus. Fine adjustments of the normal sleep–wake cycle is regulated from the suprachiasmatic nucleus in the anterior hypothalamus, possibly via serotonergic transmission. Alertness depends on the reticular activating system, arising within the brainstem and more rostral limbic systems. Dopamine from the ventral tegmentum has a role in the control of alertness. The brainstem generates components of REM sleep in a homeostatic collection of REM-activating and REM-deactivating systems. Cholinergic neurones in the tegmental area enhance REM sleep; conversely, noradrenergic and serotonergic neurones in the locus ceruleus and dorsal raphe nucleus may inhibit REM sleep. This may have particular importance in Alzheimer's disease. Lesions of cholinergic neurones in the nucleus basalis of Meynert causes EEG slowing and loss of sustained REM sleep in animal models in dementia. Furthermore, kainate antagonists, but not NMDA antagonists, appear to block glutamate-induced REM sleep (Datta 2002).

Muscle atonia of REM sleep may have a specific anatomical basis via descending inhibition from pedunculopontine nucleus to the medullary reticular formation. Non-REM sleep is controlled by diffuse areas, including the basal forebrain area, the

---

Box 34.3 Variables recorded during polysomnography

- EEG
- ECG
- EMG
- Electro-oculogram
- End-tidal pCO_2
- Leg movement
- Nasal airflow
- Oxygen saturation
- Respiratory effort

Clinical Pointer 34.1

Distinguishing sleep terrors, nightmares and nocturnal panic attacks and nocturnal seizures

One-third of a patients with panic disorder experience nocturnal panic attacks. Patients describe severe anxiety at any time during the night that occurs in a state of wakefulness and with symptoms identical to the daytime panic attack.

Nightmares also occur at any time of the night (associated with REM sleep) but often in the later stages of sleep. The fear is present on waking and related to detailed recall of a dream. Occasionally, the normal state of atonia is lost during REM sleep and dreams are enacted, with unfortunate consequences.

In sleep terrors there is usually incomplete wakening from sleep within the first couple of hours. There is intense fear, sometimes heralded by crying out, but no recollection why on waking. Episodes last for 5–15 minutes and are associated with autonomic overactivity.

Certain types of epilepsy have a predilection for sleep and others can occur at night by chance. About 20% of patients will only experience seizures at night. Short, frequent episodes associated with automatisms, vocalizations and posturing suggest frontal lobe seizures. Temporal lobe epilepsy is increasingly recognized as a cause of nocturnal anxiety and is indicated by post-ictal confusion and an abnormal EEG.

Further reading   *Culebras A 1999 Sleep disorders and neurological disease. Marcel Dekker, New York*

thalamus, the hypothalamus, the dorsal raphe nucleus and the nucleus tractus solitarius of the medulla. Tumours of the posterolateral hypothalamus, bilateral thalamus, pineal gland and upper brainstem can cause pathological hypersomnia. Bilateral paramedian thalamic infarcts cause hypersomnia and coma (see familial fatal insomnia, above) (Culebras 1992).

SUMMARY

Often taken for granted, and more often than not overlooked by clinicians, sleep disorders are a problematic complication of most neurological and psychiatric disorders. There is good evidence that poor sleep is associated with a higher than expected morbidity and mortality, and insomnia alone can be a maintaining factor in psychiatric illness. Recent advances in the pathogenesis and treatment of narcolepsy has renewed interest in these fascinating conditions.

REFERENCES AND FURTHER READING

Boeve BF, Silber MH, Ferman TJ et al 2001 Association of REM sleep behavior disorder and neurodegenerative disease may reflect an underlying synucleinopathy. Movement Disorders 16:622–630

Coren S 1996 Sleep thieves: an eye-opening exploration into the science and mysteries of sleep. The Free Press, New York

Culebras A 1992 Neuroanatomical and neurologic correlates of sleep disturbances. Neurology 42(suppl 6):19–27

Datta S 2002 Evidence that REM sleep is controlled by the activation of brain stem pedunculopontine tegmental kainate receptor. Journal of Neurophysiology 87:1790–1798

De Lecea L, Kilduff TS, Peyron C et al 1998 The hypocretins: hypothalamus-specific peptides with neuroexcitatory activity. Proceedings of the National Academy of Sciences 95:322–327

Fish DR, Sawyers D, Allen PJ et al 1991 The effect of sleep on the dyskinetic movements of Parkinson's disease, Gilles de la Tourette syndrome, Huntington's disease, and torsion dystonia. Archives of Neurology 48:210–214

Gelineau J 1880 De la narcolepsie. Gazette des Hositaux 55:635–637

Hakkanen J, Summala H 2000 Sleepiness at work among commercial truck drivers. Sleep 23:49–57

Petit D, Montplaisir J, Riekkinen P Sr et al 2000 Electrophysiological tests. In: Gauthier S (ed) Clinical diagnosis and management of Alzheimer's disease, 2nd edn. Martin Dunitz , London, p 133–154

Sandberg O, Franklin KA, Bucht G et al 2001 Sleep apnea, delirium, depressed mood, cognition, and ADL ability after stroke. Journal of the American Geriatrics Society 49:391–397

Swaab DF 1997 Prader–Willi syndrome and the hypothalamus. Acta Paediatrica 86(Suppl 423):50–54

Thannickal TC, Moore RY, Nienhius R et al 2000 Reduced number of hypocretin neurons in human narcolepsy. Neuron 27:469–474

35

Alcohol

Strong, and more especially, spirituous liquors, are a certain, though slow, poison. (John Wesley 1747)

BACKGROUND

Alcohol, more correctly called ethanol (or ethyl alcohol), is a non-specific, low potency, ubiquitous, colourless, odourless liquid that is both water-soluble and lipid-soluble. Alcohol problems are those of abuse, dependency, intoxication and withdrawal. In the US Epidemiological Catchment Area Study there was a 14% lifetime prevalence alcoholism. The point prevalence in males is about 4% and in females about 1%. Alcohol-related disorders are estimated to be the reason for assessment in one-quarter of cases presenting to accident and emergency centres and one-third of cases presenting to psychiatrists (Table 35.1).

CLINICAL FEATURES

Clinical features attributed to alcohol can be divided in those of intoxication, dependency (Box 35.1) and withdrawal.

The effects of mild intoxication (blood alcohol level 20–100 mg/ml) are mild euphoria and increased confidence (disinhibition). Above levels of 100 mg/ml there is dysarthria, ataxia and a reduced attention span. As the blood level rises above 200 mg/ml, there is increasing sedation, nausea and anterograde amnesia. Levels above 400 mg/ml can cause death from cardiovascular and CNS depression.

When withdrawing from alcohol, dependent patients experience a sudden loss of the anxiolytic and sedative effects of alcohol causing rebound insomnia and overarousal. In addition, any underlying problems that were masked by alcohol will resurface. Withdrawal phenomena begin within 12 hours but usually diminish by the fourth day (Table 35.2). The severity of withdrawal symptoms is tremendously variable. About 95% of withdrawals are limited to mild or moderate symptoms, but 5% of patients experience delirium or convulsions, or both (even when medicated). Predictors of severe withdrawal reactions include a high quantity of alcohol consumption, sudden abstinence, a history of epileptic seizures, a history of delirious episodes and previous severe withdrawals (Palmstierna 2001). It is important to distinguish psychotic features that occur in withdrawal from those that occur during intoxication and those that are due to an alcohol-induced psychotic disorder.

PATHOGENESIS

The aetiology of alcoholism is much investigated but poorly understood. Genetic factors appear to play a role, but the effect of culture, peer learning and parental roles must be the predominant influence. Genetic factors are stronger in males than females. Concordance for monozygous twins is 70% in males and 50% in females. Concordance for dizygous twins in 43% in males and 30% in females. One interesting finding is that in adoption studies an elevated risk of alcoholism is seen in biological relatives only and in men more clearly than women.

Various mechanisms have been proposed to explain the effects of alcohol on the brain. In the early 1800s, Schmiedeberg proposed that alcohol produced a global depression of neural activity (White

Table 35.1 Frequency of alcohol-related presentations to accident and emergency centres	
Presentation	Frequency (%)
Proportion of all admissions	15.7
Proportion of patients aged <65 years	24.4
Proportion of self-harm cases	34.5
Adapted from Kratzer et al (1998)	

Table 35.2 Clinical features of alcohol withdrawal

	Mild to moderate withdrawal	Severe withdrawal (delirium tremens)
Onset and duration	Onset 1–2 days, duration 1–2 days	Onset 2–5 days, duration 3–14 days
Psychological symptoms	Fearful, aroused or low mood	As mild, plus over overarousal
Somatic symptoms	Tremor, nausea, sweating, sleep disturbance, muscle cramps, tachycardia, anorexia	As mild, plus convulsions (in 10%)
Psychiatric symptoms	Perceptual distortions	Clouding of consciousness, hallucinations or illusions, delusions
Prognosis	Full recovery, but may resume drinking	Mortality of 10%

Box 35.1 Clinical markers of severe alcohol use

Alcohol dependency features
Stereotyped drinking
Primacy of drinking
Increased tolerance
Withdrawal symptoms
Compensatory or morning drinking
Compulsion to drink
Reinstatement after abstinence

Non-dependency features
Excessive drinking
Long duration of excessive use
Psychological sequelae
Binge drinking
Physical sequelae, especially blackouts, fits, cirrhosis
Cognitive disturbance
Social sequelae

After Edwards & Gross (1976)

Table 35.3 Proposed neurochemical changes in alcoholism

Chemical increased	Effect
GABA	Anxiolytic
Serotonin	Nausea
Glutamate (*N*-methyl-D-aspartate)	Amnesia
Endogenous opioids	Craving
Acetylcholine (chronically)	Unknown
Noradrenaline (norepinephrine)	Alerting and arousal effects
Dopamine	Reinforcement and craving
Hypothalamus–pituitary–adrenal axis (cortisol)	Neurotoxicity, pseudo-Cushing's syndrome

et al 2000). Simplistic theories relying on one neurotransmitter have been embarrassed by more complex data. Lipid theories postulate that alcohol acts via perturbation of the membrane lipids of CNS neurones, whereas protein theories propose that alcohol interferes with neurotransmitters and neuropeptides (Table 35.3). Both of these mechanisms, and others, could act in concert.

OUTCOME

Several large multicentre studies show a mixed picture for those undergoing treatment for alcohol dependency. About one-third of detoxified patients will complete an abstinence programme lasting over 6 months. Of those not lost to follow-up, abstinence rates at 1 year are about 25%, with help. Nevertheless, even those that relapse may have improved drinking patterns and lower mortality rates that could justify treatment (Miller et al 2001) (for further information see Ch. 45).

NEUROPSYCHIATRIC COMPLICATIONS OF ALCOHOL USE

Affective disorder and alcohol

The Epidemiological Catchment Area Study found that among subjects with a lifetime history of alcohol abuse, 13% had a history of affective disorder. Conversely, among those with a lifetime history of affective disorder, 22% also met criteria for alcohol abuse. There are also higher rates of anxiety disorder and bipolar disorder in alcoholic patients. There is a significant effect of sex: alcoholic men have only slightly higher rates of depression than non-alcoholic men (5% versus 3%) whereas women have dramatically higher rates (20% versus 7%).

There are two likely reasons for this association. The first is that alcohol causes affective disorders either directly or indirectly. Some evidence suggests that in two-thirds of men with current alcohol dependency and depression, the alcoholism came first. The second is that patients with affective symptoms use alcohol to self-medicate. This appears to be the case in women, since in two-thirds of cases depression precedes the alcohol use (Helzer & Pryzbeck 1988). Depression in current drinkers is hard to assess,

partly for the reasons discussed above. If patients achieve abstinence, many depressions will remit within weeks, even without the use of antidepressants. Conversely, if patients fail to achieve abstinence, depression continues and the risk of suicide may be up to 5% per year. Alcohol, depression and suicidality are a dangerous combination.

Does alcohol directly cause depression? Alcohol certainly causes social drift, isolation, financial hardship, loss of other interests and health problems that are sufficient to result in depression indirectly through 'non-biological' means. Acutely, alcohol causes disinhibition and mild euphoria in those with normal baseline mood. Alcohol causes disinhibited behaviour such as self-harm and suicide in patients with low baseline mood, but it is not certain that

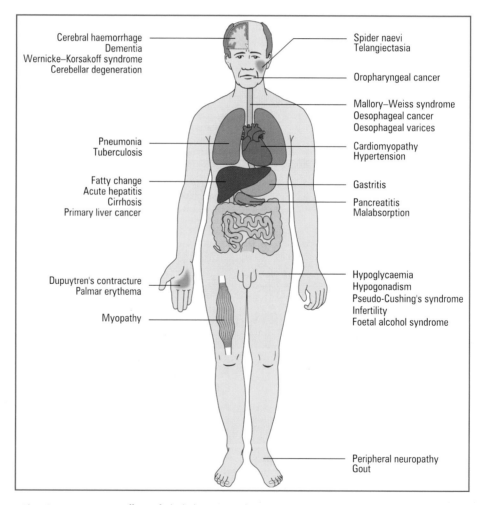

Fig. 35.1 Systemic effects of alcohol. From Haslett (1999).

Table 35.4 Clinical features of alcohol-related neuropsychiatric syndromes

Symptom or sign	Korsakoff's psychosis	Wernicke's encephalopathy	Delirium tremens	Hepatic encephalopathy	Alcoholic dementia	Alcoholic hallucinosis	Central pontine myelinolysis
Acute confusion	0	++	++++	++++	±	0	+++
Residual cognitive impairment	++	++	±	0	++++	±	±
Impaired registration	++	+	+++	++	++	±	0
Impaired short-term memory	++++	+	+++	+++	+	±	±
Visual hallucinations	0	0	++++	±	0	++	±
Auditory hallucinations	0	0		0	±	++++	0
Opthalmoplegia	0	++++	++	++	0	0	0
Ataxia	+	++++	++	++	±	0	+
Motor weakness	0	0	0	+	0	0	++++
Peripheral neuropathy	++	+++	0	0	0	0	0
Autonomic hyperactivity	0	0	++++	0	0	0	0
MRI findings	Mammillary degeneration, cortical atrophy	Mammillary degeneration	None	None	Cortical atrophy	Cortical atrophy	Demyelination in pons

0, absent; ±, variable feature; +, ++, +++, occurs with increasing commonness
Adapted from Arciniegas & Beresford (2001)

alcohol actually lowers mood for a sustained period as is popularly reported. It is simply not sufficient to say that alcohol causes depression of neuronal activity and hence depression of mood. No study has linked the effects of alcohol at the cellular level with alterations in mood (as opposed to alertness).

As with depressive disorders, anxiety disorders are now recognized to have a complex relationship with alcohol use. Established anxiety disorder increases the probability of problem drinking and increases the chances of relapse after initial abstinence. Alcohol dependency seems to cause anxiety itself, most commonly as a withdrawal effect. Eighty per cent of alcoholic people report panic attacks during acute withdrawal. Thus, the powerful anxiolytic and sedative properties of alcohol and its wide availability make it a common choice for patients with dis-

abling affective symptoms. Unfortunately, when alcohol is self-prescribed the effects of tolerance, dependency and multiple complications make it a particularly unfortunate choice.

Psychotic disorder and alcohol

Alcohol causes transient psychotic symptoms during withdrawal, usually in the form of a delirium tremens. Hallucinations occurring in clear consciousness are rare, occurring in roughly 2% of alcoholics. Diagnostically, such hallucinations cause problems in terms of differentiation from delirium tremens. The term *alcohol (or alcoholic) hallucinosis* is usually reserved for cases that occur following reduction or cessation of alcohol in someone who was previously alcohol-dependent. The hallucinations are

Box 35.2   Neuropsychiatric syndromes associated with alcohol

- Acute alcohol intoxication
- Alcohol dependency syndrome
- Delirium tremens
- Alcoholic hallucinosis
- Alcohol-induced dementia
- Alcohol-induced mood disorder
- Alcohol-induced sleep disorder
- Alcohol-induced sexual disorder
- Wernicke–Korsakoff syndrome
- Alcoholic pellagra
- Cerebellar degeneration
- Head injury due to alcohol
- Hepatic encephalopathy
- Marchiafava–Bignami disease
- Central pontine myelinolysis
- Peripheral neuropathy due to alcohol

usually second-person auditory hallucinations, often of a paranoid nature. Delusions and other first-rank symptoms are sufficiently rare that they would raise questions about the accuracy of the diagnosis. Onset is often during acute alcohol withdrawal, although with continued abstinence the hallucinations should fade away. Duration is usually short with abstinence, but Benedetti (1952) showed that if these symptoms last longer than 6 months after abstinence 50% of diagnoses will be revised to schizophrenia and 50% will manifest cognitive impairment. This latent schizophrenia theory has been challenged in recent years. Some patients suffer predominantly delusional ideas, typically of paranoid type or morbid jealously, of long duration, suggesting that there are acute and chronic subtypes of alcoholic hallucinosis. There is much that remains to be learnt about alcohol-induced psychotic disorders.

Cognitive disorder and alcohol

Patients with high levels of alcohol use have cognitive problems but these have proven difficult to study reliably, owing to comorbidity, absence of cooperation and the clinical fluctuation of these patients. One important question that is very difficult to answer conclusively is what level or duration of alcohol consumption is required to produce cognitive deficits? This area has been reviewed with the finding that the literature is split 50:50 into those studies that demonstrate a relationship between the amount of alcohol consumed and cognitive deterioration and

those that do not (Parsons & Nixon 1998). Some evidence suggests that people with low levels of alcohol use perform better than abstainers. More importantly, it is safe to conclude that drinking more than 28 units a week over a sustained period is very likely to have cognitive and anatomical consequences, but that very high levels over a considerable period are required to induce severe deficits (dementia).

There does not appear to be a robust set of impairments that characterize alcohol-related cognitive impairment. On tests of general intelligence, persons with chronic alcohol histories have, on average, a performance between 0.5 and 1 standard deviation below that of age-matched controls. Problems with executive function and memory are most often involved. Abstinence will bring about substantial improvements in the majority, although some patients continue with a below-average baseline function. Some cognitive domains (such as verbal memory) appear to improve more quickly than others. When the deficits are severe and irreversible, the term *alcohol-induced dementia* is used (see below).

Specific syndromes
Wernicke's encephalopathy
In 1881 the Polish neurologist Carl Wernicke described two cases caused by alcohol and one caused by vomiting after sulphuric acid ingestion. This acute syndrome, which may be precipitated by glucose loading without thiamine, is characterized by clouding of consciousness, ocular palsies (most often of cranial nerve VI) with or without nystagmus, ataxic gait and peripheral neuropathy.

The syndrome is seen in between 1% and 10% of alcoholics at autopsy and in approximately 15% of serious alcoholics during life. Usually the syndrome is present in partial form. Hypothermia and hypotension are also commonly seen. In the series described by Victor, 80% of patients went on to develop Korsakoff's syndrome, although 10% of patients with Korsakoff's syndrome do not show evidence of Wernicke's encephalopathy. Mortality is between 25% and 50% in patients who go untreated.

Korsakoff's syndrome
Korsakoff's syndrome was described by Sergei Korsakoff in 1887; he named it 'cerebropathia psychica toxaemica', the term 'Korsakoff's psychosis' first being used by Friedrich Jolly (1844–1904). Korsakoff described the syndrome in 30 alcoholics

Clinical Pointer 35.1

Investigation of suspected alcohol abuse

Before jumping into the deep end of medical investigations, begin by asking the patient about his or her alcohol intake. It is an exaggeration that all alcoholics are dishonest about their consumption! Take the opportunity to ask carers about drinking habits, particularly on a typical day. Consider using one of several screening questionnaires, but be aware of their limitations. A random blood, breath or urine alcohol test will reveal recent drinking – 1 unit (10 ml by volume of pure alcohol) increases blood alcohol by 20 mg/dl. The legal driving limit in the UK is 80 mg/dl (blood), 107 mg/dl (urine), 35 mg/dl (breath); >150 mg/dl (blood) is serious intoxication. Elevated γ-glutamyl transferase (GGT) (>30 U/l), aspartate aminotransferase (AST) and alanine aminotransferase (ALT) levels >45 IU/l (with AST usually more elevated than ALT) or mean corpuscular volume >96 fl is present in 95% of male alcoholics and 65% of female alcoholics. However, the sensitivity and specificity of any one test is about 50%. Other markers include uric acid, triglycerides and mitochondrial AST. Carbohydrate deficient transferrin (where available) is the most sensitive (90%) and specific (95%) test for occult alcohol use. Complications of alcohol abuse may be indicated by dehydration, nutritional or electrolyte imbalance or abnormalities of the gastrointestinal and neurological system on radiological investigation.

Further reading   Heather N, Peters TJ, Stockwell TR (eds) 2001 International handbook of alcohol dependence. Wiley, Chichester
Fiellin DA, Reid C, O'Connor PG 2000 Screening for alcohol problems in primary care – a systematic review. Archives of Internal Medicine 160:1977–1989

and 16 non-alcoholics. This chronic amnestic syndrome is characterized by:

- amnesia for new learning (anterograde episodic memory being more affected than retrograde memory, with preserved working memory)
- confabulation (not pathognomonic of the syndrome)
- preservation of other aspects of cognition (it is not a form of delirium)
- peripheral neuropathy (related to Wernicke's encephalopathy)
- hallucinations (although these were originally described, psychosis is not a defining feature).

Full recovery only occurs in less than one-quarter of patients with Korsakoff's syndrome, although more than half will show some improvement.

Mechanism of Wernicke's encephalopathy and Korsakoff's syndrome

Both syndromes are caused by thiamine depletion that disrupts glucose synthesis, neurotransmitter function and protein (DNA) synthesis via reductions in transketolase. Dietary sources of thiamine, such as vegetables, cereals, milk, liver and pork, are often replaced by alcohol in heavy drinkers. Paradoxically, the ability the absorb thiamine is reduced in thiamine-deficient alcoholics.

Pathologically, there are petechial haemorrhages and demyelination in the hypothalamic mammillary bod-

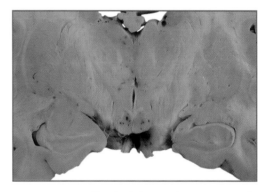

Fig. 35.2   Mammillary body haemorrhages in Wernicke's encephalopathy. From Stevens & Lowe (2000).

ies, periaqueductal grey matter and the mediodorsal thalamic nuclei in both Wernicke's encephalopathy and Korsakoff's syndrome. One study has suggested that neuronal loss in the anterior thalamic nuclei differentiates amnesic from non-amnesic alcoholics (Harding et al 2000). Cortical atrophy is also seen.

Alcohol-induced dementia

Dementia due exclusively to the direct effects of alcohol on the brain is not a clearly delineated syndrome. The cognitive deficits seen in heavy drinkers vary considerably in severity and type. They do not appear to have a characteristic regional or pathogenetic association and patients may not recover completely on abstinence. This may be because there is reduced dendritic cell arborization (a precursor of cell death). Nevertheless, the majority of chronic drinkers do show neuropsychological deficits in short- and long-term memory, visuospatial function and, to a lesser extent, executive function. Language, motor and sensory functions are usually intact. Clinicoanatomical relationships with vulnerable areas (the hippocampus, corpus callosum, medial temporal lobe and frontal lobe) have been documented. There is good evidence that changes reverse, at least in part, upon abstinence. Liver disease appears to be independent of this syndrome but nutritional compromise does exacerbate the deficits, suggesting an overlap with the Wernicke–Korsakoff syndrome. Of course, liver disease may in itself cause hepatocerebral degeneration typically following cirrhosis or chronic hepatitis. In this case, symptoms of tremor, cerebellar ataxia, dysarthria and choreoathetosis are present.

Rare alcohol-related neuropsychiatric syndromes

Alcoholic pellagra
Alcoholics with very poor nutrition may lack niacin in the diet and this eventually leads to pellagra. Pellagra can also result from a tryptophan-deficient diet, poor nutrition in the elderly and chronic diarrhoea. There is not thought to be a specific mechanism whereby alcohol per se causes pellagra.

Features are not as clearly delineated as in Wernicke–Korsakoff's syndrome. Early signs are fatigue, irritability, poor concentration and dysphoria. A clearer picture gradually emerges of confusion, hypertonia with weakness, hallucinations and possibly myoclonus, ataxia and incontinence. Catatonic signs may be present. Systemic manifestations are diarrhoea, glossitis, dermatitis and anaemia. The diagnosis may be missed, leading to further deterioration if nicotinic acid or nicotinamide is not given. Recovery is variable. Post-mortem pathology demonstrates swollen giant cells of Betz in the motor cortex and, to a lesser extent, in cranial motor nuclei and anterior horn cells.

Central pontine myelinosis
Central pontine myelinosis, or osmotic myelinosis, is a rare complication of alcohol resulting from a change in the serum osmolality that is more often recognized at post-mortem than in life. It is also seen in patients with liver disease, burns, sepsis and anorexia. The rapid correction of hyponatraemia appears to play an important role in this osmotic demyelination syndrome. Clinically, there is a spastic quadriparesis and cranial nerve paresis. The level of consciousness may be reduced and recovery is variable. Radiographic changes include involvement

---

Clinical Pointer 35.2

Management of the intoxicated patient presenting with low mood and self-harm

One of the most difficult management scenarios in psychiatry is that of patients who are currently drinking and depressed. Immediate management should be to secure the safety of staff and patient, and this may involve physical or chemical restraint. Next priority is the immediate physical needs of the intoxicated patient, because severe intoxication can be life-threatening. However, this is unlikely to be the case in someone coherent enough to complain of low mood or suicidal thoughts. Alcohol tends to exacerbate baseline mood and to cause disinhibition. Therefore complaints of dysphoria and self-harm impulses are common under the influence of alcohol, and in many cases will resolve when the person is sober. Overnight observation may be all that is required. Detailed mental state assessment is not recommended for patients who are moderately or severely intoxicated, and will need to be delayed until blood or breath alcohol levels have fallen. Patients may request acute admission for detoxification while they are intoxicated, but this is rarely indicated in an unknown patient simply because abstinence is very unlikely to be maintained without preparatory work. However, in the motivated subject, outpatient detoxification is an alternative. If depression appears to be present once the patient is assessed free of alcohol, conventional treatment is indicated, with the proviso that the contribution of alcohol to the presentation should be elicited. In the depressed patient who is currently free of alcohol, but with little real intent to remain so, treatment will be extremely difficult, perhaps impossible. Concomitant treatment of alcohol dependency, where present, is a prerequisite for helping with depression and reducing future suicide risk.

Further reading *Schuckit MA, Tipp JE, Bergman M et al 1997 Comparison of induced and independent major depressive disorders in 2,945 alcoholics. American Journal of Psychiatry 154:948–957*

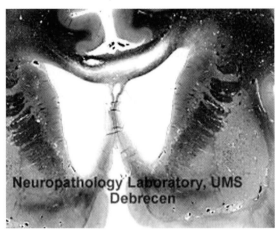

Fig. 35.3 Central pontine myelinosis. There is demyelination involving the basis pontis and pontine tegmentum (the corticospinal and corticobulbar tracts), producing an almost triangular wedge. Demyelination may interrupt lateral geniculate nuclei. It is also known as the Adams–Victor–Mancall syndrome after their original description in 1959. From Professor K Hegedüs University of Debrecen.

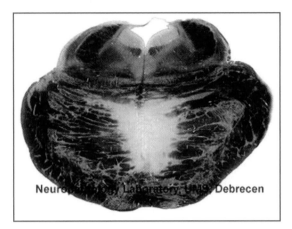

Fig. 35.4 Marchiafava–Bignami disease. Necrosis of the middle lamina of the myelinated corpus callosum occurs. The anterior and posterior commissures, centrum semiovale and other white matter tracts, such as middle cerebral peduncles, may also be involved. However, the internal capsule and corona radiata are usually spared. From Professor K Hegedüs University of Debrecen.

of the central pons, with sparing of a peripheral rim and descending corticospinal tracts. Extrapontine involvement is common.

Marchiafava–Bignami disease

The Italian pathologists Marchiafava and Bignami described three male alcoholics who died following seizures and coma. At post-mortem the middle two-thirds of the corpus callosum showed severe necrosis. Subsequent observations have shown that this is a rare complication characterized by demyelination and degeneration of the central aspect of the corpus callosum and often involving the anterior commissure.

Presenting features are a variable picture of dementia (possibly with frontal lobe features), apraxia, paresis and dysarthria. The disease is almost invariably confined to male alcoholics with 10 years or more of heavy drinking. Neuropsychiatric features can include early irritability or aggression, alteration in consciousness and an amotivational syndrome. The mechanism may be independent of malnutrition.

Acquired hepatocerebral degeneration

Acquired (non-Wilsonian) hepatocerebral degeneration is an uncommon complication of chronic hepatic cirrhosis with portosystemic shunting.

Alcohol is only one possible cause. The condition runs a chronic course interspersed with periods of acute hepatic encephalopathy. Hepatic encephalopathy has been attributed to elevated ammonia released by protein in blood and its secondary neurotransmitter effects. Clinical features include asterixis or tremor, dysarthria and ataxia, and possibly choreoathetosis and myoclonus. A spectrum of cognitive deficits can occur. Post-mortem examination reveals patchy necrosis and microcavitation with widespread hyperplasia of protoplasmic astrocytes (changes that are very similar to those seen in Wilson's disease). Pathological changes are most commonly seen in the parietal, occipital, cerebellar and basal ganglia regions. Lesions are concentrated in vascular border zones, usually sparing the hippocampus and globus pallidus, which are the sites of classical hypoxic lesions.

SUMMARY

Alcohol is the most widely available drug in the world and one that is often, regrettably, used by patients with pre-existing dysphoria and anxiety as a form of self-medication. With chronic use, a person experiences few of the positive effects but an accumulating number of hazardous effects of the drug. Alcohol is often stated to be a CNS depressant – that is, it has more inhibitory than stimulatory actions on neurones. However, the cellular actions of alcohol are not fully understood and vary from one part of the brain to another. There is no direct evidence that links the cellular actions of alcohol with its effects on mood. The actions of alcohol vary dramatically, according to the dose consumed. At high doses it is a CNS toxin, and it can be lethal in overdose. Alcohol is responsible for many neuropsychiatric problems in adults, including head injury, road traffic accidents, disruption of supportive relationships and various neuropsychiatric syndromes.

REFERENCES AND FURTHER READING

Arciniegas DB, Beresford TP 2001 Neuropsychiatry. An introductory approach. Cambridge University Press, Cambridge

Adams RD, Mancall EL, Victor M 1959 Central pontine myelosis. Archives of Neurology and Psychiatry 81:154–161

Benedetti G 1952 Die Alkoholhalluzinosen. Thieme, Stuggart

Edwards G, Gross MM 1976 Alcohol dependence: provisional description of a clinical syndrome. British Medical Journal 1:1058–1061

Harding A, Halliday G, Caine D et al 2000 Degeneration of anterior thalamic nuclei differentiates alcoholics with amnesia. Brain 123:141–154

Helzer JE, Pryzbeck TR 1988 The co-occurrence of alcoholism with other psychiatric disorders in the general population and its impact on treatment. Journal of Studies on Alcohol 49: 219–224

Koob GF, Roberts AJ, Schulteis G et al 1998 Neurocircuitry targets in ethanol reward and dependence. Alcoholism and Clinical and Experimental Research 22:3–9

Kratzer W, Blum P, Mason R et al 1998 Alcohol-associated diseases in internal medicine: a screening study on 1494 medical emergency patients. Leber Magen Darm 28:115–121

Miller WR, Walters ST, Bennett ME 2001 How effective is alcoholism treatment in the United States? Journal of Studies on Alcohol 62:211–220

Palmstierna T 2001 A model for predicting alcohol withdrawal delirium. Psychiatric Services 52:820–823

Parsons OA, Nixon SJ 1998 Cognitive functioning in sober social drinkers: a review of the research since 1986. Journal of Studies on Alcohol 59:180–190

Wesley J 1747 The iliac passion. Reprinted by Epworth Press, London, 1960, pp 29–32

White AM, Matthews DB, Best P J 2000 Ethanol, memory, and hippocampal function: a review of recent findings. Hippocampus 10:88–93

36

Illicit Drug Use

NEUROLOGY OF ILLICIT DRUG USE

Illicit drug use is increasingly recognized as an important cause of seizures, stroke, delirium, peripheral neuropathy and coma in young people. In addition, drug abusers are prone to traumatic injuries and infectious diseases.

CNS infections

Intravenous injection carries the risk of the direct introduction of pathogens into the systemic circulation. Typically these collect on heart valves as endocarditis, later being carried to the lungs, periphery or CNS. There is also the ever-present risk of HIV infection.

Encephalopathy

Severe and occasionally permanent brain damage can result from the toxic effects of several illicit drugs. This is akin to the state of acute poisoning induced by neurotoxins (see Ch. 37). Abuse of organic solvents causes an encephalopathy with both acute high-dose and chronic low-dose exposure. Organic solvents are highly lipophilic and have powerful CNS effects, including cerebral oedema and damage to white matter. This is thought to cause cognitive impairment and eventually dementia in heavy toluene users. Inhaled heroin vapour can cause a toxic form of progressive spongiform leukoencephalopathy, although this is rare. In opiate users there are often small white matter lesions, although their clinical significance is uncertain. MRI scans of cocaine abusers demonstrate cerebral atrophy.

Movement disorders

The best-known association is the role of the illicit drug contaminant MPTP (1-methyl-4-phenyl-1,2,3,6-tetrahydropyridine) in parkinsonism. Approximately 400 intravenous drug abusers who injected the meperidine analogue MPPP (1-methyl-4-phenyl-4-propionoxypiperidine) were exposed to the by-product MPTP. A small proportion developed rapidly progressive parkinsonian symptoms within 2 weeks of exposure. In this case, the mechanism is well described. MPTP is actually a pro-toxin that is converted by monoamine oxidase-B into MPP^+ (1-methyl-4-phenylpyridine). MPP^+ rapidly destroys neurones in the substantia nigra by targeting complex I (NADH coenzyme Q reductase) in the mitochondrial electron transport chain. In contrast with Parkinson's disease, other areas outside the substantia nigra are not affected. However, this observation has triggered huge interest in the oxidative stress hypothesis of Parkinson's disease and the finding that a defect in mitochondrial oxidative phosphorylation, more specifically a reduction in the activity of complex I, occurs in the striatum of patients with idiopathic Parkinson's disease. Cocaine is also well known to produce dyskinesia, usually in the form of choreoathetosis, akathisia and tremor. Less commonly, dystonia and tics emerge. Rarely, amphetamine users develop an involuntary but reversible chorea.

Seizures

Drug intoxication with cocaine and amphetamines and withdrawal of CNS depressants such as alcohol, barbiturates, benzodiazepines and opiates is associated with generalized seizures. In alcoholic patients, it is usually heavy abuse followed by sudden absti-

Table 36.1 Lifetime prevalence of drug abuse

Drug	Prevalence (%)
Caffeine	40
Tobacco	35
Alcohol	14
Cannabis	5
Stimulants	2
Sedatives	2
Opioids	1
Hallucinogens	0.5
Cocaine	0.2

nence that produces seizures in the first 48 hours of stopping drinking. Seizures occur during intoxication with cocaine, regardless of seizure history; these are usually single episodes with no lasting damage, although they can be refractory to treatment. Intravenous drug users can develop seizures as a result of brain abscess, meningitis or emboli.

Stroke

Illicit drug use should be suspected if a person aged under 40 years suffers a stroke. Cocaine (both alkaloid 'crack' cocaine and cocaine hydrochloride) causes cerebral hypertension, which can lead to haemorrhagic stroke (Fig. 36.1). This occurs within 3 days of cocaine use, at points of vascular weakness (e.g. arteriovenous malformations, occult aneurysms) and also in the thalamus and basal ganglia. Abuse of other stimulants, such as amphetamine (usually methamphetamine) and ephedrine, can also cause haemorrhagic stroke. Intravenous heroin use has been linked with ischaemic border zone infarctions. Alcohol causes hypertension and can result in haemorrhagic stroke, although the effect is a chronic rather than acute one. Embolism in intravenous drug users is another cause of stroke, although pulmonary embolus is much more likely.

NEUROPSYCHIATRIC COMPLICATIONS OF ILLICIT DRUG USE

Depression

Depression is seen about three times more commonly in those with a history of substance abuse. It is not certain whether mood disorder can be attributed directly to lasting CNS effects of the drug. Because most depression is relatively enduring while most drug abuse is periodic, the relationship is likely to be complex and to involve significant social and personality variables. Dysphoria is well recognized in conjunction with intoxication with alcohol and benzodiazepines. Intoxication with benzodiazepines or barbiturates causes drowsiness, lethargy and impaired memory. Withdrawal effects include restlessness, insomnia and anxiety with panic attacks, often compounded by the re-emergence of underlying psychiatric symptoms (for which the drugs were first taken). More severe withdrawal states can include feelings of unreality, perceptual distortions

or hallucinations and, occasionally, acute psychoses. Depression following withdrawal from cocaine may be protracted, lasting up to 3 months, but it usually subsides while craving is still present. Withdrawal from amphetamines produces a syndrome of lethargy and dysphoria, which may last for days or weeks.

Constant use of opioids and cannabis produces a persistent state of dysphoria, apathy and social withdrawal that is relieved (only to a point of near normality) by the next hit. Relatives of depressed opioid addicts have higher rates of depression, anxiety and drug abuse than normal controls and relatives of non-depressed abusers (Rounsaville et al 1991). Suicide is common in those with illicit drug problems, but is often misreported as a drug-related fatality.

Euphoria

Euphoria is the desired state of addicts using cocaine, heroin, cannabis and amphetamines. These states are transient and subject to tolerance. People describe being hyperalert and may experience visual, tactile and auditory hallucinations. Panic attacks and extreme paranoia may occur.

Psychosis

Psychosis is characteristic of chronic amphetamine abuse. Hallucinations in all sensory modalities occur during intoxication. Paranoid overvalued ideas are very common, progressing to delusions. Changes in thought content may last longer and per-

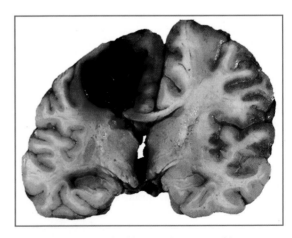

Fig. 36.1 Intracerebral haemorrhage caused by cocaine usage. From Professor Edward C Klatt, Florida State University, College of Medicine.

Table 36.2 Neuropsychiatric disorders induced by illicit drugs

Drug	Dependence syndrome	Withdrawal syndrome	Intoxication delirium	Depression or dysphoria	Anxiety	Psychosis	Cognitive deficit
Alcohol	✓	✓	✓	✓ (W)	✓ (W)	✓ (W)	✓
Amphetamine (as illicit drug)	✓	✓	✓	✓ (W)	✓	✓	✗
Caffeine	✗	✓	✗	✗	✓	✗	✗
Cannabis	✓	✗	✓	✗	✓	✓	✗
Cocaine	✓	✓	✓	✓ (W)	✓ (W)	✓	✗
Hallucinogens	✓	✗	✓	✓	✓	✓	✗
Inhalants	✓	✗	✓	✓	✓	✓	✓
Nicotine	✓	✓	✗	✗	✗	✗	✗
Opioids	✓	✓	✓	✓		✓	✗
Phencyclidine	✓	✗	✓	✓	✓	✓	✗
Sedatives	✓	✓	✓	✓ (W)	✓ (W)	✓ (W)	✓
Polysubstance abuse	✓	✓	✓	✓	✓	✓	✓

W, withdrawal effect; ✓, recognized association; ✗, no association
Adapted from Kaplan & Sadock (1995)

haps evolve over several days or weeks. Rapid resolution is typical with discontinuation, and therefore chronic delusions imply continued use. Episodes of violence fuelled by paranoid beliefs are seen. Amphetamine reproduces the positive syndrome of schizophrenia but without formal thought disorder and negative symptoms. Phencyclidine can mimic the negative syndrome. Similar positive symptoms are seen in cocaine users who, paradoxically, can become sensitized to the drug with chronic use. With cocaine, tactile hallucinations and visual hallucinations are particularly common. Psychotic disorder associated with cannabis use is controversial. Intoxication with high doses produces hallucinations, and occasionally paranoid fears, perplexity and terror may be experienced along with depersonalization and derealization. Long-term provocation of a schizophrenia-like syndrome has not been proven.

Cognition

Relatively few studies have examined the cognitive characteristics of patients at various meaningful stages of an illicit drug habit and in comparison with a control group. Studies are also confounded by polysubstance abuse histories, HIV infection, depression and difficulties obtaining accurate information. Grant et al (1978) studied 151 polysubstance abusers in comparison with psychiatric patients and healthy volunteers. Patients with a history of opiate abuse were most likely to have deficits. Thirty-seven per cent had impairment on the Halstead–Reitan

Battery compared with 26% of psychiatric patients and 8% of healthy controls. Ardila et al (1991) assessed 37 free-base cocaine abusers. After 1 month of abstinence there were still deficits in attention and recent verbal and visual memory. Heavy cocaine use for a sustained period appears to be capable of impairing cognition globally, even in subjects who are currently abstinent. However, Beatty et al (1995) found only mild and diffuse deficits in both heavy cocaine users and alcoholics. Conversely, a recent study from Robbins' group showed that chronic amphetamine and cocaine abusers have significant impairments in attention, planning and spatial working memory, which, it is suggested, indicates frontal lobe involvement (Ornstein et al 2000).

Abusers of inhalants appear to be at particular risk of neurological and cognitive deficits. Such users may have globally worse cognitive function than abusers of other drugs, and as many as two-thirds may be affected. The amount, duration and recency of the abuse appear to mediate the effects on cognitive function, and several studies have reported a dose–response relationship. Guerra et al (1987) found that cognitive performance in 93 opiate addicts before detoxification was more impaired than controls but not significantly different 1 week after detoxification. Maruff et al (1998) reported that length of time of petrol sniffing (and blood lead levels) correlated significantly with the magnitude of neurological and cognitive deficits. Cognitive functions affected by cannabis include attention, memory and verbal expression. In a well-designed study of

---

Clinical Pointer 36.1

How to identify and engage patients with illicit drug use

As with people who are abusing alcohol, illicit drug users may be hesitant about admitting their habits, at least until trust is built up. A good starting place, therefore, is to explain the purpose of an assessment and the types of help available. Involving a family member is often advantageous, both at the information-gathering stage and later to help with support and relapse prevention. When engaging a person in a treatment regimen it is invariably best to be honest about what can and cannot be offered. Drawing up clear goals and boundaries helps people with chaotic lifestyles.

The illicit drug history establishes the pattern, extent and complications of abuse. Problems with dependency, severe intoxication and neurological, psychological and social complications should be open to enquiry. Physical examination is important. In intravenous users, there is the risk of infection (including with HIV), thrombophlebitis and pulmonary embolism. In those inhaling, there is the risk of asthma, bronchitis and, in those using the nasal route, perforated nasal septum, bleeding and rhinitis.

General signs of drug use include recent needle tracks, disorientation and mood alterations. More specific indicators of acute intoxication include:

- euphoria, drowsiness, miosis, constipation, pruritis and nausea (with opioids)
- hyperactivity, hallucinations, mydriasis, tremor, tachycardia and fever (with amphetamines)
- depersonalization, hallucinations mydriasis, ataxia, conjunctivitis and tachycardia (with hallucinogens and phenylcyclidine)
- drowsiness, diaphoresis, ataxia, delirium, hypotension and miosis (with sedatives).

Urine toxicology is often the cornerstone of drug assessment and monitoring, although there are other forms of substance screening (e.g. blood, hair). However, toxicology is not a substitute for clinical skills.

Further reading   Perrone J, De Roos F, Jayaraman S et al 2001 Drug screening versus history in detection of substance use in ED psychiatric patients. American Journal of Emergency Medicine 19:49–51
Wolff K, Farrell M, Marsden J et al 1999 A review of biological indicators of illicit drug use, practical considerations and clinical usefulness. Addiction 94:1279–1298

---

current and former cannabis users, Pope et al (2001) found that the relatively subtle deficits induced by heavy cannabis use were entirely reversible. In general, subjects with MRI abnormalities have worse cognitive and behavioural function than those without, although specific clinicoanatomical relationships have not been well established.

Personality

Chronic cannabis use has been associated with an insidious change of personality, with social and intellectual decline. This is often described as an amotivational syndrome. This is a complex interaction between the changes in lifestyle associated with the priority for regular drug use and direct effects of the drug.

SUMMARY

Four per cent of the world's population use drugs illegally, half of which is accounted for by cannabis products. In the USA and Europe, one-third of the population have used an illicit drug in their lifetime. Stimulants are abused by 30 million people worldwide and use has recently been escalating. In the USA however, cocaine is the second most widely abused drug (2% of the population) and the most common drug related to overdose. Eight million people worldwide (with a concentration in Asia) abuse opiates, and this is linked with significant medical complications. In the USA, 1% of the population admit to non-medical use of prescribed psychotropics, but this has fallen from a rate of 4% in 1985. In the USA and Europe, about 10,000 deaths per year are attributed to illicit drugs. Often multiple drugs are involved, and in about 60% of cases an accidental overdose is the cause. The remainder of non-accidental cases are largely accounted for by suicide.

REFERENCES AND FURTHER READING

Ardila A, Rosselli M, Strumwasser S 1991 Neuropsychological deficits in chronic cocaine abusers. International

Journal of Neuroscience 57:73–79

Beatty WW, Katzung VM, Moreland VJ et al 1995 Neuropsychological performance of recently abstinent alcoholics and cocaine abusers. Drug and Alcohol Dependence 37:247–253

Grant I, Adams KM, Carlin AS et al 1978 The collaborative neuropsychological study of polydrug users. Archives of General Psychiatry 35:1063–1074

Guerra D, Sole A, Cami J, Tobena A 1987 Neuropsychological performance in opiate addict after rapid detoxification. Drug and Alcohol Dependence 20:261–270

Kaplan HI, Sadock BJ 1995 Pocket handbook of psychiatry,

2nd edn. Williams & Wilkins, Baltimore

Maruff P, Burns CB, Tyler P et al 1998 Neurological and cognitive abnormalities associated with chronic petrol sniffing. Brain 121:1903–1917

Ornstein TJ, Iddon JL, Baldacchino AM et al 2000 Profiles of cognitive dysfunction in chronic amphetamine and heroin abusers. Neuropsychopharmacology 23:113–126

Pope HG, Gruber AJ, Hudson JI et al 2001 Neuropsychological performance in long-term cannabis users. Archives of General Psychiatry 58:909–915

Rounsaville BJ, Weissman MM, Kleber HD 1991 Psychiatric disorders in relatives of probands with opiate addiction. Archives of General Psychiatry 48:33–42

37

Environmental Toxins

BACKGROUND

A wide range of substances can cause damage to the CNS. These include drugs, chemicals (occupational and household poisons), heavy metals, environmental pollutants (pesticides, wastes), natural plant and animal toxins, and food additives (preservatives dyes, food contaminants). The effects of occupational exposure to toxic chemicals are far from trivial. Each year 120 million people worldwide are injured or disabled after occupational accidents or exposure. In the developed world, occupational hazards account for 2% of all years of life lost and 1.7% of DALYs (total years of healthy life lost due to a disease; see Ch. 1). Eighty per cent of this exposure occurs in men. Cancers are thought to be the most common complication, followed by injury and poisoning.

Homeostatic mechanisms usually maintain essential vitamins, minerals and trace elements within acceptable limits, but these mechanisms break down in an environment of persistently high or low environmental toxin concentrations. Toxic effects of various chemicals are most commonly seen in the context of occupations such as chemical manufacture and mining, but they are also seen following deliberate ingestion in a suicide attempt. Carbon monoxide, heavy metals, organic solvents and pesticides are the usual suspects, although establishing the exact causative agent can be a challenge.

EFFECT OF CHEMICALS ON THE NERVOUS SYSTEM

Toxic substances can alter both the structure and the function of cells. The nervous system is vulnerable to toxins, partly because of the priority of continuous electrochemical signals and partly because of the inability of neurones to regenerate. In addition, neurones require relatively large quantities of oxygen to maintain their high metabolic rate and hence are especially vulnerable to anoxia. The developing nerv-

---

Clinical Pointer 37.1

Establishing the cause of suspected neurotoxicity in the workplace

There is no golden rule that can establish whether a particular agent is neurotoxic in the workplace. A list of chemicals used should be obtained from the employer. Details of exposure, including method of contamination, and of washing facilities, should also be obtained. Clinical features may or may not be helpful. Objective evidence of exposure should be obtained where possible. This may include photographs of any sign, neuropsychological assessment and possibly EEG, EMG or evoked potentials where indicated. Heavy metals are excreted in the urine and can be assayed directly. Establishing that a particular agent was neurotoxic in a particular case in often a question of judgement. However, Schaumberg & Spencer (1987) have suggested guidelines to help with this problem:

- there is a consistent pattern of neurological dysfunction
- the neurotoxic syndrome can be reproduced in animals
- there are reproducible pathological or pathophysiological findings
- the demonstrable pathological and pathophysiological findings can account for the clinical findings
- there is a temporal relationship between the intoxication and onset of the clinical syndrome
- the disorder is non-focal.

Further reading Parry GJ 2001 Neurological complications of toxin exposure in the workplace. In: Aminoff MJ (ed) Neurology and general medicine, 3rd edn. Churchill Livingstone, Edinburgh, p 645–664
Schaumberg HH, Spencer PS 1987 Recognizing neurotoxic disease. Neurology 37:276–278

Table 37.1 Neuropsychiatric effects of toxins

Drug name (mechanism)	Cerebellar syndrome	Depression and irritability	Dementia	Encephalopathy and delirium	Neuropathy (cranial)	Neuropathy (peripheral)	Parkinsonism	Seizures
Aluminium (metal)	✓		✓	✓			✓	✓
Arsenic (metal)			✓			✓		
Bismuth (metal)	✓	✓		✓	✓		✓	✓
Carbon monoxide (gas)	✓		✓		✓	✓	✓	
Carbon disulphide (solvent)				✓	✓	✓	✓	
Cyanide (solvent/gas)	✓			✓				✓
Ethylene glycol (solvent)	✓			✓			✓	✓
Hydrogen disulphide (gas)				✓				✓
Lead (metal)	✓	✓	✓	✓	✓	✓	✓	✓
Manganese (metal)	✓	✓	✓	✓	✓	✓	✓	
Mercury (metal)	✓	✓	✓	✓			✓	✓
Methanol (solvent)	✓	✓			✓		✓	
Methyl chloride (gas)	✓	✓		✓				✓
Organochlorines (pesticide)	✓	✓		✓	✓	✓	✓	✓
Organophosphate (pesticide)	✓	✓				✓		✓
Thallium (metal)	✓		✓		✓	✓	✓	
Trichlorethylene (solvent)	✓			✓	✓	✓		
Tin (metal)	✓		✓	✓				

ous system is especially vulnerable to certain toxic substances. Toxic substances seem to act selectively on the various components of the nervous system, damaging the neuronal bodies (neuropathy), axons (axonopathy) and myelin sheaths (myelinopathy).

Most potentially harmful chemicals exist in several forms that may differ radically in neurotoxic effect. For example, alkylmercury compounds are generally more toxic than elemental mercury, especially in the methylmercury form, which completely crosses the blood–brain barrier. Similarly, elemental arsenic does not cross the blood–brain barrier but is toxic to peripheral nerves. Arsenic in trivalent and pentavalent forms will readily cross into the brain. Arsenic gas is the most toxic form. The adverse effects of most compounds differ by degree of exposure. Acute exposure to high concentrations (typical of self-poisoning) is often followed by delirium, seizures and change in consciousness. Death can occur without treatment. Toxins that produce characteristic features after acute exposure include methanol (methylalcohol; associated with retinal blindness), organophosphates (associated with cholinergic syndrome) and trichlorethylene and hexacarbons (associated with narcosis). The effects of chronic exposure to lower doses (typical of accidental occupation exposure) are a wider variety of toxic features that usually accumulate with time. The common complications are illustrated in Table 37.1. Cognitive impairment is a feature common to most cases of chronic poisoning, although the specific deficits are not well characterized in general. Differential diagnosis can be difficult, since few compounds are associated with characteristic symptoms or signs (Clinical Pointer 37.1).

NEUROTOXICOLOGY OF SPECIFIC CNS TOXINS

Lead poisoning

Lead poisoning is one of the best-described toxic syndromes. It is usually caused by occupational exposure. Acute exposure may produce delirium with seizures. Long-term overexposure is also a frequent finding in inner city environments. Mildly elevated levels (above the recommended maximum of 10 μg/dl) are associated with fatigue, sleepiness, apathy and dysphoria, although over a sustained period even lower levels damage cognition in children. High blood levels above 70 μg/dl are indica-

tive of severe poisoning and prompt urgent treatment. Motor neuropathy is the classic sign, along with a gingival lead line and a white line in the epiphyses. Poor concentration is more common than dementia. Ataxia, inattention and agitation are seen in children. Elevated red blood cell protoporphyrin can be used as a screening test.

Carbon monoxide

Carbon monoxide toxicity is commonly encountered as self-poisoning with car exhaust fumes. It accounts for over 1000 deaths per year in the UK and 5000 deaths per year in the USA, and carbon monoxide is the most common cause of toxic morbidity and death in the western world. Chronic low levels of exposure may present with flu-like symptoms that are more often than not overlooked. The mechanism of damage is mainly hypoxia, since carbon monoxide combines with haemoglobin preferentially over oxygen to form carboxyhaemoglobin. Areas that are vulnerable to hypoxia are the most affected, including the periventricular white matter, the hippocampus and the basal ganglia (particularly the globus pallidus). Acute effects are delirium and coma. Delayed neurological effects (2–40 days after exposure result from damage to the hippocampus (producing memory deficits), basal ganglia (producing parkinsonism), midbrain (producing akinetic mutism), frontal cortex (producing cognitive impairment) and cerebellum (producing ataxia). The nature and severity of complications is difficult to predict and extremely variable. Markers of severity

Table 37.2 Carbon monoxide poisoning by level of carboxyhaemoglobin

Carboxyhaemoglobin (%)	Symptoms
10	Asymptomatic or may have headaches
20	Dizziness, nausea, syncope
30	Visual disturbances
40	Confusion, syncope
50	Seizures, coma
60	Cardiopulmonary dysfunction and death

Adapted from Varon & Marik (1997)

Table 37.3 Neuropsychiatric effects of chronic heavy metal poisoning

Metal	Main symptoms	Pathology	Characteristic sign (if any)	Main treatment	Common sources
Lead	Gastrointestinal symptoms, motor polyneuropathy (organic lead), widespread cognitive effects including dementia, seizures	Petechial haemorrhage, neuronal loss, micronecrosis, cerebral oedema	Blue tint to gums, motor neuropathy	Chelation therapy	Paints, petrol, pottery, batteries, pipes, solder, illicit whiskey
Mercury*	Tremor, agitation, gingivitis, cognitive deficits (dementia, especially in children), peripheral neuropathy, cerebellar and basal ganglia symptoms, chorea, scotomas, nephropathy, personality change	Neuronal loss in cerebrum and cerebellum	Fine tremor	Chelation therapy with penicillamine[†]	Elemental and organic mercury in factories, fungicides
Arsenic	Acute gastrointestinal symptoms, progressive weakness, painful sensorimotor polyneuropathy, acute tubular necrosis, marrow suppression, cognitive deficits leading to dementia, hearing loss	Metabolic disruption	Hyperkeratosis of soles, garlic halitosis, Mee's lines in nailbed	Dimercaprol or succimer or unithiol, dialysis	Weed killer, pest control, ore refineries, various industries
Thallium	Gastrointestinal symptoms, sensorimotor polyneuropathy, optic neuritis, cranial nerve palsies, ataxia, tremor, dementia, personality change	Cerebral oedema, axonal white matter lesions, neuronal loss in basal ganglia and thalamus	Alopecia	Prussian blue and haemodialysis	Pest control
Manganese	Slowly progressive cognitive impairment, lability of mood and behaviour, impaired consciousness, personality change, dementia, apathy, anorexia, insomnia, psychosis	Neuronal loss in globus pallidus, caudate, putamen, thalamus and cortex	Parkinsonism with dystonic features	Calcium versenate	Mining and iron industry, battery manufacture, steel mills, fireworks
Aluminium	Gradual onset after at least 3 years of dialysis. Aphasia, myoclonus, seizures and dementia, occasional psychotic symptoms	Neuronal loss in cortex	Dementia after dialysis	Largely symptomatic	Aluminium in dialysate
Tin	Delirium and dementia accompanied by ataxia	White matter lesions	None	Symptomatic	Canning industry, electronics, solder

*Clinical features vary depending on exposure to organic mercury or elemental mercury
[†]Not effective for organic mercury poisoning

Table 37.4 Historical examples of environmental neurotoxicity

Year(s)	Location	Substance	Comments
1930s	USA	Triorthocresyl phosphate	Bootleggers contaminated the alcoholic beverage 'Ginger-Jake' with a varnish additive (Lyndol) that contained an organophosphorus compound, leading to neuronal death in the peripheral nervous system and CNS. It is estimated that 5000 were paralysed and 20 000–100 000 were affected
1950s	Minamata Bay, Japan	Methylmercury	From the 1930s to the 1960s, a chemical company released many tonnes of mercury into Minamata Bay. People living around the bay developed methylmercury poisoning through the consumption of contaminated fish. The victims suffered from severe neurological damage, known as Minamata disease. By March 1989 there had been 2217 cases and 46 confirmed deaths
1950s	France	Tin	Contamination of stallinon with triethyltin resulted in more than 100 deaths
1950s	Morocco	Manganese	150 ore miners suffered chronic manganese intoxication involving a severe parkinsonian syndrome
1956	Turkey	Hexachlorobenzene	Hexachlorobenzene, a seed grain fungicide, poisoned 3000–4000 people, with a 10% mortality rate
1959	Morocco	Tri-o-cresyl phosphate	Cooking oil contaminated with lubricating oil affected approximately 10 000 people
1960	Iraq	Mercury	Mercury was used as a fungicide to treat seed grain used in bread; more than 1000 were people affected
1964–1965	Niigata City, Japan	Methylmercury	Methylmercury poisoning affected 911 people after its release into the Agano River, Niigata Prefecture. The main symptoms were dysaesthesia, ataxia, dysarthria, hearing disturbance and tremor
1968	Japan	Polychlorinated biphenyls	In western Japan, the consumption of rice bran oil contaminated with polychlorinated biphenyls affected 1665 people ('yusho,' or 'oil disease'). Subsequent analysis showed that the presence of toxic thermal degradation products in the oil may have been responsible for the observed health effects
1971	Iraq	Mercury	Wheat seed treated with an alkylmercury fungicide and intended for planting was mistakenly used to prepare bread. More than 6500 Iraqis were hospitalized with neurological symptoms, and 459 died
1973	USA	Methyl-n-butyl-ketone	Fabric production plant employees were exposed to the organic solvent methyl-n-butylketone. More than 80 workers suffered polyneuropathy; 180 had less severe effects
1980s	California, USA	N-Methyl-4-phenyl-1,2,3,6-tetrahydropyridine	An impurity in the synthesis of the illicit meperidine analogue MPPP caused symptoms identical to those of Parkinson's disease, but without the autonomic features or dementia

Table 37.4 *Contd*

Year(s)	Location	Substance	Comments
1981	Madrid, Spain	Toxic rape seed oil	An extensive outbreak of severe respiratory illness occurred in Madrid and the north-west regions, affecting 20 000 people. Many suffered severe pneumonia and neuropathy, and 500 people died. Investigations showed that olive oil used in cooking had been adulterated with an illegally marketed and contaminated rape seed oil containing a toxic substance
1985	USA and Canada	Aldicarb	More than 1000 people from California to British Columbia experience neuromuscular and cardiac problems following ingestion of melons contaminated with the pesticide Aldicarb

Adapted from US Congress, Office of Technology Assessment (1990)

of poisoning, such as elevated carboxyhaemoglobin levels and loss of consciousness, do not appear to be particularly predictive.

Some degree of cognitive disturbance is seen in the majority of patients, including those without evidence of damage on neuroimaging, but deficits can be subtle. Domains affected include memory and executive dysfunction (in 75% of patients) as well as attention and visuospatial skills (50% of patients) (Gale et al 1999). More than two-thirds of patients have elevated rates of depression, anxiety and frustration early after exposure, and high rates are detectable several years later. This can influence cognitive performance. Unsurprisingly, rates of depression after self-poisoning are higher than after accidental exposure and tend to improve with time, arguing against a depressogenic effect of poisoning per se (Hay et al 2002)

Organophosphorus compounds

Organophosphorus compounds were developed as chemical weapons in World Wars I and II. Their current use is as pesticides, and thus exposure typically occurs in agricultural workers. Exposure results in inhibition of acetylcholinesterase, producing a cholinergic syndrome with muscarinic effects, nicotinic effects and effects related to the dysfunction of the neuromuscular junction. Acutely, hypoxia and respiratory failure are most dangerous and result from the lack of central drive compounded with excessive bronchial secretions, bronchospasm and respiratory muscle paralysis. Secondary complications are characterized by fatigue, irritability and poor concentration. Chronically, effects begin with peripheral nerve involvement and progress to corticospinal tract signs with ataxia and myelopathy. Cognitive impairment can occur, along with drowsiness and chronic fatigue. Atropine is the specific anticholinergic treatment, although oximes can regenerate cholinesterases.

Organic solvents

Ethers, hydrocarbons, ketones and alcohols are commonly used industrial chemicals. Examples are the hydrocarbons benzene, toluene and trichlorethylene. They result in chronic toxic encephalopathy and ataxia after long-term exposure. Organic solvents are a major component of paints, glues and cleaning liquids. Toluene (methylbenzene) is one of the most widely used solvents. It can cause headaches, neuropathy, ataxia, hallucinations and coma. Carbon disulphide (used as a fumigant and solvent) is thought to be particularly toxic, producing irritability, insomnia, hallucinations and, later, sensorimotor neuropathy and parkinsonism. Inhalation of toluene, trichlorethylene and butane (from glues, cleaning fluids and lighter fuels) occurs in drug abusers. Acutely, abusers desire the euphoriant effects (which are associated with giddiness and transient disorientation and perceptual distortions). Chronic use of toluene can lead to diffuse brain damage.

Methanol

Methanol (methylalcohol) is widely available as a component of de-icers, antifreeze, paints, varnishes and paint thinners. Ingestion of 100 ml or more is likely to have toxic effects. Methanol is metabolized by alcohol dehydrogenase to formaldehyde and then to formic acid. Complications may be due to metabolic acidosis from high formic acid concentrations. The overall mortality of methanol poisoning is approximately 20%, and among survivors the rate of permanent visual impairment is 25%. Early visual disturbances are common and include blurred vision, photophobia and visual distortions. The pupils may be fixed and dilated, with fundoscopic examination revealing retinal oedema or papilloedema and engorged retinal vessels. Severe complications are seizures, blindness, oligouric renal failure, cardiac failure and pulmonary oedema. Death may be rapid with or without coma. Treatment is to decrease the metabolic degradation of the methanol into its toxic degradation products via co-administration of alcohol (which competes for alcohol dehydrogenase), dialysis and forced alkaline diuresis.

SUMMARY

Toxic quantities of heavy metals lead to an encephalopathy and, often to seizures and delirium following acute exposure. Toxic quantities accumulated slowly lead to a more mixed picture of poor concentration, parkinsonism, ataxia, neuropathy, mood alterations (often irritability) and, possibly, dementia. The syndrome may or may not be reversible. Carbon monoxide poisoning is a common cause of hypoxic brain damage, causing cognitive impairment. Organic solvents and methanol (and ethanol) are strongly neurotoxic, but are also widely available, and hence these substances are frequently abused.

REFERENCES AND FURTHER READING

Gale SD, Hopkins RO, Weaver LK et al 1999 MRI, quantitative MRI, SPECT and neuropsychological findings following carbon monoxide poisoning. Brain Injury 13:229–243

Hay PJ, Denson LA, van Hoof M et al 2002 The neuropsychiatry of carbon monoxide poisoning in attempted suicide A prospective controlled study. Journal of Psychosomatic Research 53:699–708

Portera SS, Hopkins RO, Weaver LK et al 2002 Corpus callosum atrophy and neuropsychological outcome following carbon monoxide poisoning. Archives of Clinical Neuropsychology 17:195–204

US Congress, Office of Technology Assessment 1990 Neurotoxicity: identifying and controlling poisons of the nervous system, OTA-BA-436. US Government Printing Office, Washington, DC

Varon J, Marik PE 1997 Carbon monoxide poisoning. Internet Journal of Emergency and Intensive Care Medicine 11

Delirium and Dementia

Delirium and dementia are two of the most common syndromes in medicine. At first glance, the standard textbook definitions offer a clear method of separating the two. Delirium is usually defined as an acute, reversible cognitive syndrome characterized by clouding of consciousness. Dementia is usually defined as a disorder characterized by chronic global cognitive decline. Closer observation highlights several insufficiencies in these definitions.

Reconsider delirium. In the majority of cases, delirium begins suddenly as a manifestation of disturbance of brain metabolism or oxygenation. However, in some cases, the underlying disorder evolves slowly and the higher functions wax and wane over weeks before any diagnosis is made. In most cases once a diagnosis of delirium is recognized the underlying cause is identified and the condition is reversed. But in some cases no cause is found, the cause is not reversible or the delirium continues unabated despite removal of the likely cause. In cases where delirium is irreversible, mortality is very high. There is also the question of clouding of consciousness. Again, a reduced level of consciousness is seen in many delirious patients, but so is overarousal with no stupor. The term *confusion* is often used instead, but this is unsatisfactory because it implies 'uncertainty' in everyday language, and therefore *inattention* is preferable.

Now consider dementia. In the absence of neuropathological data, both ICD-10 and DSM-IV require a 6-month minimum period before dementia can be confidently diagnosed. Of course, in bio-logical terms, the patient who develops a rapid and severe cognitive decline shortly after stroke may have an irreversible condition, even though 6 months have not yet passed. Patients with dementia without delirium also present with *disorientation* (in 92% of cases), inattention (in 45%) and *altered consciousness* (in 20%), symptoms considered hallmarks of delirium. The recent interest in Lewy body dementia has prompted rediscovery of the symptom of fluctuating cognition (particularly attention) in patients with Parkinson's dementia and Alzheimer's disease. Perhaps the main difference between dementia and delirium is that, in dementia, inattention occurs in the context of other deteriorating cognitive deficits, at least some of which are permanent. The other aspect of dementia that has recently been questioned is that of a global cognitive decline. While most patients with established Alzheimer's disease or Lewy body dementia have multiple areas of cognitive impairment, in early cases or in certain conditions (e.g. semantic dementia) specific cognitive domains are affected. The research criteria of ICD-10 recognize this by allowing separate grading of severity of memory and global cognitive performance.

There is clearly a clinical overlap of dementia and delirium, but there is also an aetiological and epidemiological overlap. For this reason, they are both considered in this section. Remember that dementia is a risk factor for delirium, but delirium is also a risk factor for dementia. In a recent systematic review, delirium occurred in 60% of patients with dementia. Many important aspects of care are the same for both conditions.

38

The Delirium Syndrome

When in acute fevers, pneumonia, phrenitis, or headache, the hands are waved before the face, hunting through empty space, as if gathering bits of straw, picking the nap from the coverlet, or tearing chaff from the wall – all such symptoms are bad and deadly. Hippocrates (460–375 BC)

BACKGROUND

Delirium (also known as 'acute confusional state') is an organic mental syndrome of acute or subacute onset, characterized by cognitive impairment (typically disorientation and inattention), fluctuating level of arousal and disturbance of the sleep–wake cycle. It is not a disease but a syndrome of acutely disturbed brain function that occurs when a serious condition affecting the CNS impairs the ability accurately to perceive the environment. The hallmark is said to be *confusion* or *clouding of consciousness*, but these terms are ill-defined and are not synonymous with delirium. The accuracy of diagnosis is enhanced if either clouding of consciousness or inattention are considered the defining characteristics (Cole et al 2003). The condition is both common and life-threatening. On average, 10% of hospitalized patients suffer delirium, but a more important figure is that delirium is seen in 25% of high-risk groups such as postoperative patients or burns victims. Cognitive and psychiatric disturbance are fundamentally related in delirium, since reduced attention processes disturb reality testing, causing an erosion of boundaries between the self and the world. Furthermore, because the patient feels unwell as a result of the underlying medical illness it is under-

standable that beliefs take on a threatening tone. Several questionnaires are available to rate delirium such as the Delirium Rating Scale (DRS) and the Confusion Assessment Method (CAM) (see Appendix V). Demonstration of cognitive impairment alone is not sufficient to make the diagnosis.

Key features of delirium

The key features of delirium include:

- reduced and variable attention (and sometimes consciousness)
- reduced perceptual discrimination, leading to hallucination and illusions
- reduced orientation to the environment
- disturbed behaviour and arousal, leading to over-activity or underactivity, or a mixed picture
- altered mood, leading to irritability, anger or disinhibition
- disordered sleep–wake cycle
- global cognitive impairment
- evidence of organic disease
- neurological signs such as tremor, ataxia and apraxia
- an acute onset and a short and fluctuant course.

PATHOGENESIS

Pathology

There is no clear unifying pathology seen in delirium, although brain electrical activity is disturbed.

Aetiology

A huge range of systemic conditions can cause delirium, particularly those that affect brain oxygenation or metabolism (see Boxes 38.1 and 46.1). Relatively minor changes may precipitate delirium in patients with pre-existing brain disease. In 15% of cases the cause of delirium is not found. In these situations an EEG may assist in confirming the diagnosis and in isolating the underlying cause (Clinical Pointer 38.1). Multiple problems may contribute to delirium in a patient, and in this situation resolution of one underlying cause will not necessarily lead to a cure. Although the nature of the presentation does not normal signify a specific causative agent, certain syndromes are recognizable (e.g. poisoning with opiates or anticholinergics) (Table 38.1).

Vulnerability factors for delirium include existing brain disease (e.g. dementia), old age, alcohol use and sensory impairment. Perpetuating factors include sensory deprivation, sleep deprivation and unfamiliarity of the environment.

OUTCOME

Prognosis

In most cases there is full recovery, but in a minority the prognosis is poor. The mortality rate in delirium is 15% at 1 month and between 20% and 50% at 6 months, higher than in non-delirious medically ill patients or in patients with dementia. There is also a

higher rate of institutional care (Cole & Primaeu 1993). Thus, the prognosis is one of extremes. Patients either do very well with complete recovery, or very badly, often going on to dementia or death (Fernandez et al 1989). The most critical factor determining outcome is whether the underlying cause is recognized and treated. The management of delirium is discussed in Chapter 46.

NEUROPSYCHIATRIC COMPLICATIONS OF DELIRIUM

Mood in delirium

Most patients feel 'unwell' or 'on-edge' but only a minority are able to vocalize clearly how they feel. Probably the most common emotional reactions are anger and a spectrum of anxiety–fearfulness–irritability. Typically, emotions are fluctuant and respond to familiar reassuring people or objects. A minority of people are behaviourally withdrawn and

---

Box 38.1 The ten most frequent causes of delirium

- Postoperative (10% of major elective procedures)
- Occult systemic disease:
  - infection
  - hypoxia
  - metabolic disorder
  - cardiovascular disorder
- Alcohol withdrawal
- Dementia
- Prescribed drug side effect
- New vascular lesion
- New fracture
- Illicit drug intoxication/withdrawal
- Terminal illness
- Unknown cause(s)

Box 38.2 Occult infections that present with delirium

- Chest infection
- Dental abscess
- Endocarditis
- Meningitis
- Osteomyelitis
- Sinusitis
- Tuberculosis
- Urinary tract infection

Clinical Pointer 38.1

The EEG in delirium

It can be difficult to distinguish milder cases of organic cognitive impairment from functional causes of disorientation. In these circumstances, the EEG can detect subtle CNS disease that would not otherwise be seen. For example, the EEG can reveal problems after cardiac surgery not seen on neuropsychological testing or neurological examination. In systemic and neurological disease, an EEG can detect changes that are subclinical on physical examination but that may present as subtle changes in the mental state. For example, Evans et al (1983) found two-thirds of patients with pernicious anaemia had both an abnormal EEG and cognitive impairment. In most cases of delirium, the EEG shows diffuse slowing of the α-rhythm background activity with or without superimposed fast waves (in proportion to the encephalopathy). This picture can also occur in Alzheimer's disease, in patients who are taking sedative medication and, occasionally, in the normal elderly. The exception to slowed EEG activity is seen in delirium caused by alcohol withdrawal, benzodiazepine withdrawal and anticholinergic toxicity, in which low-amplitude, fast activity may be seen. In mild cases of delirium the EEG may be normal. Quantitative EEG is a technique that aims to improve on the value of the routine EEG.

Further reading *Evans DL, Hall H, Ehrin E et al 1983 Organic psychoses without anaemia or spinal cord symptoms in patients with vitamin B$_{12}$ deficiency. American Journal of Psychiatry 140:218–221*
Lipowski ZJ 1990 Delirium: acute confusional states. Oxford University Press, Oxford

Table 38.1 Clues to the aetiology of delirium

Cause	Clinical features	Recommended investigation(s)
Anticholinergic poisoning	Tachycardia, dry mouth, mydriasis, urinary retention, myoclonus	History of exposure
Cholinergic agonist poisoning	Salivation, lacrimation, sweating, incontinence, gastrointestinal cramps, miosis, seizures	History of exposure
Hepatic encephalopathy	Asterixis, fetor hepaticus, sedation	EEG, arterial ammonia
Hypercalcaemia	Weakness, stupor, polyuria, headache, anorexia, vomiting, constipation	Serum calcium, parathyroid hormone, ECG
Hypocalcaemia hormone, ECG	Paraesthesia, spasms, dystonia, tetany, papilloedema, calcification	Serum calcium, parathyroid
Hypokalaemia	Weakness, hypotonia, hyporeflexia, arrhythmias, polyuria, polydipsia	Serum potassium
Hyponatraemia	Oedema, dyspnoea, pulmonary effusions, seizures	Serum sodium
Lithium overdose	Coarse tremor, nausea and vomiting, cramps, myoclonus, seizures	Serum lithium level, ECG
Opiate poisoning	Sedation, miosis, hypotension, pulmonary oedema, rhabdomyolysis, hyporeflexia	History of exposure, myoglobulin in urine
Renal failure (uraemia)	Anorexia, nausea, pruritis, epistaxis, seizures, myoclonus, stupor	Urea and creatinine
Tricyclic antidepressant overdose	Stupor, dry mouth, mydriasis, urinary retention, arrhythmias, myoclonus, seizures	Serum or urine drug level, history of overdose, ECG

apathetic (Fig. 38.1). From another perspective, a substantial number of patients who are referred to liaison psychiatry services with depression or for behavioural problems actually have delirium. There is no evidence that depression directly predisposes to delirium, except in the elderly with vascular brain lesions (where both have a common aetiology).

Cognition in delirium

Reduced or fluctuating arousal and attention are the hallmarks of delirium and influence all other cognitive functions. Orientation in time and place is usually impaired and is often used as a quick bedside diagnostic test. Reliance on this alone, however, will lead to error. There is amnesia, prominently for new material, with a minority of patients displaying confabulation. Patients have difficulty with logical thoughts, concepts and judgement. Language functions are usually temporarily impaired and speech may be absent or excessive, reflecting chaotic underlying thoughts. Tests for visual attention span and recognition memory for pictures may differentiate delirium from dementia and functional psychiatric illness (Hart et al 1997).

Psychotic features seen in delirium

At least 50% of delirious patients have hallucinations. Perceptual disturbances can affect all senses, although visual hallucinations are more common than auditory ones. There may also be disturbances in the passage of time and of body image. Illusions are probably more common than true hallucinations, but they are often misdiagnosed as hallucinations. This distinction is one of degree only. Where delusions and overvalued ideas occur these are typically fleeting, unsystematized, paranoid beliefs. Persecutory delusions are particularly common and may be troublesome for staff–patient relationships.

SUMMARY

Delirium is a acute organic brain disorder characterized by alteration in attention, arousal and distur-

Box 38.3 Prescribed medication causing delirium

High risk
Analgesics and anaesthetics:
- opioids (including withdrawal)
- nitrous oxide

Cytotoxics:
- cyclophophomide
- chlorambucil
- tamoxifen

Endocrine drugs:
- corticosteroids
- hypoglycaemic agents
- sex hormones
- thyroid hormones

Neurological drugs:
- amantadine (including withdrawal)
- anticholinergic agents
- barbiturates (including withdrawal)
- bromocriptine
- levodopa (including withdrawal)

Medium risk
Cardiovascular drugs:
- angiotensin-converting enzyme inhibitors
- alpha blockers
- antiarrhythmics (including digoxin)
- antihistamines (H_1 and H_2 agents)

Psychotropics:
- benzodiazepines
- beta blockers
- disulfiram
- lithium
- tricyclic antidepressants

Rheumatological drugs:
- interferons
- quinine

Lower risk
Anti-asthmatics:
- aminophylline
- theophylline

Antibiotics:
- cephalosporins
- isoniazid
- penicillins
- rifampicin
- sulphonamides

Antispasmodics:
- dicycloverine
- hyoscine
- probanthine

Psychotropics:
- new antidepressants

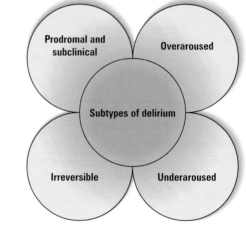

Inattentive
Fluctuating alertness
Agitation or retardation
Near-normal EEG activity

Inattentive
Hyperalert
Psychomotor agitation
Fast EEG activity

Prodromal and subclinical — Overaroused — Subtypes of delirium — Irreversible — Underaroused

Inattentive
Disturbed consciousness
Agitation or retardation
Abnormal EEG activity

Inattentive
Hypoalert
Psychomotor retardation
Slow EEG activity

Fig. 38.1 In 1980, Lipowski proposed that delirium could present in hyperactive and hypoactive forms. Hypoactive (underaroused) presentations are probably more common, but up to 50% of patients fluctuate between the two. Seventy-five per cent of patients have slow EEG activity and 10% have fast activity. The latter may be linked with the hyperactive subtype.

bance of the sleep–wake cycle, with secondary behavioural disturbance and often transient psychotic experiences. Delirium is probably due to subtle neuronal metabolic debt in oxidative metabolism, caused by a wide range of insults. Occasionally, patients with psychiatric disorders may present with disorientation, under- or overarousal and behavioural change that is phenomenologically very similar to delirium. Dementia can be very difficult to distinguish from delirium on a cross-sectional assessment, although longitudinal investigation will reveal the diagnosis in most cases.

Delirium is often avoidable, usually reversible and always controllable by sensible care of the physical environment, relationships with staff, maintenance of metabolic and nutritional state and clear explanation. Because pharmacological management is essentially symptomatic, great effort should be put into finding and treating the underlying cause.

Clinical Pointer 38.2

Ageing and neurodegenerative disease

Psychologists, pathologists, radiologists and clinicians have attempted to differentiate normal ageing from the early stages of dementia. All have met with little success. If one takes a random cohort of elderly people from the general population it is a simple matter to separate those with clear evidence of cognitive impairment plus neurological, psychiatric or pathological anomalies supporting a diagnosis of degenerative dementia. However, this leaves those with pure cognitive impairments (ranging in severity from barely detectable change to moderate change). Such patients have evidence of plaques and tangles, perhaps starting with the vulnerable hippocampus and susceptible large neurones in the second layer of the entorhinal cortex (i.e. the ventromedial portion of the temporal lobe rostral to the hippocampus) (Kordower et al 2001). Indeed, there is persuasive evidence that all the major features of Alzheimer's disease increase linearly with age. However, elderly patients with cognitive deficits at baseline are at increased risk of Alzheimer's disease, and perhaps half of such patients will eventually develop it.

Does this mean that there are two groups of elderly patients with isolated cognitive impairment, one group who will develop Alzheimer's disease and one group that will not? This is not certain, as it can be argued that the 'not' group would have developed Alzheimer's disease if they had not died from something else! The counter-position is that Alzheimer's disease is an extreme form of normal ageing. This can only be countered by the discovery of a specific anomaly separating normal ageing and Alzheimer's disease (and, it is to be hoped, defining the two purely cognitively impaired groups). The critical factor to bear in mind here is that the diagnosis is still very important prognostically, since once diagnosed with Alzheimer's disease a person is on very steep rate of cognitive decline, the rate of which is proportional to the degree of cognitive impairment.

Further reading   Brayne C, Calloway P 1988 Normal aging, impaired cognitive function, and senile dementia of the Alzheimer's type – a continuum. Lancet i:1265–1267
Kordower JH, Chu YP, Stebbins GT et al 2001 Loss and atrophy of layer II entorhinal cortex neurones in elderly people with mild cognitive impairment. Annals of Neurology 49:202–213

Delirium should be considered to be a sensitive, but non-specific, maker of systemic life-threatening illness.

REFERENCES AND FURTHER READING

Cole MG, Primaeu FJ 1993 Prognosis of delirium in elderly hospital patients. Canadian Medical Association Journal 149:41–46

Cole MG, Dendukuri N, McCusker J et al 2003 An empirical study of different diagnostic criteria for delirium among elderly medical inpatients. Journal of Neuropsychiatry 15:200–207

Fernandez F, Levy JK, Mansell PWA 1989 Management of delirium in terminally ill AIDS patients. International Journal of Psychiatry in Medicine 19:165–172

Hart RP, Best AM, Sessler CN et al 1997 Abbreviated cognitive test for delirium. Journal of Psychosomatic Research 43:417–423

Hippocrates 400 BC The book of prognostics (Adams F (ed) 1849 The genuine works of Hippocrates. C and J Adlard, London)

Jain KK 2001 Drug induced neuropsychiatric disorders, 2nd edn. Hogrefe and Huber, Gottingen

39

The Dementia Syndrome

BACKGROUND

Lishman (1998) defined dementia as 'an acquired global impairment of intellect, memory and personality but without impairment of consciousness'. This definition holds true for most common situations. In essence dementia is a syndrome of chronic, progressive and severe cognitive impairment that is caused by multiple individual diseases. As with a diagnosis of delirium, a diagnosis of dementia is incomplete without further investigation for a specific cause.

As longevity increases, so does the percentage of people who succumb to degenerative conditions. In 1900, about 1% of the population was older than 65 years of age. In 1992 that figure was 6% and by 2050 it will have risen to an incredible 25%. What is more, the world population has been rapidly increasing from 5 billion in 1988 to 6 billion in 2000. By the year 2050 there is expected to have been a five-fold increase in the number of sufferers of dementia worldwide, to an astonishing 100 million. By the year 2025, two-thirds of the world's population aged over 65 years (about 275 million people) will be residing in developing countries. Dementia in devel-

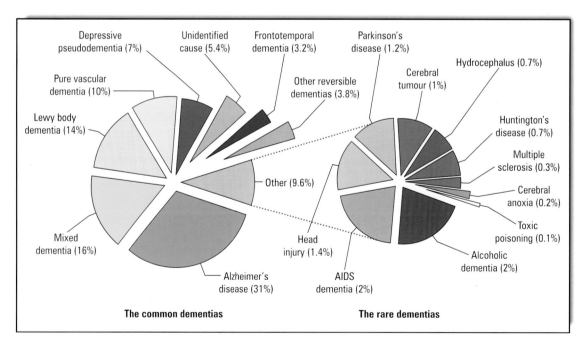

Fig. 39.1   Causes of dementia, defined clinically. Using data from multiple series of clinically defined dementia cohorts, the approximate proportion of patients with each diagnosis is presented. Figures from post-mortem series or selected populations may disagree.

oping countries is terribly overlooked, despite its rising importance. Preliminary evidence suggests it may have some unique features (Chandra et al 1998).

Dementia is equally common in men and women at any given age but, importantly, the dementia burden is greater in women, because women live longer. A Swedish study of 85 year olds found a 30% prevalence of dementia (succinctly divided into one-third with mild, one-third with moderate and one-third with severe dementia), and half of these dementias were due to Alzheimer's disease (Skoog et al 1993). The incidence of dementia is about 1% per year. The mean age of onset is 74 years. Dementia is associated with reduced life expectancy, with some dementias such as vascular dementia running a more malignant course than Alzheimer's disease. Equally importantly, dementia is associated with reduced health expectancy, and over the next 20 years this burden is expected to increase in men to move from the eleventh to the fifth most frequent cause, and in

women from the fourth to the first most significant cause of years lost through disability.

CLASSIFICATION

There have been over a hundred primary research papers that have examined the epidemiology of dementia subtypes. Making sense of these findings can be difficult. One problem is that reported rates vary according to the population studied and method of diagnosis used. There is an interesting phenomenon whereby groups interested in a particular type of dementia report higher rates of that form of dementia than most other comparative studies.

Of elderly people complaining of memory loss, the four big causes are normal or subsyndromal disorders, depression, Alzheimer's disease and vascular dementia (Andreasen et al 1999). Dementias may be classified according to whether the primary pathology originates in the CNS (these are usually neurodegenerative conditions), or whether the pathology is acquired from an extrinsic source (these are often reversible dementias (Box 39.2).

The subsyndromal disorders include *age-associated memory impairment* (AAMI), named by the National Institute of Mental Health (1986). AAMI can be defined as cognition one standard deviation below expected, whereas *mild cognitive impairment* is an intermediate position in the continuum between normality and Alzheimer's disease, with cognition one and a half standard deviations below expected. It is increasingly recognized that dementias of

---

Box 39.2 Potentially reversible dementias

Cranial
CNS tumours
Haematoma
Head injury
Hydrocephalus

Drug induced (see Box 2.9)

Endocrine and metabolic
Addison's disease
Vitamin B_1, vitamin B_{12} or folate deficiency, pellagra,
    hypocalcaemia, hypercalcaemia
Cushing's disease
Dialysis induced
Hypopituitarism
Hypothyroidism
Porphyria

Infective
Encephalitis (including HIV infection and borreliosis)
Meningitis
Syphilitic general paralysis of the insane
Whipple's disease

Psychiatric
Depression
Dissociative disorder
Factitious disorder

Toxic
Alcohol
Carbon monoxide
Heavy metals

Box 39.3 Neuroanatomical classification of dementias

Intrinsic cortical
Alzheimer's disease
Frontotemporal

Intrinsic subcortical
Parkinson's dementia
Huntington's disease
Dementia in multiple sclerosis

Intrinsic multifocal
Lewy body dementia
Vascular dementia
Mixed dementia
Prion disease

Extrinsic (see Box 39.2)

Box 39.4 Summary of diagnostic criteria for common dementias

DSM-IV criteria for dementia

I. Development of multiple cognitive deficits that include memory impairment and at least one of:

   A. aphasia
   B. apraxia
   C. agnosia
   D. disturbance of executive function.

II. The cognitive deficits must be sufficiently severe to cause impairment in occupational or social functioning and must represent a decline from a previously higher level of functioning.

III. A diagnosis of dementia should not be made if the cognitive deficits occur exclusively during the course of a delirium.

IV. Dementia may be aetiologically related to a general medical condition, to the persisting effects of substance use (including toxin exposure), or to a combination of these factors.

NINCDS/ADRDA criteria for Alzheimer's disease

Probable Alzheimer's disease

   A. Presence of dementia.
   B. Deficits in at least two areas of cognition.
   C. Progressive deterioration.
   D. No clouding of consciousness.
   E. Age 40–90 years.
   F. Absence of systemic disorders.

II. Diagnosis supported by:

   A. progressive deterioration of individual cognitive function
   B. impaired activities of daily living
   C. family history of dementia
   D. normal lumbar puncture, EEG, and evidence of atrophy on CT.

III. Features consistent with the diagnosis:

   A. plateaux in the course of the disease
   B. associated psychiatric symptoms
   C. neurological signs
   D. seizures
   E. normal CT scan.

Consensus criteria for diagnosis of probable dementia with Lewy bodies

I. Progressive cognitive decline of sufficient magnitude to interfere with normal social or occupational function. Prominent memory impairment may not occur in the early stages but is evident with progression of the disease. Deficits on tests of attention and of frontal subcortical skills and visuospatial ability may be especially prominent.

II. Two of the following core features are essential for a diagnosis of probable dementia with Lewy bodies:

   A. fluctuating cognition with pronounced variations in attention and alertness
   B. visual hallucinations which are typically well formed and detailed
   C. motor features of parkinsonism.

III. Features supportive of the diagnosis include:

   A. repeated falls
   B. syncope
   C. transient disturbances of consciousness

NINDS-AIREN criteria for vascular dementia

I. For probable vascular dementia:

   A. dementia defined by deficits in multiple domains of cognitive function, confirmed clinically and neuropsychologically, and interfering with everyday life
   B. cerebrovascular disease confirmed by focal neurological signs and evidence of vascular disease on CT or MRI
   C. a temporal relationship between IA and IB.

II. Features consistent with a probable diagnosis include:

   A. early gait disturbance
   B. unsteadiness or falls
   C. urinary symptoms
   D. pseudobulbar palsy
   E. personality and mood changes

III. Features that make the diagnosis unlikely include:

   A. early memory deficit and progressive worsening of specific cognitive deficits without evidence of focal brain lesions on neuroimaging

IV. Diagnosis of Alzheimer's disease is unlikely if:

A. sudden onset
B. focal neurological signs
C. seizures or gait disturbance early in the disease

Possible Alzheimer's disease
A. In the presence of atypical features.
B. In the presence of systemic disease (not considered to be the cause of dementia).
C. In the presence of a single progressive cognitive deficit.

Definite Alzheimer's disease
A. Clinical criteria for probable Alzheimer's disease and
B. histopathological evidence of the disorder.

D. neuroleptic sensitivity
E. systematised delusions
F. hallucinations in other modalities.

IV. A diagnosis of DLB is less likely in the presence of:

A. stroke disease, evident as local neurological signs or on brain imaging
B. evidence on physical examination and investigation of any physical illness, or other brain disorder, sufficient to account for the clinical picture.

B. absence of focal neurological signs
C. the absence of vascular lesions on CT or MRI.

IV. Clinical features of possible vascular dementia include:

A. features of section IA, with focal neurological signs, but where neuroimaging has not been performed to confirm the presence of vascular lesions
B. the absence of a temporal relationship between IA and IB
C. the presence of a subtle and variable course in the disease.

V. Criteria for definite vascular dementia are:

A. clinical criteria for probable vascular dementia
B. histopathological evidence from biopsy or autopsy
C. absence of neuropathological features of Alzheimer's disease
D. absence of other clinical or pathological cause for the disease.

NINDS–AIREN, National Institute of Neurological Disorders and Stroke–Association Internationale pour la Recherche et l'Enseignement en Neurosciences; NINCDS/ADRDA, National Institute of Neurological and Communicative Disorders and Stroke–Alzheimer's Disease and Related Disorders Associateion

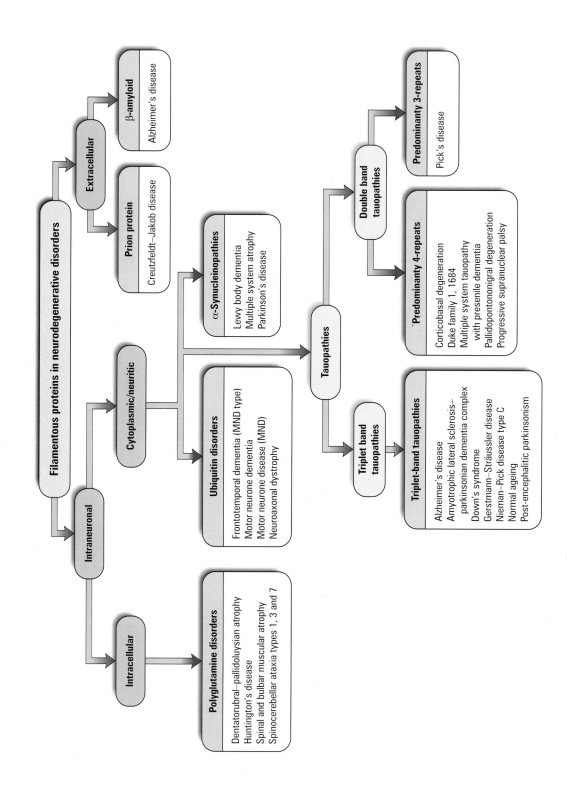

Filamentous proteins in neurodegenerative disorders

Intraneuronal

Extracellular

β-amyloid

Alzheimer's disease

Prion protein

Creutzfeldt–Jakob disease

Cytoplasmic/neuritic

α-Synucleinopathies

Lewy body dementia
Multiple system atrophy
Parkinson's disease

Ubiquitin disorders

Frontotemporal dementia (MND type)
Motor neurone dementia
Motor neurone disease (MND)
Neuroaxonal dystrophy

Intracellular

Polyglutamine disorders

Dentatorubral–pallidoluysian atrophy
Huntington's disease
Spinal and bulbar muscular atrophy
Spinocerebellar ataxia types 1, 3 and 7

Tauopathies

Double band tauopathies

Predominanty 3-repeats

Pick's disease

Predominanty 4-repeats

Corticobasal degeneration
Duke family 1, 1684
Multiple system tauopathy
  with presenile dementia
Pallidopontonigral degeneration
Progressive supranuclear palsy

Triplet band tauopathies

Triplet-band tauopathies

Alzheimer's disease
Amyotrophic lateral sclerosis–
  parkinsonian dementia complex
Down's syndrome
Gerstmann–Sträussler disease
Nieman–Pick disease type C
Normal ageing
Post-encephalitic parkinsonism

mixed pathologies are very important and also very common (see Ch. 43). It is these types of dementias that are most commonly misdiagnosed as something else. The most common mixed dementia is a combination of Alzheimer's disease and vascular dementia (see Fig. 39.1).

Table 39.1 The microscopic pathology of various degenerative dementias

Dementia	Lewy bodies	Tau tangles	Senile plaques
Alzheimer's disease (classical)	✗	✓	✓
Alzheimer's disease (early onset)	✓	✓	✓
Ataxia telangiectasia	✓	✗	✗
Corticobasal degeneration	✓	✗	✗
Creutzfeldt–Jakob disease	✗	✓	✓
Dementia pugilistica	✗	✓	✗
Down's syndrome dementia	✓	✓	✓
Frontotemporal dementias	✗	✓	✗
Hellervorden–Spatz disease	✓	✓	✗
Lewy body dementia	✓	✗	✓
Motor neurone disease dementia	✗	✓	✗
Multiple system atrophy	✓	✓	✗
Parkinson's dementia	✓	✓	✓
Progressive supranuclear palsy	✓	✓	✗
Subacute sclerosing panecephalitis	✓	✓	✗

Fig. 39.2 (opposite) Dementias can be classified on three different levels. At the most superficial is the phenotypical presentation of a condition (i.e. the symptoms and signs). Although this method is the one most commonly used in current practice, it is also the most inaccurate. We are now beginning to understand much about the pathophysiology of many diseases that cause dementia, and this has generated the classification based on abnormal protein products, as illustrated here. Arguably, the most fundamental classification would operate on the level of the genetics. It is of both clinical and theoretical importance to understand how these three systems are interrelated.

DIFFERENTIAL DIAGNOSIS

Dementia characteristically has a gradual onset and protracted course. In neurodegenerative diseases, the patient invariably deteriorates with time. Delirium, learning disability and conditions that cause focal cognitive deficits do not usually pose a problem in differential diagnosis, particularly if repeated assessments are performed. More of a problem are the so-called reversible 'pseudodementias' in which an external cause presents with dementia. The term 'pseudodementia' may be a misnomer, since many of the alleged pseudodementia syndromes can cause a very real dementia if the responsible agent continues unabated. What is more, even in cases where an external agent is identified, full resolution only occurs in a small minority of cases. The term 'pseudodementia' should be reserved for presentations of apparent sustained global cognitive impairment in which problems with consciousness, cooperation, attention, concentration or volition are actually the cause.

PRODROMAL PHASES OF DEMENTIA

In most cases, severe cognitive impairment takes some years to develop, which raises the question of what the earliest indicators of dementia are. One method of examining this question is to look prospectively at the proportion of people who per-

Box 39.5 Inherited disorders of metabolism that can cause dementia in adults

Glycolipid disorders
Gaucher's disease
Gm2 gangliosidosis
Krabbe's leukodystrophy
Metachromatic leukodystrophy
Mucosulphatidosis
Niemann–Pick disease types I and II

Glycosominoglycan disorders
α-Mannosidosis
Neuraminidase or β-galactosidase deficiency

Lipopigment disorders
Kuf's disease (adult Batten's disease)

Adrenoleukodystrophy
Adult form
Adrenomyeloneuropathy

Clinical Pointer 39.1

Validity of early onset versus senile onset dementia

Bondareff (1983) described type I Alzheimer's disease, referring to late-onset disease (over the age of 65 years), and type II Alzheimer's disease as early-onset disease (as originally described by Alzheimer). Early-onset dementia is sometimes considered to have a more rapid deterioration than classical dementia (possibly with aphasia, apraxia, alexia and agraphia). Subsequently, many clinical, neuroimaging, neuropathological and neurochemical studies have attempted to identify differences between early- and late-onset cases, without much success. Developments in services for the elderly in the UK have reinforced the distinction between those aged under 65 years and those aged over 65 years, without a firm scientific foundation. However, recent advances in the molecular genetics of familial Alzheimer's disease have reawakened interest in this field and perhaps added weight to the need for specialized services for young people with degenerative cognitive impairment.

Further reading   *Bondareff W 1983 Age and Alzheimer's disease. Lancet i:1447–1447*
Harvey RJ, Rossor MN 1995 Does early-onset Alzheimer's disease constitute a distinct subtype – the contribution of molecular genetics. Alzheimer's Disease and Associated Disorders 9(Suppl 1):S7–S13
Hodges J 2001 Early-onset dementia: a multidisciplinary approach. Oxford University Press, Oxford

form poorly on baseline cognitive tests and who go on to develop Alzheimer's disease. Chen et al (2001) at the University of Pittsburgh found that the cognitive functions most likely to show early decline (up to 3.5 years before diagnosis) were Trails b and Trails a and word list recognition and recall (Fig. 39.3).

Of course, any degree of permanent focal cognitive impairment will increase the risk of developing dementia. In the case of AAMI (affecting between 30% and 40% of the elderly population) the risk of Alzheimer's disease has been quantified as 20% over 3 years (Waite et al 2001). When cognitive

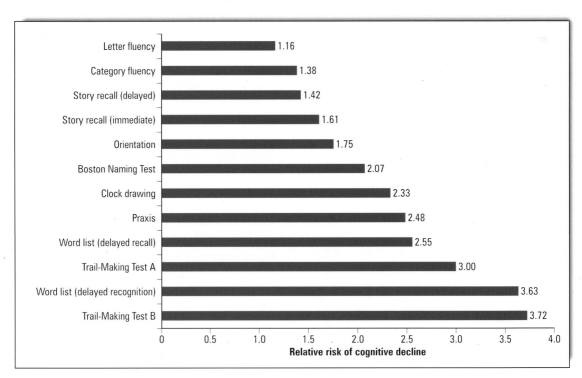

Fig. 39.3   Relative risk of cognitive decline in 68 presymptomatic Alzheimer's disease patients versus 483 controls, by neuropsychological test.

Clinical Pointer 39.2

The status of mild cognitive impairment

Patients with mild cognitive impairment (MCI) tend to lose about 1.5 points per year on the Mini-Mental State Examination (compared with 3 points for those with Alzheimer's disease). Of great interest is the prediction of deterioration to Alzheimer's disease in this group. Whereas healthy elderly controls develop Alzheimer's disease at a rate of about 1% per year (this figure is highly age dependent), the rate of progression in MCI is 10–15% per year. However, not all patients will develop Alzheimer's disease; in fact up to a third recover normal cognitive function within 5 years. In preliminary work, baseline cognitive performance, poor function, poor performance on delayed recall or paired-associate learning, hippocampal atrophy, atrophy of the superior temporal gyri and entorhinal cortices, smaller volume of the posterior cingulate cortex and apolipoprotein E4 have all been found to predict deterioration (Visser et al 2002). Several studies have suggested that depressive symptoms predict cognitive decline in MCI. There may be some merit in dividing patients with MCI into those with Alzheimer-like clinical features and those with vascular features, since in one study the former deteriorated to dementia at a rate of 40% over 2 years and the latter at a rate of 10% over 2 years (Duara et al 2002). Mortality is also higher in vascular subtypes. Early pathological findings suggest that most, if not all, patients with MCI have evidence of temporal lobe degeneration and about half also have Alzheimer-like neocortical abnormalities. Several studies have failed to find evidence of reduced acetylcholine function in MCI patients, although abnormalities in supportive trophic factors may exist (DeKosky et al 2002). In spite of this shortcoming, phase III trials of acetylcholinesterase inhibitors in preventing the deterioration of MCI are soon to be reported, including a three-arm trial of donepezil, vitamin E and placebo in 720 patients.

Further reading Bartrés-Faz D, Junqué C, López-Alomar A et al 2001 Neuropsychological and genetic difference between age-associated memory impairment and mild cognitive impairment entities. Journal of the American Geriatric Society 49:985–990

Blackwell A, Sahakian B, Veset R et al 2002 Early detection of Alzheimer's disease using neuropsychological assessment: paired associates learning and graded naming. 8th International Conference on Alzheimer's Disease and Related Disorders, Stockholm, 20–25 July

DeKosky ST, Ikonomovic MD, Styren SD et al 2002 Upregulation of choline acetyltransferase activity in hippocampus and frontal cortex of elderly subjects with mild cognitive impairment. Annals of Neurology 51:145–155

Duara R, Barker WW, Loewenstein DA et al 2002 Factors affecting the conversion to dementia of subjects with cognitive impairment. Presented at the American Academy of Neurology 54th Annual Meeting, Denver, 13–20 April

Kaye JA, Swihart T, Howieson D et al 1996 Volume loss of the hippocampus and temporal lobe in healthy elderly persons destined to develop dementia. Neurology 48:1297–1304

Visser P, Verhey F, Kester A et al 2002 Predictors of dementia in subjects with mild cognitive impairment: a quantitative meta-analysis. Neurobiology of Aging 23(suppl 1):s138

impairment is combined with extrapyramidal symptoms, vascular symptoms or clear evidence of hippocampal atrophy, the risk doubles. The syndrome of MCI is even more closely affiliated with dementia (Clinical Pointer 39.2). In the elderly with both subjective and objective memory complaints who have deficits in either verbal fluency or episodic recall, the likelihood of developing Alzheimer's disease is above 75% (Palmer et al 2003). Aside from cognitive symptoms, subtle changes in the highest of the higher functions will be noticeable in the prodromal phase of dementia. Examples include changes in social skills, fluency of communication, problem solving and occupational functions (see Tables 40.3 and 40.4). It is possible that future diagnostic tests will reveal the significance of these objectively mild but subjectively important complaints.

SUMMARY

The number of elderly people roughly doubled between the years of 1975 and 2000. This is a snapshot of a global trend in longevity that parallels improvements in social conditions in the 20th century. The same revolution is underway in the developing world and, as a result, we shall see massive increases in elderly people who have survived perinatal injury, nutritional disorders, infectious diseases and trauma in early life. This unprecedented cohort will then have to combat the three big killers of the 21st century: vascular disease, cancer and degenerative disease. There can be no doubt that the continuing excesses of Western society (poor diet, smoking, lack of exercise and, to a lesser extent, alcohol consumption) significantly contribute to current mortality figures. There are signs that these lifestyle influences are slowly improving, but that will still leave the psychiatric and neurodegenerative diseases as the scourge of the 22nd century. Dementia is the second most significant cause of poor quality of life in developed countries (after unipolar depression), but will become the most important cause within the next 20 years.

REFERENCES AND FURTHER READING

Andreasen N, Blennow K, Sjodin C et al 1999 Prevalence and incidence of clinically diagnosed memory impairments in a geographically defined general population in Sweden: the Pitea Dementia Project. Neuroepidemiology 18:144–155

Chandra V, DeKosky ST, Pandav R et al 1998 Neurologic factors associated with cognitive impairment in a rural elderly population in India: the Indo–US Cross-National Dementia Epidemiology Study. Journal of Geriatric Psychiatry and Neurology 11:11–17

Chen P, Ratcliff G, Belle SH et al 2001 Patterns of cognitive decline in presymptomatic Alzheimer's disease. Archives of General Psychiatry 58:853–858

Lishman WA 1998 Organic psychiatry. The psychological consequences of cerebral disorder. Blackwell, Oxford

Palmer K, Bäckman L, Winblad B et al 2003 Detection of Alzheimer's disease and dementia in the preclinical phase: population based cohort study. British Medical Journal 326:245–250

Skoog I, Nilsson L, Palmertz B et al 1993 A population based study of dementia in 85 year olds. New England Journal of Medicine 328:153–158

Tolnay M, Probst A 1999 Review: tau protein pathology in Alzheimer's disease and related disorders. Neuropathology and Applied Neurobiology 25:171–187

Waite LM, Broe GA, Grayson DA et al 2001 Preclinical syndromes predict dementia: the Sydney older persons study. Journal of Neurology, Neurosurgery and Psychiatry 71:296–302

40

Alzheimer's Disease

A woman, 51 years old, showed jealousy toward her husband as the first noticeable sign ... Soon a rapidly increasing loss of memory could be noticed. She could not find her way around in her own apartment ... Her entire behavior bore the stamp of utter perplexity. She was totally disoriented to time and place ... The generalized dementia progressed ... After 4½ years ... death occurred ... The autopsy revealed a generally atrophic brain without macroscopic lesions ... Scattered through the ... cortex ... one found miliary foci that were caused by the deposition of a peculiar substance. Alois Alzheimer (1864–1915)

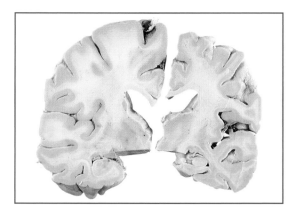

Fig. 40.1 Adjacent coronal slices from two brains. On the left is a normal brain from a 70-year-old; on the right is the same region from a 70-year-old with Alzheimer's disease. The diseased brain is atrophic, with loss of cortex and white matter, which is most marked in the hippocampal region. From Stevens & Lowe (2000).

BACKGROUND

Alzheimer's disease (defined by Kraepelin after Alois Alzheimer's observations in 1907) accounts for roughly half of all dementias. About 5 million people in the USA and perhaps 10 million people worldwide have Alzheimer's disease. These figures are predicted to increase five-fold by 2050. On this basis alone, it is probably the most important of the neuropsychiatric disorders. It is a degenerative condition in which the average survival time is about 10 years. Alzheimer's disease has a strong genetic component in early-onset cases but, in truth, the cause is not well known. The pathogenesis of this dementia is probably best understood in terms of neurone loss in the acetylcholine-rich areas of the brain (see Figs 56.1 and 56.2). This has led to recent developments in the drug treatment for dementia (see Ch. 56).

GENETICS

Genetic factors, but not necessarily single gene mutations, are probably the single most important risk factor in Alzheimer's disease (other than ageing itself). The genetic risk is polygenic and multifactorial in most cases. In about 5% of all cases of Alzheimer's disease (higher in very early-onset dementia), an autosomal-dominant inheritance is recognized. The strongest link is with chromosome 14, which codes for a transmembrane protein of uncertain function. The gene responsible has been designated presenilin-1 and it may be involved in

Table 40.1 Genetic factors in Alzheimer's disease

	Gene defect	Phenotype
Early-onset cases		
Chromosome 14	Presenilin 1 (S182 mutation)	β-Amyloid 42 peptide
Chromosome 21	Amyloid precursor protein	Amyloid
Late-onset cases		
Chromosome 1	Presenilin 2 (E5-1 mutation)	β-Amyloid 42 peptide
Chromosome 19	Atherogenic apoliprotein E ε4 homozygotes	Vascular defects

two-thirds of early-onset cases. In the remaining third, most often no genetic association is apparent. Rarely, if families do recall an autosomal-dominant inheritance then the amyloid precursor protein gene or the presenilin-2 gene may be involved. There are no clear phenotype differences between familial and sporadic cases. Certain other degenerative dementias have an autosomal-dominant inheritance, including Huntington's disease, dentatorubral–pallidoluysian atrophy, tau-associated frontotemporal disorder and the CADASIL syndrome. In late-onset cases of Alzheimer's disease, patients who are homozygous for apolipoprotein E ε4 genotype are likely to develop the condition 7 years earlier than average (see Clinical Pointer 40.2).

PATHOLOGY

A firm diagnosis of Alzheimer's disease rests on the neuropathological findings. Yet, none are pathognomonic of Alzheimer's disease. Eva Braak and Heiko Braak described six pathological stages of progression in Alzheimer's disease in 1995. This was expanded into 10 categories by André Delacourte et al in 1999. However, there is considerable individual variation (Braak & Braak 1991). Neurofibrillary tangles (NFTs) start in the medial temporal lobe structures of the enthorinal cortex and hippocampus (area CA1 before CA3, in turn before CA2), spreading to high-order association cortices and, somewhat

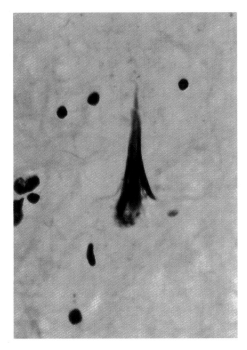

Fig. 40.2 Neurofibrillary tangles are intraneuronal inclusions in pyramidal neurones consisting of an abnormal form of the microtubular association protein tau. Eventually the neurone dies, leaving a ghost tangle. From Schmitt (1999).

later, involving the primary motor and sensory neocortex. This suggests that certain neurones are vulnerable to degeneration in Alzheimer's disease (just

---

Clinical Pointer 40.1

Genetic testing for dementia

As mentioned elsewhere, the presenilins are thought to be the cause of 50% of early-onset Alzheimer's disease (although this accounts for only 5–10% of presentations altogether). Important (but rare) mutations have also been discovered in the amyloid precursor protein genes (which lead to Alzheimer's disease) and in the tau genes (which lead to chromosome 17 dementias), in prion protein genes (which lead to prion disease) and in the specific NOTCH 3 gene on chromosome 19q12 (which leads to cerebral autosomal-dominant arteriopathy with subcortical infarcts and leukoencephalopathy (CADSIL)). Furthermore, mutations in synuclein (which lead to Lewy body dementia), Huntington gene (Huntington's disease), superoxide dismutase (which leads to motor neurone disease), and ubiquitin hydrolase and ataxin genes (which lead to spinocerebellar ataxia) have a role is disorders that feature cognitive impairment. Rather than causative genes, the apoprotein E genotype is associated with an increased risk of Alzheimer's disease and vascular dementia (see Clinical Pointer 40.2).

Thus, few genetic screening tests are currently clinically useful in adult-onset dementia. When they are considered for either presymptomatic screening or for diagnosis in affected individuals, consent and counselling are required (see Clinical Pointer 22.3). In childhood-onset learning disability and congenital cognitive impairment ('amentia'), referral for genetic screening will yield more useful results.

Further reading   *Flint J 1999 The genetic basis of cognition. Brain 122:2015–2031*
Tolmie J 1998 The genetics of mental retardation. Current Opinion in Psychiatry 11:507–513

Clinical Pointer 40.2

The significance of apolipoprotein E in Alzheimer's disease

Apolipoprotein E (ApoE) is a lipid transport molecule that is involved in lipid regulation and coded for by a single gene of the long arm of chromosome 19. There may be a link between amyloid precursor protein and ApoE as amyloid precursor protein is cleared by low-density lipoprotein lipids and ApoE is involved in cholesterol regulation. The ApoE gene is strongly expressed in the hippocampus. Of the three common variants of apoE, the ApoE ε4 allele is a risk factor for Alzheimer's disease (or perhaps more accurately, for earlier onset of dementia occurring in those aged over 65 years), whereas ApoE ε2 is a protective factor. However, the size of this effect of ApoE is modest, either doubling (when present) or halving (when absent) the standard risk of dementia at the age of 65 years from 15%; ApoE4 is neither necessary nor sufficient to cause Alzheimer's disease, because half of sufferers do not carry this gene. Furthermore, increased E4 allele frequency is not confined to Alzheimer's disease but is also seen in Lewy body dementia, Parkinson's dementia, amyloid angiopathy, stroke, mesial temporal sclerosis and Down's syndrome. The ε4 allele can be used as a marker of dementia to improve the specificity of clinical diagnosis (from 55% to 71%, according to Mayeux et al (1998)). Patients with mild cognitive impairment and the E4 allele are at increased risk of progression to Alzheimer's disease.

Further reading *Farrer LA, Cupples LA, Haines JL et al 1997 Effects of age, sex, and ethnicity on the association between apolipoprotein E genotype and Alzheimer's disease. A meta-analysis. Journal of the American Medical Association 278:1349–1356*

Mayeux R, Sanders AM, Shea S et al 1998 Utility of the apolipoprotein E genotype in the diagnosis of Alzheimer's disease. New England Journal of Medicine 338:506–511

as the pigmented neurones of the substantia nigra are vulnerable in Parkinson's disease). In the cortex, globular deposition of β-amyloid occurs in large glutamatergic pyramidal neurones of layers III and V.

The 'holy grail' of Alzheimer's disease research is a specific pathological finding that correlates highly with cognitive impairment and represents a final common pathway in the expression of the disease. Martin Roth was the first to publish an association between pathological markers and clinical severity, although this particular association has not proven

particularly robust (Roth et al 1966). One candidate area that is affected very early in the disease, perhaps preclinically, is the hippocampus (Ball et al 1985). This has been further refined by the use of the synapse density marker, synaptophysin (Fig. 40.3) (Sze et al 1997). Ultimately, the cause of neuronal death in Alzheimer's disease is not yet understood. There are many clues, but no firm conclusions. For example, in embryonic rat hippocampus, β-amyloid phosphorylates tau and leads to disruption of axonal transportation and cell death (Imahori & Uchida 1997). It is widely thought that understanding the pathogenesis of neuronal death is the key to understanding the cause of Alzheimer's dis-

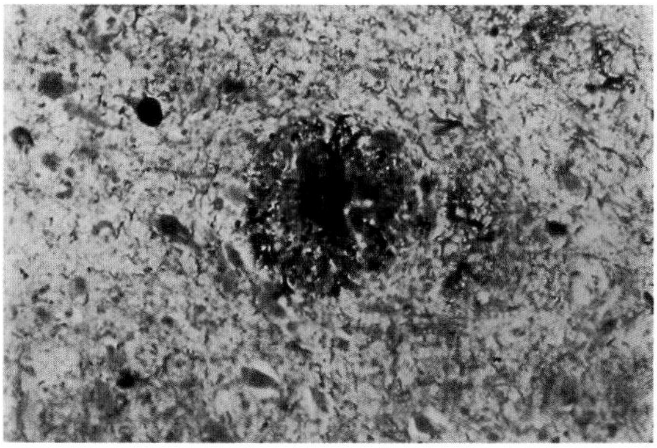

Fig. 40.3 Plaques are extracellular deposits with a core of fibrillary amyloid protein in a dense β-pleated sheet surrounded by neurite of phosphorylated tau. Certain diffuse plaques that are not visualized on silver staining may represent an early stage of plaque development. From Schmitt (1999).

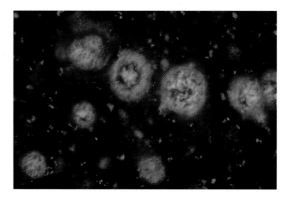

Fig. 40.4 Amyloid in Alzheimer's disease. Thioflavin and fluorescence. From Professor Edward C Klatt, Florida State University, College of Medicine.

ease and, although this seems logical, the two events may prove surprisingly difficult to pin together.

Biological markers of Alzheimer's disease

Neuroimaging markers

With the acknowledged difficulty of distinguishing early Alzheimer's disease from normal ageing, mild cognitive impairment and other forms of dementia, there has been considerable interest in identifying an in vivo diagnostic test of Alzheimer's disease. MRI, SPECT and PET have all been extensively investigated in this regard, with the rather disappointing result that an abnormal test adds weight to the diagnosis but does not prove it (it has moderate *positive predictive value*) and, conversely, that a negative test does not help in either direction (it has a low *negative predictive value*). A useful way of evaluating the utility of a biomarker is to calculate the *differential predictive value* (i.e. the positive predictive value plus the negative predictive value minus one). Unfortunately, few studies of biological markers report the necessary data in meaningful samples (including patients with early Alzheimer's disease) and provide neuropathological confirmation of diagnosis. In fact, only five studies to date have examined patients with Alzheimer's disease using MRI, SPECT or PET and collected neuropathological confirmation (Table 40.2). The results show that SPECT and PET have inadequate specificity as standard diagnostic tools but that they can be used in early cases if there is diagnostic doubt. This may be because the changes seen on functional neuroimaging predate the changes seen on structural imaging, and predate some of the neuropsychological changes. In cases of possible early Alzheimer's dis-

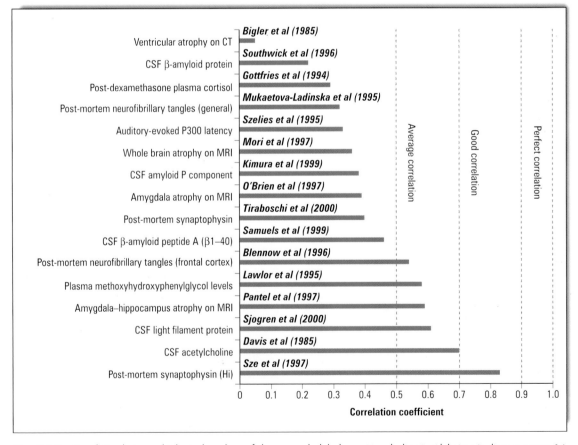

Fig. 40.5 Correlation between biological markers of disease and global cognitive decline in Alzheimer's disease across 16 studies. Hi, hippocampus.

Table 40.2 Accuracy of diagnostic tests in Alzheimer's disease

Criterion	Gold standard diagnosis	Sample	Sensitivity (%)	Specificity (%)	Positive predictive value (%)	Negative predictive value (%)	Reference
Apoliprotein E ε4 allele	Neuropathology	2188	65	68	90	31	Mayeux et al (1998)
Clinical diagnosis and apoliprotein E ε4 allele	Neuropathology	2188	94	71	94	72	Mayeux et al (1998)
CSF total tau	Clinical	413	81	62	55	85	Hulstaert et al (1999)
Combined CSF total tau and β-amyloid 42	Clinical	413	81	86	67	88	Hulstaert et al (1999)
CSF phosphorylated tau	Clinical	570	85	85	80	89	Itoh et al (2001)
Neuropsychological tests	Clinical	385	85	96	68	88	Masur et al (1994)
CT of the temporal Lobe	Neuropathology	86	95	Not presented	75	Not presented	Nagy et al (1999)
Clinical diagnosis and SPECT	Neuropathology	86	61	89	88	65	Jagust et al (2001)
SPECT	Neuropathology	54	86	73	92	57	Bonte et al (1997)
PET (bilateral temporoparietal hypometabolism)	Neuropathology	22	93	63	74	86	Hoffman et al (1996)
Clinical diagnosis	Neuropathology	2188	93	55	90	64	Mayeux et al (1998)

The accuracy of a diagnostic test requires a gold standard. Studies that have compared a diagnostic test against clinical diagnosis are limited by the fact that clinical diagnosis is not good at identifying non-Alzheimer causes of dementia. In the study by Mayeux et al (1998), of all cases thought not to be Alzheimer's disease, clinical diagnosis was wrong 45% of the time (and 77% of the time in those over 79 years of age). In the above studies, investigators compared Alzheimer's disease with clinically meaningful comparison groups, such as non-Alzheimer dementia. The clinical utility of a diagnostic test can be measured by the balance between sensitivity and specificity, in diagnostically difficult situations, such as distinguishing patients with mild Alzheimer's disease from the elderly with a similar degree of cognitive impairment. Diagnostic tests can be used to rule out or rule in suspicious cases

ease, a positive SPECT result would be expected to increase the probability of Alzheimer's disease from 67% to 84% and, conversely, a negative SPECT reduces the chances to 52% (Jagust et al 2001).

Biochemical markers

CSF levels of tau protein and β-amyloid (1–42) peptide, together with the presence of an apolipoprotein E ε4 allele, also increase confidence in an early positive diagnosis of Alzheimer's disease. β-Amyloid 42 is a free-floating protein in the CSF that accumulates in the CNS and forms amyloid plaques in the brain. Abnormally phosphorylated tau protein is the main component of helical filaments that make up neurofibrillary tangles and neuropil threads. Recent data from a large number of studies suggest that elevated CSF levels of tau protein and low CSF levels of β-amyloid 42 protein may have diagnostic significance and hold promise for minimally invasive diagnostic tests of Alzheimer's disease during life (see Table 40.2). The most exciting results have been found using assays for the phosphorylated form of

tau, rather than the less specific total taus. The best study to date published by Itoh et al (2001), was a multicentre Japanese study of 236 Alzheimer's disease patients (using the criteria of NINCDS-ADRDA (National Institute of Neurological and Communicative Disorders and Stroke–Alzheimer's Disease and Related Disorders Association)), 239 patients with other neurological diseases (including vascular dementia, frontotemporal dementia and Lewy body dementia) and 95 controls. Levels of CSF tau protein phosphorylated at serine 199 above

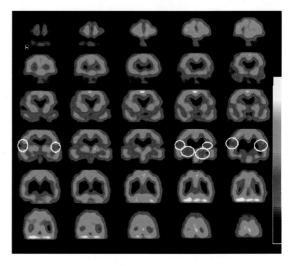

Fig. 40.6 Coronal SPECT scan in a patient with Alzheimer's disease. From Dr PK Chandak, Department of Radiology, Brigham and Women's Hospital, Harvard Medical School.

Box 40.1   Proposed biochemical markers of Alzheimer's disease

Decreased levels
Acetylcholine
Acetylcholinesterase
Choline acetyl transferase
Corticotrophin releasing factor and neuropeptide Y (in cortex)
Dopamine
GABA
Glutamate
Muscarinic M2 receptor
Nicotinic receptor
Noradrenaline (norepinephrine)
Serotonin
Somatostatin

Increased levels
Cortisol
Corticotrophin releasing factor (in hippocampus)
GH response to pyridostigmine (early stage)

Normal levels
Cholecystokinin
Excitatory amino acids
Postsynaptic acetylcholine M1 receptor
Substance P
Thyrotrophin-releasing hormone
Vasopressin
Vasointestinal peptide

Box 40.2   Risk factors and protective factors for Alzheimer's disease

Risk factors
Age
Family history (dementia, Down's syndrome or Parkinson's disease)
Mild cognitive or age-associated memory impairment
Down's syndrome
Head injury
Aluminium hypothyroidism
Systemic vascular disease or risk factors

Protective factors
Smoking
High level of education
Oestrogens
Non-steroidal anti-inflammatory drugs

1.05 fmol/ml yielded excellent differentiation of subjects with Alzheimer's disease from all other subjects (see Fig. 40.7). The high sensitivity and specificity may also hold for the earliest cases (e.g. individuals with mild cognitive impairment destined to develop Alzheimer's disease). CSF phospho-tau could be the first truly presymptomatic diagnostic test for Alzheimer's disease, if the findings hold true in studies with post-mortem confirmation (Mitchell et al 2002).

PROGNOSIS

De Ajuriaguerra et al (1964) cleverly observed that the deterioration in dementia is analogous to Piaget's developmental stages in reverse. This is also illustrated in the hierarchical dementia scale. Predictors of prognosis have been studied in 224 early Alzheimer's disease patients in New York,

Baltimore and Boston (Richards et al 1993). The independent variables of extrapyramidal symptoms and slowing of the posterior dominant EEG rhythm were associated with cognitive decline, whereas delusions were primarily associated with impaired functional capacity.

The mortality rate is approximately five times greater in patients with dementia than in healthy age-matched controls. The disease can be grouped into various types based on rapidity of progression:

- 'rapidly progressive' normally means death within 5 years
- 'normally progressive' means death within 12 years
- 'slowly progressive' means death in more than 12 years.

Crude predictors of rapid death include an early onset, aphasia, psychotic symptoms, depression and severe cognitive impairment.

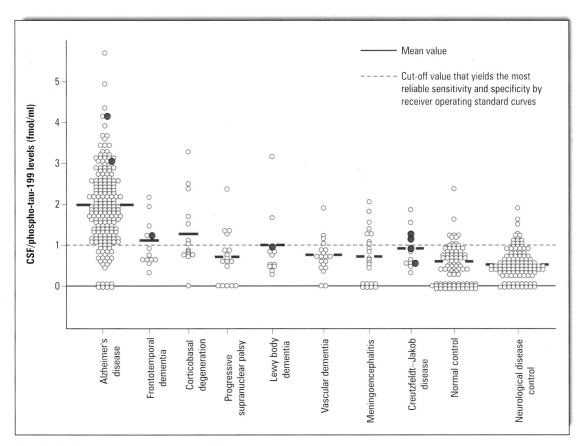

Fig. 40.7 Phospho-tau-199 levels in the CSF of patients with Alzheimer's disease and other dementias.

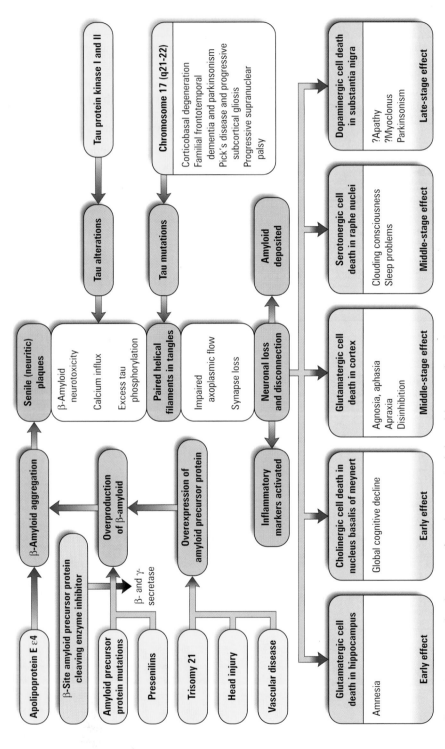

Fig. 40.8 Suggested pathogenesis of tau dementias (including Alzheimer's disease).

Table 40.3 Clinical stages of Alzheimer's disease

	Memory	Psychiatric features	Cortical features	Neurological features
Preclinical prodrome	Forgetfulness	Often none	None	None
Early (1–3 years) Stage I	Recent memory	Loss of interest	Anomia	None or subtle
Intermediate Stage II	Propagnosia, autobiographical	Anxiety, depression	Aphasia	Apraxia, agnosia, acalculia
Late (8–12 years) Stage III	Remote memory	Agitation, apathy	Echolalia	Seizures, incontinence

Box 40.3 Summary of the pathology of Alzheimer's disease

Gross pathology
Reduction in brain mass by about 10%
Cortical atrophy
Ventricular enlargement

Microscopic pathology
Loss of large pyramidal (III and IV) neurones
Loss of dendrites and synaptic markers

Molecular pathology
Senile plaques (amyloid precursor protein converted to β-amyloid protein)
Neurofibrillary tangles (microtubular association protein (tau) in paired helical filament)
Neuropil threads (cortical dendrites or axons containing the neurofibrillary tangles)
Granulovacuolar change (cytoplasmic degeneration)
Hirano bodies (eosinophilic intracytoplasmic bodies)
Amyloid (congophilic) angiopathy (accumulation of β-A4 amyloid in cerebral vessels)
Synaptic loss (up to 50% loss of synapses in the cortex)

NEUROPSYCHIATRIC COMPLICATIONS OF ALZHEIMER'S DISEASE

Neuropsychiatric problems are extremely common in Alzheimer's disease, with a point prevalence of 80% in nursing home residents and a 2-month prevalence of 75% in community-dwelling patients (Lykestos et al 2002). Such problems are sometimes referred to by the American term 'behavioural and psychological symptoms of dementia' (BPSD). Aside from the cognitive symptoms, agitation and aggression, apathy, mood disturbance, agitation, irritability/agression and sleep disturbance are the most common complaints (see Box 40.5 and Fig. 40.9) (Aarsland et al 2001). Whilst common, depression and dysthymia actually occur less frequently than in many neurological diseases (such as Parkinson's disease and stroke). Mood and psychosis fluctuate during the course of illness more than apathy and behavioural problems do. There is a weak but nonetheless interesting relationship between the complication and its peak onset in the disease process (Margallo-Lana et al 2001). In general, depression and anxiety occur early while insight is retained; irritability, distress, dysphoria and psychosis occur mid-stage; and apathy and frank behavioural disturbance occur relatively late. It is as interesting to ask why some patients do not develop certain neuropsychiatric complications as it is to ask why some do, given that Alzheimer's disease is a devastating irreversible brain disease. No doubt the influence of insight and self-awareness has much to do with how psychiatric symptoms manifest themselves (see also Clinical Pointer 56.4).

Depression in Alzheimer's disease

Cognitive impairment is an important risk factor for depression, and vice versa. A large Spanish study of 1460 elderly subjects showed that the rate of depression in the cognitively unimpaired elderly was about 5%, whereas in those with mild or moderate cognitive decline it was 12%; in those patients with dementia the rate of depression was at least 27% (Vilalta-Franch et al 1999). This has been replicated in the large Cache County Cardiovascular Health Study. There may also be an association with mania (Nilsson et al 2002). Studies in Alzheimer's disease suggest that *symptoms* of depression occur in half of patients, although a depressive *syndrome* (as defined by DSM-IV) is present in less than a quarter. Dysthymia is also recognized, more often as a consequence rather than an antecedent of dementia. When depression occurs in Alzheimer's disease

Table 40.4 Neuropsychological stages of decline in dementia

Stage	MMSE	CDR	GDS	ADAS-Cog	Cognitive performance: deficits beyond previous stage	Pathological spread: Braak staging	Functional status: functional assessment staging
Healthy elderly	30	0	1	0	No problems	I (transentorhinal area)	1. Asymptomatic
Age-associated memory impairment	24–29	0.5	2	1–12	Verbal episodic memory (extended recall)	II (CA1 field of hippocampus)	2. Word finding difficulty
Mild cognitive impairment and prodromal phase of Alzheimer's disease	21–29	0.5	3	1–13	Verbal episodic memory (delayed recall)	II (CA1 field of hippocampus)	3. Deficits in demanding settings (e.g. employment) (reduced interactiveness, loss of confidence)
Early Alzheimer's disease	21–23	1	4	13–20	Recognition memory; Spatial episodic memory; Executive dysfunction	III/IV (amygdala and thalamus)	4. Requires assistance with complex tasks (reduced time outside house, reduced time reading, difficulty with finances)
Moderate Alzheimer's disease	12–20	2	5	21–37	Semantic memory; Visuospatial awareness; Attention > vigilance; Orientation to time	V (basal cortex)	5. Requires assistance choosing proper attire; 6a. Requires assistance dressing; 6b. Requires assistance with bathing; 6d. Requires assistance with mechanics of toileting
Severe Alzheimer's disease	0–11	3	6–7	≥38	Orientation to place and person; Orbitofrontal and medial frontal deficits; Cortical and subcortical deficits	VI (cortical association areas)	6d. Urinary incontinence; 6e. Faecal incontinence; 7a. Speech limited to half a dozen words; 7b. Intelligible speech limited to single words; 7c. Ambulatory ability lost; 7d. Ability to sit up lost; 7e. Ability to smile lost; 7f. Ability to hold head up lost

Adapted from Almkvist (2000) and Reisberg (1988)
MMSE, Mini-Mental State Examination; CDR, Clinical Dementia Rating Scale; GDS, Global Deterioration Scale; ADAS-Cog, Alzheimer's disease Assessment Cognitive Subscale

Clinical Pointer 40.3

Depression and the course of Alzheimer's disease

There has been much confusion about the status of depression, or more specifically depression-related cognitive impairment, and Alzheimer's disease. This is not surprising, since depression causes significant subjective memory complaints in most sufferers and thus is an important diagnosis to rule out in elderly patients presenting to memory clinics. However, depression also causes neuropsychological deficits that are neither imaginary nor driven entirely by apathy or indecisiveness (the classic and overquoted 'don't know' answers). Depression-related cognitive impairment in the elderly is less severe than in clear Alzheimer's disease, but it is not easily distinguished from the early stages of Alzheimer's disease or from mild cognitive impairment. Indeed, depression occurs in about 50% of such patients. Visser et al (2000) compared a small group of subjects with primary depression plus cognitive impairment with depressed patients with early Alzheimer's disease. At baseline and follow-up the depressed patients with preclinical Alzheimer's disease had significantly poorer scores on the Mini-Mental State Examination, delayed recall and fluency than did the depressed subjects without preclinical Alzheimer's disease.

Following several small-scale follow-up studies, a series of epidemiological studies have suggested that depression is also a risk factor for cognitive decline. Furthermore, certain depressive symptoms, such as anhedonia, loss of interest and withdrawal, may be particularly predictive. In the largest study, involving 5781 elderly women in California, depressive symptoms were linearly related to 4-year cognitive decline. A smaller study of 1600 inhabitants in France failed to find a similar effect over 3 years, but noted a cross-sectional effect of depression on cognition at follow-up. Other studies have suggested that the effect might be confined to educated people or be limited to the domain of attention rather than global cognitive function. Predictors of cognitive decline in depressed patients are only just now being examined, but fascinating early work points towards older age, lower baseline cognitive performance, total cerebral volume and hippocampal volume as risk factors (Steffans et al 2002).

Further reading *Jorm AF 2000 Is depression a risk factor for dementia or cognitive decline? A review. Gerontology 46:219–227*
Rubin EH, Kinscherf DA, Grant EA et al 1991 The influence of major depression on clinical and psychometric assessment of senile dementia of the Alzheimer type. American Journal of Psychiatry 148:1164–1171
Steffans DC, Payne ME, Greenberg DL et al 2002 Hippocampal volume and incident dementia in geriatric depression. American Journal of Geriatric Psychiatry 10:62–71
Visser PJ, Verhey FRJ, Ponds RWHM et al 2000 Distinction between preclinical Alzheimer's disease and depression. Journal of the American Geriatric Society 48:479–484
Yaffe K, Blackwell T, Gore R et al 1999 Depressive symptoms and cognitive decline in nondemented elderly women: a prospective study. Archives of General Psychiatry 56:425–430

there tend to be less frequent suicidal thoughts but more psychomotor retardation than in patients with primary depression (Chemerinski et al 2001). Importantly, the typical psychological symptoms of depression may not be expressed by the patient with dementia (rather as in depressed patients who have a learning disability), and therefore clinicians should be aware of other markers such as increased behavioural problems (particularly withdrawal and self-harm), irritability, increased crying and sleep disturbance. This has led to a proposal from the National Institute of Mental Health for specific diagnostic criteria for depression in Alzheimer's disease. Depression is associated with retained insight and is thus frequently seen in the early and middle stages of the disease. Nevertheless, it is more often carers rather than patients themselves who rate the depression as most severe. Not infrequently, depression antedates the dementia. This may be the case even when patients are unaware of their cognitive loss (Chen et al 1999).

Many studies have linked a history of depression with the later development of dementia which raises interesting questions about their shared pathological basis (see Clinical Pointer 40.3). Where the delay between the development of depression and later development of dementia is very long, depression may be reasonably conceptualized as a risk factor for dementia. A family history of depression does not appear to increase the risk of dementia. Depression is also linked with reduced functional ability, higher levels of institutionalization and, ultimately, with increased mortality. Studies do not prove that depression is definitely causative in Alzheimer's disease, but data from other conditions suggest a role for depression in accelerating morbidity and mortality (Steele et al 1990). Certain clus-

Table 40.5 Frequency (%) of neuropsychiatric problems in dementia and mild cognitive impairment rated by the Neuropsychiatric Inventory over the preceding 2 months

Symptom	Dementia	MCI	Elderly controls
Apathy	36	15	3
Depression	32	20	7
Agitation	30	11	3
Irritability	27	15	5
Sleep problems	27	14	Unrecorded
Anxiety	22	10	6
Eating problems	20	10	Unrecorded
Delusions	18	3	2
Behavioural problems	16	4	0.5
Disinhibition	13	3	1
Hallucinations	11	1	0.5
Euphoria	3	0.5	0.3

Adapted from Lykestos et al (2002)
MCI, mild cognitive impairment

ters of neuropsychiatric symptoms tend to occur together. Patients with depressive symptoms are more likely also to have anxiety symptoms, apathy, aberrant motor activity, irritability and psychosis (Lykestos et al 2001).

Subsyndromal mood disorder

Mood disorder not reaching the criteria for a single episode is often present but is rarely addressed, and is probably more common than major depressive disorder itself. Presentation with distress, dysphoria and demoralization should alert carers to the fact that 'something isn't right'. Such patients may be deteriorating into depression or may have residual symptoms after recovering from depression. In either case, a close examination of the patient's environment to see what improvements can be made is indicated. A commonly cited symptom in dementia (and other conditions featuring disinhibition) is the *catastrophic reaction*, which occurs in about 15% of patients. This is an excessive emotional (and possibly behavioural) outburst in response to frustration at failing to complete a certain task. A combination of baseline distress, poor problem-solving skills and disinhibition are all contributory.

Mechanisms of depression in Alzheimer's disease

Studies of biological markers of depression in Alzheimer's disease are of particular interest given that it is possible to obtain neuropathological data. Pathological studies suggest no difference in cortical senile plaques or tangles in depressed versus non-depressed patients. Tentatively, loss of monoamine centres in subcortical areas (the locus ceruleus, substantia nigra and dorsal raphe) may be more affected in depressed sufferers of Alzheimer's disease, on the basis of small post-mortem series. This may manifest as lower CSF levels of dopamine, homovanillic acid and cortical noradrenaline (norepinephrine), all of whiach are putative markers of depression in Alzheimer's disease (Loreck & Folstein 1993). Unlike psychotic symptoms in Alzheimer's disease, depression is not associated with accelerated cognitive decline, but it may be linked with increased mortality (Zubenko et al 1991).

Other mood disorders in Alzheimer's disease

Apathy

Apathy is an important symptom in dementia and affects instrumental and social functions. Apathy is present in about one-third of patients with Alzheimer's disease, of whom two-thirds are depressed and one-third are not. In other words between 10% and 15% of sufferers have a pure apathy syndrome. The rate of apathy is even higher in depressed patients with Alzheimer's disease than in depressed patients without dementia (50% versus 35%) (Starkstein et al 2001). Severity of apathy in Alzheimer's disease modestly correlates with age, poor cognitive function and loss of insight (i.e. apathy tends to get worse as the disease progresses). Unselected patients with apathy have higher rates of anxiety, irritability and aberrant motor activity (Lykestos et al 2001). This is influenced by the subgroup of patients who have mixed depression and apathy. Putative biological correlates of apathy include prefrontal and anterior temporal perfusion deficits (Craig et al 1996).

Psychosis in Alzheimer's disease

Patients who lose the ability to process information about their environment are likely to form illogical and erroneous beliefs. Thus, overvalued ideas and delusions are about twice as common as hallucinations and illusions in Alzheimer's disease. Where perceptual disturbance occurs, visual hallucinations are about twice as common as auditory hallucinations. Cumulatively, the incidence of delusions or

Clinical Pointer 40.4

Distinguishing age-associated memory impairment from early Alzheimer's disease

It is not difficult to distinguish age-associated memory impairment (AAMI) from cases of severe dementia. On cognitive testing the healthy elderly do not have deficits on tests of orientation or semantic memory. Episodic memory can be affected by age but is invariably much worse in Alzheimer's disease. Memory is generally preserved on prompting (recognition more so than recall) in normal ageing, but both become impaired in severe dementia.

More problems arise when trying to distinguish suspected early Alzheimer's disease from normal ageing. This distinction is becoming increasingly muddied as research shows that subjective memory complaints, AAMI and mild cognitive impairment are risk factors for the development of Alzheimer's disease. The contribution of a family history of dementia, the presence of dementia risk factors and a history of decline from previous levels are helpful but not diagnostic. Formal neuropsychology is recommended and this may have to be repeated after 1 year to assess the rate of decline (which can be very slow in the earliest stages of Alzheimer's disease). The merit of delayed recall on Russel's Adaptation of the Visual Reproduction Test appears to correspond to a pathological diagnosis of Alzheimer's disease, but has yet to be tested formally against AAMI or mild cognitive impairment.

Neuroanatomical studies of the ageing brain show that grey matter volume decreases with age, and the most sensitive areas to neuronal loss are the insula, central sulci and cingulate sulci. Thus, MRI may reveal increased atrophy in the medial temporal lobe in Alzheimer's disease, but this is not a reliable diagnostic test. SPECT has been shown to differentiate the two conditions, with significant frontal, temporoparietal and occipital hypoperfusion seen only in Alzheimer's disease patients.

Further reading   Goldman WP, Morris JC 2001 Evidence that age-associated memory impairment is not a normal variant of aging. Alzheimer Disease and Associated Disorders 15:72–79
Laakso MP, Hallikainen M, Hanninen T et al 2000 Diagnosis of Alzheimer's disease: MRI of the hippocampus vs delayed recall. Neuropsychologia 38:579–584
Parnetti L, Lowenthal DT, Presciutti O et al 1996 H-1-MRS, MRI-based hippocampal volumetry, and Tc-99m-HMPAO-SPECT in normal aging, age-associated memory impairment, and probable Alzheimer's disease. Journal of the American Geriatric Society 44:133–138

hallucinations is 20% in the first year after diagnosis and 50% in the first 4 years (Paulsen et al 2000).

Delusions in Alzheimer's disease are classically simple unsystematized beliefs, often with a paranoid quality. They are often integrated with errors produced by memory problems (e.g. the patient believes someone is stealing from him or her) or by mood disturbance (e.g. 'everyone on the ward is out to poison me') or by disintegration with the environment (e.g. 'my house is not my home'). There is an association with reduced cognitive function, although there is a floor effect whereby a certain degree of cognitive function is necessary to generate abnormal beliefs. That said, some patients will initially accept reassurance about the abnormal beliefs only to forget a short time later. It can seem paradoxical that some patients cannot remember any new information but consistently recall an existing abnormal belief in spite of very poor cognition. Several psychotic syndromes, which are uncommon in primary psychosis, regularly occur in Alzheimer's disease. Delusional misidentification occurs in about 10% of patients (usually of the Capgras type, in which impostors take the appearance of familiar people), delusional misidentification of one's own mirror image (*mirror sign*) occurs in about 5%, and delusional misidentification of television images as being real (*TV sign*) also occurs in about 5% of sufferers. In general, the presence of psychotic symptoms in Alzheimer's disease heralds accelerated cognitive deterioration (and, in the case of visual hallucinations, probable reduced survival). Delusional misidentification syndromes have not been linked with poor prognosis, but this may be a failing of the studies. Delusions in Alzheimer's disease are associated with greater memory deficits, parkinsonism, bradyphrenia, disinhibition, agitation, behavioural disturbance and, in some cases, depression (Lykestos et al 2001, Paulsen et al 2000).

Mechanism of psychosis in Alzheimer's disease

Biological markers of psychosis in Alzheimer's disease have been studied, but are confounded by the effect of underlying disease severity. There has been some suggestion that delusions may be associated with temporal lobe, frontal lobe, hippocampal and dominant hemisphere disease, but these studies are not methodologically sound. One study found that psychotic patients tend to have greater cortical markers of disease (Zubenko et al 1991), but another found no difference in comparison with non-psychotic patients (Sweet et al 2000).

Cognition in Alzheimer's disease

Alzheimer's disease is the most common cause of sustained cognitive impairment. It is therefore not surprising that the cognitive profile of this condition is well established. The first and most obvious domain to deteriorate is that of memory. Whereas implicit learning is essentially spared, learning of new facts (particularly the narrative account or episodic memory) is not. Many studies show that deficits in delayed recall (accelerated forgetting) distinguish Alzheimer's disease from healthy controls.

There are also early deficits in recognition memory. As the disease progresses there is usually involvement of immediate recall (working memory), followed by gradual decline of long-term recall for overlearned material (referred to as a 'temporal gradient'). Deficits in immediate recall overlap with attentional deficits, which are also affected early in Alzheimer's disease. Expressive language is usually affected in the middle stages of dementia, progressing over years to anomia. An early sign is word-finding difficulty and a gradual loss of inflection (prosody).

Both mild cognitive impairment and age-associated memory impairment are risk factors for Alzheimer's disease (see Clinical Pointer 40.4; see also Clinical Pointer 39.2). Indeed, subjective memory impairment alone is a marker of future Alzheimer's disease. Subjective memory complaints will present

---

Clinical Pointer 40.5

Which cognitive assessment questionnaire in Alzheimer's disease and other dementias?

There are many scales available to assess cognitive function. These can be divided into brief screening instruments and more complex neuropsychological tests. Without associated clinical suspicions, few such measures perform well in differentiating early Alzheimer's disease from age-associated declines. Most studies are methodologically limited by their attempt to differentiate healthy elderly controls from clinically defined Alzheimer's disease. What is needed are more studies examining the differences between early Alzheimer's disease and age-associated memory impairment using pathological confirmation.

The Mini-Mental State Examination from Folstein's group is the most widely used assessment clinically, and the Alzheimer's Disease Assessment Scale (ADAS) from Davis's group (KL Davis, Mount Sinai School of Medicine, New York) is the most widely used in trials. The ADAS-cog and Mini-Mental State Examination are highly intercorrelated ($r = 0.76$), but each has its own limitations. The Mini-Mental State Examination is a very poor assessor of short-term memory (depending on three-item recall alone) and thus has a well-known ceiling effect that is imprecise in mild cognitive impairment. The result is that it tends to miss cases of mild dementia when relied upon alone (Petersen et al 2001). The authors of the ADAS have also recognized this problem and suggested 'add-ons' to their scale: word-list learning with delayed free recall digit cancellation tests to measure concentration. Recently, a new test for differentiation of mild Alzheimer's disease from healthy and depressed controls has been piloted (Test for the Early Detection of Dementia, with Differentiation from Depression (TE4D)). Other short scales include the 7-minute screen, Erzigkeit's Syndrom Kurztest (Short Performance Test, widely used in German studies). Longer scales, such as the Middlesex Elderly Assessment of Mental State and the Cambridge Cognitive Examination (CAMCOG), are alternatives that require further study.

Further reading Folstein MF, Folstein SE, McHugh PR 1975 Mini-Mental State: a practical method for grading the cognitive state of patients for the clinician. Journal of Psychiatric Research 12:189–198
Ihl R, Grass-Kapanke B, Lahrem P et al 2000 Development and validity of the test for the early detection of dementia with differentiation from depression (TE4D). Fortschritte der Neurologie Psychiatrie 68:413–422
Mohs RC, Knopman D, Petersen RC et al 1997 Development of cognitive instruments for use in clinical trials of antidementia drugs: additions to the Alzheimer's disease assessment scale that broaden its scope. Alzheimer's Disease and Associated Disorders 11(suppl 2):S13–S21
Petersen RC, Stevens JC, Ganguli M et al 2001 Practice parameter: early detection of dementia: mild cognitive impairment (an evidence-based review). Neurology 56:1133–1142
Rosen WG, Mohs RC, Davis KL 1984 A new rating-scale for Alzheimer's disease. American Journal of Psychiatry 141:1356–1364
Tombaugh TN, McIntyre NJ 1992 The Mini-Mental State Examination. A comprehensive review. Journal of the American Geriatric Society 40:922–935

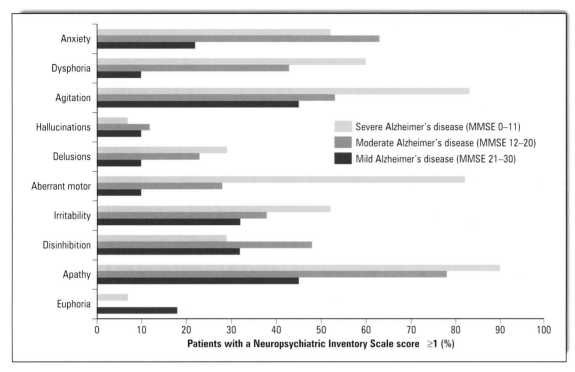

Fig. 40.9 Neuropsychiatric symptoms in Alzheimer's disease, stratified by Mini-Mental State Examination score.

much earlier than clear deficits on crude instruments such as the Mini-Mental State Examination (see Box 9.1). Subjective memory complaints are also a feature of depression, which should be ruled out in every case presenting with these problems (Jorm et al 2001). Of great interest are the specific cognitive deficits that are apparent in future sufferers of Alzheimer's disease many years before diagnosis. These deficits suddenly deteriorate close to the time at which the disease is formally diagnosed (Bäckman et al 2001). Biological abnormalities that predict conversion from mild cognitive impairment to Alzheimer's disease in the elderly are very subtle, but are just detectable in some patients. Whether these can be used clinically remains to be seen (Jack et al 1999). It is pertinent to ask what percentage of the oldest old do not have any cognitive problems on neuropsychological tests. The answer here is perhaps as many as one-third.

Behavioural and personality problems in Alzheimer's disease

Behavioural difficulties are an extremely common and often problematic feature of dementia and are

seen in up to 80% of patients with advanced dementia. Three clusters of disturbed behaviour can be defined: self-neglect behaviours, agitation-related behaviours and apathy-related behaviours (Fig. 40.9). Collectively these behavioural problems are sometimes called 'aberrant motor activity', and when they are irreversible the label 'personality change' is often used (see Ch. 77). They are inter-correlated with most other neuropsychiatric symptoms, but particularly with irritability, anxiety and disinhibition (Lykestos et al 2001). As the erosion of accurate sensory information processing occurs, patients' behaviour may become uncharacteristic and unpredictable. Such behaviour may be internally generated repetitive behaviours such as hoarding or checking as well as repetitive speech or shouting. More worryingly, patients may become a risk to themselves through poor judgement, wandering and unsafe driving. A substantial proportion become hostile, irritable or aggressive, overactive and disinhibited. Some studies have demonstrated that verbal aggression and physical aggression occurs in 5% of unselected patients, although aggression may be seen in up to 30% of those who are hospitalized. Disturbed behaviour, often with insomnia, is another recognized pattern that is difficult for carers to manage. In advanced stages of dementia, overlearned socially acceptable habits involving toileting, washing, dressing, as well as biologically driven behaviours of sleeping, eating and sexual activity can be disturbed. Socially learnt behaviours may be more amenable to environmental change than the internally driven biological behaviours, which are sometimes referred to as 'stereotyped behaviours'.

Mechanism of behavioural problems in Alzheimer's disease

Predictors of behavioural problems in dementia are not well studied. One problem behaviour may have a complex aetiology that differs from patient to patient. The effect of environmental change from familiar to unfamiliar, underlying personality and degree of cognitive impairment are all likely to play a role. The combination of behavioural problems and changes in mood, restricted motivation and activities and lack of judgement and empathy often lead relatives to complain of personality change in their loved one during the course of dementia. Regression of personality to child-like states (*retrogenesis*) and a coarsening of personality with amplification of previous traits are to be expected. There is likely to be significant involvement of the frontal and parietal lobes, but most cases will involve an admixture of multiple brain areas.

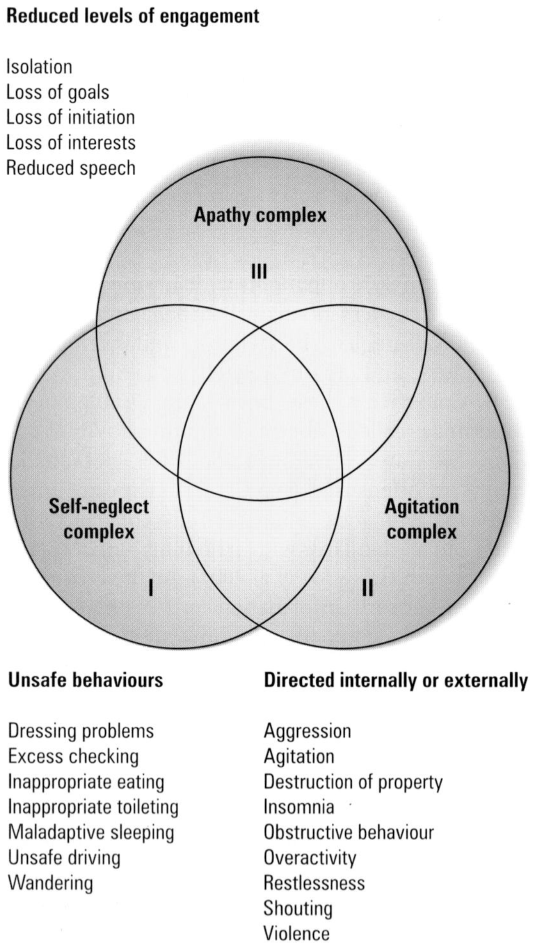

THE ROLE OF THE FAMILY IN ALZHEIMER'S DISEASE

The role of the main carer or carers cannot be overemphasized. Families are far from passive cohabitees. They strongly influence the well-being of the patient, and in turn are strongly influenced by the patient. Several studies have demonstrated that family functioning accounts for a sizeable proportion of variance in recovery from several disorders such as AIDS, cancer, cystic fibrosis and multiple sclerosis (Groom et al 1998).

Reduced levels of engagement

Isolation
Loss of goals
Loss of initiation
Loss of interests
Reduced speech

Apathy complex

III

Self-neglect complex

I

Agitation complex

II

Unsafe behaviours

Dressing problems
Excess checking
Inappropriate eating
Inappropriate toileting
Maladaptive sleeping
Unsafe driving
Wandering

Directed internally or externally

Aggression
Agitation
Destruction of property
Insomnia
Obstructive behaviour
Overactivity
Restlessness
Shouting
Violence

Fig. 40.10 Behavioural problems in dementia.

Box 40.4 Behavioural problems in Alzheimer's disease

Apparently goal-directed complex behaviour
Aggression and violence
Attempting to drive
Attempting to escape the care environment
Self-harm
Shouting, screaming
Wandering

Socially driven behaviours
Dressing
Self-care
Social skills
Toileting habit
Washing and bathing

Biologically driven behaviours
Abnormal eating
Abnormal or inappropriate sexual activity
Abnormal sleeping
Repetitive motor activity
Urination and defecation

Box 40.5 Predictors of nursing home placement in 5788 patients with advanced dementia

Patient characteristics
Male gender
Non-ethnic minority
Living alone
Functional dependence
Cognitive impairment
Difficult behaviour

Carer characteristics
Old age
Male sex
High income
High carer stress

After Yaffe et al (2002)

Carers require information, support and respite breaks. Relatives must be free to make their own decisions about what they personally can and cannot manage at home. Common questions asked by relatives are: What does the future hold? Is the patient safe to drive (see Clinical Pointer 65.1)? Am I at increased risk of Alzheimer's disease (see below)?

What to tell families about their risk

In relatives with no family history or a history of late-onset Alzheimer's disease beginning after 65 years the risk of another family member developing Alzheimer's disease is not significantly elevated. The baseline risk of Alzheimer's disease is a rate of about 8% per decade after the age of 65 years (Heston 1988). However, in a first-degree relative with a family history of early-onset Alzheimer's disease there is an increased likelihood of an early-onset dementia beginning around 60 years and again increasing by 8% per decade. Thus the risk is 16% by the age of 80 years. If two first-degree relatives have the disease starting before age 70 years, then the age at which the risk for the children begins is brought forward to 45 years. In summary, even for those with a family history of Alzheimer's disease, the chances are that they will *not* develop the disease (unless they have a rare early-onset gene).

The management of carer stress is discussed in Chapter 62.

SUMMARY

Alzheimer's disease is the most common degenerative disorder and the single most common cause of neuropsychiatric problems. Subtle neuropathological changes (loss of synapse density and neurofibrillary tangles in the entorhinal cortex and hippocampus) and neuropsychological changes (impaired delayed recall test of episodic memory) occur many years before other clinical manifestations and diagnosis. Alzheimer's disease is characterized by high rates of transient delusions and visual hallucinations that fluctuate in severity. Dysphoria is more common than major depressive disorder, and the latter is most often in the early stages. As Alzheimer's disease progresses there is an increasing tendency to develop behavioural problems, including apathy, agitation and self-neglect. Neuropsychiatric complications have a large impact on carers at home and on staff in residential care facilities. A range of pharmacological and non-pharmacological treatments have been shown to be very effective, while not significantly influencing disease course.

REFERENCES AND FURTHER READING

Aarsland D, Cummings JL, Larsen JP 2001 Neuropsychiatric differences between Parkinson's disease with dementia and Alzheimer's disease. International Journal of Geriatric Psychiatry 16:184–191

Almkvist O 2000 Neuropsychological and instrumental diagnosis of dementia: a review. In: Maj SM, Sartorius N, Okasha A et al (eds) Dementia. Wiley, Chichester, p 143–165

Alzheimer A 1907 Uber eigenartige Erkrankung der Hirnrinde. Allgemeine Zeitschrift für Psychiatrie 64:146–148

Bäckman L, Small BJ, Fratiglioni L 2001 Stability of the pre-clinical episodic memory deficit in Alzheimer's disease. Brain 124:96–102

Ball MJ, Fisman M. Hachinski V et al 1985 A new definition of Alzheimer's disease: a hippocampal dementia. Lancet i:14–16

Bigler ED, Hubler DW, Cullum CM et al 1985 Intellectual and memory impairment in dementia: computerized axial tomography volume correlations. Journal of Nervous and Mental Disease 173:347–352

Blennow K, Bogdanovic N, Alafuzoff I et al 1996 Synaptic pathology in Alzheimer's disease: relation to severity of dementia, but not to senile plaques, neurofibrillary tangles, or the ApoE4 allele. Journal of Neural Transmission

103:603–618

Bonte FJ, Weiner MF, Bigio EH et al 1997 Brain blood flow in the dementias: SPECT with histopathologic correlation in 54 patients. Radiology 202:793–797

Braak H, Braak E 1991 Neuropathological staging of Alzheimer related changes. Acta Neuropatholgica (Berlin) 182:239–259

Chemerinski E, Petracca G, Sabe L et al 2001 The specificity of depressive symptoms in patients with Alzheimer's disease. American Journal of Psychiatry 158:68–72

Chen P, Ganguli M, Mulsant BH et al 1999 The temporal relationship between depressive symptoms and dementia: a community-based prospective study. Archives of General Psychiatry 56:261–266

Craig AH, Cummings JL, Fairbanks L et al 1996 Cerebral blood flow correlates of apathy in Alzheimer's disease. Archives of Neurology 53:1116–1120

Davis BM, Mohs RC, Greenwald BS et al 1985 Clinical studies of the cholinergic deficit in Alzheimer's disease. I. Neurochemical and neuroendocrine studies. Journal of the American Geriatrics Society 33:741–748

de Ajuriaguerra J, Rey-Bellet M, Tissot R 1964 A propos de quelques problèmes posés par le déficit opératoire de veillards atteints de démence dégénérative en début d'évolution. Cortex 1:103–132, 232–256

Gottfries CG, Balldin J, Blennow K et al 1994 Regulation of the hypothalamic–pituitary–adrenal axis in dementia disorders. Annals of the New York Academy of Sciences 746:336–343

Groom KN, Shaw TG, O'Connor ME et al 1998 Neurobehavioral symptoms and family functioning in traumatically brain-injured adults. Archives of Clinical Neuropsychology 13:695–711

Heininger K 1999 A unifying hypothesis of Alzheimer's disease. II. Pathophysiological processes. Human Psychopharmacology 14:525–581

Heininger K 2000 A unifying hypothesis of Alzheimer's disease. IV. Causation and sequence of events. Reviews of Neuroscience 11:213–328

Heston L 1988 Morbid risk in first-degree relatives of persons with Alzheimer's disease. Archives of General Psychiatry 45:97–98

Hoffman JM, Hanson MW, Welsh KA et al 1996 Interpretation variability of (18)FDG-positron emission tomography studies in dementia. Investigative Radiology 31:316–322

Hulstaert F, Blennow K, Ivanoiu A et al 1999 Improved discrimination of AD patients using β-amyloid (1–42) and tau levels in CSF. Neurology 52:1555–1562

Imahori K, Uchida T 1997 Physiology and pathology of tau protein kinases in relation to Alzheimer's disease. Journal of Biochemistry 121:179–188

Itoh N, Arai H, Urakami K et al 2001 Large-scale, multicenter study of cerebrospinal fluid tau protein phosphorylated at serine 199 for the ante mortem diagnosis of Alzheimer's disease. Annals of Neurology 50:150–156

Jack CR, Petersen RC, Xu YC et al 1999 Prediction of AD with MRI-based hippocampal volume in mild cognitive impairment. Neurology 52:1397–1403

Jagust W, Thisted R, Devous MD et al 2001 SPECT perfusion imaging in the diagnosis of Alzheimer's disease: a clinical–pathologic study. Neurology 56: 950–956

Jorm AF, Christensen H, Korten AE et al 2001 Memory complaints as a precursor of memory impairment in older people: a longitudinal analysis over 7–8 years. Psychological Medicine 31:441–449

Kimura M, Asada T, Uno M et al 1999 Assessment of cerebrospinal fluid levels of serum amyloid P component in patients with Alzheimer's disease. Neuroscience Letters 273:137–139

Lawlor BA, Bierer LM, Ryan TM et al 1995 Plasma 3-methoxy-4-hydroxyphenylglycol (MHPG) and clinical symptoms in Alzheimer's disease. Biological Psychiatry 38:185–188

Loreck DJ, Folstein MF 1993 Depression in Alzheimer's disease. In: Starkstein S E, Robinson R G (eds) Depression in neurological disease. Johns Hopkins Press, Baltimore, p 50–62

Lykestos CG, Sheppard J-ME, Steinberg M et al 2001 Neuropsychiatric disturbance in Alzheimer's disease clusters into three groups: the Cache County study. International Journal of Geriatric Psychiatry 16:1043–1053

Lykestos CG, Lopez O, Jones B et al 2002 Prevalence of neuropsychiatric symptoms in dementia and mild cognitive impairment: results from the cardiovascular health study. JAMA 288:1475–1483

Margallo-Lana M, Swann A, O'Brien J et al 2001 Prevalence and pharmacological management of behavioural and psychological symptoms amongst dementia sufferers living in care environments. International Journal of Geriatric Psychiatry 16: 39–44

Markesbery WR 1998 Neuropathology of dementing disorders. Edward Arnold, London

Masur DM, Sliwinski M, Lipton RB et al 1994 Neuropsychological prediction of dementia and the absence of dementia in healthy elderly persons. Neurology 44:1427–1432

Mayeux R, Saunders AM, Shea S et al (for the Alzheimer's disease Centers Consortium on Apolipoprotein E in Alzheimer's disease) 1998 Utility of the apolipoprotein E genotype in the diagnosis of Alzheimer's disease. New England Journal of Medicine 338:506–511

Mega MS, Cummings JL, Fiorello T et al 1996 The spectrum of behavioral changes in Alzheimer's disease. Neurology 46:130–135

Mitchell TW, Mufson EJ and Schneider JA et al 2002 Parahippocampal tau pathology in healthy aging, mild cognitive impairment, and early Alzheimer's disease. Annals of Neurology 51:82–189

Mori E, Hirono N, Yamashita H et al 1997 Premorbid brain size as a determinant of reserve capacity against intellectual decline in Alzheimer's disease. American Journal of Psychiatry 154:18–24

Mukaetova-Ladinska EB, Hurt J, Wischik CM 1995 Biological determinants of cognitive change in normal aging and dementia. International Review of Psychiatry 7:399–417

Nagy Z, Hindley NJ, Braak H et al 1999 Relationship between clinical and radiological diagnostic criteria for Alzheimer's disease and the extent of neuropathology as reflected by 'stages': a prospective study. Dementia and Geriatric Cognition 10:109–114

Nilsson FM, Kessing LV, Sorensen TM et al 2002 Enduring increased risk of developing depression and mania in patients with dementia. Journal of Neurology Neurosurgery and Psychiatry 73:40–44

O'Brien JT, Desmond P, Ames D et al 1997 Temporal lobe magnetic resonance imaging can differentiate Alzheimer's disease from normal ageing, depression, vascular dementia and other causes of cognitive impairment. Psychological Medicine 27:1267–1275

Pantel J, Schroder J, Shad LR et al 1997 Quantitative magnetic resonance imaging and neuropsychological functions in dementia of the Alzheimer type. Psychological Medicine 27:221–229

Paulsen JS, Salmon DP, Thal LJ et al 2000 Incidence of and risk factors for hallucinations and delusions in patients with probable AD. Neurology 54:1965–1971

Perl DP 2000 Neuropathology of Alzheimer's disease and related disorders. Neurologic Clinics 18:847–871

Petersen RC, Stevens JC, Ganguli M et al 2001 Practice parameter: early detection of dementia: mild cognitive impairment (an evidence-based review). Report of the Quality Standards Subcommittee of the American Academy of Neurology. Neurology 56:1133–1142

Reisberg B 1988 Functional assessment staging (FAST). Psychopharmacology Bulletin 24:653–659

Richards M, Folstein M, Albert M et al 1993 Multicenter study of predictors of disease course in Alzheimer-disease (the predictors study) 2. Neurological, psychiatric, and demographic influences on baseline measures of disease severity. Alzheimer's Disease and Associated Disorders 7:22–32

Roth M, Tomlinson BE, Blessed G 1966 Correlation between scores for dementia and counts of senile plaques in cerebral grey matter of elderly subjects. Nature 209:109–100

Samuels SC, Silverman JM, Marin DB et al 1999 CSF beta-amyloid, cognition, and APOE genotype in Alzheimer's disease. Neurology 52:547–551

Sjogren M, Rosengren L, Minthon L et al 2000 Cytoskeleton proteins in CSF distinguish frontotemporal dementia from AD. Neurology 54:1960–1964

Southwick PC, Yamagata SK, Echols CL et al 1996 Assessment of amyloid beta protein in cerebrospinal fluid as an aid in the diagnosis of Alzheimer's disease. Journal of Neurochemistry 66:259–265

Starkstein SE, Petracca G, Chemerinski E et al 2001 Syndromic validity of apathy in Alzheimer's disease. American Journal of Psychiatry 158:872–877

Steele C, Rovner B, Chase GA et al 1990 Psychiatric symptoms and nursing home placement of patients with Alzheimer's disease. American Journal of Psychiatry 147:1049–1051

Stevens A, Lowe J 2000 Pathology, 2nd edn. Harcourt, St Louis

Sweet RA, Hamilton RL, Lopez SL et al 2000 Psychotic symptoms in Alzheimer's disease are not associated with more severe neuropathologic features. International Psychogeriatrics 12:547–558

Sze CI, Troncoso JC, Kawas C et al 1997 Loss of the presynaptic vesicle protein synaptophysin in hippocampus correlates with cognitive decline in Alzheimer disease. Journal of Neuropathology and Experimental Neurology 56:933–944

Szelies B, Mielke R, Grond M et al 1995 P300 in Alzheimer's disease: relationships to dementia severity and glucose metabolism. Journal of the Neurological Sciences 130:77–81

Tiraboschi P, Hansen LA, Alford M et al 2000 The decline in synapses and cholinergic activity is asynchronous in Alzheimer's disease. Neurology 55:1278–1283

Vilalta-Franch J, Llinas-Regla J, Lopez-Pousa S 1999 Depression and dementia: case–control study. Revue Neurologique 29:599–603

Yaffe K, Fox P, Sands L et al 2002 Predictors of nursing home placement in patients with dementia: importance of both patient and caregiver characteristics. Presented at the American Academy of Neurology 54th Annual Meeting, Denver, 13–20 April

Zubenko GS, Moossy J, Martinez J et al 1991 Neuropathological and neurochemical correlates of psychosis in primary dementia. Archives of Neurology 48:619–624

41

Fronto-temporal and Focal Dementias

BACKGROUND

In recent years the concept of dementia has moved from a homogeneous global cognitive process to one that can vary depending on the underlying pathological process and susceptibility of the individual concerned. Several focal syndromes of dementia have been described. The best known is frontotemporal dementia, or frontal lobe dementia.

Frontotemporal dementia is an early-onset dementia that affects men and women equally. Early presentation favours neuropsychiatric features, whereas neurological signs develop late (primitive reflexes are the exception). Frontotemporal dementia may account for as many as 20% of all early-onset cases. At post-mortem frontal lobe dementias account for no more than 10% of all dementias. The aetiology is unknown, although recently genetic analysis has determined that a handful of disorders, including progressive supranuclear palsy and corticobasal degeneration, are related clinically and pathologically to frontotemporal dementia. About one-third of patients with frontotemporal dementia and parkinsonism have a family history of the disorder. These disorders are aetiologically related by genetic mutations on chromosome 17 (17q21-22) which affects the structure or function of the microtubule-binding

domain of the tau gene (see Fig. 39.2). Such patients at high genetic risk of frontotemporal dementia have preclinical neuropsychological deficits years before diagnosis (Geschwind et al 2001).

Neuropathology

There is atrophy of the frontal and temporal lobe, due in part to a loss of cells from layers III and V and to a lesser extent layer II of the cortex (Fig. 41.1). Occasionally, subcortical neuronal loss is seen, with degeneration of the striatum. Where the frontal lobe

---

Box 41.1 The Manchester (Lund) criteria for frontotemporal dementia

Behavioural disorder
Insidious onset and slow progression
Early loss of insight
Early loss of social awareness
Early signs of disinhibition
Mental rigidity and inflexibility
Stereotypes, repetitive and imitating behaviour
Hyperorality and dietary changes
Distractibility and impulsivity

Affective symptoms
Depression, anxiety and sentimentality
Hypochondriasis and bizarre somatic complaints
Emotional bluntness and apathy
Amimia

Speech and cognition
Progressive reduction of speech
Stereotypy of speech
Perseveration
Echolalia
Late mutism
Preservation of spatial orientation
Preservation of receptive speech
Preservation of praxis

Physical signs
Early primitive reflexes
Early incontinence
Late akinesia, rigidity and tremor
Low and labile blood pressure

Investigations
Normal EEG
Predominant frontal and anterior temporal atrophy
Frontal lobe disorder on neuropsychology

Supportive features
Onset before 65 years of age
Positive family history
Motor neurone disease

Table 41.1 Neuropathological features of the main causes of frontotemporal dementia

Pathological feature	Alzheimer's disease	Pick's disease	Frontotemporal dementia	Motor neurone disease	Corticobasal degeneration
Neuronal inclusion	Neurofibrillary tangles	Pick body	None	Motor neurone disease inclusion	Corticobasal inclusion
Main pathology	Hippocampus and neocortex	Hippocampus and neocortex	Layers III and V frontal and temporal neocortex	Neocortex (layer II) and anterior horn cells	Neocortex (layer II) and substantia nigra
Tau immunoreactivity	✓ (tau 55, 64, 69 triplet)	✓ (tau 55, 64 doublet)	✗	✗	✓ (tau 64, 69 doublet)
Ubiquitin immunoreactivity	✓	✓	✗	✓	✗
CSF-tau level	High	Intermediate	Low	Untested	Intermediate

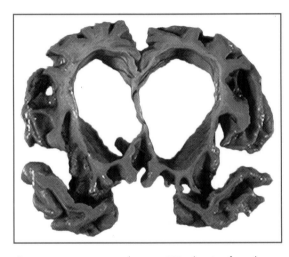

Fig. 41.1 Post-mortem brain in FTD, showing frontal atrophy. From Professor Edward C Klatt, Florida State University, College of Medicine.

tated as *non-Pick frontal lobe dementia*. This leaves a separate group of cases with well-circumscribed Pick bodies (these contain a specific 55 kDa and 64 kDa tau doublet) that can be designated *classic Pick's disease*. Rarely, patients suffer loss of large cortical neurones with involvement of the substantia nigra, hypoglossal nucleus and anterior horn cells, indicting a *frontotemporal dementia of the motor neurone type*. These patients have a rapidly progressive illness. There are inclusions in neuronal perikarya of hippocampal dendate gyrus that express ubiquitin but do not express tau or α-synuclein immunoreactivity. This is sometimes labelled 'dementia with ITSNU' (inclusions tau and synuclein negative, ubiquinated). Cases have been recorded in which the syndrome may arise as a secondary consequence of frontal projection systems and other subcortical diseases. Compared with Alzheimer's disease, acetylcholine activity appears to be normal or reduced in the nucleus basalis of Meynert only.

alone is involved, some authors prefer the term 'frontal variant of frontotemporal dementia'. Alzheimer examined microscopically the cases of frontotemporal dementia described by Pick, and noted ballooned cells, astrocyctic gliosis and neuronal argentophilic inclusions (*Pick bodies*). Pick described the 'knife-blade' macroscopic appearance of gyri transformed by focal cortical atrophy. The disorder can be highly asymmetrical, affecting only the left or right frontal or temporal region, a finding that might have clinical significance.

The majority of patients do not show gliosis, but rather a microvacuolar or spongiform appearance of the superficial layer II, which is probably best anno-

NEUROPSYCHIATRIC FEATURES OF FRONTAL LOBE DEMENTIA

Typical neuropsychiatric features are those of frontal lobe dysfunction (i.e. disinhibition, impulsivity, loss of judgement, obsessionality and apathy). There is a characteristic loss of empathy for others. Often there is a rigidity of behaviour with perseveration and sometimes hyperorality. Some patients have an irresistible urge to explore items in their visual field (*utilization behaviour*) and are said to have the human equivalent of the Klüver–Bucy syndrome.

Most patients deny any problems, despite a deteriorating course. They lack both personal and social awareness. Family members most often notice inconsiderate and inappropriate comments and behaviour. Combine this tendency with disinhibition, impulsivity and episodes of aggression, and shoplifting or sexual promiscuity can result. Relatives will often describe that the patient's personality as changed. In many ways they are correct, in that an amalgamation of deficits has caused the sufferer to act and behave differently from what he or she would otherwise have done, and this change is permanent.

Cognition

In general, memory is better preserved than in Alzheimer's disease, although patients do have retrieval problems that are often helped by prompts. Tests of abstraction and planning are typically performed poorly, but visuospatial and praxis abilities are preserved.

Occasionally, patients present with non-fluent aphasia with impaired repetition and word retrieval and relatively preserved behaviour until late in the disease process. This is often delineated as the *progressive non-fluent aphasia dementia syndrome* (see below). Speech abnormalities are characteristic of frontotemporal dementia and include progressive loss of expressive speech, stereotypy of speech (palilalia), reduced verbal fluency, echolalia and, in late stages, mutism. These features are said to help distinguish frontotemporal dementia from early-onset Alzheimer's disease, in which patients tend to suffer logoclonia of speech. Other features suggestive of early-onset Alzheimer's disease include myoclonus, seizures and an abnormal EEG. Features suggestive of frontotemporal dementia are loss of basic emotions (including loss of interest and embarrassment), overeating (especially cramming food) and preserved ability to locate objects.

On closer inspection these neat distinctions hide a more complex picture. Studies show that most patients with frontotemporal dementia confirmed at post-mortem fulfil standard criteria for Alzheimer's disease in life. Also, several types of dementia can feature frontal impairments (Box 41.2). Some neuropsychological studies suggest that impairments in the domains of attention, language, perception and memory may not contribute to the clinical differentiation of Alzheimer's disease and frontotemporal dementia, whereas deficits in problem solving (seen in frontotemporal dementia), orientation and praxis (seen in Alzheimer's disease) are more valid clinical indicators (Rascovsky et al 2002).

Mood symptoms

Emotions are shallow and quite superficial in many patients. More persistent elevation of mood and lowering of mood are also seen in a minority of sufferers. Irritability and emotional blunting are more common in the early stages, whereas apathy and withdrawal tends to develop late. Most families describe sufferers as having a loss of emotional interest in things.

Other symptoms

Many patients with severe dementia develop stereotyped repetitive behaviours that can be semi-purposeful or purposeful. Examples include collecting objects, dressing rituals and tapping or clapping. Psychotic symptoms are not well studied in frontotemporal dementia, but they can occur. They are reported as often having a bizarre quality in the absence of severe cognitive impairment and thus may occur early in the disease. Studies show that, compared with other dementias, visual hallucinations are relatively rare in frontotemporal dementia (Fig. 41.2). On the other hand, dietary changes, particularly carbohydrate cravings, are common and may result from temporal lobe damage or disinhibition. A reduced sex drive is more common than hypersexuality.

Mechanism of neuropsychiatric features in frontotemporal dementia

The pathogenesis of the psychiatric disturbances in frontotemporal dementia is assumed to relate to the regional neurodegeneration of the frontal cortex. Snowden et al (1996) divided frontotemporal dementia into three subtypes and reported distinct patterns of hypoperfusion patterns. The disinhibited subtype was associated with orbitofrontal hypoperfusion, the apathetic subtype with dorsolateral hypoperfusion of the frontal lobe, and the stereotypic subtype, which is characterized by the presence of complex compulsive behaviour, with both striatal and temporal hypoperfusion (Fig. 41.3).

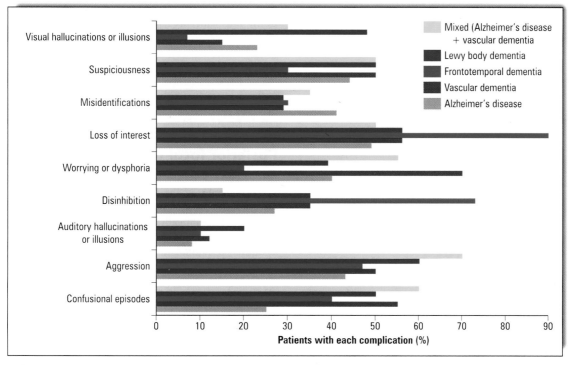

Fig. 41.2 Comparison of psychiatric symptoms in five common dementias. Data from Ballard et al (2000), Bathgate et al (2001) and Londos et al (2000).

Box 41.2 Dementia associated with frontotemporal features

- Alzheimer's disease
- Classical frontotemporal dementia
- Corticobasal degeneration
- Familial multiple system tauopathy
- Huntington's disease
- Motor neurone disease dementia
- Parkinson's disease
- Pick's disease
- Progressive supranuclear palsy
- Hydrocephalus

Few studies have attempted to replicate this provocative finding. One group measured regional cerebral glucose metabolism with PET in 12 patients with focal frontal lobe lesions and 15 patients with frontotemporal dementia. They found that impulsiveness and loss of emotional control were associated with hypometabolism in the left amygdala, whereas indifference to rules was associated with hypometabolism in the right orbitofrontal cortex (Giannakopoulos et al 2001). In the lesion-only group, executive function test performance was significantly correlated with hypometabolism in the dorsolateral prefrontal cortex. Rosso et al (2001) measured regional anatomical correlates of obsessive–compulsive behaviour in 90 patients with frontotemporal dementia. There was a significant association with temporal lobe atrophy and a trend towards significance with caudate atrophy.

OTHER RARE FOCAL CORTICAL DEMENTIAS

Semantic dementia

Semantic dementia (also known as 'progressive fluent aphasia', 'temporal variant of frontotemporal dementia' or 'hereditary dysphasic dementia') is seen with focal cortical atrophy of the dominant lateral temporal cortex, which gives rise to a decline in cognition in parallel with communication skills. Speech is grammatically correct and fluent, but with an empty quality. Patients often complain that they cannot remember the names of everyday objects

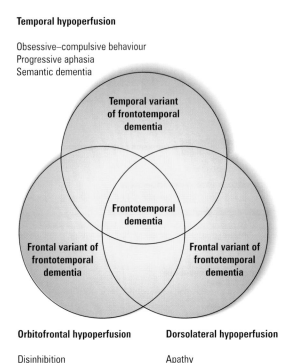

Temporal hypoperfusion

Obsessive–compulsive behaviour
Progressive aphasia
Semantic dementia

Temporal variant of frontotemporal dementia

Frontotemporal dementia

Frontal variant of frontotemporal dementia

Frontal variant of frontotemporal dementia

Orbitofrontal hypoperfusion

Disinhibition
Irritability
Lability of mood

Dorsolateral hypoperfusion

Apathy
Executive deficits
Poor abstraction
Poor judgement

Fig. 41.3 Clinical variants of frontotemporal dementia.

and, indeed, on testing there is impaired general knowledge with reduced category fluency and impaired comprehension abilities. On tests of reading, subjects are unable to read irregularly spelled words (i.e. they have surface dyslexia). Orientation, non-verbal recall, executive function and visuospatial functions are left intact. As the condition advances, patients may develop behaviours suggestive of the Klüver–Bucy syndrome. Patients with selective non-dominant temporal atrophy have not been well described, but may present with loss of knowledge of familiar faces (*agnosic prosopagnosia*), loss of empathy and emotional blunting. It is important to remember that similar clinical and pathological features can be seen in the late stages of Alzheimer's disease.

Progressive non-fluent aphasia

Focal atrophy of the dominant inferior frontal cortex causes the sister syndrome to the progressive fluent aphasia, with a gradual decline in language fluency (hesitancy, agrammatical sentences, poor repetition), but with preserved comprehension. Verbal and auditory short-term memory is impaired. Where behaviour and personality is affected, it is simply called frontotemporal dementia. Patients with non-dominant frontal atrophy may present with features similar to those with classical orbitofrontal lesions.

Posterior focal cortical dementia

Posterior focal cortical dementia, often with asymmetric atrophy of the parieto-occipital cortex, presents with visuospatial deficits, ataxia and parietal lobe signs. Specifically, there may be visual agnosia (for objects and faces), constructional apraxia, ataxia, agraphia, acalculia and transcortical sensory aphasia.

Chromosome-17-linked dementias

A number of dementias featuring amyotrophy, behavioural problems and extrapyramidal signs may be linked together by an abnormality in a one or more genes on chromosome 17. In 1994, Wilhelmsen at the University of California observed that the so-called 'disinhibition–dementia–Parkinson–amyotrophy complex' locus was localized to chromosome 17q21–22 by linkage analysis. Observations in 10 other families illustrated a chromosome 17 autosomal inheritance pattern in five other dementias (familial progressive subcortical gliosis, pallidopontonigral degeneration, hereditary Pick's disease, frontotemporal dementia and progressive fluent aphasia). Several chromosome-17-linked dementias have an abnormal tau gene product, perhaps suggesting that it is the microtubule-associated protein tau gene on chromosome 17 that is defective.

SUMMARY

The comparatively rare dementias of Pick's disease, dementia of motor neurone disease and pure frontotemporal dementia tend have an earlier age of onset than Alzheimer's disease and a less severe course. However, they feature profound impairments in judgement, empathy and responsible behaviour that have a significant effect of quality of life for patient and carers alike. In many ways the lack of insight associated with the condition makes life more difficult for carers than patients. As the condition does not appear to involve acetylcholine, the new acetylcholinesterase inhibitors may not be as effective as they are in Alzheimer's disease and Lewy body dementia. Early frontotemporal dementia may involve abnormal tau due to an aberration on chromosome 17.

REFERENCES AND FURTHER READING

Ballard C, Neill D, O'Brien J et al 2000 Anxiety, depression and psychosis in vascular dementia: prevalence and associations. Journal of Affective Disorders 592:97–106

Bathgate D, Snowden JS, Varma A et al 2001 Behaviour in frontotemporal dementia, Alzheimer's disease and vascular dementia. Acta Neurologica Scandinavica 103:367–378

Geschwind DH, Robidoux J, Alarcon M et al 2001 Dementia and neurodevelopmental predisposition: cognitive dysfunction in presymptomatic subjects precedes dementia by decades in frontotemporal dementia. Annals of Neurology 50:741–746

Giannakopoulos P, Sarazin M, Pillon B et al 2001 Metabolic correlates of behavioral deficits in frontal lobe pathologies. Presented at the 31st Annual Meeting of the Society for Neuroscience, San Diego, 13 November

Londos E, Passant U, Brun A et al 2000 Clinical Lewy body dementia and the impact of vascular components. International Journal of Geriatric Psychiatry 15:40–49

Rascovsky K, Salmon DP, Ho GJ et al 2002 Cognitive profiles differ in autopsy-confirmed frontotemporal dementia and AD. Neurology 58:1801–1808

Rosso SM, Roks G, Stevens M et al 2001 Complex compulsive behaviour in the temporal variant of frontotemporal dementia. Journal of Neurology 24811:965–970

Snowden JS, Neary D, Mann DM 1996 Frontotemporal lobar degeneration: frontotemporal dementia, progressive aphasia, semantic dementia. Clinical Neurology and Neurosurgery Monographs. Churchill Livingstone, Edinburgh

Wilhelmsen KC, Lynch T, Pavlou E et al 1994 Localization of disinhibition–dementia–parkinsonism–amyotrophy complex to 17q21-22. American Journal of Human Genetics 55:1159–1165

42

Lewy Body Dementia

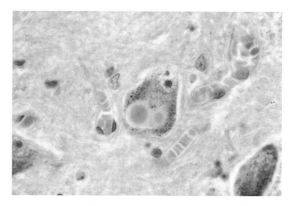

Fig. 42.1 Lewy bodies are spherical inclusions seen in the cytoplasm of melanin-containing neurones. Typically, they have a hyaline core and a pale halo. They are based on aggregated neurofilaments and α-synuclein. Lewy bodies were first identified using the haematoxylin and eosin (H&E) stain, but this does not clearly reveal cortical Lewy bodies, which require modern staining methods such as immunoperoxidase for ubiquitin, illustrated here. From Stevens & Lowe (2000).

BACKGROUND

Lewy body dementia (LBD) is a newly recognized but relatively common cause of dementia. A triad of dementia, parkinsonism and psychosis (hallucinations) is said to be characteristic of diffuse Lewy body disease. Revised criteria are shown in Box 42.1. Lewy bodies are spherical intraneuronal cytoplasmic inclusions 15–30 μm in diameter. They were originally described by Lewy in 1912 as occurring in brainstem nuclei in Parkinson's disease. Lewy bod-

---

Box 42.1 Consensus criteria for Lewy body dementia

Progressive cognitive decline of sufficient magnitude to interfere with normal social or occupational function.

Two of the following (for probable DLB) or one of the following (for possible LBD):
- fluctuating cognition
- recurrent visual hallucinations
- spontaneous parkinsonism.

Features supportive of the diagnosis:
- repeated falls
- syncope
- transient loss of consciousness
- neuroleptic sensitivity
- systematized delusions
- other hallucinations.

Diagnosis less likely in the presence of:
- stroke
- a disorder accounting for the above.

After McKeith et al (1996)

---

ies are argyrophilic and labelled by both ubiquitin and neurofilament antibodies. The degree to which Lewy bodies play a role in Parkinson's disease and LBD is not certain. In LBD, Lewy bodies are found in subcortical sites, as well as diffusely in the neocortex (although there is an unpredictable relationship between the two). Subcortical Lewy bodies tend to appear first in the substantia nigra and entorhinal cortex and later in the cingulate gyrus and hippocampus. Later, cortical Lewy bodies appear, largely in the perikarya of pyramidal neurones in layers V and VI. They are seen in about one-quarter of autopsied dementia cases using anti-ubiquitin antibody staining. This does not necessarily indicate the prevalence of LBD, since 20–40% of cases of clinically definite Alzheimer's disease also have Lewy bodies, mainly in the substantia nigra, and as many as two-thirds of Alzheimer's disease patients with parkinsonism have Lewy bodies (Gearing et al 1995). This group with mixed pathologies (Alzheimer's plus Lewy body) is important because they are more common than cases with Lewy bodies alone and also appear to have a distinct clinical profile (Del Ser et al 2001). One very basic question that is rarely asked is what percentage of patients fulfilling the clinical criteria for LBD actually have Lewy bodies at postmortem (i.e. have pathologically defined dementia with Lewy bodies (DLB)). The answer appears to be surprisingly few, perhaps less than one-quarter of patients, which raises the subsidiary question of

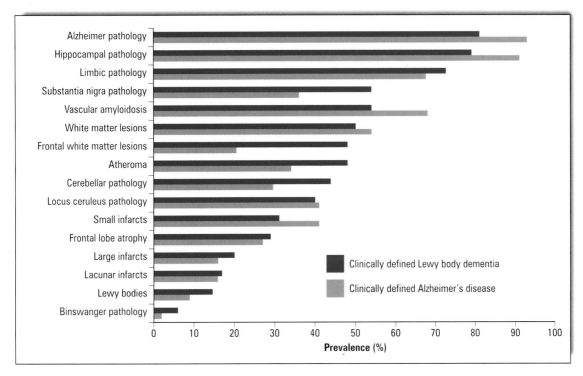

Fig. 42.2 Prevalence of neuropathological changes in clinically defined cases with Alzheimer's disease and Lewy body dementia. Data from Londos et al (2001).

what disorders this disease is frequently confused with during life (Fig. 42.2 and Clinical Pointer 42.1) (Londos et al 2001, Lopez et al 2000).

PATHOGENESIS

The pathology of pure LBD closely resembles that of idiopathic Parkinson's disease (see Clinical Pointer 42.1). Whether Lewy bodies are directly responsible for cognitive impairment is not certain. The best clinicoanatomical relationship in LBD is the link between Lewy bodies in the substantia nigra and parkinsonism. Hippocampal and parahippocampal cortical Lewy bodies probably have a major role in cognition in both Parkinson's disease and LBD (Harding & Halliday 2001).

Recent research interest has focused on markers of neuronal degeneration using antibodies against α-, β- and γ-synuclein. α-Synuclein is a nerve terminal protein that is a better marker of Lewy bodies than ubiquitin. These markers also revealed presynaptic axon terminal pathology in the hippocampus and filamentous ubiquitin-immunoreactive inclusions known as *Lewy neurites*, which are also found in the hippocampus of Parkinson's disease and multiple system atrophy. There may be clinically important reductions in choline acetyltransferase activity in the cortices, which appears at an earlier stage in LBD than in Alzheimer's disease (Tiraboschi et al 2002). That said, studies to date have only found a weak relationship between acetylcholine function and cognitive impairment. Regarding dopamine, striatal dopamine is reduced in LBD, but less extensively than in Parkinson's disease. Dopamine turnover is not significantly increased in LBD, unlike in Parkinson's disease.

NEUROPSYCHIATRIC FEATURES OF LEWY BODY DEMENTIA

LBD is characterized by both cortical and subcortical involvement and neuropsychiatric symptoms reflect this. The progressive dementia is similar to that seen in Alzheimer's disease. Compared with patients with Alzheimer's disease, those with LBD may show less temporal lobe atrophy on MRI and more hypoperfusion of occipital lobes on SPECT, but not distinctly enough for these findings to be used as a diagnostic test. Subtle differences on neuropsychological testing include a greater frequency of deficits in verbal fluency, visuospatial ability and attention in LBD, which has parallels with the dementia of Parkinson's disease. Studies comparing DLB with Alzheimer's disease have also found equivalent rates of memory problems in the two conditions. Overall, neuropsychological tests have not been able to differentiate LBD reliably from other dementias.

A day-to-day fluctuating mental state may be an important distinguishing clinical feature, and this formed a cornerstone of McKeith's original criteria (see Box 42.1). Nevertheless, differential diagnosis is difficult and presentations can be confused with delirium in patients with dementia and Parkinson's disease. Fluctuating cognition has been reported in 80% of those with DLB, 40% of those with vascular dementia and 20% of those with Alzheimer's disease. The nature of fluctuating cognition, when delirium is removed, may involve fluctuating attention as a core feature (Ballard et al 2001). The rate of fluctuating attention and reaction time is comparable in LBD (with parkinsonism) and Parkinson's dementia (Ballard et al 2002). The pathological basis of fluctuating cognition is uncertain.

Patients with diffuse LBD often suffer hallucinations, delusions and psychosis. Hallucinations are more common, being earlier and more persistent in LBD than in Alzheimer's disease, and delusions of misidentification are probably equally common. In view of the prominence of cognitive and psychotic symptoms, mood abnormalities have not been properly examined in patients with LBD. At least

---

Clinical Pointer 42.1

Distinguishing Lewy body dementia from Alzheimer's disease and Parkinson's dementia

Of the three core features of LBD (fluctuation, visual hallucinations, spontaneous parkinsonism) none is pathognomonic and all may occur in both Alzheimer's disease and Parkinson's disease, as well as in vascular dementia and delirium. At least eight studies have examined the clinical consensus criteria for LBD. Even in the larger studies, confirmation relies on an inadequate handful of pathologically confirmed cases. The best study (Londos et al 2001) was recently published from the Lund University Hospital group in Sweden. They looked at 48 cases of clinically diagnosed LBD and 45 cases of Alzheimer's disease, with fascinating results. Alzheimer pathology was found in 81% of the LBD group and 93% of the Alzheimer's disease group. Lewy body pathology (based on α-synuclein staining) was found in the same percentage of patients in both groups (40%). The clinically misdiagnosed cases of LBD, in fact, had Alzheimer's disease pathology with vascular white matter lesions in the frontal lobes. This and other studies strongly suggest that Alzheimer's disease is occasionally misdiagnosed as pure LBD or pure vascular dementia (usually when mixed pathology is present). Clinically, pure Alzheimer's disease should be indicated by a prodrome of memory loss, late appearance of hallucinations and less likelihood of parkinsonism. LBD is almost certainly incorrectly diagnosed frequently, especially when the true diagnosis is mixed dementia, Parkinson's dementia or vascular parkinsonism. Because the are no fundamental neuropathological differences between cases with Parkinson's dementia and LBD, the two conditions may be considered to be opposite ends of the same disease process. Despite this, authors continue to try to distinguish between them clinically. One suggested feature is that dementia should occur within 2 years of parkinsonism in the case of LBD. Another is that the onset of Parkinson's dementia usually begins with tremor, balance problems or other extrapyramidal sign, whereas parkinsonism at onset is said to only occur in one-quarter of cases of LBD. Other clinical pointers that may help the clinician distinguish Parkinson's dementia from DLB include an absence of tremor in the latter, along with little or no response to levodopa. The rate of rigidity, bradykinesia, and gait abnormalities is little different in the two conditions.

Further reading Harding AJ, Halliday GM 2001 Cortical Lewy body pathology in the diagnosis of dementia. Acta Neuropathologica 102:355–363
Kosunen O, Soininen H, Paljarvi L et al 1996 Diagnostic accuracy of Alzheimer's disease: a neuropathological study. Acta Neuropathologica 91:185–193
Londos E, Passant U, Gustafson L et al 2001 Neuropathological correlates to clinically defined dementia with Lewy bodies. International Journal of Geriatric Psychiatry 16:667–679
Lopez OL, Litvan I, Catt KE et al 1999 Accuracy of four clinical diagnostic criteria for the diagnosis of neurodegenerative dementias. Neurology 53:1292–1299
McKeith I, Burn D 2000 Spectrum of Parkinson's disease, Parkinson's dementia and Lewy body dementia. Neurologic Clinics 18:865–883

Table 42.1 A comparison of three related dementias that feature Lewy bodies (% of patients)

Symptom	Alzheimer's disease	Parkinson's disease	Lewy body dementia
Dementia	100	34	100
Parkinsonism at onset	5	90	25
Delusions	30	10	50
Visual hallucinations	15–30	20	40–60
Depression	30	50	40
Dopamine loss	Mild	Severe	Severe
Acetylcholine loss	Moderate and late	Mild and early	Severe
Cortical Lewy bodies	Rare	Common	Always

Box 42.2 Pathology in Lewy body dementia

- Diffuse Lewy bodies
- Lewy neurites
- Locus ceruleus neuronal loss
- Meynert nucleus neuronal loss
- Neurofibrillary tangles
- Senile plaques
- Substantia nigra neuronal loss

lines, symptoms are non-specific, occurring also in delirium and Parkinson's disease. Dementia with Lewy bodies is a neuropathological diagnosis. Lewy bodies are found in cortical and subcortical sites (the same finding is seen in Parkinson's disease). From a neuropsychiatric point of view many complications can arise, particularly visual hallucinations, which may be due to deficits in visual information processing. Exciting treatment options are emerging.

one study has suggested that depression may accompany cortical Lewy bodies (Lopez et al 2000).

Serious extrapyramidal side effects may occur with the use of standard doses of antipsychotics and have even been reported with atypical antipsychotics (see Ch. 57). From a biological perspective, cholinergic deficiency (reduced post-mortem choline acetyltransferase) may be associated with hallucinations in DLB (Perry et al 1990). Two small studies, requiring confirmation, report a biological basis for LBD hallucinations. Ballard et al (2000) suggested that delusions were associated with elevated muscarinic M1 receptor binding and that visual hallucinations are associated with significant reductions in choline acetyltransferase in Brodmann area 36 (Ballard et al 2000). Halliday et al (2002) found that visual hallucinations in patients with LBD and Parkinson's disease were related to high densities of Lewy bodies in the amygdala, parahippocampus gyrus and inferior temporal cortices.

SUMMARY

LBD is an increasingly recognized form of dementia that shares features with Alzheimer's disease and Parkinson's dementia, both clinically and pathologically. The purported core clinical features have sparked much debate and, despite consensus guide-

REFERENCES AND FURTHER READING

Ballard C, Piggott M, Johnson M et al 2000 Delusions associated with elevated muscarinic binding in dementia with Lewy bodies. Annals of Neurology 48:868–876

Ballard C, O'Brien J, Gray A et al 2001 Attention and fluctuating attention in patients with dementia with Lewy bodies and Alzheimer disease. Archives of Neurology 58:977–982

Ballard C, Aarsland D, McKeith I et al 2002 Attention and fluctuating attention in Parkinson's disease with and without dementia and dementia with Lewy bodies. Presented at the American Academy of Neurology 54th Annual Meeting, Denver, 13–20 April

Del Ser T, Hachinski V, Merskey H et al 2001 Clinical and pathologic features of two groups of patients with dementia with Lewy bodies: effect of coexisting Alzheimer-type lesion load. Alzheimer's Disease and Associated Disorders 15:31–44

Gearing M, Mirra S, Hedreen JC et al 1995 The consortium to establish a registry for Alzheimer's disease (CERAD). Part X. Neuropathology confirmation of the clinical diagnosis of Alzheimer's disease. Neurology 45:461–466

Harding AJ, Halliday GM 2001 Cortical Lewy body pathology in the diagnosis of dementia. Acta Neuropathologica 102:355–363

Harding AJ, Broe GA, Halliday GM 2002 Visual hallucinations in Lewy body disease relate to Lewy bodies in the temporal lobe. Brain 125:391–403

Lewy FH 1912 Paralysis agitans. Pathologische anatomie. In: Lewandowsky M (ed) Handbuch der Neurologie. Springer, New York, p 920–933

Londos E, Passant U, Gustafson L et al 2001 Neuropathological correlates to clinically defined dementia with Lewy bodies. International Journal of Geriatric Psychiatry 16:667–679

Lopez OL, Hamilton RL, Becker JT et al 2000 Severity of cognitive impairment and the clinical diagnosis of AD with Lewy bodies. Neurology 54:1780–1787

McKeith IG, Galasko D, Kosaka K et al 1996 Consensus guidelines for the clinical and pathologic diagnosis of dementia with Lewy bodies (DLB): report of the consor-tium on DLB international workshop. Neurology 47:1113–1124

Perry EK, Kerwin J, Perry RH et al 1990 Cerebral cholinergic activity is related to the incidence of visual hallucinations in senile dementia of Lewy body type. Dementia 1:2–4

Tiraboschi P, Hansen LA, Alford M et al 2002 Early and widespread cholinergic losses differentiate dementia with Lewy Bodies from Alzheimer disease. Archives of General Psychiatry 59:946–951

43

Vascular Dementia

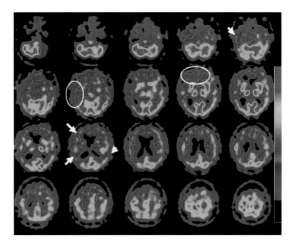

Fig. 43.1 SPECT scan in a patient with vascular dementia. In these coronal slices, high metabolic activity is shown as red and low activity by blue-black. There are multiple areas of localized hypoperfusion, particularly in the right frontal cortex and right parietal cortex (circles). From Dr PK Chandrak, Department of Radiology, Brigham and Women's Hospital, Harvard Medical School.

BACKGROUND

Vascular dementia occurs in 2.5% of people over the age of 65 years. The largest epidemiological studies suggest that it accounts for approximately one-quarter of cases of dementia in men and 10% or so of cases in women. It may be the most common form of dementia among men from Japan. Post-mortem studies suggest that a vascular contribution to dementia lies on a continuum, with some degree of vascular changes seen in one-third of the elderly and 50% of those with Alzheimer's disease (see Clinical Pointers 4.3 and 17.1). The rates of vascular dementia increase with age, but not as dramatically as the increase in the rate of Alzheimer's disease.

PATHOGENESIS

A variety of vascular lesions can cause dementia. About half of cases consist of a pure form of one of the conditions shown in Box 43.1 and the remainder are a combination of vascular pathologies. Stroke is a cause of dementia in 15–25% of patients who were cognitively intact before their stroke.

In a paper quoted over 1000 times in the last 30 years, Tomlinson et al (1970) in Newcastle showed that there was considerable overlap between Alzheimer's disease and vascular dementia. Patients with vascular dementia are often misdiagnosed with Alzheimer's disease, because vascular brain lesions may not be apparent on CT and because vascular dementia can have a gradual onset and a course sim-

> **Box 43.1 Pathology of vascular dementia**
>
> *Large-vessel disease*
> Multi-infarct dementia
> Strategic infarct dementia
> Single-vessel dementia (post-stroke)
>
> *Small-vessel disease*
> Cortical (and subcortical) disease:
> - collagen disease
> - hypertensive angiopathy
> - atherosclerotic angiopathy
>
> Subcortical disease:
> - Binswanger's disease
> - lacunar state
>
> *Hypoxic disease*
> Border zone infarcts
> White matter infarcts
>
> *Haemorrhagic disease*
> Cerebral haemorrhage
> Subarachnoid haemorrhage
> Subdural haemorrhage

ilar to Alzheimer's disease. The Hachinski Ischaemic Scale was introduced in 1975 and validated for the differentiation of *multi-infarct dementia* from Alzheimer's disease. There have subsequently been many studies attempting to test this claim. One meta-analysis of 312 patients showed that the scale is a reliable way of differentiating vascular dementia and Alzheimer's disease, but that the differential diagnosis of mixed dementias is more difficult (Table 43.1) (Moroney et al 1997). Other criteria for vascular dementia exist, including the State of California Alzheimer Disease Diagnostic and Treatment Center (ADDTC), the National Institute of Neurological Disorders and Stroke–Association Internationale pour la Recherche et l'Enseignement en Neurosciences (NINDS–AIREN), the DSM-IV and ICD-10 (see Box 39.4). They all require evidence of cerebrovascular disease, although in the case of DSM-IV and ICD-10 this does not have to be radiological evidence. There should be focal signs (not required by the ADDTC criteria) or symptoms (not required by the ADDTC or ICD-10 criteria) and a temporal relation between the pathology and the presentation. Clinicopathological validation of these scales has been attempted (Gold et al 2002).

Pathology

If a person is unlucky enough to acquire a vascular brain lesion in an area critical for dense information processing, such as the thalamus, hippocampus or cingulate gyrus, then dementia can result despite only a modest volume of tissue being damaged. This has been called 'strategic infarct dementia' (SID). One recent study found that the volume of vascular lesions in limbic areas, heteromodal-association areas, frontal cortex and white matter explained 50% of the variance in cognitive impairment in vascular and mixed dementias (Zekry et al 2003).

CLINICAL FEATURES

Compared with Alzheimer's disease, vascular dementia tends to affect younger patients, who present with complaints such as headache, dizziness or amnesia and associated localizing neurological signs. The classic picture of abrupt onset, episodic, 'step-wise' deterioration associated with focal symptoms and signs is probably seen in less than half of true cases of vascular dementia. Indeed, about half of cases in prospective series have a prodromal phase of mild cognitive impairment. Function following a vascular lesion is notoriously variable, with

---

Box 43.2   Full Hachinski Ischaemic Scale

1.	Abrupt onset	2 points
2.	Stepwise deterioration	1 point
3.	Fluctuating course	2 points
4.	Nocturnal confusion	1 point
5.	Relative preservation of personality	1 point
6.	Depression	1 point
7.	Somatic complaints	1 point
8.	Emotional incontinence	1 point
9.	History of hypertension	1 point
10.	History of stroke	2 points
11.	Evidence of atherosclerosis	1 point
12.	Focal neurological symptoms	2 points
13.	Focal neurological signs	2 points

A score ≤4 indicates Alzheimer's disease
A score ≥7 indicates vascular dementia

Table 43.1   Discriminating items on the Hachinski scale

	Vascular dementia versus Alzheimer's disease	Vascular dementia versus mixed dementia	Mixed dementia versus Alzheimer's disease
Fluctuating course	OR = 8	No effect	OR = 0.20
Stepwise deterioration	OR = 6	OR = 4	No effect
Hypertension	OR = 4	No effect	No effect
History of stroke	OR = 4.30	No effect	OR = 0.08
Focal neurological symptoms	OR = 4.40	No effect	No effect
Emotional incontinence	No effect	OR = 3	No effect

Adapted from Moroney et al (1997)
OR, odds ratio

Box 43.3   Non-localizing features of vascular dementia

- Behavioural disturbance
- Delirium
- Disorientation
- Global cognitive impairment
- Loss of insight
- Mood disorder
- Poor concentration
- Psychosis
- Sleep disturbance
- Social withdrawal

day-to-day fluctuations noted in vascular dementia. This is certain to cause diagnostic errors with Lewy body dementia.

Vascular lesions can occur entirely silently, unnoticed by patients, carers or doctors. On the other hand, presentations can be very severe, with reduced consciousness and delirium seen in up to one-third of patients. No single clinical picture is pathognomic of vascular dementia. Three-quarters of patients have involvement of the frontal lobes (and frontal–subcortical pathways) and thus present with classical frontal lobe features such as motor weakness, urinary incontinence, lack of judgement, empathy and inhibition, and primitive reflexes. The resultant shuffling gait can cause problems with the differential diagnosis of Parkinson's disease. A pure subcortical picture is seen in about 50% of patients (a combination of subcortical and cortical occurs in a further 40%). This *subcortical ischaemic vascular dementia* (or SIVD) features slowness of thought and action, upper motor neurone pyramidal signs, extrapyramidal signs and possible pseudobulbar symptoms. The dominant parietal lobes seem to be affected frequently in vascular dementia, probably in border zone areas (see Fig. 4.3). The brainstem is also vulnerable if the vertebrobasilar supply is involved; such patients present with falls, vertigo, diplopia and nystagmus.

OUTCOME

The 5-year mortality rate in vascular dementia is almost twice that of Alzheimer's disease, at about 60%. The proportion of patients entering nursing homes is also higher than in Alzheimer's disease.

Neuropsychiatric features of vascular dementia

Systematic examinations of the neuropsychiatric complications of vascular dementia are beginning to appear. Patients with vascular dementia have higher rates of delirium, anxiety and depression than are seen in any other common forms of dementia. A recent study of 92 patients with vascular dementia and 92 patients with Alzheimer's disease demonstrated higher rates of anxiety and depression, but not psychosis, in vascular dementia (Ballard et al 2000). In this study, patients who had depressive symptoms performed worse on cognitive testing than did those with vascular dementia but no depression. In addition, both anxiety and depressive symptoms were more clearly related to severity of dementia than in Alzheimer's disease. Extrapyramidal signs and frontal release signs (e.g. the grasp reflex) appear to be associated with severity of depression in vascular dementia. The specific clinical features of vascular dementia also apply to cases of mixed dementia in combination with higher rates of visual hallucinations and aggression, which are probably derived from comorbid Alzheimer pathology (see Fig. 41.2).

Cognition in vascular dementia

Several studies have compared cognitive findings in vascular dementia with those in Alzheimer's disease. One methodological weakness is that vascular dementia has a variable cognitive profile depending on the nature of the vascular deficits. Leaving that criticism to one side, patients with vascular dementia tend to have greater attentional, executive and verbal fluency problems, whereas patients with Alzheimer's disease tend to have greater short-term memory and language difficulties (repetition and naming). Vascular dementia patients with well-defined subcortical ischaemia, performed worse on the Controlled Word Association Test (executive function), but better on the Rey Auditory Verbal Learning Test (recognition memory) than did matched patients with Alzheimer's disease (Tierney et al 2001). The authors advised caution in using neuropsychological tests alone to distinguish between these common conditions. Several neuroimaging findings have been correlated with the degree of cognitive impairment in vascular dementia. These include ventricular volume, extent and type of white matter lesions, degree and site of atrophy, and multiple lesions in the dominant hemisphere and limbic structures (for a review, see Erkinjuntti et al 1999). These factors are essentially the same risk factors that predict post-stroke dementia (Pohjasvaara et al 2000).

Cognitive syndromes following strategically placed infarcts

Thalamus

Damage to the thalamus, particularly bilaterally and involving the anterior nuclei, causes cognitive deficits characterized by memory loss and poor verbal fluency. The degree to which thalamic insults cause dysphasia is debated, but a variable subcortical thalamic aphasia syndrome resembling a partial Wernicke's syndrome has been reported. The memory loss is in the domain of episodic memory for new material. Dominant lesions tend to cause the verbal and visual memory problems (possibly with dysphasia preserving repetition), whereas the non-dominant side causes visuospatial deficits and neglect.

After dorsomedial infarcts (supplied by the tubero-thalamic artery), memory defects are combined with drowsiness, abulia and vertical gaze disturbances. In these cases memory impairments may be transient unless the lesion extends rostrally to include the mammillothalamic tract or axons of the ventro-amygdalofugal pathway.

In the case of anterior thalamic infarcts (supplied by the paramedian thalamic arteries) disturbance of consciousness resolves to leave amnesia alone (anterograde more than retrograde) or amnesia in combination with apathy, language disturbances or neglect (Fig. 43.3).

Angular gyrus

Dominant lesions of the angular gyrus cause alexia with agraphia, aphasia and, possibly, Gerstmann's syndrome, without focal motor symptoms or signs.

Internal capsule

Verbal memory loss occurs when the genu is involved. Fluctuating alertness, inattention, apathy and psychomotor retardation are also seen when the lesion interrupts the inferior and anterior thalamic peduncles.

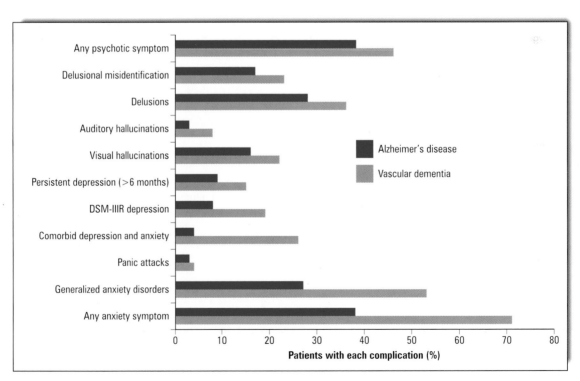

Fig. 43.2 Comparison of psychiatric disorders in 92 patients with vascular dementia and 92 patients with Alzheimer's disease. Data from Ballard et al (2000).

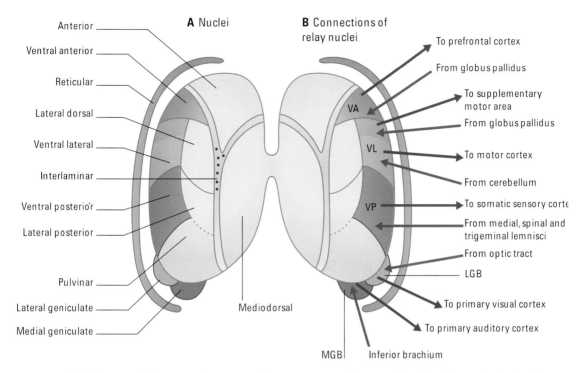

A Nuclei

Anterior
Ventral anterior
Reticular
Lateral dorsal
Ventral lateral
Interlaminar
Ventral posterior
Lateral posterior
Pulvinar
Lateral geniculate
Medial geniculate
Mediodorsal

B Connections of relay nuclei

To prefrontal cortex
From globus pallidus
VA
To supplementary motor area
From globus pallidus
VL
To motor cortex
From cerebellum
VP
To somatic sensory corte
From medial, spinal and trigeminal lemnisci
From optic tract
LGB
To primary visual cortex
To primary auditory cortex
MGB   Inferior brachium

Fig. 43.3 The thalamus is the largest nuclear mass in the nervous system. The internal medullary lamina divide the thalamus into anterior, lateral and dorsomedial groups. The anterior nucleus receives afferents from the mammillary body and sends efferents to the cingulate gyrus in the circuit of Papez. The dorsomedial nucleus receives afferents from the amygdala as part of the amygdala circuit. Lesions to a small area of the thalamus can cause a devastating strategic infarct dementia syndrome. From Fitzgerald & Folan-Curran (2001).

Basal ganglia

Lesions to the caudate can cause a range of cognitive deficits, most notably executive dysfunction and memory disturbance. Generally the frontal abnormalities are more severe than the memory difficulties. There may be difficulty in recall, even with cues, but otherwise normal immediate recognition performance.

Mood in vascular dementia

The rate of major depression in vascular dementia is about four times higher than in Alzheimer's disease (Komahashi et al 1994). At 70%, the rate of anxiety symptoms is at least twice that in Alzheimer's disease. In vascular dementia, depression can occur at all stages of dementia. Both anxiety and depression appear to be more severe (as well as frequent) in vascular dementia. Apathy also appears to be more common in the early and medium stages of demen-

tia. Other behavioural and emotional changes, such as disinhibition, loss of interest and social avoidance, tend to be slightly more common in vascular dementia than Alzheimer's disease. It is uncertain whether there is a correlation between the severity of the psychiatric complications and the severity of cognitive deficits in vascular dementia, since studies differ in their findings. It may be necessary to examine this question separately for each symptom to get an answer. The effect of regional deficits on neuropsychiatric symptoms requires close scrutiny. Provisionally, patients with frontal hypoperfusion deficits have higher rates of irritability, depression and anxiety than those without.

Psychosis in vascular dementia

Psychosis is most often seen in the context of delirium occurring after a newly acquired vascular brain lesion. These symptoms are typically fleeting paranoid (persecutory) delusions and odd visual hallucinations and misinterpretations. Sensory impairments have a large contribution to play in such patients. Occasionally, an irritative lesion in the temporal or occipital lobe will produce recurrent hallucinations that the patient describes in detail and that appear to be at odds with the patient's general demeanour. Overall, studies have not shown the rates of delusions or hallucinations to be markedly increased compared with Alzheimer's disease, although the rates of delusional misidentification may be higher in Alzheimer's disease (see Fig 43.2). Visual hallucinations are more common in Lewy body dementia than vascular dementia.

THE SPECIAL CASE OF MIXED DEMENTIA

The most common pathologies found in the brains of victims of dementia are neurofibrillary tangles in the medial temporal lobes and small vessel vascular disease (MRC CFAS 2001). As each of these is found in about 60–75% of post-mortem cases, it should be of no surprise that the chance of a combination of Alzheimer and vascular pathologies occurring together is high. For example, neurofibrillary tangles are found in 30–50% of patients with vascular dementia. In essence, this is the condition of mixed dementia (although cases with Alzheimer and Lewy body pathology should also be classified as a form of mixed dementia). Unfortunately, these pathological data are not available during life, and we must rely on imperfect markers of disease such as clinical criteria or MRI findings. Post-mortem studies show that MRI scans detect about 50% of the vascular lesion load seen histologically in aged brains. Furthermore, as no test can rule out the possibility of plaques or tangles during life, all cases of vascular dementia could be cases of mixed dementia. This illustrates why the clinical entity of mixed dementia remains imprecise and under-recognized. However, there is accumulating evidence that mixed dementia has features distinct from those of either pure Alzheimer's disease or pure vascular dementia. For example, in both the NUN study (Snowdon et al 1997) and the OPTIMA study (Esiri et al 1999), patients with Alzheimer's disease had poorer cognitive function if they had superadded infarcts. More provocatively, in one study (Hirono et al 2000) of patients meeting the clinical criteria for Alzheimer's disease but with MRI evidence of white matter

hyperintensities, the severity of hyperintensities correlated with the likelihood of urinary incontinence, grasp reflex and aberrant motor activity, whereas whole brain volume correlated with cognitive impairment. The importance of additional vascular pathology in patients who meet the criteria for Alzheimer's disease has been replicated in the neuropathological study by Londos et al (2001). As with pure vascular dementia, there is always the hope in mixed dementia that the vascular diathesis can be modified (see Ch. 47). Given the evidence currently available, it is certainly important to attempt to distinguish between dementias with and without a significant vascular contribution, but more work needs to be done in order to delineate the natural history and response to treatment of pure vascular dementia from that in mixed dementia.

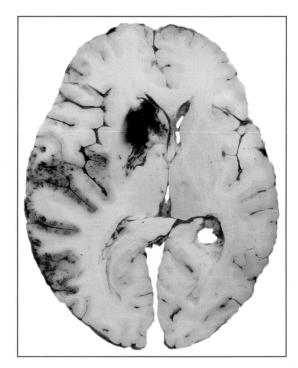

Fig. 43.4 Brain lesions of vascular origin may be produced through ischaemia, haemorrhage or oedema as a result of many different diseases. The vascular pathology in vascular dementia is varied. Lipohyalinosis and microatheroma are thought to be the most common mechanisms underlying arterial occlusion, although amyloid angiopathy and senile arteriosclerosis probably also have a role. From Peter Rochford, Museum Curator, James Vincent Duhig Pathology Museum, University of Queensland.

SUMMARY

In men, vascular dementia is the second most common form of dementia, presenting with more mood problems and more delirium than in Alzheimer's disease. In men and women, vascular factors are the most common pathology contributing to the dementias. The classic stepwise episodic course is seen in only half of patients, although day-to-day fluctuations are seen. The frontal and parietal lobes appear to suffer vascular damage disproportionately in this condition.

Diagnostically, neuroimaging helps confirm the clinical history and examination, allowing a more accurate diagnosis during life. Mixed cases of dementia, particularly vascular dementia with Alzheimer's disease, poses a particular challenge for clinicians, as it regularly mimics other conditions such as pure Alzheimer'' disease and Lewy body dementia.

Vascular dementia, more than any other dementia, holds most promise for preventive measures.

REFERENCES AND FURTHER READING

Ballard C, Neill D, O'Brien J et al 2000 Anxiety, depression and psychosis in vascular dementia: prevalence and associations. Journal of Affective Disorders 59:97–106

Erkinjuntti T, Bowler JV, DeCarli CS et al 1999 Imaging of static brain lesions in vascular dementia: implications for clinical trials. Alzheimer's Disease and Associated Disorders 13(suppl 3):S81–S90

Esiri MM, Nagy Z, Smith MZ et al 1999 Cerebrovascular disease and threshold for dementia in the early stages of Alzheimer's disease. Lancet 354:919–920

Gold G, Bouras C, Canuto A et al 2002 Clinicopathological validation study of four sets of clinical criteria for vascular dementia. American Journal of Psychiatry 159:82–87

Hirono N, Kitagaki H, Kazui H et al 2000 Impact of white matter changes on clinical manifestation of Alzheimer's disease: a quantitative study. Stroke 31:2182–2188

Komahashi T, Ohmori K, Nakano T et al 1994 Epidemiological survey of dementia and depression among the aged living in the community in Japan. Japanese Journal of Psychiatry and Neurology 48:517–552

Londos E, Passant U, Gustafson L et al 2001 Neuropathological correlates to clinically defined dementia with Lewy bodies. International Journal of Geriatric Psychiatry 16:667–679

Moroney JT, Bagiella E, Desmond DW et al 1997 Meta-analysis of the Hachinski ischemic score in pathologically verified dementias. Neurology 49:1096–1105

MRC CFAS (Neuropathology Group of the Medical Research Council Cognitive Function and Ageing Study) 2001 Pathological correlates of late-onset dementia in a multi-centre, community-based population in England and Wales. Lancet 357:169–175

Snowdon DA, Greiner LH, Mortimer JA et al 1997 Brain infarction and the clinical expression of Alzheimer disease: the NUN study. JAMA 277:813–817

Tierney MC, Black SE, Szalai JP et al 2001 Recognition, memory and verbal fluency differentiate probable Alzheimer's disease from subcortical ischaemic vascular disease. Archives of Neurology 58:1654–1659

Tomlinson BE, Blessed G, Roth M 1970 Observations on the brains of demented old people. Journal of Neurological Science 11:205–242

Pohjasvaara T, Mantyla R, Salonen O et al 2000 How complex interactions of ischemic brain infarcts, white matter lesions, and atrophy relate to poststroke dementia. Archives of Neurology 57:1295–1300

Wade JPH, Mirsen T, Hachinski VC et al 1987 The clinical diagnosis of Alzheimer's disease. Archives of Neurology 44:24–29

Zekry D, Duyckaerts C, Belmin J et al 2003 The vascular lesions in vascular and mixed dementia: the weight of functional neuroanatomy. Neurobiology of Aging 24:213–219

Evidence-based Review of Treatments in Neuropsychiatry

This review of treatments in neuropsychiatry uses levels 1a–2b shown in Table IV.1.

Table IV.1   Hierarchy of evidence in the medical literature

Grade of recommendation	Level of evidence	Study methodology
A	1a	Systematic review (with homogeneity)* of randomized controlled trials
	1b	Individual randomized controlled trial (with narrow confidence interval)
	1c	All patients died before treatment introduced or none die now that treatment is used
B	2a	Systematic review (with homogeneity)* of cohort studies
	2b	Individual cohort study (including low-quality randomized controlled trial (e.g. <80% follow-up)
	2c	'Outcomes' research
	3a	Systematic review (with homogeneity)* of case–control studies
	3b	Individual case–control study
C	4	Case series (and poor-quality cohort and case–control studies)†
D	5	Expert opinion without explicit critical appraisal, or based on physiology, bench research or 'first principles'

*Homogeneity is a systematic review that is free of variations (heterogeneity) in the results of individual studies
†A poor-quality cohort study is one that failed to define comparison groups or failed to measure exposure and outcomes measures in the same objective way in both exposed and non-exposed subjects and/or failed to identify or appropriately to control known confounders and/or failed to carry out a sufficiently long and complete follow-up of patients. A poor-quality case–control study is one that failed to clearly define comparison groups and/or failed to measure exposures and outcomes in the same objective way in both cases and controls and/or failed to identify or appropriately to control known confounders

44

Principles of Treatment in Neuro-psychiatry

The basic principles of treatment in neuropsychiatry are really no different from good-quality practice in mainstream psychiatry or neurology (Box 44.1). Patients with neuropsychiatric presentations often require symptomatic treatment with agents that specifically help with the problem areas of sleep, agitation, abnormal movements, motivation or irritability. It is important to concentrate on treating the most distressing and disabling complaints as rated by patients and carers, rather than to attempt to correct biological markers of disease in isolation. Many neuropsychiatric disorders are less common than those seen in general adult psychiatry. For this reason, it is necessary to accept that double-blind randomized controlled trials (RCTs) do not exist for every presenting problem. Instead, clinicians must use a more basic level of evidence rather than take the nihilistic approach of not treating the distressed patient at all. This level of evidence based on experience is sometimes referred to as 'medicine-based evidence'. For brevity, I shall outline only good-quality evidence from RCTs (see Table IV.1 and Appendix VI) pertaining to treatments in neuropsychiatry. The reader may choose to appraise the evidence presented critically, since even the quality of the 'good' studies cited varies enormously.

One of the main principles of drug therapy is that patients with CNS disease are unusually sensitive to many psychotropic drugs, and therefore it is wise to begin with a low dose (perhaps in the form of a test dose) and increase it gradually thereafter. Where possible, use the simplest regimen to manage the patient. However, do not undertreat for fear of possible side effects when actual illness-related problems are present and require attention (Box 44.2). Be prepared to take into account comorbid physical disease and consider drug–drug interactions (see Ch. 64).

COMPLIANCE

Compliance is a good place to start talking about treatments in neuropsychiatry. Compliance can be crudely divided into good and bad, but is better represented on a continuum. It is often assumed that poor compliance is a fault of the patient alone. Many patients discontinue medication because of side effects or a breakdown in the doctor–patient rela-

---

Box 44.1   Ten aims of treatment in neuropsychiatry

- Engage the patient in a therapeutic relationship
- Explain the diagnosis, prognosis and treatment to the patient and family in a considered manner
- Treat clinical features symptomatically
- Prevent or minimize further deterioration
- Use the minimum level of care necessary for the patient's best interests
- Encourage maximum quality of life for patient and carers
- Offer continuing care to the patient and family as the condition progresses
- Use specialist services and a multidisciplinary approach where indicated
- Maintain the dignity of the patient and family up to and beyond the patient's death

---

Box 44.2   Five golden rules for drug treatment

- Use an effective dose for an effective period
- Use the minimum effective regimen
- Monitor closely for adverse effects
- Withdraw the agent with caution
- Offer other kinds of help

Clinical Pointer 44.1

Dealing with non-compliance in neuropsychiatry

A good rule of thumb is that one-third of patients are fully compliant, one-third show partial compliance and one-third have poor or no compliance.

Examination of RCTs in neurology and psychiatry reveals that a substantial proportion of patients suffer drug-induced side effects. In a prospective study, Hoge et al (1990) found that 35% refused medication on the basis of adverse effects, but surprisingly physicians recognized this as the reason for non-compliance only 7% of the time. In the case of HIV dementia, Alzheimer's disease, Lewy body dementia and Parkinson's disease, the rates of adverse medication effects are even higher.

Therefore the first step in addressing non-compliance is prevention via appropriate prescribing. Factors associated with non-compliance include severity of illness (with loss of insight), a history of medication non-compliance, substance use, a chaotic lifestyle and an unsupportive family or friends.

The second step is forming a therapeutic relationship, because the patient needs to be able to reveal embarrassing problems such as sexual dysfunction, should they occur.

The third step is regular risk–benefit reviews. The patient needs to feel that there is a reason for continuing the medication and minimal reasons for discontinuing medication.

The fourth step in dealing with non-compliance is to discuss the issue fully with the patient and their family. If the patient has sensible reasons for refusing, then offer an alternative or offer a compromise; if the patient is refusing irrationally or because of fear, try to persuade the patient or give the patient time to think about the options. In the rare cases where medication must be given against the patient's wishes then capacity will have to be assessed for the treatment of a physical disorder, and the Mental Health Act (involuntary treatment) may be appropriate in the case of psychiatric treatment.

Further reading   Hoge SK, Appelbaum PS, Lawlor T et al 1990 A prospective, multicenter study of patients' refusal of antipsychotic medication. Archives of General Psychiatry 47:949–956
Olfson M, Mechanic D, Hansell S et al 2000 Predicting medication noncompliance after hospital discharge among patients with schizophrenia. Psychiatric Services 51:216–222

Box 44.3   Reasons for non-compliance

Patient-related reasons
Psychological characteristics (e.g. illness beliefs)
Sociodemographic factors
Substance use

Illness-related reasons
Cognitive impairment
Poor insight
Psychosis

Medication-related reasons
Cost
Frequency
Inconvenience or availability
Side effects

Environment-related reasons
Professional support
Social support
Stigma

Medical-team-related reasons
Attitudes
Doctor–patient relationship
Education

tionship. For example, Chadwick's group found that non-compliance with antiepileptic drugs was associated with how important patients felt it was to take medication, whether patients reported feelings of stigma, whether patients were experiencing any side effects and how easy they found their primary care physician to talk to (Buck et al 1997). This serves as a good reminder that therapy begins with first contact with the patient and the patient's family and that time spent eliciting their fears about the illness and its consequences will invariably reap rewards in the long term.

REFERENCES AND FURTHER READING

Buck D, Jacoby A, Baker GA et al 1997 Factors influencing compliance with antiepileptic drug regimes. Seizure 6:87–93

Clinical Pointer 44.2

Coping with the burden of chronic disease: adjustment to disability

Understanding how people cope with the significant threats imposed by illness is difficult. This is partly because there are a wide range of coping styles and partly because these are difficult and sometimes impossible for a patient to describe in detail. The medical profession has also developed rather simplistic and fixed coping categories, whereas in reality a person may use different strategies at different times in response to particular stressors. In trying to understand these we may consider illness-related factors (severity of disease), cognitive factors (appraisal of the disability, coping strategies) and external factors (social and professional support). These have been extensively reviewed by Lazarus & Folkman (1984).

Expectations of sufferers and carers that are appropriate in acute illness often cause problems in chronic illness. In the acute disease model it is considered culturally appropriate to relinquish responsibilities, volunteer any difficult symptoms and complain of what cannot be done on account of illness. When these styles of coping prevail in chronic illness, individuals may become more handicapped by their psychology than their medical impairments. Sufferers often develop cognitive distortions in an attempt to understand or justify their need. Thus common attitudes to illness that have an understandable origin may easily develop to excess. Examples are: 'I am a burden to my family', 'I am powerless to the effects of the illness', 'I cannot do anything whilst being unwell', 'No one wants to see me, now I am ill', 'My family is only involved because they have to be' and 'The illness is much more serious than the doctors let on'. These attitudes are quite complex and are not easily summarized in one particular coping style, yet they probably predispose to poor outcomes. Psychological influences on physical and emotional health have been particularly well described in the field of cancer care. Certain coping styles may impact negatively on family, friends and health professionals. There is also good evidence that coping styles such as hopelessness and stoic acceptance reduce the quality of life and survival of patients with bowel resection, cancer, haemodialysis, HIV and stroke. Avoidant or passive coping styles are also associated with clinical depression. However, in some circumstances denial has been linked with good outcomes. This contradiction suggests that it is not really the coping style per se that is predictive, but whether it alleviates or exacerbates distress in that person. Recognizing maladaptive attitudes is important in improving adjustment to illness, but this must be assessed on a case-by-case basis. Patients should not be criticized for having the 'wrong attitude', but rather encouraged to take more control of and responsibility for their situation, to look for opportunities to improve their day-to-day quality of life and to think in terms of 'what can I do' rather than 'what can't I do'.

Further reading Lazarus RS, Folkman S 1984 Stress, appraisal, and coping. Springer, New York
Lee M, Rotheram-Borus MJ 2001 Challenges associated with increased survival among parents living with HIV. American Journal of Public Health 91:1303–1309
Lewis SC, Dennis MS, O'Rourke SJ et al 2001 Negative attitudes among short-term stroke survivors predict worse long-term survival. Stroke 32:1640-1645

45

Treatment in Patients Abusing Alcohol or Illicit Drugs

INTOXICATION AND WITHDRAWAL

Intoxication with alcohol poses considerable problems for staff in A&E departments. One frequent dilemma is whether it is safe to assume that the intoxicated patient is behaviourally disturbed because of alcohol alone. Not only are intoxicated people more likely to sustain a head injury, but even moderate intoxication at the time of a head injury is predictive of poor head injury outcome (Gurney et al 1992). Patients who are not a danger to themselves or others can be reassessed after 'sleeping it off'. Severe intoxication can cause respiratory depression and aspiration and, in the most severe cases, may justify treatment with dialysis. Poisoning with other alcohol-related substances (e.g. ethylene glycol, methanol, isopropanol) can also be treated with dialysis (Abramson & Singh 2000). In an ideal world, an alcohol antagonist would be available to reverse the effects and bring an unpredictable situation rapidly under control. The benzodiazepine antagonist flumazenil has been investigated in this regard and may have some efficacy at high doses (Lheureux & Askensai 1991).

Withdrawal from occult alcohol dependence is a major problem in hospitalized patients. Typically, patients admitted for other reasons undergo withdrawal beginning 24 hours or so after admission to hospital. Medical treatment includes rehydration, electrolyte replacement and vitamin supplementation. Parenteral thiamine must be given because oral thiamine is poorly absorbed in those who are already malnourished (Thomson & Cook 1997). Treatment is by slow intravenous infusion because of the small but recognized risk of an anaphylactic reaction. Treatment should be continued for 3–5 days in those with signs of thiamine deficiency. Withdrawal should be suspected in all middle-aged patients developing delirium or seizures shortly after admission.

The American Society of Addiction Medicine Working Group conducted a meta-analysis of 65 studies concerned with the pharmacological management of alcohol withdrawal (Mayo-Smith 1997). Six placebo-controlled trials of benzodiazepines showed benefits over placebo in reducing delirium and seizures. There was a trend toward fewer seizures when using long-acting benzodiazepines compared with short-acting benzodiazepines. Antipsychotics, including phenothiazines and haloperidol, were less effective than benzodiazepines in reducing delirium and seizures. Beta blockers, clonidine, chlormethiazole and meprobamate have been shown to reduce peripheral signs and symptoms of alcohol withdrawal, but not necessarily seizures or delirium.

ABSTINENCE AND PREVENTION OF RELAPSES

Pharmacological approaches to relapse prevention include blocking the effect of the abused drug, substituting a safer alternative and reducing the central mechanisms involved in addiction itself. Gaul et al (1999) conducted a prospective, multicentre, naturalistic study of an established treatment programme in 850 alcohol-dependent patients. After 5 years, 44% of drinkers were abstinent and 38% remained heavy drinkers; 7.6% had died. Those who were abstinent fared better in terms of medical, psychological and social outcomes than those who continued drinking. The drug treatments used to enhance abstinence have been recently reviewed. Garbutt et al (1999) examined 41 studies, including 11 follow-up or subgroup studies, and found evidence for benefit with acamprosate, disulfiram and naltrexone.

Acamprosate is thought to act mainly on the GABA system, reducing the supersensitivity induced by alcohol. Whitworth et al (1996) conducted a randomized controlled trial (RCT) of acamprosate versus placebo in 455 people hospitalized with chronic or episodic alcohol dependence. This study used five criteria for relapse: self-reported alcohol consumption, physical signs of alcoholism, tremor index, mean corpuscular volume, and γ-glutamyl-transpeptidase. Although 60% of subjects dropped out over the course of the study, in an intention-to-treat analysis showed that at 1 year 20% of patients who received acamprosate were abstinent compared with 7% of patients who received placebo (number needed to treat, 9). The mean cumulative duration of abstinence was higher in the acamprosate group. In a conflicting study, Chick et al (2000b) enrolled 581 alcoholics into a double-blind RCT of acamprosate versus placebo. One-third were episodic drinkers and 84% were male. The 6-month study period was completed by only 35% of patients and there was a 14% excess drop-out rate on active treatment. Compliance was poor – only 57% of patients were judged to be taking at least 90% of their tablets. The mean total of abstinent days achieved was not significantly different, nor were rates of complete abstinence, although patients on the active drug rated less craving and less anxiety than those on the placebo. In comparison with other trials, patients in this study began taking medication a longer time after detoxification and recommenced drinking more often before medication was started. Overall, the data suggest that acamprosate reduces drinking frequency, although its effects on enhancing abstinence or reducing time to first drink are less clear.

Disulfiram inhibits the hepatic metabolism of alcohol, leading to an unpleasant flushing sensation induced by acetaldehyde. The effect is an aversive behavioural intervention. There is some evidence that disulfiram reduces drinking frequency, but there is minimal evidence to support improved continuous abstinence rates.

The effect of naltrexone on drinking behaviour is particularly interesting. It is thought to reduce the positive reinforcing effects of acute alcohol consumption (euphoria and disinhibition) by blocking opioid-dependent dopamine release. Eight double-blind RCTs have demonstrated the safety and efficacy of naltrexone in alcoholism. Most recently, Chick et al (2000a) randomized 175 patients who met criteria for alcohol dependence or abuse to oral naltrexone 50 mg/day or placebo for 12 weeks as an adjunct to psychosocial treatment. Intention-to-treat analysis revealed no differences between groups, but patients who were compliant with naltrexone reported consuming half the amount of alcohol as those on placebo. This and other studies demonstrate that naltrexone reduces the risk of deterioration to heavy drinking and the frequency of drinking compared with placebo, but does not substantially enhance complete abstinence (or time to first drink after detoxification). Evidence also suggests that in patients with a history of failed abstinences (i.e. most patients) the most successful strategy is cognitive therapy, to cope with small relapses, plus naltrexone rather than the more common strategy of aiming for complete abstinence once more (Sinclair 2001).

Following the success of naltrexone, nalmefene is under investigation. Nalmefene is a new opioid antagonist that is structurally similar to naltrexone but with the advantage of no dose-dependent hepatotoxic effects, greater oral bioavailability, longer duration of antagonist action and more competitive binding with the opioid receptor subtypes that are thought to reinforce drinking (Mason et al 1999).

TREATMENT OF THE NEUROPSYCHIATRIC COMPLICATIONS OF ALCOHOL ABUSE

Depression and antidepressants

The treatment of depression in patients with alcohol problems has been the subject of several RCTs. McGrath et al (1996) conducted a randomized, placebo-controlled, 12-week trial of imipramine hydrochloride combined with weekly relapse prevention psychotherapy in 69 actively drinking depressed alcoholics. Improvement in mood more than alcohol consumption was shown.

Mason et al (1996) conducted a 6-month study of desipramine versus placebo in 71 patients with primary alcohol dependence (including 28 with depression) who had been abstinent for a median of 8 days before randomization. Alleviation of depression and duration of abstinence were both significantly better in those taking the active drug.

Cornelius et al (1997) enrolled 51 patients with comorbid major depressive disorder and alcohol dependence and randomized them to fluoxetine ($n = 25$) or placebo ($n = 26$) in a 12-week, double-blind trial. Improvement in depressive symptoms was significantly greater in the fluoxetine group, as was reduction in total alcohol consumption. This replicated an earlier study that demonstrated a positive effect of fluoxetine over placebo on mood but not abstinence (Kranzler et al 1995).

Roy-Byrne et al (2000) studied 64 subjects with major depressive disorder and alcohol dependence using 12 weeks of nefazadone versus placebo plus a weekly psycho-educational group on alcoholism. Although depression improved significantly more in the nefazadone group, reduction in drinking was not different between groups.

Pettinati et al (2001) examined the use of sertraline in alcoholic patients. A total of 100 alcohol-dependent subjects with ($n = 53$) or without ($n = 47$) a lifetime diagnosis of comorbid depression enrolled in a 14-week RCT of sertraline 200 mg/day or placebo. Sertraline seemed to provide an advantage in reducing drinking in alcohol-dependent patients without lifetime depression, this being illustrated best by the measure of drinking frequency during treatment. However, sertraline was no better than placebo in patients with a diagnosis of lifetime comorbid depression.

Anxiety and anxiolytics

The importance of treating anxiety disorder in the context of alcoholism is not reflected in the number of trials on this subject. Malcolm et al (1992) randomized 67 alcoholics to 45–60 mg/day of buspirone or placebo. Anxiety scores, as measured by the Hamilton Anxiety Scale, declined significantly in both groups, but there was no advantage of buspirone over placebo in terms of anxiety or abstinence. Kranzler et al (1994) at the University of Connecticut repeated this study using a 12-week, placebo-controlled design in 61 anxious alcoholics, all of whom also received weekly relapse prevention psychotherapy. Outcomes were measured at the end of treatment and at a 6-month follow-up evaluation. In this study, buspirone therapy was associated with reduced anxiety and fewer drinking days during the follow-up period.

Clinical Pointer 45.1

Non-pharmacological strategies in the prevention of alcoholic relapse

Patients who are dependent on alcohol often have reasons for continuing to drink as well as reasons for wanting to give up. Overcoming the withdrawal symptoms is only a small step in the process. Preparatory steps before detoxification include exploring the patient's motivation ('stages of change'), level of support, understanding of likely difficulties and problem-solving ability. Having achieved abstinence, patients must learn to recognize and manage high-risk situations, use self-help and support resources, and attend for supervision. The availability of alcohol and social instability are likely to be important risk factors in relapse, and thus patients should be motivated to change their home circumstances, as well as being motivated to give up alcohol. In addition, services should be available to influence and support friends and family of the patient, since these people will have a key role in successful relapse prevention.

Unfortunately, even with a good package the chances of maintaining abstinent for more than 1 year are probably no more than 50:50. Several non-pharmacological treatment strategies have been compared. In Project MATCH (Matching Alcoholism Treatments to Client Heterogeneity), 1726 alcohol-dependent participants at 10 sites were randomized to three treatments: cognitive–behavioural treatment, motivational enhancement therapy and 12-step facilitation. Outpatients were interviewed 1 and 3 years after treatment. There were negligible differences between the three treatments, but there were differences based on individual patient variables. Patients high in anger fared better in motivational enhancement therapy than in the other two MATCH treatments. Conversely, 12-step facilitation was more effective than motivational enhancement therapy for patients with networks that were supportive of drinking. Readiness-to-change and self-efficacy emerged as the strongest predictors of long-term drinking outcome. A second large study of motivational enhancement therapy versus social behaviour and network therapy is now under way in The United Kingdom Alcohol Treatment Trial (UKATT).

Further reading   Allen J, Anton RF, Babor TF et al 1998 Matching alcoholism treatments to client heterogeneity: Project MATCH three-year drinking outcomes. Alcoholism – Clinical and Experimental Research 22:1300–1311
Friedmann PD, Saitz R, Samet JH 1998 Management of adults recovering from alcohol or other drug problems – relapse prevention in primary care. JAMA 279:1227–1231

Psychosis and antipsychotics

Treatments for psychosis in alcohol abuse, namely alcoholic hallucinosis, have not yet been subject to RCTs, with one obscure exception (Kabes et al 1985). Case series have supported the use of antipsychotics.

Cognition and antidementia drugs

One small study examined the sympatheticolytic substance dihydroergocristine in comparison with placebo in augmenting withdrawal regimens (Rainer et al 1996). There was a modest effect on improved cognitive function. Two studies have looked at the merit of selective serotonin reuptake inhibitors (SSRIs) in alcohol-related Korsakoff's syndrome. Martin et al (1995) studied the effects of fluvoxamine in a small randomized, placebo-controlled, double-blind crossover study. Cognitive function and concentration of the CSF monoamines were measured. Fluvoxamine decreased 5-hydroxy-indoleacetic acid levels, and this correlated with an improvement on the Wechsler Memory Scale Memory Quotient, independent of effects on attention or depression. The second SSRI study, which examined fluoxetine for the treatment of Korsakoff's syndrome, had inadequate methodology (O'Carroll et al 1994).

Khan et al (1993) at the University of Washington, Seattle, studied the cognitive effects of a low dose of thyrotropin releasing hormone (2.0 mg intravenously) in 18 chronic alcoholic patients who exhibited memory deficits. Patients with a shorter duration of alcohol use (mean 16 years) performed significantly better with thyrotropin releasing hormone than with placebo on a test involving verbal learning and memory. Those with a more chronic history of alcohol abuse (mean 27 years) did not show a response.

TREATMENT OF THE NEUROPSYCHIATRIC COMPLICATIONS OF ILLICIT DRUG ABUSE

There is a very limited literature addressing the treatment of illicit drug-induced psychiatric syndromes. Hernandez-Avila et al (1998) from Mexico City published the only RCT to date, in which 40 men admitted to an acute psychiatric unit for inhalant dependence were randomized to 5 weeks

of carbamazepine or haloperidol in identical-appearing capsules. There was comparable response in both groups, with approximately half the patients considered treatment responders. Adverse effects were more common and more severe in the haloperidol group.

SUMMARY

The management of substance abuse can be summarized as follows:

- control disruptive behaviour in intoxicated patients if safety is an issue
- examine for concomitant physical injury and complications
- delay psychiatric examination until the patient is not intoxicated
- where dependency is present, use an appropriate detoxification regimen
- administer nutrition and fluid support as required
- screen for anxiety and depression
- consider SSRIs as first-line therapy
- document residual cognitive deficits
- offer a package of care to help prevent relapse
- remember that controlled use may be an important achievement for some people.

REFERENCES AND FURTHER READING

Abramson S, Singh AK 2000 Treatment of the alcohol intoxications: ethylene glycol, methanol and isopropanol. Current Opinion in Nephrology and Hypertension 9:695–701

Chick J, Anton R, Checinski K et al 2000a A multicentre, randomized, double-blind, placebo-controlled trial of naltrexone in the treatment of alcohol dependence or abuse. Alcohol and Alcoholism 35:587–593

Chick J, Howlett H, Morgan MY et al 2000b United Kingdom multicentre acamprosate study (UKMAS): a 6-month prospective study of acamprosate versus placebo in preventing relapse after withdrawal from alcohol. Alcohol and Alcoholism 35:176–187

Cornelius JR, Salloum IM, Ehler JG et al 1997 Fluoxetine in depressed alcoholics – a double-blind, placebo-controlled trial. Archives of General Psychiatry 54:700–705

Garbutt JC, West SL, Carey TS et al 1999 Pharmacological treatment of alcohol dependence – a review of the evidence. JAMA 281:1318–1325

Gaul A, Lligona A, Colom J 1999 Five-year outcome in alcohol dependence: a naturalistic study of 850 patients in

Catalonia. Alcohol and Alcoholism 34:183–192

Gurney JG, Rivara FP, Mueller BA et al 1992 The effects of alcohol intoxication on the initial treatment and hospital course of patients with acute brain injury. Journal of Trauma – Injury, Infection and Critical Care 3:709–713

Hernandez-Avila CA, Ortega-Soto HA, Jasso A et al 1998 Treatment of inhalant-induced psychotic disorder with carbamazepine versus haloperidol. Psychiatric Services 49:812–815

Kabes J, Skondia V, Marholdova K et al 1985 Piracetam effectivity in alcoholic psychosis – double-blind crossover placebo controlled comparison. Activitas Nervosa Superior 27:66–67

Khan A, Mirolo MH, Claypoole K et al 1993 Low-dose thyrotropin-releasing hormone effects in cognitively impaired alcoholics. Alcohol – Clinical and Experimental Research 17:791–796

Kranzler HR, Burleson JA, Delboca FK et al 1994 Buspirone treatment of anxious alcoholics – a placebo-controlled trial. Archives of General Psychiatry 51:720–731

Kranzler HR, Burleson JA, Korner P et al 1995 Placebo-controlled trial of fluoxetine as an adjunct to relapse prevention in alcoholics. American Journal of Psychiatry 152:391–397

Lheureux P, Askenasi R 1991 Efficacy of flumazenil in acute alcohol intoxication – double-blind placebo-controlled evaluation. Human and Experimental Toxicology 10:235–239

McGrath PJ, Nunes EV, Stewart JW et al 1996 Imipramine treatment of alcoholics with primary depression – a placebo-controlled clinical trial. Archives of General Psychiatry 53:232–240

Malcolm R, Anton RF, Randall CL et al 1992 A placebo-controlled trial of buspirone in anxious inpatient alcoholics. Alcohol – Clinical and Experimental Research 16:1007–1013

Martin PR, Adinoff B, Lane E et al 1995 Fluvoxamine treatment of alcoholic amnestic disorder. European Neuropsychopharmacology 5:27–33

Mason BJ, Kocsis JH, Ritvo EC et al 1996 A double-blind, placebo-controlled trial of desipramine for primary alcohol dependence stratified on the presence or absence of major depression. JAMA 275:761–767

Mason BJ, Salvato FR, Williams LD et al 1999 A double-blind, placebo-controlled study of oral nalmefene for alcohol dependence. Archives of General Psychiatry 56:719–724

Mayo-Smith MF, for the American Society of Addiction Medicine Working Group on Pharmacological Management of Alcohol Withdrawal 1997 Pharmacological management of alcohol withdrawal. A meta-analysis and evidence-based practice guideline. JAMA 278:144–151

O'Carroll RE, Moffoot APR, Ebmeier KP et al 1994 Effects of fluvoxamine treatment on cognitive functioning in the alcoholic Korsakoff syndrome. Psychopharmacology 116:85–88

Pettinati HM, Volpicelli JR, Luck G et al 2001 Double-blind clinical trial of sertraline treatment for alcohol dependence. Journal of Clinical Psychopharmacology 21:143–153

Rainer M, Mucke HAM, Chwatal K et al 1996 Alcohol-induced organic cerebral psychosyndromes – partial reversal of cognitive impairments assisted by dihydroergocristine. Psychopharmacology 127:365–369

Roy-Byrne PP, Pages KP, Russo JE et al 2000 Nefazodone treatment of major depression in alcohol-dependent patients – a double-blind, placebo-controlled trial. Journal of Clinical Psychopharmacology 20:129–136

Sinclair JD 2001 Evidence about the use of naltrexone for different ways of using it in the treatment of alcoholism. Alcohol and Alcoholism 36:2–10

Thomson AD, Cook CHC 1997 Parenteral thiamine and Wernicke's encephalopathy: the balance of risks and perception of concern. Alcohol and Alcoholism 32:207–209

Whitworth AB, Fischer F, Lesch OM et al 1996 Comparison of acamprosate and placebo in long-term treatment of alcohol dependence. Lancet 347:1438–1442

46

Treatment in Patients with Delirium

Box 46.1 Risk factors and maintaining factors in delirium

- Alcohol
- Any form of stress
- Biochemical derangement
- Comorbid physical illness
- Dementia
- Environmental adversity and change
- Old age
- Past history of delirium
- Polypharmacy
- Preoperative use of sedatives
- Recent surgery
- Sensory impairment
- Sleep deprivation
- Vitamin deficiency (especially thiamine)

In delirium, more than in any other condition, appropriate management begins with a thorough physical examination and battery of investigations. The reason that the mortality rate in delirium is at least double the non-delirium in-hospital mortality rate is not that delirium per se kills, but that the underlying condition, if not identified, will! Six months after discharge, patients with delirium have significantly worse independent function than patients who had not experienced delirium in hospital. It is essential to begin treatment with an informant history and thorough review of the notes. Be vigilant for possible risk factors (Box 46.1) and be alert to the occurrence of multiple risk factors.

PREVENTION

As the risk factors for delirium are well known, prevention is achievable. However, because prediction is never completely accurate this approach runs the risk of missing a significant proportion of patients who develop delirium without the identified risk factors. In an interesting study, Inouye et al (1999) studied 852 elderly medical admissions and instituted standardized protocols for the management of six delirium-related risk factors:

- cognitive impairment
- sleep deprivation
- immobility
- visual impairment
- hearing impairment
- dehydration.

Delirium developed in 10% of the intervention group and 15% of the standard care group. Duration of delirium, but not its severity, was significantly improved. This confirms that sensible measures (e.g. improving oxygenation in those with cardiovascular disease, giving heparin for the immobile, rationalizing medication regimens, recognizing early infections) can affect the onset and course of delirium. Surgical procedures are strongly associated with delirium, with both the surgery and the anaesthesia contributing to acute and chronic postoperative cognitive impairment (Moller et al 1998).

Again, simple measures such as preoperative education, patient-controlled analgesia and careful postoperative care can dramatically reduce rates of delirium. An alternative approach is to medicate patients at high risk of delirium with antipsychotic medication. At the time of writing, one adequately powered study had been reported. Kalisvaart et al (2002) randomized 450 elderly patients at medium or high risk of developing postoperative delirium to 6 days of haloperidol 1.5 mg/day begun 3 days preoperatively, or placebo. Haloperidol prophylaxis reduced the rate of postoperative delirium by 40%.

NURSING CARE

Once the delirium has occurred, high-quality nursing care is vital. Patients with delirium are sensitive to their environment and deteriorate quickly. Avoid excess stimulation but use daylight and a night light to help sleep–wake cycle orientation. Use familiar cues from the patient's home, such as clothes, clocks and pictures, to reorientate the patient. Ensure that the patient has his or her own glasses, hearing aid and dentures, as required. Explain the requirements clearly to the family and, if possible, enlist their help in reassuring the patient during daylight hours. Monitor the patient carefully near the nursing station and regularly assess their fluid status and nutrition. In some cases, periods of one-to-one nursing may be needed and for this consistency of staff is helpful. Use physical restraints only when absolutely necessary, and within local guidelines. Try to ambulate patients who are not bed-bound as much as possible.

PHARMACOLOGICAL MANAGEMENT

Withdrawal regimens for illicit drugs or alcohol should be used where indicated. Clinical experience suggests that benzodiazepines or antipsychotics are the drugs of choice for symptomatic management in patients who are disturbed, distressed or psychotic as a result of delirium. Very few comparative studies are available (reviewed by Cole et al 1998). Breitbart et al (1996) conducted a small randomized controlled trial in HIV-infected patients with delirium. Eleven patients were randomly assigned to treatment with haloperidol, 13 to chlorpromazine and six to lorazepam. Treatment with either haloperidol or chlorpromazine was successful in improving delirium, but all patients who received lorazepam developed treatment-limiting adverse effects.

In fact, adverse events are one of the most important considerations in selecting a suitable agent to control delirium. Oversedation, falls, extrapyramidal side effects and worsening cognition are the most common complications. Hence, low starting doses of medication are recommended, particularly in the elderly. It is generally wise to avoid drugs with anticholinergic or anti-adrenergic properties (including chlorpromazine), since these drugs exacerbate the situation. There are several unexpected drugs with anticholinergic properties (Box 46.2). Alternatives to the haloperidol include risperidone, although hypotension can result. Atypical antipsychotics are now becoming available as intramuscular injections, with trials in schizophrenia, mania and

Box 46.2 Drugs with unexpected anticholinergic effects

- Cimetidine
- Digoxin
- Dipyramidole
- Furosemide
- Nifedipine
- Prednisolone
- Ranitidine

dementia under way (Wright et al 2001). They are also likely to be of use in delirium.

SUMMARY

The management of delirium can be summarized as follows:

- control active disruptive behaviour
- investigate intensively for the underlying cause or causes
- provide explanation and reorientation cues
- be prepared to offer intensive but not intrusive nursing
- administer low-dose antipsychotics for persistent, distressing symptoms
- augment with benzodiazepines for persistent behavioural disturbance
- expect a high likelihood of dose-related adverse effects
- consider the effects of concomitant physical illness and medication
- consider prophylactic treatment in those undergoing high-risk surgery
- keep the family informed and involved
- offer advice to prevent future recurrence.

REFERENCES AND FURTHER READING

Breitbart W, Marotta R, Platt MM et al 1996 A double-blind trial of haloperidol, chlorpromazine, and lorazepam in the treatment of delirium in hospitalized AIDS patients. American Journal of Psychiatry 153:231–237

Cole MG, Primeau FJ, Elie LM 1998 Delirium: prevention, treatment, and outcome studies. Journal of Geriatric Psychiatry and Neurology 11:126–137

Inouye SK, Bogardus ST, Charpentier PA et al 1999 A multicomponent intervention to prevent delirium in hospitalised older patients. New England Journal of Medicine

340:669–676

Kalisvaart K, de Jonghe J, Alkmaar A et al 2002 A placebo-controlled post-operative delirium study of haloperidol-prophylaxis in elderly hip-surgery patients. Neurobiology of Aging 23(suppl 1):s85

Litaker D, Locala J, Franco K 2001 Preoperative risk factors for postoperative delirium. General Hospital Psychiatry 23:84–89

Moller JT, Cluitmans P, Rasmussen LS et al 1998 Long term postoperative cognitive dysfunction in the elderly ISPOCD1 study. Lancet 351:857–861

Wright P, Birkett M, David SR et al 2001 Double-blind, placebo-controlled comparison of intramuscular olanzapine and intramuscular haloperidol in the treatment of acute agitation in schizophrenia. American Journal of Psychiatry 158:1149–1151

47

Treatment in Patients with Cerebro-vascular Disease

STROKE

Rehabilitation following stroke

Rather than review acute treatment of stroke, let us consider how the longer term outcome is influenced by neuropsychiatric disorders. Stroke is a serious medical condition in which one-quarter of patients will die within the first month. Although mortality reduces with time, roughly another quarter will die over the ensuing 5 years. At 6 months post-stroke, half of patients have not regained independence (Speech & Dombovy 1995). Although improvements tend to plateau after 1 year, there is some evidence that motor recovery occurs earlier than cognitive recovery (Roth et al 1998). Over this period, admission to a stroke unit and a structured rehabilitation influences long-term outcome (Cifu & Stewart 1999, Gubitz & Sandercock 2001). Stroke unit rehabilitation covers a complex package of care that increasingly includes neuropsychiatric status (Indredavik et al 1999).

Principles of stroke rehabilitation include:

- education
- physical treatment (e.g. oxygen, intravenous saline solution)
- physical rehabilitation (e.g. early mobilization)
- support and encouragement (e.g. motivational techniques)
- prevention of avoidable complications (e.g. by using antibiotics and antipyretics)
- early recognition and treatment of non-avoidable complications
- neuropsychiatric assessment and intervention.

Depression and rehabilitation following stroke

Depression is an important influence on stroke outcome. This area is worth examining in some detail, since depression is likely to affect the rehabilitation outcomes of most neuropsychiatric diseases, if the effect is a true one. Two early uncontrolled studies reported an association between the presence of low mood and slow recovery following stroke (Feibel & Springer 1982, Kotilla et al 1984). Subsequently, Robinson's group (Morris et al 1992, Parikh et al 1990, Shimoda & Robinson 1998) reported the same association when comparing patients with mood disorder with matched stroke patients without mood disorder. In the first small study, 25 patients with both minor and major depression had more impaired function at 2 years than 38 non-depressed stroke patients (Parikh et al 1990). In the second small study, 20 depressed patients had worse function (on the Karnofsky scale but not the Barthel scale) at 1 year compared with 29 non-depressed sufferers. There was a trend in this study towards greater improvement in cognitive performance in the non-depressed patients (Morris et al 1992). In the third study, 27 patients with depression were shown to have impaired social function, activities of daily living and cognitive function compared with 100 controls at either 12 or 24 months post-stroke (Shimoda & Robinson 1998). In addition, patients with generalized anxiety disorder post-stroke ($n = 15$) had worse social function and activities of daily living, but not cognitive function at follow-up. The fact that these small studies showed any relationship could be taken as an indication of the possible strength of that relationship.

Angeleri et al (1993) looked at the long-term outcome of 180 consecutive stroke patients who had been admitted at least 1 year previously (mean duration post-stroke, 37 months). Depression significantly correlated with long-term disability and reduced social activities. Ramasubbu et al (1998) asked 626 patients to complete the Center for Epidemiological Studies Depression Scale (CES-D) at 7–10 days post-stroke. A moderately strong correlation was found between CES-D and Barthel scores. In multifactorial analysis, depression remained an independent predictor of function, along with age, medical illness, weakness, exercise and total neurological symptoms. The magnitude of the effect of depression on function was the same as the influence of total neurological symptoms on function (only age and weakness were more highly correlated). Van de Weg et al (1999) assessed 85 patients admitted for rehabilitation after stroke. Depressed patients had significantly lower functional status at baseline. Improvement was better in the depressed patients treated with antidepressants, but not between depressed and non-depressed patients. The result is difficult to interpret because the study was underpowered. Pohjasvaara et al (2001) found that DSM-IIIR major depression, but not minor depression, at 3 months post-stroke correlated with functional status 12 months later. There was a bi-directional relationship in that early functional impairment also influenced the development of later depression. In two groups of post-stroke patients, one with cognitive impairment and one consecutive series, Gillen et al (1999) found that depressed patients had a slower rate of recovery than the non-depressed patients. In their larger study of 243 patients, a history of depression was associated with a longer length of stay (Gillen et al 2001).

Antidepressant treatment of depressed patients post-stroke should help the rehabilitation outcomes of treated patients (providing that the treatment successfully alleviates mood symptoms). Nevertheless, even when treated, depressed patients are only half as likely to show functional recovery as non-depressed patients (Paolucci et al 2001). Whether antidepressant treatment improves rehabilitation outcome of non-depressed stroke patients is not clear. In a fascinating study, Dam et al (1996) found that fluoxetine improved neurological deficits and Barthel scores more than both maprotiline and placebo (Dam et al 1996). This result has been replicated by some groups (Miyai & Reding 1998), but not others Robinson et al (2000). Interestingly, an improvement in rehabilitation has been reported with levodopa (Scheidtmann et al 2001).

Depression and mortality following stroke

Unselected community studies have demonstrated that depressed patients in nursing homes have elevated mortality rates compared with non-depressed patients (Rovner et al 1991). Strong evidence suggests that patients with ischaemic heart disease are more likely to die after myocardial infarction if they are depressed (Glassman & Shapiro 1998), and isolated studies suggest a similar effect in patients with cancer (Kaplan & Reynolds 1988) and AIDS (Mayne et al 1996). A recent large-scale study of 3529 acutely ill hospitalized patients (not including stroke patients) assessed the relationship between mood (within 1 week of admission), severity of illness, functional status and 6-month mortality (Roach et al 1998). Although low mood correlated weakly with function and severity, low mood also independently predicted survival time. This suggests than the influence of mood on mortality is not an effect of illness severity alone. Morris et al (1993a) examined 91 patients at 2 weeks post-stroke and diagnosed depression in 37 of them. Overall, depressed patients were 1.7 times more likely to die over the subsequent 10 years. This effect was independent of comorbidity and cognitive impairment. In this sample, social isolation was an added risk factor for mortality in conjunction with depression. In a parallel study, the same group looked at the relationship between depression at 2 months post-stroke and mortality at 15 months post-stroke

(Morris et al 1993b). Depression and the personality variable introversion were both significantly associated with mortality, although the effect was not a powerful one.

Treatment of the neuropsychiatric complications of stroke

Patients with cerebrovascular disease are particularly sensitive to the dose-related side effects of psychotropic drugs. There is also a theoretical risk of further haemorrhage when using selective serotonin reuptake inhibitors (SSRIs) in patients who have sustained a haemorrhagic stroke. Both animal and human studies lend some support for the use of antidepressants in stroke patients, regardless of the presence of depression (see above). There have been few controlled trials of antidepressants in stroke and none to date of antipsychotics. The most recent antidepressant trial compared fluoxetine and nortriptyline in 104 stroke patients and found an advantage for fluoxetine (Robinson et al 2000). ECT is not recommended within 3 months of stroke, owing to changes in intracerebral pressure and blood flow. There is also the important issue of co-existing cardiovascular disease in patients with cerebrovascular disease (see Clinical Pointer 47.2). Treatments in stroke patients with cognitive deficits must be informed from the literature on vascular dementia (see below).

Depression, emotionalism and antidepressants

Lipsey et al (1984) randomized 34 patients to receive placebo or nortriptyline 6 months post-stroke. Patients were treated for a mean duration of 42 days. Significantly more patients in the nortriptyline group achieved remission, although no differences in cognitive status or functional status were evident. Reding et al (1986) studied 27 patients with depression at 6 weeks post-stroke. Patients were randomized to trazadone or placebo and received treatment for 4 weeks. Although no statistically significant differences in depression were evident, patients who were either depressed or positive on the dexamethasone suppression test had a greater functional improvement on trazodone than placebo. In the largest study to date, Andersen et al (1994) randomized 66 patients to placebo or citalopram for 42 days. Both intention-to-treat and completor analysis showed significantly greater improvement in the active treatment arm.

In a 6-week randomized controlled trial (RCT), Laruitzen et al (1994) compared imipramine plus mianserin with desipramine plus mianserin in 20 stroke patients. There was a trend towards greater improvement in the imipramine-treated group. Two other RCTs have directly compared two antidepressants post-stroke. Dam et al (1996) enrolled 52 hemiplegic patients an average of 3 months post-stroke. Although many patients were depressed this was not a prerequisite for entry into the study. Patients were then randomly assigned to 3 months treatment with placebo, maprotiline or fluoxetine. All patients received physiotherapy. Baseline depression scores were higher in the active treatment arms than the placebo arm (significantly so for maprotyline only), but patients who received either maprotyline or fluoxetine showed significant improvement in mood. Interestingly, patients who received fluoxetine showed greater improvements in neurological deficits and Barthel scores than did maprotiline-treated patients. Robinson et al (2000) compared nortriptyline ($n = 16$), fluoxetine ($n = 23$) and placebo ($n = 17$) in a 12-week RCT at 6 weeks post-stroke. Nortriptyline produced a more favourable outcome in depression and anxiety symptoms, but the fact that twice as many patients dropped out of the study on fluoxetine must be taken into account. Raffaele et al (1996) at the University of Catania, Italy, conducted a randomized, placebo-controlled trial of trazodone 30 days post-stroke. Improvements were noted in Barthel scores. One group has examined the effectiveness of methylphenidate in a RCT in stroke patients (Grade et al 1998). Ten patients received methylphenidate for 3 weeks and 11 patients received placebo. Patients were not necessarily depressed but were undergoing community rehabilitation an average of 18 days post-stroke. There were no significant differences between the groups at baseline but after 3 weeks the methylphenidate-treated patients had lower scores on mood and higher functional independence. In addition, greater motor recovery was apparent in this group when those with motor abnormalities at baseline were considered. No differences in cognitive performance were noted.

In one open-label study of note, Gonzalez-Torrecillas et al (1995) compared fluoxetine and nortriptyline in 37 patients. Eleven patients were also given placebo. Patients with major or minor depression were treated for 6 weeks. Both antidepressant arms were equally effective and more effective than placebo. Patients who received antidepressants

---

Clinical Pointer 47.1

Non-pharmacological treatment of distress following stroke

Although the majority of RCTs concerning treatment of psychosocial difficulties post-stroke are pharmacological, a small literature exists on non-drug treatment (Knapp et al 2000). Several types of intervention have been examined. The least time consuming is the provision of information. However, simply handing out leaflets, no matter how informative they are, is least likely to have beneficial effects – although the patient may like the extra personal contact involved. A more intensive educational programme has been shown in one study to improve knowledge and distress for a sustained period (Evans et al 1988). Provision of support is one of the most common interventions although, probably as anticipated, gains in function or mood are usually modest. A related approach is to concentrate on helping the patient develop his or her own social support network, although patients with significant disability find this difficult. Patient support groups are liked by some patients but not others. They can help by reducing isolation and allowing sharing of common problems and resources; they can also act as a source of informal support and encouraging function out of the house. More specialized cognitive–behavioural therapy (CBT) has been tried. In one study involving ten sessions of CBT over 3 months, CBT wsas ineffective (Lincoln & Flannigan 2003).

Further reading *Evans RL, Matlock AL, Bishop DS et al 1988 Family intervention after stroke: does counseling or education help? Stroke 19:1243–1249*
Knapp P, Young J, House A et al 2000 Non-drug strategies to resolve psychosocial difficulties after stroke. Age and Ageing 29:23–30
Lincoln NB, Flannigan T 2003 Cognitive–behavioural therapy for depression following stroke: a randomized controlled trial. Stroke 34:111–115

---

showed a significantly greater improvement in functional status, neurological impairment and cognitive impairment. A positive effect on cognition after treating depression has also been found by other groups (Kimura et al 2000). Of great future interest is the use of well-tolerated antidepressants in the prophylaxis of post-stroke depression. In a key publication, Rasmussen et al (2003) found a significant benefit for sertraline over placebo in preventing depression in the 12 months after stroke (number needed to treat = 7), with additional benefits on cardiovascular complications.

Several RCTs have attempted to treat patients with post-stroke emotionalism with antidepressants. Andersen et al (1993) compared citalopram with placebo in a crossover study involving 16 consecutive patients. Although the treatment protocol was brief (3 weeks) and the study underpowered, in 13 patients in whom frequency of crying could be assessed, the number of daily crying episodes decreased by at least 50% in all patients treated with citalopram and two treated with placebo. In a larger study, Robinson et al (1993) randomly assigned 82 stroke patients to nortriptyline or placebo for 6 weeks. There was significantly greater improvement in patients given nortriptyline than placebo, including those rated on the Pathological Laughter and Crying Scale (which was developed by the group at the same time). Improvement in emotional lability was independent of depression status.

Also, treatment was not affected by lesion location or time since stroke, although numbers in the study may have been too small to demonstrate an underlying effect.

In a small RCT involving 20 stroke patients with emotionalism, fluoxetine appeared to be an effective treatment of emotionalism (Brown et al 1998). More recently, Burns et al (1999) in Manchester asked 28 patients with post-stroke emotionalism to participate in an 8-week, randomized double-blind, placebo-controlled trial of low-dose sertraline. In contrast to previous studies, patients were excluded if they were depressed. The authors reported a statistically significant improvement in emotionalism, especially tearfulness.

In conclusion, post-stroke depression responds to conventional antidepressant treatment, with the proviso that patients are sensitive to dose-related side effects. No direct comparisons of treatment response in post-stroke depression compared with primary depression are available, but depression associated with occult cerebrovascular disease is often more refractory to treatment. Studies examining early interventions for and prevention of post-stroke depression are under way (Palomäki et al 1999). Studies in patients with post-stroke emotionalism demonstrate that conventional antidepressants are effective, often with a response that can be seen in days rather than weeks. The improvement is accompanied by an improvement in depression, but the therapeutic effect appears to be at least partially independent of this. Further work is required to discover whether conventional antidepressants are equally successful in treating emotionalism in other neurological diseases.

Summary

The management of the neuropsychiatric complications of stroke can be summarized as follows:

- screen for mood changes, apathy and irritability at 1 month and 6 months post-stroke
- screen for cognitive deficits and delirium at 1 week and 3 months post-stroke (use secondary prevention and treatment evidence from vascular dementia)
- consider SSRIs as first-line treatment for depression, anxiety and emotionalism, and begin treatment as early as possible and continue for at least 1 year
- offer a package of care for apathy (see Clinical Pointer 52.1)
- be prepared to involve the patient's family in therapy that is designed to help adjustment to living with disability
- offer continuing multidisciplinary care and support
- consider the effects of concomitant cardiovascular disease.

VASCULAR DEMENTIA

Patients with vascular dementia are a challenging group for medical management. On average they have three comorbid medical disorders (the disorder most likely to be co-existing is cardiovascular disease) and are prescribed six or more types of drugs (Gambassi et al 1999). They are at high risk of further stroke and cardiovascular-related morbidity and mortality.

Prevention of vascular dementia

Perhaps the most exciting prospect is that of significant primary prevention. 'Primary prevention' refers to the reduction of population exposure to causal agents and risk factors. Given that most known vascular risk factors are risk factors for both vascular depression and vascular dementia, identifi-

cation and control of these factors is likely to be of benefit. People with a history of stroke or transient ischaemic attack are at high risk of all vascular events, but they are at particular risk of subsequent stroke, with a rate of about 5% a year. People with atrial fibrillation (treated with aspirin) also have an elevated risk of about 3% a year.

Hypertension is the largest influence on stroke, with a 10 mmHg decrease in systolic pressure and a 5 mmHg decrease in diastolic pressure conferring a risk reduction in stroke incidence of 15–30% in the population (Sudlow et al 2001). Hypertension and hypotension have been associated with later cognitive impairment in cross-sectional and prospective studies (Stewart 1999). Some data on the efficacy of blood pressure reduction on cognitive function in vascular dementia is available (Meyer et al 1986). The Syst-Eur trial demonstrated that treatment of isolated systolic hypertension reduced the incidence of dementia by 50% (Forette et al 1998).

Lipid-lowering strategies prevent deaths from myocardial infarction but are not so helpful in stroke prevention. One study of more than 2000 patients noted a small benefit (Scandinavian Simastatin Survival Study Group 1994), but another with over 3000 patients did not (Shepherd et al 1995). A recent meta-analysis of 16 large statin trials demonstrated an overall reduction in risk of stroke by 29%, with most benefit in reduction of non-fatal stroke (Herbert et al 1997). The effect of statins on stroke is clearest in the presence of coronary heart disease.

Anticoagulation does not appear to be effective following a transient ischaemic attack or for the secondary prevention of stroke and, furthermore, it can cause cerebral haemorrhage. Even so, in those with atrial fibrillation in whom the risk of stroke is high, benefits may outweigh the risks (Sudlow et al 2001).

The intensive treatment of type 2 diabetes can reduce complications but has not been shown to influence stroke per se (UK Prospective Diabetes Study Group 1998). Once the disease is established, it is still likely that control of such risk factors will influence disease recurrence. The problem here is that measures such as reducing blood pressure may be deleterious in the acute phase of stroke disorders, and therefore need to be applied with caution (Skoog 1994).

The American Heart Association guidelines on the use of carotid endarterectomy distinguish between

Clinical Pointer 47.2

Psychotropic prescribing in patients with cardiovascular disease

Given the importance of cerebrovascular disease in neuropsychiatry, it is relevant to consider the effect of systemic vascular disease on psychotropic drugs. Ninety per cent of patients with vascular dementia also have cardiovascular disease.

Tricyclic antidepressants, via sodium channel blockade (which is also caused by phenothiazine antipsychotics), produce quinidine-like antiarrhythmic actions in healthy tissue but proarrhythmic action within a hypoxic environment. Antiadrenergic effects of psychotropics include postural (orthostatic) hypotension and reflex tachycardia. The rate of hypotension in otherwise healthy depressed patients is about 8%, but in those with heart failure this rises to an alarming 50% (Glassman et al 1983). Critical left ventricular function does not seem to be significantly compromised by tricyclic antidepressants, on the basis of radionuclide angiographic studies (Roose et al 1987). SSRIs have few of the cardiovascular problems associated with the tricyclics. In studies from Glassman and colleagues, fluoxetine, paroxetine and sertraline all demonstrated no effect on blood pressure, conduction disturbance, ionotropic function or arrhythmogenesis in healthy patients and in those with cardiac disease (Glassman 1997).

Monoamine oxidase inhibitors can cause changes in blood pressure, particularly when given with other drugs that affect catecholamines. Venlafaxine produces a dose-dependent increase in blood pressure, particularly at doses above 300 mg/day. Psychostimulants are generally well tolerated.

There is increasing recognition of cardiac conduction abnormalities with older antipsychotics, including haloperidol, chlorpromazine, pimozide and thioridazine. However, following the suspension of sertindole for QT prolongation, the safety of atypical antipsychotics is still under scrutiny.

Lithium appears to be relatively safe cardiovascularly, although it is usually not prescribed in cardiovascular disease owing to its propensity to cause T-wave abnormalities and sinus node dysfunction. Carbamazepine can produce atrioventricular conduction disturbances, although this is rare.

Disulfiram can be dangerous when taken with alcohol in relapsing alcoholics, since it has been associated with cardiac arrest in the antabuse reaction. Benzodiazepines and buspirone are usually well tolerated.

Further reading   *Glassman AH 1997 Death, depression and heart disease in late-life. Biological Psychiatry 42(suppl 1):3S*
Glassman AH, Bigger JT 2001 Antipsychotic drugs: prolonged QTc interval, torsade de pointes, and sudden death. American Journal of Psychiatry 158:1774–1782
Glassman AH, Johnson LL, Giardina EGV et al 1983 The use of imipramine in depressed patients with congestive heart failure. JAMA 250:1997–2001
Roose SP, Glassman AH, Giardina EGV et al 1987 Cardiovascular effects of imipramine and bupropion in depressed patients with congestive heart failure. Journal of Clinical Psychopharmacology 7:247–251

neurologically asymptomatic and symptomatic patients. Based on several large-scale studies, endarterectomy out-performs medical treatment in most circumstances when stenosis is moderate (50–69%) or severe (≥70%). Of particular interest here is the literature concerning the effect of endarterectomy on cognition. Given that carotid stenosis is associated with cognitive deficits, intervention might be expected to improve performance (Bakker et al 2000). One systematic review identified 28 studies, but found only a trend favouring improvement in long-term cognitive outcomes (Lunn et al 1999). This may be because the surgical procedure itself can prejudice cognitive function in one-quarter of patients in the first 30 days postoperatively (Heyer et al 2002).

Early intervention in vascular dementia

Modification of the vascular pathogenesis is another therapeutic avenue of attack. Supportive therapy is the simplest but perhaps most effective early intervention in stroke. Once the infarct has occurred, the cellular effects may be minimized by neuroprotective strategies. Environmental variables have been shown to be important in animal models of stroke. For example, hypothermia is neuroprotective and hyperthermia in human stroke is probably detrimental. Furthermore, normoglycaemia is important, since both hyperglycaemia and hypoglycaemia are associated with a worse stroke outcome. If one accepts that it is the vascular lesion that influences cognition directly, then these methods may help. It should be emphasized that no direct work on vascular depression has been done at all.

Of particular interest are the *N*-methyl-D-aspartate (NMDA), excitatory amino acid and calcium channel antagonists. Nimodipine is a calcium channel antagonist that aims to minimize the final common pathway of calcium-induced cellular damage. In several trials, nimodipine was shown to possess anti-ischaemic properties. In addition, it may improve stroke or vascular dementia outcome, particularly in mild to moderate cases (Tobares et al 1989). It is associated with side effects, which include psychotic symptoms. Drugs that modulate the neurotransmitter or neuroendocrine consequences of vascular events may, in theory, help the long-term course of vascular dementia and vascular depression. Nootropics appear to improve cerebral metabolism via a novel mechanism (possible neurotransmitter actions) (Gouliaev & Senning 1994). The neuroendocrine stress response itself, although acutely physiological, can have deleterious consequences if persistent. From animal models of stroke, late stress hormone reduction holds further promise (Smith-Swintosky et al 1996), as does the prospect of stem cell implantation (Riess et al 2002).

Late intervention in vascular dementia

Realistically, the majority of intervention will be offered once the vascular damage has been done. To what extent can this type of treatment modify the extent of future complications? One small study examined the use of aspirin in vascular dementia. Daily use aspirin 325 mg stabilized or improved the cerebral perfusion and cognition in 66 patients with multi-infarct dementia over a 2-year follow-up period (Meyer et al 1989). Other antiplatelet drugs, such as ticlopidine, clopidogrel and dipyridamole, have been shown to be effective in the secondary prevention of stroke, but have not been examined in vascular dementia.

A placebo-controlled trial of pentoxifylline (oxpentifylline), which aims to improve microcirculation, in vascular dementia showed significantly less cognitive deterioration over a 36-week period (Black et al 1992).

Naftidrofuryl is a 5-hydroxytryptamine-2 receptor antagonist that inhibits smooth muscle contraction and platelet inhibition. It has an established place in the treatment of peripheral vascular disease. Two studies have recently reported beneficial effects in patients with vascular dementia or mixed dementia. The largest of these studies recruited 339 patients aged 50–85 years from 40 centres across Europe. The patients fulfilled National Institute of Neurological Disorders and Stroke–Association Internationale pour la Recherche et l'Enseignement en NeuroSciences (NINDS–AIREN) criteria for vascular dementia. After 6 months treatment with 400 or 600 mg of naftidrofuryl, 16% deteriorated, compared with 33% who were treated with placebo. Benefits were more noticeable with the lower dose and in patients with mild dementia at baseline (Möller et al 2001). The second, smaller study, found similar benefits in a 1-year RCT (Emeriau et al 2000).

The ergot alkaloid derivatives hydergine and nicergoline have been studied in view of their possible vasodilatory effects. Nicergoline has a track record in cerebrovascular disorders. A recent Cochrane Review found that in trials involving 921 patients, the Peto odds ratio for improvement in the subjects treated with nicergoline was 3.33 based on clinicians' clinical impression (Fioravanti & Flicker 2002). However, only three of the reviewed studies considered vascular dementia exclusively. Hydergine is licensed for use in dementia by the Food and Drug Administration in the USA. From a review of 47 trials, it appears to have modestly beneficial actions in dementia and may be even more effective in vascular dementia subtypes (Schneider & Olin 1994).

One important line of investigation concerns calcium channel blockers, such as nimodipine and nicardipine. In a multicentre study from Spain, nicardipine 20 mg three times daily delayed cognitive decline in a randomized placebo-controlled trial of 156 patients with vascular dementia (Frank et al 1999). In a 26-week double-blind, placebo-controlled study of nimodipine, 259 patients were recruited (128 for nimodipine, 131 for placebo), and 251 were available for the intention-to-treat analysis. There was no demonstrable advantage of nimodipine on cognitive, social or global assessments, although a positive trend favouring nimodipine was shown in a subgroup of 92 patients with subcortical (small vessel) vascular dementia (Pantoni et al 2000). An international multicentre RCT with nimodipine given orally for 12 months that included only patients with subcortical vascular dementia is due to report soon.

The drug cyclandelate (which is related to papaverine) has vasodilatory actions similar to those of the calcium antagonists, perhaps via inhibition of phosphodiesterase. In a 24-week, double-blind, multicentre, randomized parallel-group study the efficacy and safety of cyclandelate 800 mg twice daily was evaluated in 147 patients with probable Alzheimer's disease or vascular dementia. The effect size was small and significant only in those with higher ADAS-cog scores (Weyer et al 2000).

A new line of investigation is the value of acetylcholinesterase inhibitors in vascular dementia. The first acetylcholinesterase inhibitor to be investigated in a double-blind RCT was galantamine. Erkinjuntti et al (2002) randomized 396 patients with vascular dementia (or Alzheimer's disease with cerebrovascular disease) to galantamine 24 mg/day and 196 patients to placebo. Fives times as many patients on galantamine withdrew because of adverse effects, although this was accounted for in an intention-to-treat analysis. After 6 months, those receiving the active drug showed significant improvements in cognition over those taking placebo. Secondary neuropsychiatry outcomes on Neuropsychiatric Inventory scores, including anxiety, apathy and delusions, were also improved with the active drug. The cognitive benefits were maintained in a 12-month, open-label extension study involving 124 patients. This result has now been replicated in a larger sample (Kaufer et al 2002). This was closely followed by the results of two similar sized multicentre, 24-week, double-blind RCTs, the first involving 404 patients with probable or possible vascular dementia who were treated with donepezil and 199 who were treated with placebo (Pratt 2002). Cognition and global function showed significant improvements in the active-treatment group compared with the placebo group. Eleven per cent of patients on placebo or 5 mg donepezil discontinued because of adverse events, and 22% on 10 mg donepezil discontinued. Results were identical when this study was combined with the second study, a cumulative total of 1219 patients.

Several drugs with novel mechanisms of action have been studied in vascular dementia. These include the antiadrenergic agent buflomedil, denbufylline a cyclic AMP phosphodiesterase inhibitor, the NMDA receptor antagonist memantine, and the neuroprotective agent propentofylline. In a preliminary study of 73 patients suffering from mild vascular dementia, buflomedil 300 mg was more effective than placebo over 90 days in patients with vascular dementia (Cucinotta et al 1992). The xanthine derivative denbufylline was evaluated in 110 patients with vascular or mixed dementia and in 226 patients with Alzheimer's disease. Patients who received denbufylline showed a trend towards improved cognitive scores, but the effects were not statistically significant. There was no difference in responses between patients with Alzheimer's disease and those with vascular dementia (Treves & Korczyn 1999). Memantine is a non-competitive antagonist of NMDA receptors, which, in contrast to competitive NMDA antagonists, is well tolerated. Following a successful phase III trial in vascular dementia and Alzheimer's disease, two 6-month prospective, double-blind RCTs have been completed in the UK ($n = 581$) and France ($n = 321$), specifically in vascular dementia (Orgogozo et al 2002). In both the UK and the French trials, patients on memantine improved significantly relative to placebo in their ADAS-cog total scores. Stronger treatment effects were seen in patients with low baseline scores on the Mini-Mental State Examination. Memantine tended to stabilize cognitive function, in contrast to a worsening on placebo. Just as importantly, adverse effects were minimal.

Propentofylline is a drug that inhibits microglial proliferation. Rother et al (1998) reviewed the evidence from four double-blind RCTs, involving 901 patients with Alzheimer's disease and 359 patients with mild to moderate vascular dementia. The maximum study duration was 56 weeks. The authors suggested that propentofylline provided consistent improvements over placebo in both Alzheimer's disease and vascular dementia, and that it potentially slowed disease progression after the drug was withdrawn.

Summary

The management of vascular dementia can be summarized as follows:

- Offer primary prevention to those at risk:
  - control atrial fibrillation with or without warfarin or aspirin
  - reduce hyperlipidaemia
  - control hypertension
  - encourage smoking cessation
  - recommend lifestyle changes
  - carotid endarterectomy for moderate to severe carotid stenosis
  - aspirin following myocardial infarction.

- Offer secondary prevention in those with early changes:
  - consider early antiplatelet therapy
  - consider subcutaneous heparin.
- Prevent further deterioration in those with established vascular dementia:
  - continue antiplatelet therapy
  - consider acetylcholinesterase inhibitors
  - consider ergot alkaloids or calcium channel blockers
  - consider memantine
  - consider naftidrofuryl
  - consider pentoxifylline (oxpentifylline).
- Screen regularly for depression, anxiety, apathy, delirium and irritability, and offer conventional treatment if these conditions are found.
- Beware of co-existing cardiovascular disease.
- Maximize quality of life by continuing care, support and structured activities.

VASCULAR DEPRESSION

Although vascular depression is a new and not widely accepted concept, one double-blind RCT has been reported. Taragano et al (2001) examined adjuvant treatment with either the calcium channel blocker nimodipine or an inactive comparator (vitamin C) in 84 patients with vascular depression (Alexopoulos criteria). Nimodipine is licensed by the Food and Drug Administration in the USA for neurological outcome of subarachnoid haemorrhage. Patients were also treated with antidepressants at standard doses. At 60 days, 45% of patients on nimodipine plus antidepressants entered full remission compared with 25% on antidepressants alone, although the percentage who showed any response was similar in both groups. Among early responders, fewer patients on the combination treatment relapsed than did patients on antidepressants alone. This study is of interest, given that calcium channel blockers are associated with a small increased risk of suicide and perhaps depression when used for cardiovascular disease (Sorensen et al 2001).

REFERENCES AND FURTHER READING

Andersen G, Vestergaard K, Riis JO 1993 Citalopram for poststroke pathological crying. Lancet 342:837–839

Andersen G, Vestergaard K, Laruitzen L 1994 Effective treatment of post-stroke depression with selective serotonin reuptake inhibitor citalopram. Stroke 25:1099–1104

Angeleri F, Angeleri VA, Foschi N et al 1993 The influence of depression, social activity, and family stress on functional outcome after stroke. Stroke 24:1478–1483

Bakker FC, Klijn CJM, Jennekens-Schinkel A et al 2000 Cognitive disorders in patients with occlusive disease of the carotid artery: a systematic review of the literature. Journal of Neurology 247:669–676

Black RS, Barclay LL, Nolan KA et al 1992 Pentoxifylline in cerebrovascular dementia. Journal of the American Geriatric Society 40:237–244

Brown KW, Sloan RL, Pentland B 1998 Fluoxetine as a treatment for post-stroke emotionalism. Acta Psychiatrica Scandinavica 98:455–458

Burns A, Russell E, Stratton-Powell H et al 1999 Sertraline in stroke-associated lability of mood. International Journal of Geriatric Psychiatry 14:681–685

Cifu DX, Stewart DG 1999 Factors affecting functional outcome after stroke: a critical review of rehabilitation interventions. Archives of Physical Medicine and Rehabilitation 80(suppl 1):S35–S39

Cucinotta D, Casucci MAA, Pedrazzi F et al 1992 Multicenter clinical placebo-controlled study with buflomedil in the treatment of mild dementia of vascular origin. Journal of International Medical Research 20:136–149

Dam M, Tonin P, De Boni A et al 1996 Effects of fluoxetine and maprotiline on functional recovery in poststroke hemiplegic patients undergoing rehabilitation therapy. Stroke 27:1211–1214

Emeriau JP, Lehert P, Mosnier M 2000 Efficacy of naftidrofuryl in patients with vascular or mixed dementia: results of a multicenter, double-blind trial. Clinical Therapeutics 22:834–844

Erkinjuntti T, Kurz A, Gauthier S et al 2002 Efficacy of galantamine in probable vascular dementia and Alzheimer's disease combined with cerebrovascular disease: a randomised trial. Lancet 359:1283–1290

Feibel JH, Springer CJ 1982 Depression and failure to resume social activities after stroke. Archives of Physical Medicine and Rehabilitation 63:276–278

Fioravanti M, Flicker L 2002 Efficacy of nicergoline in dementia and other age associated forms of cognitive impairment (Cochrane Review). Cochrane Library, issue 1. Oxford: Update Software

Forette F, Seux M-L, Staessen JA et al 1998 Prevention of dementia in randomized double-blind placebo-controlled systolic hypertension in Europe (Syst-Eur) trial. Lancet 352:1347–1351

Frank A, Diez-Tejedor E, Barrerio P et al 1999 An experimental, randomized, double-blind placebo-controlled clinical trial to investigate the effect of nicardipine on cognitive function in patients with vascular dementia. Revista De Neurologia 28:835–845

Gambassi G, Landi F, Lapane KL et al 1999 Is drug use by the elderly with cognitive impairment influenced by type of dementia? Pharmacotherapy 19:430–436

Gillen R, Eberhardt TL, Tennen H et al 1999 Screening for depression in stroke: relationship to rehabilitation efficiency. Journal of Stroke and Cerebrovascular Disease 8:300–306

Gillen R, Tennen H, Eberhardt McKee T et al 2001 Depressive symptoms and history of depression predict rehabilitation efficiency in stroke patients. Archives of Physical Medicine and Rehabilitation 82:1645–1649

Glassman AH, Shapiro PA 1998 Depression and the course of coronary artery disease. American Journal of Psychiatry 155:4–11

Gonzalez-Torrecilaas JL, Hildebrand J, Medlewicz J et al 1995 Effects of early treatment of post-stroke depression on neuropsychological rehabilitation. International Journal of Psychogeriatrics 78:547–560

Gouliaev AH, Senning A 1994 Piracetam and other structurally related nootropics. Brain Research Review 19:180–222

Grade C, Redford B, Chrostowski J et al 1998 Methylphenidate in early poststroke recovery: a double blind placebo-controlled study. Archives of Physical Medicine and Rehabilitation 79:1047–1050

Gubitz G, Sandercock P 2001 Stroke management. In: Barton S (ed) Clinical evidence. Issue 6, BMJ Publishing Group, London, p146–159

Herbert PR, Gaziano JM, Chan KS et al 1997 Cholesterol lowering with statin drugs, risk of stroke and total mortality. An overview of randomized trials. JAMA 278:313–321

Heyer EJ, Sharma R, Rampersad A et al 2002 A controlled prospective study of neuropsychological dysfunction following carotid endarterectomy. Archives of Neurology 59:217–222

Indredavik B, Bakke RPT, Slordahl SA et al 1999 Treatment in a combined acute and rehabilitation stroke unit. Which aspects are most important? Stroke 30:917–923

Kaplan GA, Reynolds P 1988 Depression and cancer mortality and morbidity: prospective evidence from the Alameda County Study. Journal of Behavioural Medicine 11:1–13

Kaufer D, Lilienfeld S, Schwalen S et al 2002 Beneficial effects of galantamine on patient behaviour and caregiver distress in Alzheimer's disease and dementia associated with cerebrovascular disease. Twelfth Meeting of the European Neurological Society, 22–26 June 2002, Berlin. Journal of Neurology 249(suppl 1/130)

Kimura M, Robinson RG, Kosier JT 2000 Treatment of cognitive impairment after poststroke depression: a double-blind treatment trial. Stroke 31:1482–1486

Kotila M, Waltimo O, Niemi ML et al 1984 The profile of recovery from stroke and factors influencing outcome. Stroke 15:1039–1044

Laruitzen L, Bendsen BB, Vilmar T et al 1994 Post-stroke depression: combined treatment with imipramine or desipramine and mianserin: a controlled study. Psychopharmacology 114:119–122

Lipsey JR, Robinson RG, Pearlson GD et al 1984 Nortriptyline treatment of post-stroke depression: a double-blind treatment trial. Lancet i:297–300

Lunn S, Crawley F, Harrison MJG et al 1999 Impact of carotid endarterectomy upon cognitive functioning: a systematic review of the literature. Cerebrovascular Diseases 9:74–81

Mayne TJ, Vittinghoff E, Chesney MA et al 1996 Depressive affect and survival among gay and bisexual men infected with HIV. Archives of Internal Medicine 156:2233–2238

Meyer JS, Judd BW, Tawakina T et al 1986 Improved cognition after control of risk factors for multi-infarct dementia. JAMA 256:2203–2209

Meyer JS, Rogers RL, McClintic K et al 1989 Randomized clinical trial of daily aspirin therapy in multi-infarct dementia: a pilot study. Journal of the American Geriatric Society 37:549–555

Miyai I, Reding MJ 1998 Effects of antidepressants on functional recovery following stroke: a double blind study. Journal of Neurological Rehabilitation 12:5–13

Möller HJ, Hartmann A, Kessler C et al 2001 Naftidrofuryl in the treatment of vascular dementia. European Archives of Psychiatry and Clinical Neurosciences 251:247–254

Morris PL, Raphael B, Robinson RG 1992 Clinical depression is associated with impaired recovery from stroke. Medical Journal of Australia 157:239–242

Morris PLP, Robinson RG, Andrzejewski P et al 1993a Association of depression with 10-year poststroke mortality. American Journal of Psychiatry 150:124–129

Morris PLP, Robinson RG, Samuels J 1993b Depression, introversion and mortality following stroke. Australian and New Zealand Journal of Psychiatry 27:443–449

Orgogozo J, Forette F, Wilcock G et al 2002 Memantine in vascular dementia. Presented at the Second International Congress on Vascular Dementia, Salzburg

Palomäki H, Kaste M, Berg A et al 1999 Prevention of poststroke depression: 1 year randomised placebo controlled double blind trial of mianserin with 6 month follow up therapy. Journal of Neurology, Neurosurgery and Psychiatry 66:490–494

Pantoni L, Bianchi C, Beneke M et al 2000 The Scandinavian Multi-Infarct Dementia Trial: a double-blind, placebo-controlled trial on nimodipine in multi-infarct dementia. Journal of Neurological Sciences 175:116–123

Paolucci S, Antonucci G, Grasso MG et al 2001 Post-stroke depression, antidepressant treatment and rehabilitation results: a case–control study. Cerebrovascular Diseases 12:264–271

Parikh RM, Robinson RG, Lipsey JR et al 1990 The impact of poststroke depression on recovery in activities of daily living over a 2-year follow-up. Archives of Neurology 47:785–789

Pohjasvaara T, Vataja R, Leppävuori A et al 2001 Depression is an independent predictor of poor long-term functional outcome post-stroke. European Journal of Neurology 8:315–319

Pratt R 2002 Results of clinical studies with donepezil in VaD. Presented at the Second International Congress on Vascular Dementia, Salzburg, Austria

Raffaele R, Rampello L, Veccchio I et al 1996 Trazodone therapy of the post-stroke depression. Archives of Gerontology and Geriatrics 23(suppl 5):217–220

Ramasubbu R, Robinson RG, Flint AJ et al 1998 Functional impairment associated with acute post-stroke depression: the stroke data bank study. Journal of Neuropsychiatry and Clinical Neuroscience 10:26–33

Rasmussen A, Lunde M, Poulsen DL et al 2003 A double-blind placebo controlled study of sertraline in the prevention of depression in stroke patients. Psychosomatics 44:216–221

Reding JJ, Orto LA, Winter SW et al 1986 Antidepressant therapy after stroke: a double-blind trial. Archives of Neurology 43:763–765

Riess P, Zhang C, Saatman KE 2002 Transplanted neural stem cells survive, differentiate, and improve neurological motor function after experimental traumatic brain injury. Neurosurgery 51:1043–1052

Roach MJ, Conners AF, Dawson NV et al 1998 Depressed mood and survival in seriously ill hospitalized adults. Archives of Internal Medicine 158:397–404

Robinson RG, Parikh RM, Lipsey JR et al 1993 Pathological laughing and crying following stroke: validation of a measurement scale and a double-blind treatment study. American Journal of Psychiatry 150:286–293

Robinson RG, Schultz SK, Castillo C et al 2000 Nortriptyline versus fluoxetine in the treatment of depression and in short-term recovery after stroke: a placebo-controlled, double-blind study. American Journal of Psychiatry 157:351–359

Roth EJ, Heinemann AW, Lovell LL et al 1998 Impairment and disability: their relation during stroke rehabilitation. Archives of Physical Medicine and Rehabilitation 79:329–335

Rother M, Erkinjuntti T, Roessner M et al 1998 Propentofylline in the treatment of Alzheimer's disease and vascular dementia: a review of phase III trials. Dementia and Geriatric Cognitive Disorders 9(suppl 1): 36–43

Rovner BW, German PS, Brant LJ et al 1991 Depression and mortality in nursing homes. JAMA 265:993–996

Scandinavian Simastatin Survival Study Group 1994 Randomised trial of cholesterol lowering in 4444 patients with coronary heart disease. Lancet 344:1384–1389

Scheidtmann K, Fries W, Muller F 2001 Effect of levodopa in combination with physiotherapy on functional motor recovery after stroke: a prospective, randomised, double-blind study. Lancet 358:787–790

Schneider LS, Olin JT 1994 Overview of clinical trials of hydergine in dementia. Archives of Neurology 51:787–798

Shepherd J, Cobbe S M, Ford I et al for the West of Scotland Coronary Prevention Study Group 1995 Prevention of coronary heart-disease with pravastatin in men with hyper-cholesterolemia. New England Journal of Medicine 333:1301–1307

Shimoda K, Robinson RG 1998 Effect of anxiety disorder on impairment and recovery from stroke. Journal of Neuropsychiatry 10:34–40

Skoog I 1994 Risk factors for vascular dementia: a review. Dementia 5:137–144

Smith-Swintosky VL, Pettigrew LC, Sapolsky RM et al 1996 Metyrapone, an inhibitor of glucocorticoid production, reduces brain injury induced by focal and global ischemia and seizures. Journal of Cerebral Blood Flow and Metabolism 16:585–598

Sorensen HT, Mellemkjaer L, Olsen JH 2001 Risk of suicide in users of beta-adrenoceptor blockers, calcium channel blockers and angiotensin converting enzyme inhibitors. British Journal of Clinical Pharmacology 52:313–318

Speech DP, Dombovy ML 1995 Recovery from stroke: rehabilitation. Baillière's Clinical Neurology 4:317–338

Stewart R 1999 Hypertension and cognitive decline. British Journal of Psychiatry 174:286–287

Sudlow C, Sandercock P, Gubitz G et al 2001 Stroke prevention. In: Barton S (ed) Clinical evidence, Issue 6. BMJ Publishing Group, London, p 160–177

Tarangano FE, Allegri R, Vicario A et al 2001 A double-blind randomized clinical trial assessing the efficacy and safety of augmenting standard antidepressant therapy with nimodipine in the treatment of 'vascular depression'. International Journal of Geriatric Psychiatry 16:254–260

Tobares N, Pedromingo A, Bigorra J 1989 Nimodipine treatment improves cognitive functions in vascular dementia. In: Bergener M, Reisberg B (eds) Diagnosis and treatment of senile dementia. Springer-Verlag, Berlin, p 360–365

Treves TA, Korczyn AD 1999 Denbufylline in dementia: a double-blind controlled study. Dementia and Geriatric Cognitive Disorders 10:505–510

UK Prospective Diabetes Study Group 1998 Tight blood pressure control and risk of macrovascular and microvascular complications in type 2 diabetes: UKPDS 38. BMJ 317:703–713

Van de Weg FB, Kuik DJ, Lankhorst GJ 1999 Post-stroke depression and functional outcome: a cohort study investigating the influence of depression on functional recovery from stroke. Clinical Rehabilitation 13:268–272

Weyer G, Eul A, Milde K et al 2000 Cyclandelate in the treatment of patients with mild to moderate primary degenerative dementia of the Alzheimer type or vascular dementia: experience from a placebo controlled multi-center study. Pharmacopsychiatry 33:89–97

48

Treatment in Patients with Epilepsy

NEUROLOGICAL MANAGEMENT OF EPILEPSY

It is not usual to start anticonvulsants after the first seizure unless there are clear risk factors for recurrence, such as penetrating head injury, ongoing EEG changes or learning disability. On average, 50% of patients will have a second seizure following a first non-febrile seizure, but the risk diminishes markedly with time. The risk of recurrence after a second unprovoked seizure is about 80%. Nevertheless, two-thirds of patients will become free of seizures if correctly treated. Historically, epilepsy has been treated with one of four common drugs: sodium valproate, carbamazepine, phenytoin and phenobarbitone. Many would now replace phenobarbitone with lamotrigine as suggested first-line treatment, since about twice as many patients can tolerate lamotrigine as the older antiepileptic drugs (AEDs).

Partial seizures

Lamotrigine is one of a series of new AEDs licensed primarily for add-on treatment of drug-refractory partial seizures. These new AEDs include gabapentin, lamotrigine, levetiracetam, oxcarbazepine, tiagabine, topiramate and, outside the UK, zonisamide (Fig. 48.1). One meta-analysis examined 20 trials in drug-resistant partial epilepsy (Marson et al 1997). Gabapentin and lamotrigine,

topiramate and vigabatrin were more effective than placebo. Phenytoin and lamotrigine have the advantage of a once-daily administration, whereas carbamazepine and valproate are given twice a day (in slow-release form). Sodium valproate is now available in a combination with valproic acid (as divalproex sodium), but the once-daily extended-release formulation has not been approved in the UK or the USA for either epilepsy or bipolar disorder. Carbamazepine probably remains the drug of choice in partial seizures and is considered to be safer than valproate in pregnancy (see Ch. 63) (Marsden 2001).

Generalized seizures

Although there have been few, if any, placebo-controlled studies in generalized epilepsy and no studies have definitively demonstrated a difference in efficacy between AEDs, sodium valproate is probably the drug of choice in generalized seizures, partly because only about 10% of people discontinue it because of side effects, compared with 20% on carbamazepine (Matterson et al 1985). Carbamazepine is ineffective in the treatment of absence and myoclonic epilepsies and in children with absence seizures (ethosuximide is an alternative). Lamotrigine, levetiracetam and oxycarbazepine may be effective as monotherapy for generalized tonic–clonic seizures (McAuley et al 2002).

Epilepsy and learning disability

The treatment of epilepsy in people with learning disability is challenging. Outcomes are poorer than in patients with epilepsy alone, for several reasons:

- baseline function is already impaired
- there is often a structural basis for epileptogenesis that is not amenable to surgery
- medication compliance and therapeutic monitoring may vary
- the epilepsy is often long-standing
- adverse effects are heightened in those with established brain pathology.

For these reasons, sodium valproate, gabapentin and lamotrigine are favoured over phenytoin and barbiturates. Oxcarbazepine may be preferred over carbamazepine, and the newer AEDs are useful, particularly as add-on therapy (Deb 2000). Several modest-sized randomized controlled trials (RCTs) have been conducted in specific learning disability syndromes. These include vigabatrin in West's syndrome (Elterman et al 2001) and lamotrigine, felbamate and topiramate in Lennox–Gastaut syndrome (Kerr & Bowley 2001). The other factor to consider is the effect of any psychotropic drug on the seizure disorder (see below).

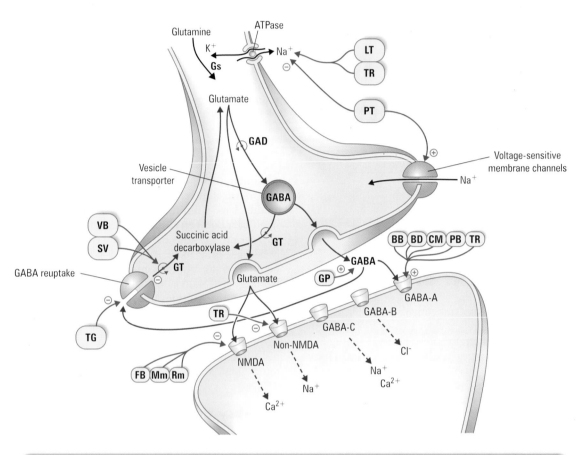

Key	Enzymes			Drugs			
	GABA	γ-Aminobutyric acid		**BB**	Barbiturates	**PB**	Phenobarbital
	GAD	Glutamic acid decarboxylase		**BD**	Benzodiazepines	**PT**	Phenytoin
	Gs	Glutamate synthetase		**CM**	Carbamazepine	**Rm**	Remacemide
	GT	GABA transaminase		**FB**	Felbamate	**SV**	Sodium valproate
				GP	Gabapentin	**TG**	Tiagabine
				LT	Lamotrigine	**TR**	Topiramate
				Mm	Memantine		

Fig. 48.1   The GABA synapse. GABA is the main inhibitory neurotransmitter, with rich concentrations in the basal ganglia and cerebellum. GABA is formed via a metabolic pathway called the GABA shunt. The reuptake of GABA occurs via a highly specific transmembrane transporter. GABA-A receptors are ionotropic receptors that activate a ligand-gated chloride channel. This raises the membrane potential, causing inhibition. GABA-B receptors are metabotropic, coupled to G proteins. Glutamate acts on ionotropic N-methyl-D-aspartate (NMDA) receptors and non-NMDA receptors (kainic acid and α-amino-3-hydroxy-5-methyl-4-isoxazole propionic acid). NMDA receptors may have a pivotal role in long-term potentiation (memory). NMDA receptors are highly permeable to calcium; this is normally regulated by magnesium ions. Magnesium and memantine are selective antagonists at this receptor and are both under investigation in terms of possible neuroprotective benefits.

Adverse effects on the CNS of AEDs

There is a hierarchy of CNS adverse effects which is, from least to most toxic, lamotrigine, topiramate, sodium valproate, carbamazepine, phenytoin, phenobarbitone (see also Table 48.3). Cognitive side effects are discussed in Chapter 18 and summarized in Table 48.1. Certain AEDs have been associated with depression, psychosis and disinhibition (see Table 48.3) (Besag 2001). Plasma monitoring is really useful only for checking compliance and in cases of suspected pharmacological interactions (Jannuzzi et al 2000). Valproate, gabapentin, lamotrigine and vigabatrin do not induce liver enzymes and confer an advantage to women taking the oral contraceptive.

Refractory epilepsy and emergency treatment

Approximately 20% of those with epilepsy are refractory to treatment. Environmental factors can have an influence. Fatigue, stress, flashing lights and hypoglycaemia can precipitate seizures, at least in some patients, as can drugs that lower the seizure threshold, such as xanthine derivatives and ciprofloxacin. These should be avoided wherever possible. Seizure control may be improved by changing to an alternative first-line AED (carbamazepine instead of sodium valproate, or vice versa). The original drug is gradually withdrawn after the new drug has reached a therapeutic dose. A high (but tolerated) dose is the usual target in these circumstances. Consideration of a third AED is the next step, along with re-investigation and review of compliance. If this does not help, then two first-line drugs can be given together. If seizure control remains a problem on a second-line AED, the addition of a newer drug such as vigabatrin, lamotrigine, zonisamide or gabapentin (or the intermittent use of clobazam) can be tried. There is some concern that vigabatrin causes irreversible concentric visual field damage in

Table 48.1 Summary of cognitive effects of anticonvulsant drugs

Drug	Area affected
High risk	
Phenobarbitone*	IQ, memory, attention
Benzodiazepines*	Memory, attention, speed
Medium risk	
Phenytoin	Memory, attention, speed
Carbamazepine*	Attention, speed
Sodium valproate	Speed
Topiramate*	Attention, verbal fluency
Low risk	
Gabapentin	
Lamotrigine	
Vigabatrin	
Oxcarbazepine	

*Effects are dose-dependent

Table 48.2 Summary of seizure type and associated antiepileptic drugs

Seizure pattern	First-line drug	Second-line alternative	Third-line alternative
Absence seizure	Ethosuximide	Sodium valproate	Clonazepam
Atonic	Clonazepam	Sodium valproate	Vigabatrin
Atypical absence seizure	Sodium valproate	Acetazolamide	Clonazepam
Infantile spasms	ACTH	Sodium valproate	Topiramate
Lennox–Gestaut syndrome	Sodium valproate	Topiramate	Lamotrigine
Myoclonic seizures	Sodium valproate or clonazepam	Lamotrigine	Topiramate or lamotrigine
Partial seizure with or without secondarily generalization	Carbamazepine or sodium valproate	Phenytoin	Topiramate or lamotrigine
Primary generalized tonic–clonic seizure	Sodium valproate or carbamazepine	Phenytoin	Topiramate or lamotrigine
Rolandic seizures	Carbamazepine	Gabapentin	Phenytoin

Table 48.3 Summary of AEDs

Drug and mechanism of action	Indications	Side-effects	Preparations	Serum monitoring
Carbamazepine (sodium channel blocker, GABA-A agonist)	√ Partial and generalized seizures × Absence, myoclonus	Sedation, gastrointestinal upset, dizziness, headache, tremor, insomnia, diplopia, hyponatraemia, leukopenia, allergic reactions	Tablets, chewable tablets, slow-release liquid, suppositories	Useful (hepatic excretion) 20–50 μmol/l
Clonazepam (GABA-A agonist)	√ Augmentation of partial seizures × Limited by side effects	Sedation, confusion, cognitive impairment, disinhibition, hypersalivation	Tablets, liquid	Not useful (hepatic excretion)
Clobazam (GABA-A agonist)	√ Second-line treatment × Limited by side effects	Sedation, blurred vision, ataxia, disinhibition, minimal cognitive effects	Tablets, capsules	Not useful (hepatic excretion)
Ethosuximide (calcium channel blocker)	√ Absence seizures × Generalized seizures	Gastrointestinal upset, sedation, ataxia, allergic reactions, extrapyramidal side effects	Capsules, syrup	Useful (hepatic excretion) 300 0150700 μmol/l
Gabapentin (potentiates GABA synthesis, blocks calcium influx)	√ Augmentation of partial seizures × Generalized and absence seizures	Sedation, dizziness, headache, fatigue, tremor, gastrointestinal upset, rhinitis	Capsules	Not useful (renal excretion)
Lamotrigine (sodium channel blocker, glutamate antagonist)	√ Partial and generalized seizures × Myoclonic epilepsy	Rash, headache, dizziness, diplopia, ataxia, nausea, sedation, tremor	Tablets, chewable tablets	Not known (hepatic excretion) 4–60 μmol/l

Drug (mechanism)	Indications	Side effects	Formulation	Drug level monitoring
Oxcarbazepine (analogue of carbamazepine)	√ Partial and generalized seizures	Fatigue, sedation, dizziness	Tablets	Not known (hepatic excretion)
Phenobarbital (GABA-A agonist)	√ Partial and generalized seizures × Limited by side effects	Sedation, cognitive deficits, sexual dysfunction, vitamin deficiency, connective tissue problems	Tablets, elixir, injection	Useful (hepatic excretion) 40–170 μmol/l
Phenytoin (sodium channel blocker)	√ Partial and generalized seizures × Absence and myoclonus	Ataxia, sedation, headache, hypersensitivity, gingival hyperplasia, vitamin deficiency, others	Capsules, chewable tablets, liquid, injection	Useful (hepatic excretion) 40–80 μmol/l
Topiramate (sodium channel blocker, GABA-A agonist)	√ Partial and generalized seizures × Limited by side effects	Headache, paraesthesiae, tremor, sedation, fatigue, weight change, ataxia, cognitive deficits	Tablets	Not useful (renal excretion) 6–74 μmol/l
Sodium valproate (reduces catabolism of GABA)	√ Most epilepsies (broad spectrum) × Mild enzyme inhibitor	Weight gain, fatigue, rash, nausea, tremor, alopecia, bone marrow suppression	Tablets, capsules, syrup, slow release, injection	Not useful (hepatic excretion) 300–600 μmol/l
Vigabatrin (inhibitor of GABA transaminase)	√ Infantile spasms × Monotherapy	Sedation, weight gain, headache, paraesthesiae, depression, confusion, visual disturbance	Tablets, powder	Not useful (renal excretion)
Zonisamide (possible GABA action)	√ Augmentation of partial seizures × Monotherapy	Ataxia, agitation, somnolence, anorexia, psychosis	Tablets	Not known (hepatic excretion)

about one-third of patients, and zonisamide has been associated with agitation and psychosis.

About 10% of patients will have intractable epilepsy despite these steps. Attempts to control the seizures should still continue, usually under the supervision of a specialist unit. Anterior temporal lobectomy is an option, particularly for those whose seizures are caused by mesial temporal sclerosis or tumours of the temporal lobe. However, the 5-year recurrence rate of seizures after anterior temporal lobectomy is 50%.

Refractory seizures should not be confused with status epilepticus, which refers to continuous seizures for 30 minutes or more. The significance is that after 30 minutes there is a physiological stage of decompensation. Hyperglycaemia turns to hypoglycaemia and cerebral blood flow falls, in part owing to hypotension and failing cerebral autoregulation. The consequences may be recurrent epilepsy in those without a prior history and, in 5%, death from tonic–clonic seizures. This is one of the few indications for 'emergency dosing'– that is, rapid dose escalation. Few AEDs can be given intramuscularly. Exceptions are phenobarbital and midazolam. Special preparation of diazepam and phenytoin minimize inflammation when given intravenously. Occasionally, resistant status epilepticus requires intervention from an anaesthetist.

TREATMENT OF THE NEUROPSYCHIATRIC COMPLICATIONS OF EPILEPSY

Mood disorders, antidepressants and mood stabilizers

Before antidepressants are used, attempt to elucidate what factors are contributing to depression in this particular case. Is it the stigma of seizures in the workplace, the disabling effects on lifestyle, disturbances in sleep or cognition, or does it seem to be related directly to ictal seizures? In most cases, improved seizure control will bring about improved mood. Most AEDs (with the possible exceptions of phenobarbitone and vigabatrin) do not cause depression directly but may do so indirectly, via distress from other unrecognized adverse effects. Some authors suggest that AEDs with possible antidepressant properties should be used as first-line treatment of depression in epilepsy. The evidence that either carbamazepine or sodium valproate are anti-depressant (when used alone) is very weak, despite their clear antimanic properties. Recently, investigators in one AED trial had the foresight to measure mood in 133 epileptic patients randomized to lamotrigine or valproate (Edwards et al 2001). Although patients had only mild depressive symptoms at baseline, significantly more beneficial effects on mood were apparent with lamotrigine than valproate. When this study is examined closely, it seems that this effect may have been due to the more favourable side-effect profile of lamotrigine (which nevertheless does not detract from the results).

In terms of specific antidepressant drugs, some literature suggests that monoamine oxidase inhibitors (MAOIs) may be anticonvulsant, although they can cause myoclonic jerks. Serotonin is not crucial to the pathophysiology of seizures, and hence selective serotonin reuptake inhibitors (SSRIs) do not significantly alter seizure threshold. Reboxetine also appears to be well tolerated. Seizures have been reported with amoxapine, maprotiline and most tricyclic antidepressants. Carbamazepine is structurally related to tricyclic antidepressants and this may be used to advantage. ECT can be safely used in epileptic patients. After the induced seizure has occurred, the seizure threshold may be raised (i.e. ECT has anticonvulsant properties). Robertson & Trimble (1985) attempted an ambitious three-arm RCT of amitriptyline, nomifensine (no longer available) and placebo in 39 depressed patients with epilepsy. The study was underpowered and failed to demonstrate clear differences between the groups.

No RCTs of mania or hypomania in patients with epilepsy have been conducted but treatment here is usually straightforward, at least initially. Carbamazepine or sodium valproate are used, and they can

---

Box 48.1 Predictors of poor outcome in epilepsy

Clear EEG spike and wave activity
Established CNS disease
Extremes of age
Family history of epilepsy
Learning disability
Longer duration of remission to date
Low IQ
Multiple seizures before therapy
Partial seizures
Poor compliance
Structural brain disease

be combined in refractory cases. The duration of treatment has not been addressed, and therefore must be guided by the severity and frequency of episodes, along with the implications of relapse.

Psychosis and antipsychotics

Most clinicians express concern when prescribing antipsychotics to patients with a history of seizures. This concern must not prevent the appropriate treatment of psychotic symptoms. Even when seizures appear to worsen with a psychotropic prescription, the anticonvulsant dose can be titrated higher. In patients complaining of low-grade or infrequent delusions or hallucinations, the interference with the patient's life may be such that no drug treatment is necessary. As with depression, improvement in seizure control, where possible, is a sensible first step. In terms of specific antipsychotics, sulpiride and amisulpride may be the safest, since there have been only a handful of reports of seizures with these drugs and they have minimal effects on the EEG. Drugs that cause seizures in more than 1% of healthy controls are usually considered inappropriate in epilepsy (Table 48.4). These include clozapine, loxapine, zotepine (above 300 mg/day) and chlorpromazine (above 1 g/day). Drugs with an intermediate risk of between 0.5% and 1% include olanzapine and quetiapine. Risperidone appears to be in the low-risk category.

A very similar psychopharmacology question arises in patients with established schizophrenia who develop epilepsy. The difference here is that psychosis may be more refractory to treatment. Thus, more combinations of antipsychotics may be required, and there is the problem of effective treatment of any negative syndrome.

EFFECT OF PSYCHOTROPICS ON SEIZURE THRESHOLD

In animal models, serotonin and noradrenaline (norepinephrine), as well as SSRIs and low-dose imipramine, have been shown to be mildly anticonvulsant (imipramine and carbamazepine share the same action on sodium channels). MAOIs also appear to have anticonvulsant properties, which makes them a good choice in patients with unstable epilepsy. Several studies have examined the effect of psychotropic drugs on seizure threshold in epileptic

Table 48.4 Risk of seizures from common psychotropic agents

Drug	Risk (%)
High risk	
High-dose chlorpromazine	9
Clozapine	5
Zotepine	10–20
Medium risk	
Olanzapine	1
Quetiapine	1
Bupropion	0.5
Low risk	
Risperidone	0.3
SSRIs	0.1
Venlafaxine	0.3
Mirtazepine	0.05

patients. In general, the effect of psychotropics is less than is generally thought. However, certain drugs can cause seizures; particularly chlorpromazine (in 10% on the maximum dose), clozapine (in 5% on the maximum dose) and bupropion. Some clinicians advocate prescribing such drugs alongside an anticonvulsant for patients at high risk of seizures.

Peck et al (1983) conducted a meta-analysis of 98 studies with imipramine and found the seizure incidence to be 0.33% with a dose-related effect. For patients prescribed less than 200 mg/day there was almost no appreciable increased risk. Bupropion has a seizure risk of 0.5% in those receiving less than 450 mg/day. Studying the effects of psychotropics on the EEG in healthy patients is one way of assessing the potential for seizures. Clozapine affects the EEG rhythm in the majority of people, with paroxysmal discharges noted in 40%. In pre-marketing studies, the risk of seizures approached 5% with 900 mg/day but was probably nearer 1% with low doses (Devinsky et al 1991). Both tonic–clonic and myoclonic seizures were observed. Buspirone and lithium probably have proconvulsant activity.

A valuable source of information about drug-related seizure risk is the incidence of seizures that follows an overdose with that particular drug. A review of seizures after tricyclic antidepressant overdoses in 2500 patients demonstrated seizures in about 8% of cases (Frommer et al 1987). Such seizures tend to occur 3–6 hours after ingestion. Particularly implicated in this regard are amoxapine and maprotiline, whereas trazadone appears relatively safe. Fewer reports indicate seizures after SSRIs (although case reports do exist), but overall evidence to date shows that, as a class, the SSRIs are much less likely to cause seizures than are the tricyclic antidepressants. Antipsychotics as a class also appear to be safer than tricyclic antidepressants, with a rate of seizures after overdose of 1% (Alldredge 1999). An incidence of up to 9% has been recorded for those taking high doses of phenothiazines (>1000 mg/day chlorpromazine equivalents).

Few studies can claim to comment on the effect of psychotropics on seizure threshold in an adequate sample of patients with epilepsy. One old study recorded the effect on seizures of starting thioridazine in 100 patients with epilepsy. Interestingly, seizure frequency was reported to be improved in 40% of patients and unchanged in 20% (Pauig et al 1961).

SUMMARY

The management of neuropsychiatric complications of epilepsy can be summarized as follows:

- screen for mood changes, anxiety, psychosis and cognitive impairment
- elucidate whether complications are seizure-related
- elucidate whether complications are pre-ictal, ictal, post-ictal or interictal
- review existing antiepileptic medication for efficacy and adverse effects
- avoid psychotropics with a high risk of drug-induced seizures
- SSRIs or MAOIs are the preferred first-line treatments for depression and anxiety
- amisulpride or risperidone are the preferred first-line treatments for psychosis and delirium
- carbamazepine or sodium valproate are the preferred first-line treatments for mania
- do not withhold necessary psychotropic medication out of fear of precipitating future seizures
- consider possible drug interactions.

REFERENCES AND FURTHER READING

Alldredge B 1999 Seizure risk associated with psychotropic drugs: clinical and pharmacokinetic considerations. Neurology 53(suppl 2):69–75

Besag FMC 2001 Behavioural effects of the new anticonvulsants. Drug Safety 24:513–536

Deb S 2000 Epidemiology and treatment of epilepsy in patients who are mentally retarded. CNS Drugs 13:117–128

Devinsky O, Honigfeld G, Patin J 1991 Clozapine-related seizures. Neurology 41:369–371

Edwards KR, Sackellares JC, Vuong A et al 2001 Lamotrigine monotherapy improves depressive symptoms in epilepsy: a double-blind comparison with valproate. Epilepsy and Behaviour 2:28–36

Elterman RD, Shields WD, Mansfield KA et al 2001 Randomized trial of vigabatrin in patients with infantile spasms. Neurology 57:1416–1421

Frommer DA, Kulig KW, Rumack B 1987 Tricyclic antidepressant overdose: a review. JAMA 257:521–526

Jannuzzi G, Cian P, Fattore C et al 2000 A multicenter randomized controlled trial on the clinical impact of therapeutic drug monitoring in patients with newly diagnosed epilepsy. Epilepsia 41:222–230

Kerr M, Bowley C 2001 Evidence-based prescribing in adults with learning disability and epilepsy. Epilepsia 42(suppl 1): 44–45

McAuley JW, Biederman TS, Smith JC et al 2002 Newer therapies in the drug treatment of epilepsy. Annals of Pharmacotherapy 36:119–129

Marsden A 2001 Epilepsy. In: Barton S (ed) Clinical evidence, issue 6. BMJ Publishing Group, London, p 972–981

Marson A G, Kadir ZA, Hutton JL et al 1997 The new antiepileptic drugs: a systematic review of their efficacy and tolerability. Epilepsia 38:859–880

Matterson R, Cramer J, Collins JF et al 1985 Comparison of carbamazepine, phenobarbital, phenytoin, and primidone in partial and secondarily generalized tonic–clonic seizures. New England Journal of Medicine 313:145–151

Pauig PM, Deluca MA, Osterheld RG 1961 Thioridazine hydrochloride in the treatment of behaviour disorders in epileptics. American Journal of Psychiatry 117:832–833

Peck AW, Stern WC, Watkinson C 1983 Incidence of seizures during treatment with tricyclic antidepressant drugs and bupropion. Journal of Clinical Psychiatry 44:197–201

Roberston MM, Trimble MR 1985 The treatment of depression in patients with epilepsy: a double-blind trial. Journal of Affective Disorders 9:127–136

49

Treatment in Patients with Post-acute Head Injury

NEUROLOGICAL TREATMENTS IN HEAD INJURY

Logically, both the medical and neuropsychiatric management of the head-injured patient can be divided into acute and post-acute (rehabilitation) stages. Acute medical and neurosurgical treatment of patients with serious head injuries are difficult to study in a randomised controlled trial (RCT) and results from existing studies have been disappointing (Table 49.1) (Roberts et al 1998). Nevertheless, available information has been incorporated in the new National Institute of Clinical Excellence (NICE) guidelines 'Head Injury in Infants, Children and Adults: Triage, Assessment, Investigation and Early Management', and this aspect of treatment is therefore not reviewed here.

Post-traumatic seizures

Early unblinded studies using older anticonvulsants led to the widespread prophylactic use of these drugs early after severe head injury. Recently, this evidence has been critically re-examined in one systematic review and one meta-analysis (Schierhout & Roberts 1998, Temkin 2001). The consensus is that early use of phenytoin or carbamazepine does indeed prevent

Table 49.1 Trials involving interventions following mild, moderate and severe head injury

Category	No. of trials	No. of participants
Aminosteroid	3	1331
Anaesthetics	27	1010
Antidepressant	3	26
Antiseizure	8	1212
Antispasticity	2	12
Anti-ulcer	5	354
Beta blockers	2	135
Calcium antagonists	5	1405
Cognitive therapy	8	406
Corticosteroids	23	2515
Dimethyl sulfoxide	1	35
Endocrine	5	258
Fluid therapy	4	127
Hypothermia	9	364
Management and information	7	2280
N-Methyl-D-aspartate antagonists	2	485
Nootropics	3	123
Nutrition	24	854
Osmotic diuretics	3	140
Polyethylene glycol superoxide dismutase	2	567
Phospholipids	4	350
Pyritinol hydrochloride	3	370
Physical therapy	8	364
Stimulants	10	215
TRIS	4	411
Vasopressin	3	36
Ventilation	10	563
Others	20	665

Adapted from Dickinson et al (2000)

'provoked' seizures within the first 7 days of injury. However, the story is more complex than it first appears. The evidence that antiepileptic drugs (AEDs) prevent later seizures is not convincing. Furthermore, it is these later 'unprovoked' seizures that have prognostic significance. In other words, early seizure control is not accompanied by a reduction in mortality or neurological disability, or even by a reduction in late seizures. In addition, the risks as well as the benefits of long-term treatment with AEDs must be considered (Dikmen et al 1991). For these reasons, treatment with older AEDs beyond the initial week of injury in patients with no history of seizures following a non-penetrating traumatic head injury is not recommended (Yablon et al 1998).

Studies with new anticonvulsants are urgently needed to see if these recommendations hold true.

Rehabilitation

There is a large literature on the impact of medical treatment on long-term outcomes. This area is of particular importance, given that approximately 50% of head-injury victims (including mild head injury) are left with significant disability (Thornhill et al 2000).

Dickinson et al (2000) reviewed 126 trials that examined modification of disability after head injury in adults. The authors felt that the primary data were inadequate and prevented the drawing of clear conclusions. However, this review has itself been criticized because it did not distinguish between heterogeneous patient groups and did not consider a representative range of outcome measures (Murray & Teasdale 2000). Similar methodological problems were reported by The American Academy of Pediatrics in an extensive review of studies of the management of minor head injury in children (Homer & Kleinman 1999).

Well-designed studies of non-pharmacological interventions in the rehabilitation stage of recovery are not common. RCTs (usually comparing different levels of rehabilitation for ethical reasons) are even rarer (Chesnut et al 1999). The handful of studies done to date suggest a definite advantage for intensive neurorehabilitation in the early phase of recovery, but the effect becomes increasingly difficult to demonstrate with time. Yet, surprisingly, quite simple interventions may be effective. Wade et al (1998) randomized over 1000 head-injury patients

(with mixed injuries) to routine care or additional information and advice 1 week later. At 6-months follow-up the intervention produced a small reduction in everyday difficulties, reduction in social disability and less severe post-concussion symptoms in the moderate or severely injured group. It is likely that the provision of support, through personal contact, is more important than the information given out (Powell et al 2002).

TREATMENT OF THE NEUROPSYCHIATRIC COMPLICATIONS OF HEAD INJURY

Early intervention and prevention

Although there is no literature in this area, it is worth mentioning if only to encourage future research. There is accumulating evidence on the prediction of neuropsychiatric complications after head injury. It may soon be possible to screen A&E attenders with mild head injury and offer those at risk of complications some form of early intervention. Treatment possibilities may be informed from a parallel literature in which the development of post-traumatic stress disorder (PTSD) symptoms was prevented by the early administration of a short course of propranolol (Pitman et al 2002). Antidepressants, already shown to be effective in preventing relapse of PTSD, may also confer the same benefits. Non-pharmacological strategies, including advice and monitoring, should also be considered.

Treatment of cognitive problems

Cognitive dysfunction is such an integral part of head injury that it is usually addressed as part of a rehabilitation programme. Such difficulties are also a feature of the post-concussional syndrome (see below). Although much has been written about this aspect of treatment (see Clinical Pointer 50.2), good-quality evidence for effectiveness is hard to find (Carney et al 1999, Park & Ingles 2001). Two RCTs suggest that specific forms of cognitive rehabilitation reduce memory failures together with a number of secondary benefits (Carney et al 1999). Studies investigating whether pharmacological strategies improve memory or concentration after head injury are very much in their infancy. Plenger

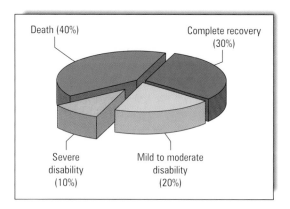

Fig. 49.1 Outcomes after severe head injury with coma.

et al (1996) conducted an RCT of methylphenidate versus placebo in 23 patients with closed head injury. Those treated with methylphenidate showed significantly better improvement in motor performance, global disability and attention at 30 days, although differences were not sustained at 90 days. An underpowered study of patients given amantadine or placebo in a crossover design, unsurprisingly failed to detect any treatment effects (Schneider et al 1999).

Treatment of mood problems and post-concussional symptoms

Mooney & Haas (1993) conducted a placebo-controlled, single-blind RCT of methylphenidate in 38 men with head injuries. Methylphenidate was globally superior to placebo, with a noticeable effect on alleviation of anger. Mood symptoms following head injury have been treated with desipramine in a randomized study of 10 patients with 'severe traumatic brain injury and long-standing depression' (Wroblewski et al 1996). In this study desipramine was superior to placebo. Brooke et al (1992) conducted a small placebo-controlled trial of propranolol (up to 420 mg/day) for agitation in 21 patients with head injury. Although there was no difference in the frequency of episodes of agitation, the severity of episodes was diminished in those receiving propranolol. One study has examined the value of carbamazepine versus placebo in aggressive patients who had sustained frontal lobe injury from a variety of causes (Foster et al 1989). Patients in the intervention group were significantly improved on both affective and behavioural outcome measures. With only limited research evidence, experience from other conditions and clinical experience has led clinicians to use carbamazepine to treat agitation and aggression, dopamine-elevating drugs (with or without noradrenergic properties) to treat apathy and SSRIs to treat impulse-control disorders, possibly with the addition of beta blockers and other anticonvulsants where indicated.

Several studies have examined whether interventions might reduce post-concussional symptoms after head injury. As post-concussional symptoms are not specific to head-injured patients but are also seen, albeit less frequently, in non-head-injured accident victims and in depressed patients, interventions are unlikely to be applicable only to the head-injured patient. One of the more rigorous studies (but not strictly randomized) compared 79

patients seen at 1 week and 3 months after a mild head injury, with 123 patients seen only at 3 months. Those given information early on had lower levels of distress, anxiety, hostility and sleep disturbance (Cameron et al 2002).

Patients who have sustained a head injury often require lengthy periods of rehabilitation for physical, cognitive and psychological needs. Patients are usually frustrated at their inability to perform simple tasks, and more realistic goal setting and education often helps. There is a danger that neuropsychiatric symptoms may be overlooked when other pressing problems dominate the clinical picture. Furthermore, the assessment of neuropsychiatric problems in patients with communication difficulties poses a particular challenge (see Ch. 70). As a rule of thumb, emotional problems after head injury can be usefully divided into: depression, emotionalism and anxiety, which tend to respond to conventional antidepressant treatment (Fann et al 2000); irritability and anger generated by frustration, which may also respond to antidepressants; and anger generated by disinhibition, which is best treated by slow titration of a mood stabilizer such as carbamazepine as first-line treatment.

SUMMARY

The following management is recommended for neuropsychiatric complications of head injury:

- After severe injuries, screen for agitation and delirium in the first 7 days.
- In the absence of a first seizure, prophylactic use of older anticonvulsants is not recommended for preventing late post-traumatic seizures following severe head injury (but they may be used to prevent seizures in the first 7 days).
- Screen for apathy, irritability, depression, anxiety and cognitive impairment within the first 3 months.
- Screen for adjustment difficulties, post-concussional syndrome and poor residual quality of life within the first 6 months.
- Document cognitive deficits using a standardised tool.
- Offer continuing care and support for those who require it.
- Consider written information for all head-injured patients attending A&E and specific advice and/or support for those with risk factors

for poor outcome.

- Consider carbamazepine as first-line treatment for agitation and aggression where disinhibition is present, and sodium valproate, beta blockers and antipsychotics as alternatives.
- Consider receptor-specific antidepressants (second and third generation) as first-line treatment for depression, apathy, irritability or anxiety.
- Consider methylphenidate as first-line treatment for apathy.

REFERENCES AND FURTHER READING

Brooke MM, Patterson DR, Questad KA et al 1992 The treatment of agitation during initial hospitalization after traumatic brain injury. Archives of Physical Medicine and Rehabilitation 73:917–921

Cameron P, Kelly AM, Nelms R et al 2002 Impact of early intervention on outcome following mild head injury in adults. Journal of Neurology, Neurosurgery and Psychiatry 73:330–332

Carney N, Chesnut RM, Maynard H et al 1999 Effect of cognitive rehabilitation on outcomes for persons with traumatic brain injury: a systematic review. Journal of Head Trauma Rehabilitation 14:277–307

Chesnut RM, Carney N, Maynard H et al 1999 Summary report: evidence for the effectiveness of rehabilitation for persons with traumatic brain injury. Journal of Head Trauma Rehabilitation 14:176–188

Dickinson K, Bunn F, Wentz R et al 2000 Size and quality of randomised controlled trials in head injury: review of published studies. BMJ 320:1308–1311

Dikmen SS, Temkin NR, Miller B et al 1991 Neurobehavioral effects of phenytoin prophylaxis of post-traumatic seizures. JAMA 265:1271–1277

Fann JR, Uomoto JM, Katon WJ 2000 Sertraline in the treatment of major depression following mild traumatic brain injury. Journal of Neuropsychiatry and Clinical Neuroscience 12:226–232

Foster HG, Hillbrand M, Chi CC 1989 Efficacy of carbamazepine in assaultive patients with frontal-lobe dysfunction. Progress in Neuro-Psychopharmacology 13:865–874

Homer CL, Kleinman L 1999 Technical report: minor head injury in children. Pediatrics 104:78

Mooney GF, Haas LJ 1993 Effect of methylphenidate on brain injury-related anger. Archives of Physical Medicine and Rehabilitation 74:153–160

Murray GD, Teasdale GM 2000 Quality of randomised controlled trials in head injury. BMJ 321:1223–1223

Park NW, Ingles JL 2001 Effectiveness of attention rehabilitation after an acquired brain injury: a meta-analysis. Neuropsychology 15:199–210

Pitman RK, Sanders KM, Zusman RM et al 2002 Pilot study of secondary prevention of posttraumatic stress disorder with propranolol. Biological Psychiatry 51:189–192

Plenger PM, Dixon CE, Castillo RM et al 1996 Subacute methylphenidate treatment for moderate to moderately severe traumatic brain injury: a preliminary double-blind placebo-controlled study. Archives of Physical Medicine and Rehabilitation 77:536–540

Powell J, Heslin J, Greenwood R 2002 Community based rehabilitation after severe traumatic brain injury: a randomised controlled trial. Journal of Neurology, Neurosurgery and Psychiatry 72:193–202

Roberts I, Schierhout G, Alderson P 1998 Absence of evidence for the effectiveness of five interventions routinely used in the intensive care management of severe head injury: a systematic review. Journal of Neurology, Neurosurgery and Psychiatry 65:729–733

Schierhout G, Roberts I 1998 Prophylactic antiepileptic agents after head injury: a systematic review. Journal of Neurology, Neurosurgery and Psychiatry 64:108–112

Schneider WN, Drew-Cates J, Wong TM et al 1999 Cognitive and behavioural efficacy of amantadine in acute traumatic brain injury: an initial double-blind placebo-controlled study. Brain Injury 13:863–872

Temkin NR 2001 Antiepileptogenesis and seizure prevention trials with antiepileptic drugs: meta-analysis of controlled trials. Epilepsia 42:515–524

Thornhill S, Teasdale GM, Murray GD et al 2000 Disability in young people and adults one year after head injury: prospective cohort study. BMJ 320:1631–1635

Wade DT, King NS, Wenden FJ et al 1998 Routine follow up after head injury: a second randomised controlled trial. Journal of Neurology, Neurosurgery and Psychiatry 65:177–183

Wroblewski BA, Joseph AB, Cornblatt RR 1996 Antidepressant pharmacotherapy and the treatment of depression in patients with severe traumatic brain injury: a controlled, prospective study. Journal of Clinical Psychiatry 57:582–587

Yablon SA, Jackson MS, Meythaler JM et al for the Brain Injury Special Interest Group of American Academy of Physical Medicine and Rehabilitation 1998 Practice parameter: antiepileptic drug treatment of post-traumatic seizures. Archives of Physical Medicine and Rehabilitation 79:594–597

50

Treatment in Patients with Multiple Sclerosis

NEUROLOGICAL TREATMENTS IN MULTIPLE SCLEROSIS

In order to retard the natural history of multiple sclerosis (MS), a treatment must combat disease-related axonal degeneration. Since MS pathology usually accumulates gradually, there is ample opportunity to begin treatment early in the disease course. On the other hand, there is persuasive evidence that axonal degeneration continues after the acute inflammation has resolved. The effectiveness of a disease-modifying treatment is likely to be influenced by the stage of disease when the treatment is initiated as well as by the aggressiveness of the disease itself.

The mainstay of treatment for MS has been glucocorticoids since they were first used in 1950. Although glucocorticoids work well as symptomatic relief, they do not appear to alter the long-term course of the disease (Andersson & Goodkin 1998). ACTH and oral prednisolone are effective, but intravenous methylprednisolone is much better tolerated and perhaps faster acting (Tremlett et al 1998). A recent Cochrane Review of six modest-sized trials of methylprednisolone versus ACTH showed a non-significant advantage for methylprednisolone in establishing an acute remission, but no long-term

benefits (Filippini et al 2001). Many other specific symptomatic treatments are available, including antispastic agents (baclofen), drugs to reduce tremor (clonazepam), anticholinergics to relieve urinary symptoms, anticonvulsants to control neuralgia and stimulants to reduce fatigue (amantadine, modafinil). However, most interest has concentrated on drugs that potentially alter the disease course.

Classical relapsing–remitting multiple sclerosis

Much interest surrounds immunosuppressive treatments, exemplified by the β-interferons (interferon-β-1a and interferon-β-1b). Interferon-β inhibits the phagocytosis of myelin. The landmark study was the 1993 IFNB MS Study Group trial of relapsing–remitting MS (IFNB Multiple Sclerosis Study Group 1993). Beneficial effects of interferon-β-1b were seen at 2 years as measured by severity of relapses and specific MRI findings. After 3 years, however, advantages of treatment were gradually lost. Nevertheless, interferon-β-1b became the first non-cytotoxic drug approved in the USA for MS, followed by interferon-β-1a in 1996. The large PRISM study (Prevention of Relapses and disability by Interferon-[β]-1a Subcutaneously in MS) reported that, after 2 years, not only were relapses reduced but the rates of disability and re-admissions were improved (PRISMS 1998).

An alternative to the interferons is glatiramer acetate. Glatiramer acetate (also known as copolymer 1) is a synthetic substance with properties similar to those of myelin basic protein. It was approved for use in MS in the USA in 1996 (Johnson et al

---

Box 50.1 Drugs for multiple sclerosis

Symptomatic treatment
Glucocorticoids (see Filippini et al (2001))

Early intervention
Interferon-β-1b (see ETOMS study (Comi et al 2001))
Interferon-β-1a (see CHAMPS study (Jacobs et al 2000))

Relapsing–remitting MS
Interferon-β-1b (see IFNB Multiple Sclerosis Study Group 1993)
Interferon-β-1a (see Jacobs et al 1996, PRISMS 1998)
Glatiramer acetate (see Johnson et al 1995)

Secondary progressive MS
Interferon-β-1b (see European Study Group 1998)

1995). It has gained approval in 16 European countries but has not been recommended for use in the UK by the National Institute of Clinical Excellence (NICE) on the grounds of lack of cost-effectiveness (see below).

What is not so clear is the magnitude of the therapeutic effect in relapsing–remitting MS. As a guide, these treatments tend to reduce the number of relapses from three in 3 years to two in 3 years, a modest effect at best. Given that these drugs reduce the frequency of relapses in established MS, it is to be expected that they increase the latency to first relapse if given early after first onset of the disease. Two recent studies – CHAMPS (the Controlled High-Risk Subjects Avonex MS Prevention Study) (Jacobs et al 2000) and ETOMS (the Early Treatment of Multiple Sclerosis Study) (Comi et al 2001) – have confirmed that this is so. In real terms, both studies are disappointing because they did not examine the effect of delaying the first relapse on subsequent disease progression.

Chronic progressive multiple sclerosis

Several trials are now under way to examine the effects of interferons in secondary progressive MS. So far, only the European Study Group trial (1998) has convincingly shown that the drug can decrease the development of disability in secondary progressive MS. A total of 358 patients were allocated to placebo and 360 were allocated to interferon-β-1b. Over 2–3 years, the proportion of treated patients who had worsening of disability was 20% lower than the proportion of patients who received placebo. However, two large studies provisionally reported as showing no benefit of treatment in secondary progressive MS have yet to be published.

Other therapeutic options that are potentially disease modifying in chronic progressive MS include methotrexate, azathioprine and intermittent cyclophosphamide. These traditional immunosuppressive regimens may be more cost-effective and easier to administer, but they can be toxic, and further research is required in terms of a direct comparison of these drugs with the interferons.

Guidelines from NICE (UK)

Summarizing the evidence, interferons offer a modestly beneficial effect on the course of MS, an effect demonstrable from the earliest stages of the disease. The most important question, of whether they help long-term outcome by influencing disease progression, is currently certain. Data on quality of life and neuropsychiatric complications are sparse.

On this basis, and amid some confusion, the National Institute of Clinical Evidence (NICE) in the UK released (February 2002) guidelines stating that 'on the balance of their clinical and cost effectiveness neither β-interferon nor glatiramer acetate is recommended for the treatment of MS in the NHS in England and Wales.'

The current position is that the NHS has entered into an arrangement with manufacturers which means that both glatiramer acetate and interferon-β will be available to all patients with relapsing–remit-

---

Clinical Pointer 50.1

Rehabilitation for multiple sclerosis

Rehabilitation for sufferers from MS is often multidisciplinary, involving occupational therapists, physiotherapists, speech therapists, nurses and doctors. The aim is usually to improve disability rather than neurological impairment. Secondary effects may include improvement in distress and emotional problems and perhaps also in fatigue. Intervention can be carried out on an inpatient or an outpatient basis, although realistically many centres lack the necessary resources. Accompanying medical treatment for muscle spasticity and urinary tract problems are recommended.

Cognitive rehabilitation employs both basic and advanced measures. Basic measures include using a problem-solving approach, avoiding unnecessary problems, focusing attention, allowing extra time, making links with known material, anticipating difficulties and being systematic.

Further reading Burks J, Johnson K (eds) 2000 Multiple sclerosis, diagnosis, medical management and rehabilitation Demos Medical, New York
Kalla T, Downes JJ, van den Broek M 2001 The pre-exposure technique: enhancing the effects of errorless learning in the acquisition of face–name associations. Neuropsychology and Rehabilitation 11:1–16

ting MS and those with relapse-predominant secondary progressive MS.

ADVERSE NEUROPSYCHIATRIC EFFECTS OF GLUCOCORTICOIDS

Corticosteroids are used widely in medicine, in both acute and chronic illnesses. Prednisolone is most commonly prescribed owing to its predominant glucocorticoid activity. High doses are used in certain conditions, such as polymyalgia rheumatica and temporal arteritis. Corticosteroids are used in a variety of dermatological conditions, although topical applications usually limit systemic complications. Long-term use of corticosteroids is common in ulcerative colitis and Crohn's disease. Other conditions such as MS, ankylosing spondylitis and asthma may show symptomatic improvement with short-term use of corticosteroids, and therefore long-term use is usually avoided. Hydrocortisone (synthetic cortisol) and cortisone (which is converted to hydrocortisone in the liver) have mineralocorticoid activity that makes them unsuitable for adrenal replacement therapy. Hydrocortisone is used for emergency corticosteroid treatment and as a topical corticosteroid. The synthetic corticosteroids betamethasone and dexamethasone have very high glucocorticoid activity with insignificant mineralocorticoid activity, which is used to advantage in cerebral oedema. Deflazacort is a newly introduced corticosteroid with high glucocorticoid activity; it is derived from prednisolone.

Intravenous methylprednisolone is the treatment of choice for acute relapses of MS. It is usually given as an infusion over 3 hours each day, for between 3 and 15 days (depending on response). Cardiac arrhythmias, seizures and anaphylactic reactions are very rare. Predictable and reversible side effects include new or worsening minor infections, insomnia, hyperglycaemia, a metallic taste, weight gain and gastrointestinal complaints.

Psychiatric complications of glucocorticoid therapy have been recognized for over 45 years (Rome & Braceland 1952). Disturbances in mood are most often cited but, increasingly, cognitive deficits are recognized (Belanoff et al 2001). Epidemiological, prospective and placebo-controlled studies report that approximately one-third of patients taking glucocorticoids experience significant mood distur-

bance and sleep disruption, three times the rate in matched controls (Chrousos et al 1993, Patten 2000). Up to 20% of patients taking high-dose glucocorticoids report more severe but short-lived psychiatric disorders that closely resemble psychotic depression, mania or paranoid psychosis. Authors who have closely observed these incipient mood changes suggest that hypomania or mixed affective states are the most common forms of altered mood, developing in 20–30% of subjects (Boston Collaborative Drug Surveillance Program 1972, Minden et al 1988, Naber et al 1996). A recent double-blind, placebo-controlled trial of brief corticosteroid administration in healthy subjects demonstrated that the majority of people develop subtle disturbances in mood and cognition, which reverse upon cessation of therapy (Wolkowitz 1994). This observation is also seen clinically, since patients treated with long-term prednisone have explicit memory deficits not seen in matched controls (Keenan et al 1996). Unlike the cushingoid features (e.g. obesity, acne, hirsutism, striae), the neuropsy-

---

Box 50.2 Adverse effects of glucocorticoids

Psychiatric
Cognitive impairment (chronic use)
Dysphoria and depression
Irritability
Mania and hypomania
Mixed affective states
Pathological emotionalism
Psychosis (any type)

Neurological
Insomnia
Peripheral myopathy

Dermatological
Acne
Purpura
Thin skin

Orthopaedic
Osteoporosis
Pathological fractures

Endocrine
Adrenal suppression
Hyperglycaemia
Short stature (in children)
Weight gain

Metabolic
Hypokalaemia
Immune suppression
Neutropenia

chiatric effects are less dose-dependent. Unlike the metabolic effects of glucocorticoids (e.g. hypertension, sodium retention, potassium loss, hyperglycaemia, lipid changes) the neuropsychiatric features are less duration-dependent. Nevertheless, brief pulses of corticosteroids appear to be much safer than continuous dosing, even when the dose of each pulse is very high. To date, no satisfactory predictors of steroid-induced psychiatric complications have been found, although some evidence supports different neuropsychiatric effects with synthetic versus natural steroids.

TREATMENT OF THE NEURO-PSYCHIATRIC COMPLICATIONS OF MULTIPLE SCLEROSIS

Effective treatment of MS is likely to benefit both the physical and mental symptoms of MS. Few of the large trials of primary treatments have included neuropsychiatric measures as secondary endpoints. Several studies have included functional assessments, often using the Kurtzke Functional Status Scale and the Kurtzke Extended Disability Scale (see Appendix V). Quality of life is disproportionately affected in MS (Murphy et al 1998). Fischer et al (2000) recently reported a reasonably large study of 166 relapsing–remitting MS patients who under-

went cognitive testing at baseline and at 6 months (to 2 years) after treatment with interferon-β-1a. In this prospective study, the patients acted as their own controls. The authors found improvements in learning and memory and, to a lesser extent, in visuospatial abilities, problem solving and processing speed.

The effect of interferon treatment on mood is of interest given that one of the most common reasons for discontinuation of therapy in the pivotal IFNB MS Study was depression. Recently, Patten & Metz (2002) re-analysed safety data from 4469 MS patients treated with interferon-β-1a. At 2 years, 27% of placebo-treated patients and 27% of high-dose interferon-β-1a treated patients had experienced depression. Drop-outs because of depression were more common in the interferon groups. Mohr et al (1999) examined the effect of interferon treatment on depression in 50 patients with MS. The measure of mood was Profile of Mood States, which may be better thought of as measuring dysphoria rather than depression in this cohort. Patients who were dysphoric before initiation of treatment had some relief when treatment was started but returned to their baseline levels 2 weeks later. In a related study, the same group found that 41% of patients starting interferon treatment for MS experienced worsening depression within 6 months of starting treatment. When depression was treated, 86% continued with interferon treatment, com-

---

Clinical Pointer 50.2

Cognitive rehabilitation for neuropsychiatric disease

Cognitive rehabilitation (non-pharmacological therapy to improve cognition) has been examined in the context of head injury, MS, stroke and Alzheimer's disease. Mostly, effects are modest, but nevertheless can be clinically significant. Barriers to cognitive rehabilitation include poor motivation, depression, lack of support and unavailability of services.

Patients with Alzheimer's disease generally do not benefit from simple rehearsal (repetition) and, furthermore, may become frustrated at these exercises. Other methods sometimes used include use of visual imagery, face–name association and verbal mnemonic strategies. Patients with stroke and head injury may improve most when deficits are moderate. Learning by association, for example pairing a bleep with exit from a ward, can be a useful technique. On a larger scale, specialized units should be designed with these kind of difficulties in mind. Patients with memory problems are still able to acquire implicit memory (procedural information) on training, which can be useful. Furthermore, the use of partial cues can resurrect a memory that the person is not consciously aware of. Rehabilitation of cognitive deficits (aphasia and unilateral neglect) delivered by specialists is more effective than treatment delivered by non-specialist therapists, including family members. External aids are often valuable and can be categorized as follows:

- time reminders (e.g. alarm calls, diary, calendar)
- person and place reminders (e.g. name tags, symbols, colour coded clothes)
- external reminders (e.g. prompts from others, post-it notes, tape recorder, video, radio pager)
- internal reminders (e.g. visual imagery, association recall, grouping items).

Further reading   Cicerone KD, Dahlberg C, Kalmar K et al 2000 Evidence-based cognitive rehabilitation: recommendations for clinical practice. Archives of Physical Medicine and Rehabilitation 81:1596–1615

pared with 38% of the patients who received no therapy for depression (Mohr et al 1997). This effect of mental state symptoms on compliance with physical treatments is a common theme in neuropsychiatry and also in other medical specialties such as cardiology (Carney et al 1995). From these data, it is possible that interferon treatment can adversely influence mood, despite positive effects on MS itself, and therefore mood should be monitored in this group.

Fatigue is a major problem in about one-third of patients with MS; it has both physical and psychological components (Comi et al 2001). Patient-rated mental and physical fatigue appears to overlap closely with disability, motivation and depression in most patients (Kroencke et al 2000). One modest-sized three-arm study examined the value of amantadine and pemoline versus placebo in treating fatigue in MS (Krupp et al 1995). In 119 patients, amantadine significantly reduced fatigue compared with placebo, but pemoline did not. Neither amantadine nor pemoline affected the secondary outcome measures of sleep or depression.

Depression and antidepressants

In a small double-blind randomized controlled trial, desipramine was compared with placebo in 28 patients with MS and depression (Schiffer & Wineman 1990). Both groups also received individual psychotherapy. A significantly greater number of patients improved on active drug compared with placebo, and this was unrelated to degree of disability. About half of the desipramine-treated patients experienced side effects.

Larcombe & Wilson (1984) examined the use of cognitive–behavioural therapy (CBT) for depression in MS in an open-label study. This has been replicated in a further 40 patients (Jonnsson et al 1993). Mohr et al (2000) recently reported the results of an 8-week trial of telephone-administered CBT versus usual care in 32 patients. Results suggested a significant benefit for telephone CBT in improving depression and adherence to interferon treatment. Also of interest, one study has examined the treatment of emotionalism in patients with MS. Schiffer et al (1985) piloted low-dose amitriptyline in comparison with placebo in 12 patients. Amitriptyline was significantly more effective than placebo. Several recent reviews of the treatment of mood disorders in MS are available, but they are limited by the paucity of original research in this area.

Cognitive enhancement

Several groups have begun to explore the value of cognitive training for patients with MS who have cognitive deficits. Jonnsson et al (1993) compared so-called 'usual care' in 20 patients with a structured cognitive rehabilitation programme in 20 patients, described as 'direct training, compensatory strategies and neuropsychotherapy'. Modest gains in both cognitive function and mood were reported, although the study was neither randomized nor blinded. Mendozzi et al (1998) compared a specific computer-assisted memory retraining programme with a non-specific programme and no treatment in 60 patients with MS, matched at baseline. Significantly greater improvements were noted in the advanced group. Recently, one group has reported positive results of donepezil in the treatment of cognitive disturbance of MS (Greene et al 2000). The open-label study involved only 17 patients, but nevertheless is worth highlighting since other studies of the acetylcholinesterase inhibitors are sure to follow.

SUMMARY

The management of neuropsychiatric complications of MS can be summarized as follows:

- assess perceived disability, support, quality of life and prognosis in relation to neuropsychiatric complications
- use a sensitive and standardized cognitive assessment tool or consider referral for neuropsychological testing
- expect the unexpected – almost any psychiatric complication can occur in MS
- consider MRI for patients with persistent psychosis or cognitive impairment, but do not dismiss patients with 'normal appearing white matter'
- attempt to maximize quality of life in any person presenting with mental health problems – treatment of the underlying MS is a valid approach to mental health problems
- use conventional treatments for depression, anxiety and psychosis in MS, but be aware of possible steroid-induced syndromes
- monitor patients treated with interferons for an adverse effect on mood
- use a multidisciplinary approach to ongoing treatment.

REFERENCES AND FURTHER READING

Andersson PB, Goodkin DE 1998 Glucocorticosteroid therapy for multiple sclerosis: a critical review. Journal of Neurological Science 160:16–25

Belanoff JK, Gross K, Yager A et al 2001 Corticosteroids and cognition. Journal of Psychiatric Research 35:127–145

Boston Collaborative Drug Surveillance Program 1972 Acute adverse reactions to prednisone in relation to dosage. Clinical Pharmacology 13:694–698

Carney RM, Freedland KE, Eisen SA et al 1995 Major depression and medication adherence in coronary artery disease. Health Psychology 14:88–90

Chrousos GA, Kattah JC, Beck RW et al 1993 Side effects of glucocorticoid treatment: experience of the optic neuritis treatment trial. JAMA 269:2110–2112

Comi G, Filipi M, Barkhof F et al 2001 Effect of early interferon treatment on conversion to definitive multiple sclerosis. Lancet 357:1576–1582

European Study Group on Interferon β-1b in Secondary Progressive MS 1998 Placebo-controlled multicentre randomised trial of interferon β-1b in treatment of secondary progressive multiple sclerosis. Lancet 352:1491–1497

Filippini G, Brusaferri F, Sibley WA et al 2001 Corticosteroids or ACTH for acute exacerbations in multiple sclerosis (Cochrane Review). In: The Cochrane Library, Issue 2. Update Software, Oxford

Fischer JS, Priore RL, Jacobs LD et al 2000 Neuropsychological effects of interferon β-1a in relapsing multiple sclerosis. Multiple Sclerosis Collaborative Research Group. Annals of Neurology 48:885–892

Greene YM, Tariot PN, Wishart H et al 2000 A 12-week, open trial of donepezil hydrochloride in patients with multiple sclerosis and associated cognitive impairments. Journal of Clinical Psychopharmacology 20:350–356

IFNB Multiple Sclerosis Study Group 1993 Interferon β-1b is effective in relapsing–remitting multiple sclerosis. I: Clinical results of a multicenter, randomized, double-blind, placebo-controlled trial. Neurology 43:655–661

Jacobs LD, Cookfair DL, Ruckick RA et al for the Multiple Sclerosis Collaborative Research Group (MSCRG) 1996 Intramuscular interferon β-1α for disease progression in relapsing multiple sclerosis. Annals of Neurology 39:285–294

Jacobs LD, Back RW, Simon JH et al 2000 Intramuscular interferon β-1a therapy initiated during a first demyelinating event in multiple sclerosis. CHAMPS Study Group. New England Journal of Medicine 343:898–904

Johnson KP, Brooks BR, Cohen JA et al 1995 Copolymer 1 reduced relapse rate and improves disability in relapsing–remitting multiple sclerosis: results of a phase III multicenter, double-blind placebo-controlled trial. Neurology 45:1268–1276

Jonnsson A, Korfitzen EM, Heltberg A et al 1993 Effects of neuropsychological treatment in patients with multiple sclerosis. Acta Neurologica Scandinavica 88:394–400

Keenan PA, Jacobson MW, Soleymani RM et al 1996 The effect on memory of chronic prednisone treatment in patients with systemic disease. Neurology 47:1396–1402

Kroencke DC, Lynch SG, Denney DR 2000 Fatigue in multiple sclerosis: relationship to depression, disability, and disease pattern. Multiple Sclerosis 6:131–136

Krupp LB, Coyle PK, Doscher C et al 1995 Fatigue therapy in multiple sclerosis: results of a double-blind, randomised parallel trial of amantadine, pemoline and placebo. Neurology 45:1956–1961

Larcombe NA, Wilson PH 1984 An evaluation of cognitive–behavioural therapy for depression in patients with multiple sclerosis. British Journal of Psychiatry 145:366–371

Mendozzi L, Pugnetti L, Motta A et al 1998 Computer-assisted memory retraining of patients with multiple sclerosis. Italian Journal of Neurological Sciences 19(suppl S):S431–S438

Minden SL, Orav J, Schildkraut JJ 1988 Hypomanic reactions to ACTH and prednisolone treatment for multiple sclerosis. Neurology 38:1631–1634

Mohr DC, Goodkin DE, Likosky W et al 1997 Treatment of depression improves adherence to interferon β-1b therapy for multiple sclerosis. Archives of Neurology 54:531–533

Mohr DC, Likosky W, Dwyer P et al 1999 Course of depression during the initiation of interferon β-1a treatment for multiple sclerosis. Archives of Neurology 56:1263–1265

Mohr DC, Likosky W, Bertagnolli A et al 2000 Telephone-administered cognitive–behavioral therapy for the treatment of depressive symptoms in multiple sclerosis. Journal of Consulting Clinical Psychology 68:356–361

Murphy N, Confavreux C, Haas J et al 1998 Quality of life in multiple sclerosis in France, Germany, and the United Kingdom. Cost of Multiple Sclerosis Study Group. Journal of Neurology, Neurosurgery and Psychiatry 65:460–466

Naber D, Sand P, Heigl B 1996 Psychopathological and neuropsychological effects of 8-days' corticosteroid treatment. A prospective study. Psychoneuroendocrinology 21:25–31

Patten SB 2000 Exogenous corticosteroids and major depression in the general population. Journal of Psychosomatic Research 49:447–449

Patten SB, Metz LM 2002 Interferon-β-1a and depression in secondary progressive MS: data from the Spectrims trial. Neurology 59:744–746

PRISMS (Prevention of Relapses and Disability by Interferon β-1a Subcutaneously) in Multiple Sclerosis Study Group 1998 Randomised double-blind placebo-controlled study of interferon β-1a in relapsing/remitting multiple sclerosis. Lancet 352:1498–1504

Rome HP, Braceland FL 1952 The psychological response to ACTH, cortisone, hydrocortisone, and related steroid substances. American Journal of Psychiatry 108:641–651

Schiffer RB, Wineman NM 1990 Antidepressant pharmacology of depression associated with multiple sclerosis. American Journal of Psychiatry 147:1493–1497

Schiffer RB, Herndon RM, Rudick RA 1985 Treatment of pathological laughing and weeping with amitriptyline.

New England Journal of Medicine 312:1480–1482

Tremlett HL, Luscombe DK, Wiles CM 1998 Use of corticosteroids in multiple sclerosis by consultant neurologists in the United Kingdom. Journal of Neurology, Neurosurgery and Psychiatry 65:362–365

Wolkowitz OM 1994 Prospective controlled studies of the behavioural and biological effects of exogenous corticosteroids. Psychoneuroendocrinology 19:233–255

Treatment in Patients with Parkinson's Disease

NEUROLOGICAL TREATMENTS IN PARKINSON'S DISEASE

The pharmacological treatment of Parkinson's disease is a major challenge even for the most experienced clinician. This area has been comprehensively reviewed and guidelines have been produced (Olanow et al 2001).

Levodopa

Levodopa is a precursor of dopamine, which, unlike dopamine itself, can cross the blood–brain barrier. Levodopa is prescribed with an inhibitor of peripheral dopa decarboxylase, which reduces peripheral metabolism from 99% to 90%. Levodopa plus carbidopa (sinamet) or levodopa plus benserazide (madopar) are the common combinations. Domperidone may be necessary to control nausea and vomiting during dose titration.

Levodopa is the most effective drug for alleviating symptoms of Parkinson's disease, but this statement has to be tempered by the knowledge that levodopa effectively 'burns out' after 3–8 years of continuous use. In addition, undertreating and overtreating the patient are associated with adverse consequences, mainly periods of immobility and

dyskinesias, respectively (Miyasaki et al 2002). For these reasons, clinicians tend to reserve levodopa for when it is most needed, although in the elderly levodopa may be first-line treatment.

Levodopa-sparing strategies in the newly diagnosed patient

For the patient with mild symptoms it may not be necessary to use drug treatment at all. Instead, support and education together with advice about coping with symptoms and maintaining a good quality of life is sufficient. In patients complaining primarily of tremor, antimuscarinic drugs that block cholinergic receptors in the corpus striatum are an option. Selegiline is the classic treatment in early Parkinson's disease, but it is subject to considerable controversy. Selegiline selectively inhibits monoamine oxidase B, irreversibly reducing the central breakdown of dopamine. It also inhibits the re-uptake of dopamine at the presynaptic dopamine receptor. Results of the widely quoted Deprenyl and Tocopherol Anti-oxidative Therapy of Parkinsonism (DATATOP) study, involving 800 patients, showed that selegiline could delay the need for levodopa by up to a year, but thereafter its advantage wore off. Furthermore, a secondary randomization involving selegiline or placebo in patients taking levodopa was not convincing (Shoulson et al 2002). A shadow has been cast over selegiline after a study involving 500 patients (randomized to levodopa, bromocriptine or levodopa plus selegiline) showed a 35% increased mortality in the selegiline arm (Lees 1995). Note this was not found in the DATATOP extension study.

The other main levodopa-sparing strategy involves the dopamine agonists. Dopamine agonists include the ergot derivatives bromocriptine, lysuride and pergolide, which are thought to act directly on post-synaptic dopaminergic receptors (Fig. 51.1). All three can cause nausea and vomiting without domperidone cover. Evidence supporting three new drugs (cabergoline, pramipexole and ropinirole) has recently become available (Olanow et al 2001). Ropinirole and pramipexole are licensed for both monotherapy and augmentation, whereas cabergoline is licensed only as adjunctive therapy. A recent multicentre double-blind randomized controlled trial (RCT) of ropinirole versus levodopa in mild to moderate early Parkinson's disease revealed that dyskinesias developed three times more slowly in the ropinirole group than the levodopa group (Rascol et al 2000).

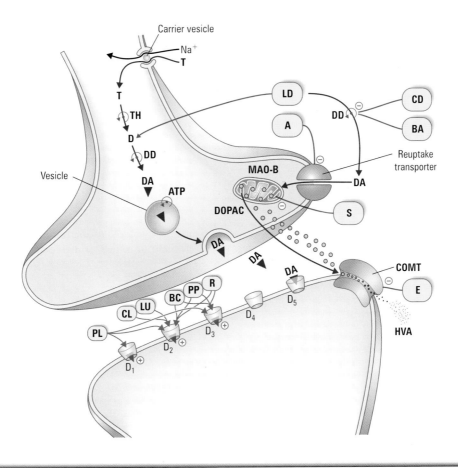

Fig. 51.1 The dopaminergic synapse.

Key	A	Amantadine	DA	Dopamine	MAO-B	Monoamine oxidase type B
	ATP	Adenosine triphosphate	DD	Dopa decarboxylase	PL	Pergolide
	BA	Benserazide	DOPAC	3,4-Dihydroxyphenylacetic acid	PP	Pramipexole
	BC	Bromocriptine	E	Entacapone	R	Ropinirole
	CL	Cabergoline	HVA	Homovanillic acid	S	Selegiline
	CD	Carbidopa	LD	Levodopa	T	Tyrosine
	COMT	Catechol-*o*-methyl transferase	LU	Lysuride	TH	Tyrosine hydroxylase
	D	Dopa	MAO	Monoamine oxidase		

Levodopa augmentation strategies in the late-stage Parkinson's patient

Catechol-*o*-methyl transferase (COMT) converts levodopa to dopamine before it crosses the blood–brain barrier and assists in the breakdown of levodopa peripherally. New COMT inhibitors have been trialed in late Parkinson's disease, with some success. Tolcapone has been withdrawn after three hepatotoxic deaths, but entacapone is used as an augmentation to levodopa in patients experiencing 'end-of-

dose' motor fluctuations. Apomorphine is a potent D_1 and D_2 dopamine agonist that is usually given subcutaneously; it is licensed for the management of refractory motor fluctuations in patients who are inadequately controlled by levodopa.

Surgery

Surgery for Parkinson's disease continues to be a source of controversy. Surgery refers to ablative procedures, deep brain (electrical) stimulation of the subthalamic nucleus (it is interesting to note that ECT is beneficial for patients with Parkinson's disease, although the duration of benefit is short) and

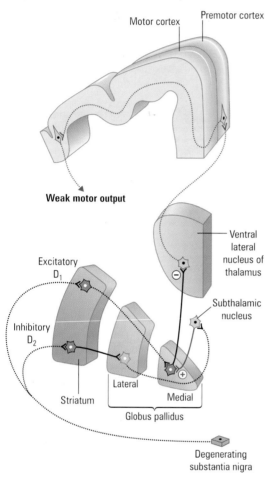

Fig. 51.2 Degeneration of the dopaminergic signal from the substantia nigra impacts on the striatum. Loss of tonic facilitation of spiny striatal neurons (D_1 receptors) and loss of tonic facilitation of those bearing D_2 receptors causes bias from the 'direct' to the 'indirect' pathways. The disinhibited subthalamic nucleus activates the GABA neurones projecting to the ventral lateral nucleus of the thalamus. Thus the weakly discharging thalamocortical neurones fail to excite the motor neurones.

foetal transplantation. Pallidotomy (a lesion to the globus pallidus) reduces contralateral tremor and rigidity during 'off' periods and dyskinesia during 'on' periods. Thalamotomy has also been shown to alleviate tremor in some cases. Bilateral surgery runs the risk of damage to motor tracts, producing mutism, dysarthria, dysphonia and gait disturbances, and there is a significant risk of permanent adverse effects in 3–10% of patients (Moore & Clark 2001). Unilateral posteroventral internal globus pallidus ablation is associated with minor cognitive change, but extension into the anterior portion or the external globus pallidus is more problematic. There has been considerable controversy concerning grafts of foetal dopaminergic cells intro the striatum. Preliminary evidence suggests that the treatment is effective, at least up until 1 year post-surgery (Clarkson 2001). However, some studies indicate that, to be effective, mesencephalic tissue from 3–5 human embryos is required for each hemisphere, and therefore for ethical reasons this treatment is still highly experimental.

TREATMENT OF THE NEUROPSYCHIATRIC COMPLICATIONS OF PARKINSON'S DISEASE

Unfortunately, the most common psychiatric complications of Parkinson's disease are the most difficult to treat successfully. This is largely because patients with Parkinson's disease are sensitive to the antidopaminergic and antiadrenergic effects that are common with antidepressants and antipsychotics.

Depression and antidepressants

Klassen et al (1995) reviewed 12 antidepressant trials in Parkinson's disease that had used reasonable methodology. Tricyclic antidepressants, either alone or in combination with levodopa, can cause hypotension. Monoamine oxidase inhibitors (MAOIs) can be problematic in the treatment of depression in Parkinson's disease because concomitant use of dopaminergic agonists can cause a hypertensive crisis. Problems are more likely with the irreversible type A MAOIs (both selective (clorgyline) and non-selective (tranylcypromine, phenelzine and iproniazid)). Continuing work with selective reversible MAOIs is promising, although caution should be exercised with selegiline (Jansen-Steur & Ballering 1999). It is generally recommended that selegiline should be discontinued 2 weeks before a serotonergic antidepressant is started.

Newer generations of drugs are therefore of particular interest. Caution should still be exercised, because there is a possibility of exacerbating tremor, bradykinesia and akathisia, even with the selective serotonin reuptake inhibitors (SSRIs) (Richard et al 1999). Of the SSRIs, sertraline may be the drug of choice, since it has some properties of inhibiting dopamine reuptake and it has a low propensity to cause extrapyramidal side effects. Of interest, selegiline may improve mood in depressed patients with Parkinson's disease (Allain et al 1991), although several smaller negative RCTs exist (Klassen et al 1995). Caution is needed when combining the MAOI selegiline with SSRIs, since there is a risk of precipitating the serotonin syndrome (the incidence is reported as 0.24%) (Toyama & Iacono 1994), but just as non-selective type A MAOIs can be used with SSRIs, the interactions reported with type B MAOIs and SSRIs are very rare (Richard et al 1997). One RCT has also documented mood-elevating effects of pramipexole (Corrigan et al 2000). Several other small RCTs have suggested antidepressant effects of novel (non-antidepressant) agents such as S-adenosylmethionine (Carrieri et al 1990).

Unfortunately, there is no good scientific evidence to guide treatment of apathy in Parkinson's disease. Increasing dopamine agonism using higher doses of existing antiparkinsonian medication, adding amantadine, or using an antidepressant with dopaminergic properties, such as methylphenidate or bupropion, have been suggested.

Mood stabilizers

Sodium valproate has rarely been noted to cause extrapyramidal side effects, and both lithium and valproate are well known to cause tremor. Care is needed with carbamazepine because of sedation and drug interactions.

Anxiety and anxiolytics

The treatment of anxiety symptoms in Parkinson's disease has not yet been systematically studied. Fortunately, SSRIs are better tolerated in Parkinson's disease than the tricyclics antidepressants are,

Table 51.1 Summary of drugs for motor symptoms in Parkinson's disease

Drug	Efficacy as monotherapy
Dopamine agonists	
Levodopa	Good
Bromocriptine	Moderate
Pergolide	Moderate
Pramipexole	Moderate
Ropinirole	Moderate
COMT inhibitors	
Entacapone	Nil
Type B MAOIs	
Selegiline	Slight
Glutamate N-methyl-D-aspartate antagonists	
Amantadine	Mild
Anticholinergics	
Trihexyphenidyl	Mild
Benztropine	Mild

Adapted from Ahlskog (2001)

and SSRIs are therefore the treatment of choice. Very rarely SSRIs can cause or exacerbate a tremor; anecdotally this may be most often the case with paroxetine. Some patients complain of panic attacks after levodopa treatment, but in most there is no association (Vazquez et al 1993). Conventional psychological therapies for anxiety disorders are an important option, although these have not been examined in Parkinson's disease per se.

Psychosis and antipsychotics

In the event of psychosis, a review of antiparkinsonian medication is indicated because dopaminergic agents are well recognized as causing hallucinations, delusions and delirium (see Ch. 21). True drug-induced psychosis can be reversed quickly in most cases. Recent studies have suggested that the dose, duration and frequency of levodopa treatment may have little association with psychotic symptoms. One possible mechanism is drug-induced sleep disturbance, particularly REM sleep behaviour disorder, which has been linked with hallucinations.

Hallucinations occur in about 6% of those treated with levodopa and 17% of those treated with ropinirole (Rascol et al 2000). Withdrawal of the likely offending agent is the most sensible first course of action, but in the absence of a clear culprit with-

Clinical Pointer 51.1

Physical rehabilitation for patients with Parkinson's disease

Reduced function in Parkinson's disease is related to impairments of bradykinesia and loss of postural reflexes, disabilities of reduced mobility and falls, and the handicaps of social isolation and loss of independence. There is a temptation for patients to accept their situation as hopeless because they feel themselves deteriorating. Rehabilitation helps both the physical aspects and the emotional aspects. Rehabilitation may improve handicap and disability more than it improves neurological impairments. Exercise is one of the simplest but most effective modalities of rehabilitation. Exercises with complex movements (e.g. dance) appear to be most effective. However, the benefits gradually diminish if the routine is stopped. Environmental cues can also be used to improve gait. Visual cues such as floor markers and auditory cues such as rhythmic sounds can increase gait velocity and stride length. Speech is another area of concern for patients. It is usually of low volume and monotonous, with or without dysarthria. Speech therapy with voice and respiratory training has been shown to be beneficial.

Further reading   de Goede CJT, Keus SHJ, Kwakkel G et al 2001 The effects of physical therapy in Parkinson's disease: a research synthesis. Archives of Physical Medicine and Rehabilitation 82:509–515
Melnick ME 2001 Basal ganglia disorders: metabolic, hereditary, and genetic disorders in adults. In: Umphred DA (ed) Neurological rehabilitation. Mosby, St. Louis, p 661–695

Clinical Pointer 51.2

Pharmacotherapy for drug-induced movement disorder

Antipsychotics and antidopaminergic antiemetics cause extrapyramidal side-effects. Dopamine agonists (levodopa) cause chorea, dystonia and, rarely, myoclonus. CNS stimulants (amphetamine, cocaine and methylphenidate) increase dopamine turnover and cause tics and chorea in some people. Lithium has weak antidopaminergic actions that may be responsible for common tremor and rare dyskinesia. Antidepressants can cause tremor, although this is relatively rare (occurring in approximately 2–5% of patients), and even less often akathisia. Myoclonus and parkinsonism has been associated with treatment with tricyclic antidepressants and SSRIs. Oral contraceptives can cause dyskinesia, presumably owing to an effect of oestrogens on dopamine. Unfortunately, drug-induced extrapyramidal side-effects are overlooked in at least 50% of patients. Reduction in dose or discontinuation of medication (where possible) is the first sensible measure. Muscarinic antagonists are often prescribed for parkinsonism, although procyclidine and orphenadrine are stimulating, whereas benzatropine is mildly sedating.

Tremor, rigidity, bradykinesia as well as impaired postural reflexes, seborrhoea and cognitive impairment are features of secondary parkinsonism. The syndrome usually manifests itself 3–30 days after treatment is started, and it is more common in older patients. A dose reduction or change from a highly antidopaminergic drug to a lower potency drug are obvious methods to reduce secondary parkinsonism. Bradykinesia may be treated with biperiden or amantadine, and tremor and rigidity usually respond to anticholinergic treatment.

Dystonia most commonly presents acutely (24–96 hours) after initiation of treatment, most often in the young. Anticholinergics or benzodiazepines are usually effective. Chronic or persistent dystonia ('tardive dystonia') may occur in 2% of cases.

Akathisia is recognized as a common (25%) adverse drug effect, especially in middle-aged female patients. In some patients without feelings of distress, the term 'pseudoakathisia' has been used. Patients may complain of paraesthesia in the legs. It is associated with aggression, suicidal behaviour and poor compliance. Chronic akathisia can occur, particularly in association with tardive dyskinesia. Treatment with clonazepam, beta blockers, anticholinergics, clonidine or cyproheptadine may be useful.

Treatment options for tardive dyskinesia include gradual withdrawal of the antipsychotic agent, avoiding anticholinergics. Dopamine depleters (tetrabenazine), GABA mimetics (valproate), calcium channel blockers, vitamin E and cholinomimetics have also been tried, but the syndrome is often irreversible, although non-progressive.

Chorea and dystonia are often combined in levodopa-induced dyskinesia. Amantadine has been shown to be an effective treatment for this presentation.

Further reading   Cunningham Owens DG 1999 A guide to the extrapyramidal side-effects of antipsychotic drugs. Cambridge University Press, Cambridge

drawal of medication in the following order is indicated: anticholinergics, amantadine, selegiline, dopamine agonists, COMT inhibitors and, lastly, levodopa. This is in order of likely hazard–benefit ratio.

If unacceptable motor deterioration occurs, then antipsychotics should be prescribed, together with an antiparkinsonian agent. The atypical antipsychotics, including clozapine and risperidone, have been successfully used in Parkinson's patients (Friedman & Factors 2000). Risperidone is the least atypical of the atypical antipsychotics and can exacerbate extrapyramidal symptoms even in low doses. Open-label studies have been conducted with olanzapine and quetiapine. Two open studies and one randomized study found an exacerbation of motor symptoms in a high proportion of patients treated with olanzapine (Gimenez-Roldan et al 2001, Goetz et al 2000). Thus, at this point, clozapine may be the drug of choice, since it may actually improve extrapyramidal symptoms (as opposed to not worsening them) and has been shown to be effective in two multicentre RCTs, one in the USA and one in France (French Clozapine Parkinson Study Group 1999, Parkinson Study Group 1999). Hypotension, weight gain and agranulocytosis are the major concerns when using clozapine in patients with Parkinson's disease. Under the terms of its UK license, clozapine should be used only for patients with refractory schizophrenia by psychiatrists registered with the manufacturer's Clozaril Patient Monitoring Services (CPMS), and therefore it may have to be prescribed 'off licence'.

Antidementia strategies

The first question is to what extent existing therapies help cognition in patients with Parkinson's disease. Open-label studies and case reports have shown a modest improvement following treatment with selegiline, levodopa and tolcapone. However, the randomized DATATOP study (see above) using selegiline and tocopherol failed to show any preventive effect (Kieburtz et al 1994). Dopaminergic agents such as methylphenidate can improve aspects of cognition (particularly attention) in controls and children with attention deficit hyperactivity disorder (Kulisevsky 2000). This could be relevant to patients with and without dementia. Kulisevsky et al (2000) examined cognitive performance in 10 patients randomized to pergolide and 10 patients randomized to levodopa. Tests were performed before treatment and every 6 months up to

24 months. Both treatments were associated with a significant improvement in motor scores and in tests assessing learning and long-term verbal and visual memory, visuospatial abilities and various frontal tasks. Cognitive benefits were not sustained past 18 months. Attention, Stroop Test performance and short-term memory were not influenced by either treatment. In a second small RCT, bromocriptine showed beneficial effects on speed of processing but not on more advanced cognitive performance (Weddell & Weiser 1995). Overall then, pharmacological strategies currently do not offer much hope for patients with Parkinson's dementia, although some improvement should be expected with conventional treatment in those with more subtle cognitive deficits. Education, support and cognitive rehabilitation are therefore empirically indicated.

The second question is whether any other strategies benefit patients with Parkinson's disease who have cognitive impairment. Unfortunately, this question has not been sufficiently examined for a clear answer to be given. New atypical antipsychotics are thought at least not to exacerbate cognition in Parkinson's disease, but an improvement has not been shown (in contrast to similar studies in schizophrenia) (Aarsland et al 1999). Anticholinergics can easily exacerbate cognitive function in the elderly, and Parkinson's disease is no exception. However, it is also possible that low doses might improve cognitive function (or at least improve motor function and not exacerbate cognitive dysfunction) and therefore clinical judgement is necessary. One very interesting report, which has a parallel with work in Alzheimer's disease, is the use of oestrogen in Parkinson's disease. Marder et al (1998) reported an open-label, but reasonably sized, study of the effects of oestrogen replacement on women with Parkinson's disease (with and without dementia). There appeared to be a protective (or delaying) effect on the development of dementia, although the authors acknowledge that an RCT is necessary to confirm this. The first RCT of an acetylcholinesterase inhibitor in patients with dementia of Parkinson's disease has been reported by Aarsland et al (2002) in Norway. In a small cross-over study of 14 patients, the authors randomized 14 patients to 10 weeks of donepezil or 10 weeks of placebo. After 10 weeks, there was an improvement in cognition in the donepezil group but not in the placebo group, with no exacerbation of motor symptoms. A soon to be reported randomized controlled trial from Laura Marsh's group involving 16 cognitively impaired patients with Parkinson's disease also showed modest effects of donepzil over placebo, although the drug was poorly tolerated.

SUMMARY

The management of neuropsychiatric complications of Parkinson's disease can be summarized as follows:

- many patients will have unacceptable symptoms of either depression or anxiety (even mild symptoms should be considered as an indication for treatment)
- evaluate patients carefully, because somatic symptoms of Parkinson's disease can overlap with depression, apathy and adverse effects of medication
- differentiate between three common presentations of psychosis – in clear consciousness, in delirium and in those with dementia
- screen for cognitive impairment in the young and for dementia in the elderly
- use psychotropics with particular care (beware of hypotension, exacerbation of motor symptoms and drug interactions)
- consider clozapine or quetiapine as first-line treatment for psychosis
- consider sertraline as first-line treatment for depression or anxiety
- consider acetylcholinesterase inhibitors in the treatment of Parkinson's dementia.

REFERENCES AND FURTHER READING

Aarsland D, Larsen JP, Lim NG et al 1999 Olanzapine for psychosis in patients with Parkinson's disease with and without dementia. Journal of Neuropsychiatry and Clinical Neuroscience 11:392–394

Aarsland D, Laake K, Larsen JP et al 2002 Donepezil for cognitive impairment in Parkinson's disease: a randomised controlled study. Journal of Neuropsychiatry, Neurosurgery and Neuropsychiatry 72:708–712

Ahlskog JE 2001 Parkinson's disease: medical and surgical treatment. Neurologic Clinics 19:579–605

Allain H, Cougnard J, Neukirch HC et al 1991 Selegiline in de novo parkinsonian patients: the French multicenter trial (FSMT). Acta Neurologica Scandanivica 84(suppl 136):73–78

Carrieri PB, Indaco A, Gentile S et al 1990 S-Adenosylmethionine treatment of depression in patients with Parkinson's disease. A double-blind, crossover study versus placebo. Current Therapies in Research and Clinical Experiments 48:154–160

Clarkson ED 2001 Fetal tissue transplantation for patients with Parkinson's disease: a database of published clinical results. Drugs and Aging 18:773–785

Corrigan MH, Denahan AQ, Wright CE et al 2000 Comparison of pramipexole, fluoxetine, and placebo in patients with major depression. Depression and Anxiety 11:58–65

French Clozapine Parkinson Study Group 1999 Clozapine in drug induced psychosis in Parkinson's disease. Lancet 353:2041–2042

Friedman JH, Factors SA 2000 Atypical antipsychotics in the treatment of drug-induced psychosis in Parkinson's disease. Movement Disorders 15:201–211

Gimenez-Roldan S, Mateo D, Navarro E et al 2001 Efficacy and safety of clozapine and olanzapine: an open-label study comparing two groups of Parkinson's disease patients with dopaminergic-induced psychosis. Parkinsonism and Related Disorders 7:121–127

Goetz CG, Blasucci LM, Leurgans S et al 2000 Olanzapine and clozapine: comparative effects on motor function in hallucinating PD patients. Neurology 55:789–794

Jansen-Steur ENH, Ballering LAP 1999 Combined and selective monoamine oxidase inhibition in the treatment of depression in Parkinson's disease. Advances in Neurology 80:505–508

Kieburtz K, McDermott M, Como P et al 1994 The effect of deprenyl and tocopherol on cognitive performance in early untreated Parkinson's disease. Parkinson's Study Group. Neurology 44:1756–1759

Klassen T, Verhey FRJ, Sneijders GHJM et al 1995 Treatment of depression in Parkinson's disease: a meta-analysis. Journal of Neuropsychiatry and Clinical Neurosciences 7:281–286

Kulisevsky J 2000 Role of dopamine in learning and memory: implications for the treatment of cognitive dysfunction in patients with Parkinson's disease. Drugs and Aging 16:365–379

Kulisevsky J, Garcia-Sanchez C, Berthier ML et al 2000 Chronic effects of dopaminergic replacement on cognitive function in Parkinson's disease: a two-year follow-up study of previously untreated patients. Movement Disorders 15:613–626

Lees AJ 1995 Comparison of therapeutic effects and mortality data of levodopa and levodopa combined with selegiline in patients with early, mild Parkinson's disease. BMJ 311:1602–1607

Marder K, Tang M-X, Alfaro B et al 1998 Postmenopausal estrogen use and Parkinson's disease with and without dementia. Neurology 50:1141–1143

Miyasaki JM, Martin W, Suchowersky O et al 2002 Practice parameter: initiation of treatment for Parkinson's disease: an evidence-based review. Neurology 58:11–17

Moore AP, Clarke C 2001 Parkinson's disease. In: Barton S (ed) Clinical evidence, issue 6. BMJ Publishing Group, London, p 1019–1028

Olanow CW, Watts RL, Koller WC 2001 An algorithm (decision tree) for the management of Parkinson's disease: treatment guidelines. Neurology 56(suppl 5):s1–s88

Parkinson Study Group 1999 Low-dose clozapine for the treatment of drug-induced hallucinations in Parkinson's disease. New England Journal of Medicine 340:757–763

Rascol O, Brooks DJ, Korczyn AD et al for the 056 Study Group 2000 A five-year study of the incidence of dyskinesia in patients with early Parkinson's disease who were treated with ropinirole or levodopa. New England Journal of Medicine 342:1484–1491

Richard IH, Kurlan R, Tanner C et al 1997 Serotonin syndrome and the combined use of deprenyl and an antidepressant in Parkinson's disease. Neurology 48:1070–1077

Richard IH, Maughn A, Kurlan R 1999 Do serotonin reuptake inhibitor antidepressants worsen Parkinson's disease? A retrospective case series. Movement Disorders 14:155–157

Shoulson I, Oakes D, Fahn S et al 2002 Impact of sustained deprenyl (selegiline) in levodopa-treated Parkinson's disease: a randomized placebo-controlled extension of the Deprenyl and Tocopherol Antioxidative Therapy of Parkinsonism Trial. Annals of Neurology 515:604–612

Toyama SC, Iacono RP 1994 Is it safe to combine a selective serotonin reuptake inhibitor with selegiline. Annals of Pharmacotherapy 28:405–406

Vazquez A, Jimenez-Jimenez FJ, Garcia-Ruiz P et al 1993 'Panic attacks' in Parkinson's disease. A long-term complication of levodopa therapy. Acta Neurologica Scandinavica 87:14–18

Weddell RA, Weiser R 1995 A double-blind cross-over placebo-controlled trial of the effects of bromocriptine on psychomotor function, cognition, and mood in de novo patients with Parkinson's disease. Behavioral Pharmacology 6:81–91

Wichmann T, Delong MR 2002 Neurocircuitry of Parkinson's disease. In: Davis KL, Charney D, Coyle JT et al (eds) Neuropsychopharmacology: the fifth generation of progress. Lippincott Williams & Wilkins, Philadelphia, p 1761–1779

52

Treatment in Patients with Huntington's Disease and Chorea

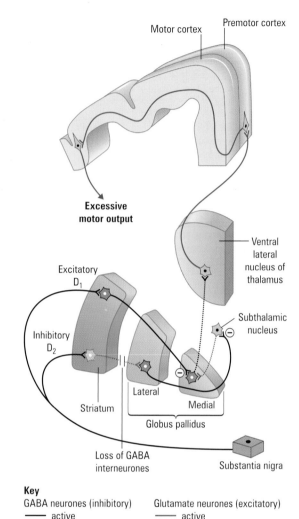

Fig. 52.1 Pathophysiology of Huntington's disease. GABA and enkephalin striatopallidal neurones projecting to the globus pallidus externus are affected in the very early grades of the disease. Loss of the GABA neurones that project from the pallidum (striatum) to the lateral or external globus pallidus disinhibits the GABA neurones that act on the subthalamic nucleus. The subthalamic nucleus becomes relatively inactive and, in turn, overactivates the lateral nucleus of the thalamus and the motor cortex. As the disease progresses, GABA and substance P striatonigral neurones (projecting to the substantia nigra) and striatopallidal neurones (projecting to the globus pallidus internus) are involved.

Huntington's disease is a neurodegenerative movement disorder that is often difficult to treat. The neuropsychiatric symptoms are so integral to the degenerative disease that it is difficult to subdivide treatments into those aimed at managing chorea and those aimed at managing cognition or mood. That said, few treatment studies of Huntington's disease have included useful psychiatric outcome measures.

TREATMENT OF THE CHOREA OF HUNTINGTON'S DISEASE

Haloperidol, fluphenazine and sulpiride are used to treat the chorea of Huntington's disease; alternatives are the monoamine depleter tetrabenazine (which can induce depression) and anticholinergics (sometimes at high doses), although these treatments are not supported by high-quality evidence-based research. Clinicians prescribing typical antipsychotics attempt to avoid extrapyramidal symptoms by beginning with a low dose and increasing it gradually. Levodopa and dopamine agonists rarely help the akinetic–rigid syndrome seen in some patients, although amantadine or an anticholinergic can be partially effective.

Clinical Pointer 52.1

A practical approach to the treatment of apathy

Apathy is one of the most difficult symptoms to treat in psychiatry. In part this is because a complex mixture of cognitive, biological and social factors influence volition. The starting place must be adequate encouragement and incentive for the patient. A person who dislikes his or her day centre is unlikely to be enthusiastic about attending! The next step is to exclude possible confounding influences on motivation. Most important is depression, but consider also any physical illness, agoraphobia, the negative syndrome of schizophrenia, chronic fatigue and tiredness, and any sleep problem. The next consideration is the adverse influence of drugs. These might be side effects of prescribed medication (e.g. parkinsonism, cognitive dysfunction, sedation) or adverse effects of non-prescribed medication (particularly cannabis, alcohol and sedatives). A general rule of thumb is to avoid high doses of conventional antipsychotics, benzodiazepines and sedative antiepileptic drugs when attempting to treat apathy empirically. When present, an underlying neuropsychiatric condition should be identified and conventionally treated. The characteristics of apathy in various neurological diseases are discussed throughout this text.

The next and arguably the most beneficial step in most cases is to institute a graded behavioural program. The basic principles are as follows. Begin with the simplest tasks, allow the patient to set the agenda for change in advance, draw up an increasing schedule of daily activities, incorporate repetition of each task until it becomes routine, and allow some variation in performance. At the same time encourage and support the patient as much as possible. If difficulties occur, the carer will often have to accompany the patient and model each step before the patient tries for himself or herself. The key point is that the progress is slow but achievable.

Finally, there is the option of specific medication to enhance drive. None has been subject to a RCT and therefore all should be used with caution. The options are dopamine-enhancing drugs and antidepressants. There are case reports of benefit with methylphenidate, levodopa, bromocriptine and possibly bupropion and reboxetine. Clinical experience suggests higher chances of success when there are few maintaining factors and few neurological deficits.

Further reading *Campbell JJ, Duffy JD 1997 Treatment strategies in amotivated patients. Psychiatric Annals 27:44–49*

An examination of the literature for randomized controlled trials in the treatment of Huntington's disease reveals one small placebo-controlled study for each of the following drugs: acetyl-L-carnitine (Goetz et al 1990), cannabidiol (Consroe et al 1991), clozapine (VanVugt et al 1997), fluoxetine (Como et al 1997), ketamine (Murman et al 1997), milacemide (Giuffra et al 1992), piracetam (Mateo & Gimenez-Roldan 1996) and tiapride (Deroover et al 1984). Although nearly all of these agents have had little effect on chorea, the small size of the studies increases the chance of a false-negative finding. Two studies have examined the glutamate receptor ion-channel blocker remacemide hydrochloride (Kieburtz et al 1996, 2001). After encouraging results from the first small trial, remacemide was compared with coenzyme Q10 in the largest multi-centre study of early Huntington's disease (2001) (Kieburtz et al 2001). A total of 347 patients were randomized to coenzyme Q10 600 mg/day, remacemide hydrochloride 200 mg/day, both treatments or neither treatment for a total of 30 months. Patients treated with coenzyme Q10 showed a trend toward slowing in functional decline, although the difference between groups was only 13%. Verhagen et al (2002) conducted a double-blind cross-over study of amantadine versus placebo in 24 patients with genetically confirmed Huntington's disease. Approximately half the group showed a response to amantadine, with a greater than 30% improvement in chorea at rest. However, there was no cognitive benefit. In an impressive study of 64 patients with early Huntington's disease (defined as less than 5 years' duration), Kremer et al (1999) examined the ability of lamotrigine to slow the deterioration of Huntington's disease. At 30 months, there was no clear evidence that lamotrigine retarded the rate of progression, but more patients on lamotrigine reported symptomatic improvement and there was a trend toward decreased chorea. Against expectations, cognitive performance improved over the study period in both drug and placebo groups.

TREATMENT OF THE NEUROPSYCHIATRIC COMPLICATIONS OF HUNTINGTON'S DISEASE

I am not aware of any good-quality therapeutic studies on the psychiatric complications of Huntington's disease. In time, such studies are certain to appear, but until then clinicians must still treat patients to the best of their ability. In early Huntington's disease, patients may reasonably opt for non-pharmacological strategies to control symptoms of anxiety or depression. That said, there no reason to consider depression or anxiety to be refractory to conventional pharmacological treatment, although maximum benefit is likely to result from a package of care. Irritability and aggression are complex symptoms that can benefit from treatment in the majority of cases. Common sense advice of avoiding stressful triggers and maximizing the quality of daily routines is the first step. Irritability is often a symptom of depression; if so, this should be addressed. Psychological interventions for irritability include anger management, relaxation strategies and family therapy. Case reports and clinical experience support the use of selective serotonin reuptake inhibitors, carbamazepine and divalproex sodium in the treatment of illness-related irritability (see Ch. 49).

In the later stages of Huntington's disease, cognitive deficits and apathy are very difficult to manage. The treatment of apathy is discussed in Clinical Pointer 52.1. Strategies for patients with failing cognitive function are largely those of simplifying the tasks that patients are required to perform so that they can manage their environment safely and with dignity.

SUMMARY

The management of the neuropsychiatric complications of Huntington's disease can be summarized as follows:

- beware of side effects of psychotropic drugs used to treat chorea
- screen for irritability, aggression, depression and anxiety early in the course of disease
- expect to find apathy, irritability or dementia late in the course of disease and offer multidisciplinary treatment if these features are present
- where possible, use non-pharmacological treatments
- differentiate between three presentations of psychosis – in clear consciousness, in delirium and in those with dementia

- consider in advance the implications of screening relatives.

REFERENCES AND FURTHER READING

Como PG, Rubin AJ, O'Brien CF et al 1997 A controlled trial of fluoxetine in nondepressed patients with Huntington's disease. Movement Disorders 12:397–401

Consroe P, Laguna J, Allender J et al 1991 Controlled clinical trial of cannabidiol in Huntington's disease. Pharmacology, Biochemistry and Behavior 40:701–708

Deroover J, Baro F, Bourguignon RP et al 1984 Tiapride versus placebo: a double-blind comparative study in the management of Huntington's chorea. Current Medical Research and Opinions 9:329–338

Giuffra ME, Mouradian MM, Chase TN 1992 Glutamatergic therapy of Huntington's chorea. Clinical Neuropharmacology 15:148–151

Glass M, Dragunow M, Faull RLM 2000 The pattern of neurodegradation in Huntington's disease: a comparative study of cannabinoid, dopamine, adenosine and GABA(A) receptor alterations in the human basal ganglia in Huntington's disease. Neuroscience 97:505–519

Goetz CG, Tanner CM, Cohen JA et al 1990 L-Acetylcarnitine in Huntington's disease: double-blind placebo controlled crossover study of drug effects on movement disorder and dementia. Movement Disorders 5:263–266

Kieburtz K, Feigin A, McDermott M et al 1996 A controlled trial of remacemide hydrochloride in Huntington's disease. Movement Disorders 11:273–277

Kieburtz K, Koroshetz W, McDermott M et al 2001 A randomized, placebo-controlled trial of coenzyme Q(10) and remacemide in Huntington's disease. Neurology 57:397–404

Kremer B, Clark CM, Almqvist EW et al 1999 Influence of lamotrigine on progression of early Huntington disease: a randomized clinical trial. Neurology 53:1000–1011

Mateo D, Gimenez-Roldan S 1996 The effect of piracetam on involuntary movements in Huntington's disease: a double-blind randomised comparative study. Journal of Neurology 11:16–19

Murman DL, Giordani B, Mellow AM et al 1997 Cognitive, behavioral, and motor effects of the NMDA antagonist ketamine in Huntington's disease. Neurology 49:153–161

VanVugt JPP, Siesling S, Vergeer M et al 1997 Clozapine versus placebo in Huntington's disease: a double blind randomised comparative study. Journal of Neurology, Neurosurgery and Psychiatry 63:35–39

Verhagen ML, Morris MJ, Farmer C et al 2002 Huntington's disease. A randomized, controlled trial using the NMDA-antagonist amantadine. Neurology 59:694–699

53

Treatment in Patients with Tourette's Syndrome and Tics

Tourette's syndrome is a chronic movement disorder that is much misunderstood and is most often manifest in children and adolescents. Provision of sensible information is vital to help patients and families cope with this socially distressing condition. In addition to tics, there is often comorbid behavioural disturbance, obsessive–compulsive disorder, attention deficit hyperactivity disorder (ADHD) and self-injurious behaviour. There is also the complicating factor of the early age of onset of this condition. Many drugs are not licensed for use in children, understandably given that the long-term implications of drugs such as typical antipsychotics have not been studied in young people. Epidemiological evidence appears to suggest that the prognosis of Tourette's syndrome is much improved when treated (Robertson 2000).

PHARMACOLOGICAL TREATMENT

There have been at least 20 double-blind randomized controlled trials (RCTs) in Tourette's syn-

drome, usually, it must be said, of very poor quality. The majority of trials have shown a consistent benefit of antidopaminergic agents on the tics of Tourette's syndrome. If one looks for trials that have enrolled more than 20 patients with Tourette's syndrome, the field is cut to a handful of studies. In a much-quoted study, Shapiro et al (1989) from the Tourette Clinic in New York 57 sufferers were randomized to haloperidol, pimozide and placebo. Beneficial effects were seen in both active arms, but the study was underpowered to detect a true difference between active drugs. Haloperidol, sulpiride and pimozide are the most commonly investigated antipsychotics, but there is no good evidence that suggests any particular drug has superior efficacy, and side effects occur in many patients (Shapiro & Shapiro 1993).

Given their safety profile, there is interest in the use of atypical antipsychotics. Early open-label studies with risperidone were somewhat encouraging, but not convincing. Recently, Bruggeman et al (2001) reported a 12-week multicentre study that enrolled 50 patients with Tourette's syndrome and randomized them to risperidone ($n = 26$, mean daily dose 3.8 mg) or pimozide ($n = 24$, mean daily dose 2.9 mg). Fifty-four per cent of the risperidone patients and 38% of the pimozide patients had only mild or no symptoms at the endpoint, and symptoms of anxiety and depressive mood improved in both groups. Improvement in obsessive–compulsive behaviour was significant only in the risperidone group, although groups were not matched for obsessive–compulsive disorder at baseline. Moreover, outcome was assessed using the Tourette's Syndrome Severity Scale, which has been criticized for its imprecise ratings.

Dopamine agonists as well as antagonists have been tried in Tourette's syndrome. Pergolide is a dopamine agonist (more active at D_2 than D_1 receptors) that is used widely in Parkinson's disease. Gilbert et al (2000) reported the first double-blind, placebo-controlled, cross-over trial of pergolide, in 24 children age 7–17 years with Tourette's syndrome. Children were randomized to receive either placebo or up to 300 µg/day of pergolide for the first 6-week treatment period, with a 1-week placebo washout, followed by cross-over to the other treatment. Compared with placebo treatment, pergolide treatment was associated with significantly improved tic severity. No patient had a serious adverse event and pergolide was well tolerated.

In a similar vein, the monoamine oxidase inhibitor selegiline has been subject to one placebo controlled trial in Tourette's syndrome. Feigin et al (1996) conducted a trial in 24 children with Tourette's syndrome and comorbid ADHD. There were two 8-week treatments periods separated by a 6-week washout, but only 15 subjects completed this course. Overall, there was not a convincing effect of selegiline on either tics or ADHD.

One group has investigated the nicotine antagonist and antihypertensive drug mecamylamine in 61 Tourette's syndrome patients aged between 8 and 17 years (Silver et al 2001). It was not shown to be effective as monotherapy in this study.

Clonidine (an α_2-adrenoceptor agonist) is thought to be effective in Tourette's syndrome following the results of a modest-quality RCT (Leckman et al 1991). Twenty-one subjects completed a 12-week trial on clonidine and were compared with 19 subjects on placebo. Both groups showed improvements, although these were greater in the clonidine group. Singer et al (1995) from Johns Hopkins Hospital in Baltimore compared clonidine with desipramine and placebo in a randomized, triple cross-over design. Thirty-four children with comorbid Tourette's syndrome and ADHD completed the protocol of 6-week medication cycles with clonidine (0.05 mg four times daily), desipramine (25 mg four times daily) and placebo. Desipramine showed global benefits, whereas clonidine was disappointing, not positively affecting tics at all. Guanfacine is another α_2-adrenoceptor agonist. It has been reported to have less hypotensive and sedative effects. Scahill et al (2001) reported the effects in a modest-sized RCT in which 17 boys with ADHD and a tic received guanfacine and 17 received placebo for 8 weeks. Guanfacine was associated with a mean improvement of 37% in a teacher-rated ADHD Rating Scale and 31% in tic severity, compared with 8% and 0%, respectively, for placebo

Castellanos et al (1997) conducted a 9-week RCT of methylphenidate, dexamphetamine and placebo in boys with both tics and ADHD. There seemed to be an advantage for methylphenidate, although there is some question whether appropriate doses were used in this trial. The Tourette's Syndrome Study Group (2002) conducted a trial of methylphenidate alone ($n = 37$), clonidine alone ($n = 34$), clonidine plus methylphenidate ($n = 33$) and placebo ($n = 32$). The combined group showed maximal benefit. Furthermore, the clonidine group improved most on measures of impulsivity and hyperactivity, whereas the methylphenidate group improved most on inattention. Methylphenidate did not exacerbate tics in this study. Focal motor tics are sometimes treated with injections of botulinum toxin, a treatment that is effective and safe and lasts for several months.

MANAGEMENT OF COMORBID CONDITIONS

In patients troubled by comorbid obsessive–compulsive disorder, conventional treatment is indicated (Soomro 2001). That is, an SSRI. Clomipramine is equally (or almost equally) effective but has more side effects, and it therefore should usually be used as a second-line treatment. Third-line options are antipsychotics and monoamine oxidase inhibitors. Cognitive therapy or behavioural therapy (or a combination) are intensive but effective forms of treatment, where local resources allow.

In those with ADHD, conventional treatment is again indicated. Ten out of 13 brief RCTs show that the amphetamine derivative methylphenidate is more effective than placebo, and three out of four studies suggest it is equally as effective as dexamphetamine. Mild side effects, including anorexia, insomnia, headaches, irritability and abdominal pain, are common. Five RCTs support the use of clonidine, although its merit compared with methylphenidate is unknown (Joughin et al 2001). One RCT shows comparable effectiveness of guanfacine and dexamphetamine (Taylor & Russo 2001). A handful of studies also support the use of tricyclic antidepressants. Stimulants may also be of use in conduct disorder, although no trials exist in cohorts with Tourette's syndrome (Baving & Schmidt 2001).

SUMMARY

Patients with Tourette's syndrome, and their relatives, always require advice and support and this may be sufficient in patients with mild symptoms and good function. Clonidine and antipsychotics are often the mainstay of conventional pharmacological treatment, and it is likely that, as more studies are reported, atypical antipsychotics will be preferred, mainly on account of their better side-effect profile. Guanfacine is particularly promising option, with few side effects, and may be the drug of choice in children, especially those with comorbid ADHD. The value of behavioural treatment, family intervention, education and support has not been discussed here, but is particularly important in children struggling to come to terms with this severe movement disorder.

The management of the neuropsychiatric complications of Tourette's syndrome can be summarized as follows:

- no pharmacological treatment may be necessary
- consider risperidone for first-line treatment of tics in adults
- consider clonidine or guanfacine for first-line treatment in children or in those with comorbid ADHD
- use conventional treatment for obsessive–compulsive disorder and mood disorder, if present
- offer support and information to all patients and their families.

REFERENCES AND FURTHER READING

Baving L, Schmidt MH 2001 Evaluated treatment approaches in child and adolescent psychiatry I. Zeitschrift fur Kinder- und Jugendpsychiatrie und Psychotherapie 29:189–205

Bruggeman R, van der Linden C, Buitelaar JK et al 2001 Risperidone versus pimozide in Tourette's disorder: a comparative double-blind parallel-group study. Journal of Clinical Psychiatry 62:50–56

Castellanos FX, Elia J, Marsh WL et al 1997 Controlled stimulant treatment of ADHD and comorbid Tourette's syndrome: effects of stimulant and dose. Journal of the American Academy of Child and Adolescent Psychiatry 36:589–596

Feigin A, Kurlan R, McDermott MP et al 1996 A controlled trial of deprenyl in children with Tourette's syndrome and attention deficit hyperactivity disorder. Neurology 46:965–968

Gilbert DL, Sethuraman G, Sine L et al 2000 Tourette's syndrome improvement with pergolide in a randomized, double-blind, crossover trial. Neurology 54:1310–1315

Joughin C, Zwi M, Ramchandani P 2001 Attention deficit hyperactivity disorder in children. In: Barton S (ed) Clinical evidence, issue 6. BMJ Publishing Group, p 234–242

Leckman JF, Hardin MT, Riddle MA et al 1991 Clonidine treatment of Gilles de la Tourette's syndrome. Archives of General Psychiatry 48:324–328

Robertson MM 2000 Tourette syndrome, associated conditions and the complexities of treatment. Brain 123:425–462

Scahill L, Chappell PB, Kim YS et al 2001 A placebo-controlled study of guanfacine in the treatment of children with tic disorders and attention deficit hyperactivity disorder. American Journal of Psychiatry 158:1067–1074

Shapiro AK, Shapiro E 1993 Neuroleptic drugs. In: Kurlan R (ed) Handbook of Tourette's syndrome and related tic and behavioural disorders. Marcel Dekker, New York, p 347–377

Shapiro E, Shapiro AK, Fulop G et al 1989 Controlled-study of haloperidol, pimozide, and placebo for the treatment of Gilles-de-la-Tourette syndrome. Archives of General Psychiatry 46:722–730

Silver AA, Shytle RD, Sheehan KH et al 2001 Multicenter, double-blind, placebo-controlled study of mecamylamine monotherapy for Tourette's disorders. Journal of the American Academy of Child and Adolescent Psychiatry 40:1103–1110

Singer HS, Brown J, Quaskey S et al 1995 The treatment of attention-deficit hyperactivity disorder in Tourette's syndrome: a double-blind placebo-controlled study with clonidine and desipramine. Pediatrics 95:74–81

Soomro GM 2001 Obsessive compulsive disorder. In: Barton S (ed) Clinical evidence, issue 6. BMJ Publishing Group, London, p 754–762

Taylor FB, Russo J 2001 Comparing guanfacine and dextroamphetamine for the treatment of adult attention-deficit/hyperactivity disorder. Journal of Clinical Psychopharmacology 21:223–228

Tourette's Syndrome Study Group 2002 Treatment of ADHD in children with tics. A randomized controlled trial. Neurology 58:527–536

54

Treatment in Patients with Wilson's Disease

Zinc acetate (Galzin) is approved by the Food and Drug Administration in the USA for presymptomatic and maintenance treatment, and it is preferred by many experts for pregnant and paediatric patients. However, it acts too slowly for initial monotherapy. Tetrathiomolybdate is an alternative depleting agent that may be the drug of choice for patients presenting with neurological symptoms. Tetrathiomolybdate is the least likely agent to cause neurological exacerbations and works more quickly than zinc alone. Such treatments may be used in conjunction with a low-copper diet. Recommendations are that urinary copper excretion should reach values below 80 mg/day. With this regimen, the outcome is generally good. Walshe & Yealland (1993) studied 137 patients with neurological complications of Wilson's disease. Two-thirds improved substantially, but 11 patients died despite adequate treatment. An improvement in clinical symptoms is often seen within 6 months and continuous therapy provides near-normal life-expectancy.

NEUROLOGICAL TREATMENT OF WILSON'S DISEASE

Although Wilson's disease was originally described in 1883, it took another half century before an effective treatment became available. The chelating agent British anti-Lewisite (BAL) was developed during World War I as an antidote to arsenic poisoning. When it was administered to patients with Wilson's disease in 1948, Mandelbrote and colleagues found increases in urinary copper excretion, which was subsequently discovered to be therapeutic by Denny-Brown & Porter (1951). The copper chelator D-penicillamine then became the standard treatment for many years. The agent is effective, but can cause disabling side effects such as hypersensitivity reactions, systemic lupus erythematosus and nephrotic syndrome, in up to one-quarter of patients. For this reason, more recent chelators, such as trientine, and copper depleters, such as tetrathiomolybdate and zinc, are preferred. The action of depleters is to induce renal and biliary copper excretion and increase synthesis of metallothionein, which detoxifies intracellular copper. Although there are currently no randomized controlled trials in this area, several are in progress and long-term prospective studies have been performed (Brewer et al 1998).

TREATMENT OF THE NEUROPSYCHIATRIC COMPLICATIONS OF WILSON'S DISEASE

The reader will not be surprised to discover there are no substantial studies concerning the treatment of neuropsychiatric complications of Wilson's disease. From first principles, many symptoms are reflections of CNS disease, and therefore the underlying disease process should be the focus of attention. Examples of psychiatric symptoms that are likely to reflect underlying CNS lesions include cognitive impairment, delirium, pure mania, emotionalism, disinhibition and personality change. Consistent with this, Dening & Berrios (1990) reported than incongruous behaviour and cognition improve more than irritability and depression following conventional treatment.

The main issue when treating psychiatric symptoms is adverse effects. The use of psychotropic medication must be considered carefully. Patients with Wilson's disease and basal ganglia involvement may tolerate antipsychotics and antidepressants poorly, owing to exacerbations of parkinsonism and tremor. In the subgroup of patients with seizures, the effect of psychotropic drugs on seizure threshold should be taken into account (see Ch. 48). Cardiac conduc-

Clinical Pointer 54.1

Prescribing psychotropic drugs in liver disease

There are three issues to consider about psychotropics and liver disease. Does the drug exacerbate pre-existing liver disease? Does the liver disease cause pharmacokinetic problems? Are interactions of particular concern?

In depression, as a rule of thumb, the dose of an antidepressant should be reduced by one-half in moderate liver disease. Irreversible monoamine oxidase inhibitors can be hepatotoxic.

In psychosis, it is worth noting that amisulpride and sulpiride do not undergo significant metabolism by the liver. Ziprasidone also appears to be well tolerated in liver disease.

Several anticonvulsants are not metabolized significantly by the liver. These include gabapentin, piracetam, topiramate and vigabatrin.

Sedative drugs should be prescribed with particular caution, since they may precipitate liver encephalopathy at the same time as masking the signs. The terminal benzodiazepine metabolites lorazepam and oxazepam are generally considered to be the benzodiazepines of choice.

Further reading   Collis I, Lloyd G 1992 Psychiatric aspects of liver disease. British Journal of Psychiatry 161:12–22

tion abnormalities may be seen in up to one-third of patients with Wilson's disease. For this reason ECG monitoring is required when tricyclic antidepressants and antipsychotics are given. Clearly, liver disease is an important complicating factor (Clinical Pointer 54.1). Impaired drug metabolism can cause drug accumulation or unexpected interactions. When present, hepatic encephalopathy may need to be treated.

SUMMARY

The management of the neuropsychiatric complications of Wilson's disease can be summarized as follows:

- investigate for Wilson's disease in all patients who present with abnormal movements and impaired liver function
- screen for irritability, depression and cognitive deficits

- offer disease-modifying treatments early
- beware of late neurological and psychiatric complications
- beware of psychotropic drugs in patients with established liver disease.

REFERENCES AND FURTHER READING

Brewer GJ, Dick RD, Johnson VD et al 1998 Treatment of Wilson's disease with zinc: XV. Long-term follow-up studies. Journal of Laboratory and Clinical Medicine 132:264–278

Dening TR, Berrios GE 1990 Wilson's disease: a longitudinal study of psychiatric symptoms. Biological Psychiatry 28:255–265

Denny-Brown D, Porter H 1951 The effect of BAL (2,3-dimercaptopropanol) on hepatolenticular degeneration (Wilson's disease). New England Journal of Medicine 245:917–925

Walshe JM, Yealland M 1993 Chelation treatment of neurological Wilson's disease. Quarterly Journal of Medicine 86:197–204

55

Treatment in Patients with Specific Movement Complaints

TREATMENTS IN PATIENTS WITH ABNORMAL MOVEMENTS

Myoclonus

Piracetam is occasionally used for myoclonus of cortical origin, its use being supported by evidence from three open trials and two double-blind trials (Genton et al 1999). Although side effects are generally infrequent, high doses often have to be used. Piracetam and levetiracetam (an (S)-enantiomer) are pyrrolidone derivatives. Piracetam is a nootropic drug used in the therapy of age-related cognitive disturbances and stroke, whereas levetiracetam is primarily an antiepileptic drug (AED), although it is under investigation for myoclonus.

Tremor

Essential tremor is usually persistent and progressive. Essential tremor and tremor from other causes is often treated with propranolol, given in a dose of 40–320 mg/day (Koller et al 2000). This is support-

ed by evidence from nine small randomized controlled trials (RCTs) (Sampaio & Ferreira 2001). Primidone is a barbiturate that is metabolized to phenobarbitone. Evidence from two cross-over RCTs and clinical experience suggests that, in some cases, this drug can provide relief from benign essential tremor, but at a cost of possible sedation, daytime sleepiness, tiredness and depression. These options are supported by reasonable evidence.

Recently, there has been interest in the possibility that new AEDs (including gabapentin) are effective in essential tremor. The evidence is not yet conclusive (Gironell et al 1999).

Tremor associated with multiple sclerosis and cerebellar disease and neuropathic tremor may respond to propranolol or clonazapam, but these tremors are in many cases resistant to treatment.

Dystonia

There is an accumulating number of studies in the treatment of dystonia. The use of botulinum toxin has improved the quality of life of patients with this painful condition compared with the older treatment with trihexyphenidyl tablets. Two forms of toxin, botulinum toxin type A and type B, have proven effective in multicentre trials in subjects with cervical dystonia. Patients who are resistant to botulinum toxin type A will often respond to type B (Brashear 2001).

TREATMENTS IN PATIENTS WITH DRUG-INDUCED ABNORMAL MOVEMENTS

Akathisia

Propranolol and other lipophilic beta blockers seem to be the most effective treatments for acute akathisia. If these are ineffective, benzodiazepines would appear to be a sensible next choice. Other agents that have been investigated include amantadine or clonidine, ritanserin, piracetam, sodium valproate and bicyclic and tricyclic antidepressants (Miller & Fleischhacker 2000).

Tardive dyskinesia

Tardive dyskinesia is one of the most unwelcome effects of prescribed medication. In two-thirds of cases it is irreversible, even following discontinuation of the suspected drug, and therefore prevention must always be the main therapeutic goal. This can be achieved by minimizing exposure to antipsychotic medication, particularly in those who develop early extrapyramidal side effects. Patients who begin to develop signs of tardive dyskinesia while taking typical antipsychotics should certainly be switched to atypical agents.

Many potential treatments for tardive dyskinesia have been suggested and several have been subject to RCT methodology. A meta-analysis showed that baclofen, deanol and diazepam were no more effective than placebo (Soares & McGrath 1999). Limited success has been achieved in RCTs of levodopa, clonidine, oxypertine, sodium valproate, tiapride and vitamin E, although further adverse effects must be considered. There is an association between the presence of tardive dyskinesia and both cognitive deficits and the negative syndrome of schizophrenia. It remains to be seen whether this is due to a shared risk factor or to a confounding effect of long-term antipsychotic medication.

The pharmacotherapy of other drug-induced movement disorders is discussed in Clinical Pointer 51.2.

SUMMARY

The management of specific movement complaints can be summarized as follows:

- always consider drug-induced causes of movement disorder, particularly agitation versus akathisia and Parkinson's disease versus parkinsonism
- consider long-term complications in those with movement disorder
- screen for neuropsychiatric complications, particularly cognitive impairment and depression
- avoid long-term exposure to typical antipsychotics, particularly in those with early extrapyramidal side effects.

REFERENCES AND FURTHER READING

Brashear A 2001 The botulinum toxins in the treatment of cervical dystonia. Seminars in Neurology 21:85–90

Genton P, Guerrini R, Remy C 1999 Piracetam in the treatment of cortical myoclonus. Pharmacopsychiatry 32(suppl 1):49–53

Gironell A, Kulisevsky J, Barbanoj M et al 1999 A randomized placebo-controlled comparative trial of gabapentin and propranolol in essential tremor. Archives of Neurology 56:475–480

Koller WC, Hristova A, Brin M 2000 Pharmacologic treatment of essential tremor. Neurology 54(suppl 4):S30–S38

Miller CH, Fleischhacker WW 2000 Managing antipsychotic-induced acute and chronic akathisia. Drug Safety 22:73–81

Sampaio C, Ferreira J 2001 Essential tremor. In: Barton S (ed) Clinical evidence, issue 6. BMJ, London, p 981–989

Soares KVS, McGrath JJ 1999 The treatment of tardive dyskinesia: a systematic review and meta-analysis. Schizophrenia Research 39:1–16

56

Treatment in Patients with Alzheimer's Disease

TREATMENTS FOR AGE-ASSOCIATED MEMORY IMPAIRMENT AND MILD COGNITIVE IMPAIRMENT

There are currently few informative studies concerning mild cognitive impairment and age-associated memory impairment. Oestrogen in the form of hormone replacement therapy for post-menopausal women has been examined, mainly in epidemiological studies, with promising results. Several randomized controlled trials (RCTs) using the herbal remedy ginkgo (*Ginkgo biloba*), an extract from the biloba tree, have been performed, but to date the effects found have been small or non-existent. Several RCTs in mild cognitive impairment are currently being conducted (see Clinical Pointer 39.2).

TREATMENT OF COGNITIVE IMPAIRMENT IN ALZHEIMER'S DISEASE

It is likely that the arrival of the antidementia drugs will be seen as a breakthrough of similar magnitude to the launch of the first generation of antipsychotics and antidepressants in the 1950s. However,

like these drugs, antidementia agents will need considerable development before their potential is realized. The pharmacological treatment of Alzheimer's disease illustrates the difficulty of treating patients with established degenerative disease. It is probably unrealistic to expect a drug (taken for a relatively short period of time) to reverse entirely the massive consequences of late degenerative disease. Early enthusiasm that the new antidementia drugs would permanently arrest the deterioration of the disease has been superseded by a more honest evaluation that they offer a temporary pause in the inevitable decline. The average annual decline in cognition in Alzheimer's disease is 3.3 points on the Mini-Mental State Examination (Han et al 2000), similar to the 'minimal clinically important difference' that clinicians report (Burback et al 1999). Studies of the new antidementia treatments rarely show a magnitude of effect as large as this, and are typically only half as effective. Furthermore, this effect 'wears-off' as the decline in cognition becomes more rapid. In two large US studies of donepezil, benefit over placebo was only maintained for 24 weeks, after an initial 12 weeks of treatment. If initial treatment was extended to 24 weeks, benefit was lost after a subsequent 6-week washout period (Doody et al 2001). Both galantamine and rivastigmine have shown advantage over placebo beyond 6 months in 12-month follow-up studies (6 months trials, 6 months open-label extensions) (Winblad et al 2001a). Donepezil is the only drug for which 52-week data have been reported, but one of the two studies was not designed to compare drug and placebo at 52 weeks, as non-responders were removed differently in the drug and placebo arms.

Given the limited data to date, a fair summary is that cognitive benefits are barely maintained for up to a maximum of 1 year and, while these cognitive changes are often statistically significant, they may not be clinically significant. Fortunately, these drugs have other key benefits – effects on function, behaviour and neuropsychiatric symptoms – which are widely acknowledged as critical to the quality of life of the patient and carer. However, again there is a catch. If maintenance, as opposed to improvement, is expected, then baseline function is highly significant. To put it simply, if quality of life is poor at baseline, preservation of this level of function is not a particularly good outcome. On the other hand, if quality of life is good, then a slowing of deterioration or the prevention of behavioural complications is valuable. Clearly, further long-term trial work is

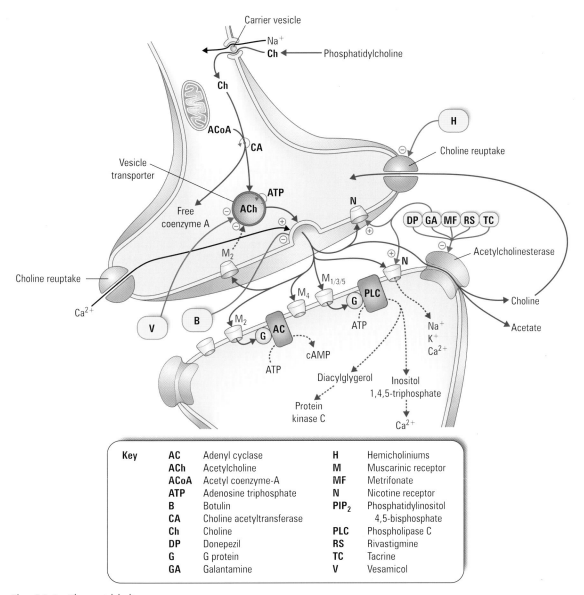

Fig. 56.1   The acetylcholine synapse.

Key					
	AC	Adenyl cyclase	**H**	Hemicholiniums
	ACh	Acetylcholine	**M**	Muscarinic receptor
	ACoA	Acetyl coenzyme-A	**MF**	Metrifonate
	ATP	Adenosine triphosphate	**N**	Nicotine receptor
	B	Botulin	**PIP$_2$**	Phosphatidylinositol
	CA	Choline acetyltransferase		4,5-bisphosphate
	Ch	Choline	**PLC**	Phospholipase C
	DP	Donepezil	**RS**	Rivastigmine
	G	G protein	**TC**	Tacrine
	GA	Galantamine	**V**	Vesamicol

required to clarify the many unanswered questions in this area. Only progress to date (August 2003) can be reviewed here.

Cholinergic therapy

Both the structure and function of the cholinergic system is affected in Alzheimer's disease. The loss seems disproportionate to general neurone loss and thus may be implicated as a cause rather than an effect. Both choline acetyltransferase and acetyl-cholinesterase (AChE) are reduced in Alzheimer's disease. The catabolic enzyme AChE breaks down acetylcholine and has been shown to correlate (using cortical biopsy) with cognitive impairment and reaction times in Alzheimer's disease. Replacement of acetylcholine using precursors such as lecithin or choline has been unsuccessful, as have cholinergic agonists such as bethanechol, pilocarpine and arecoline. Summers et al (1986) reported on the ability of tetrahydroaminoacridine (tacrine) to improve cognition in dementia and, since then, five more drugs that inhibit AChE have been investigated – donepezil, rivastigmine, galantamine, physostigmine and metrifonate. Tacrine and donepezil have been licensed by the Food and Drug Administration in the USA for use in early Alzheimer's disease. These drugs can be classified by their enzyme inhibition (reversible and short-acting or irreversible and long-acting) or by their mechanism of action (Fig. 56.3) (Nordberg & Svensson 1998).

AChE has several different isoforms, of which G4 is the dominant form in the cortex and hippocampus; this isoform is reduced in Alzheimer's disease. It has been suggested, but not proven, that the selectivity of cholinesterase inhibitors for AChE versus butylcholinesterase may influence efficacy (but not adverse effects) (Weinstock 1999).

Certain drugs also act on nicotinic receptors, enhancing the effect of endogenous acetylcholine via a mechanism called the 'allosterically potentiating ligand action' (Maelicke et al 2001). In fact, nicotinic agonists may delay (or prevent) the accumulation of β-amyloid (Nordberg et al 2002).

These drugs appear to slow the inevitable loss of acetylcholine from the brain, and initially may bring about some distinct improvement in function.

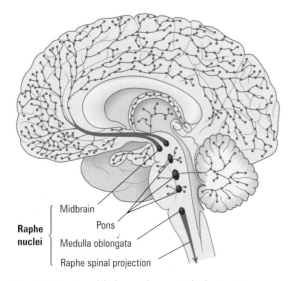

Fig. 56.2 Acetylcholine pathways in the brain. From Fitzgerald & Folan-Curran (2001).

However, these drugs are only now beginning to be tested in late-stage Alzheimer's disease.

Tacrine

Tacrine is a centrally acting, reversible AChE inhibitor that has some cognitive benefits in Alzheimer's disease when given in high doses (Knapp et al 1994). It may also improve the degree of independent living and survival (Smith et al 1996). Unfortunately, its use is limited by hepatic side effects (an increase in the alanine aminotransferase (ALT) is seen in about one-quarter of patients) and cholinergic side effects (seen in 16% of patients). Recommendations are that tacrine should be discontinued once the ALT level is five times normal, although the majority of patients are able to tolerate a re-challenge. About one-third of patients also experience gastrointestinal side effects; these can be reduced by taking the drug with food.

Raskind et al (1997) examined the effects of tacrine on 419 patients with mild to moderate Alzheimer's disease in a 30-week double-blind randomized placebo-controlled trial. About half of patients improved behaviourally, although side effects of gastrointestinal upset and hepatic enzyme elevation were seen.

Kaufer et al (1996) published the results of an open-label examination of the behavioural effects of tacrine in Alzheimer's disease, measured by the Neuropsychiatric Inventory. There was a dose–response relationship between tacrine and improvements in apathy, behaviour, anxiety and hallucinations. Knopman et al (1996) analysed the long-term outcome of almost 600 patients who had completed the double-blind 30-week study of tacrine. Fewer patients on tacrine either died or required nursing home placement for up to 2 years. Note that this study was not randomized, and therefore further studies are required to confirm its finding.

Donepezil

Donepezil was the first drug to be licensed for dementia in the UK, in March 1997. It must be used with caution in cases of sick sinus syndrome or other supraventricular conduction abnormalities, in patients at risk of developing peptic ulcers, in asthma and in obstructive airways disease. It is better tolerated than tacrine, without the need for weekly blood tests. About 10% of patients are unable to tolerate donepezil, largely because of gastrointestinal side effects.

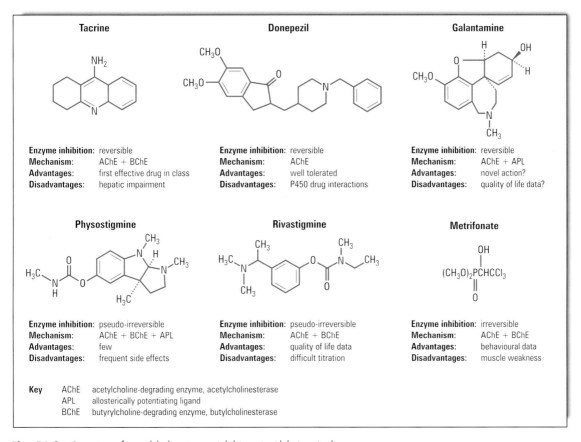

Fig. 56.3 Overview of acetylcholinesterase inhibitors in Alzheimer's disease.

Three systematic reviews have examined the effect of donepezil (and rivastigmine) on cognition. A Cochrane Review (Birks & Melzer 1998), a review by Wolfson et al (2000) and a review by Livingston & Katona (2000) all found that donepezil prevented cognitive deterioration up to 24 weeks after starting therapy (when measured using the Alzheimer's Disease Assessment Scale – cognitive subscale (ADAS-cog)), but with no significant benefits on quality of life. Adverse effects included nausea, diarrhoea, cardiovascular instability, nasal congestion and insomnia. Overall, clinical improvement was seen in 25% of those given 10 mg/day for 24 weeks, compared with 14% in the placebo group. A recent small-scale randomized controlled trial (RCT) demonstrated even more favourable global outcomes (Greenberg et al 2000). Donepezil has recently been investigated for its benefits on behaviour and mood as well as those on cognition. Cumming's group found that patients treated with donepezil were significantly less likely to be reported as threat-

ening, destroying property and talking loudly (Cummings & Askin-Edgar 2000).

In 2001, two multicentre groups have published 1-year double-blind placebo-controlled data. Both suggest that there is delay in functional decline of approximately 5 months on donepezil compared with placebo, with associated positive effects on care (Mastey et al 2001, Mohs et al 2001). Winblad et al (2001b), on behalf of the Donepezil Nordic Study Group, compared donepezil in 142 patients with mild to moderate Alzheimer's disease (Mini-Mental State Examination (MMSE) scores between 10 and 26), of whom 95 completed the study, with 144 patients randomized to placebo. On the Gottfries–Bråne–Steen Global Dementia Rating Scale, drug-treated patients declined by approximately half as much as placebo-treated patients over 52 weeks (although this was only of borderline significance in last-observation carried-forward analysis). Perhaps more importantly, 31% improved from baseline, compared with 22% in the placebo group (Fig. 56.4). Using the Mini-Mental State Examination there was no demonstrable fall from baseline in drug-treated patients, although this is partly a reflection of the lack of subtlety of this test in mild dementia. Of note, 81% of patients on donepezil and 75% on placebo experienced a treatment-emergent adverse event. Two double-blind RCTs of donepezil in severe Alzheimer's disease (MMSE scores between 5 and 17) have now been published (Feldman et al 2001, Gauthier et al 2003). In both studies, after 24 weeks of treatment there were significant benefits over placebo in cognition, function and behaviour. Neuropsychiatric items such as dysphoria, anxiety and apathy also improved and the magnitude of change was greater than comparable studies in mild Alzheimer's disease.

Galantamine

Galantamine is a tertiary alkaloid originally isolated from the bulbs of snowdrop and narcissus. This AChE inhibitor has been compared with placebo in a RCT of 650 outpatients with mild to moderate Alzheimer's disease (Wilcock et al 2000). There were significant benefits over placebo in both cognition and function over a 6-month treatment period. Patients' functional ability appears to have been improved compared with placebo for up to 12 months of treatment with galantamine. Galantamine probably benefits behavioural disturbances and carer burden.

There have been two other high-quality RCTs of galantamine treatment of Alzheimer's disease. Tariot et al (2000) conducted a double-blind RCT involving 978 patients with probable Alzheimer's disease. On flexible-dose galantamine, mid- and high doses were significantly better than placebo at preventing deterioration in cognition and quality of life (measured by activities of daily living). Raskind et al (2000), in a large study of 636 patients, found similar benefits, but could not demonstrate improvement in quality of life as measured using the Disability Assessment for Dementia Scale. Nevertheless, cognitive improvement was maintained for the entire duration of the study. Side effects of galantamine are similar to those of the other AChE inhibitors described above, but can also

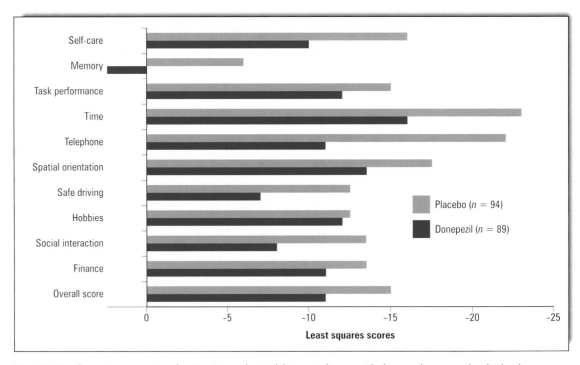

Fig. 56.4 Change in progressive deterioration scale in Alzheimer's disease with donepezil compared with placebo over 52 weeks. Data from Winblad et al (2001b).

include agitation and tremor. Recently, a 1-year head-to-head comparative study of galantamine versus donepezil in moderate to severe Alzheimer's disease showed slight advantage for galantamine in the domains of cognition and carer burden (McKeith et al 2003).

Rivastigmine

Rivastigmine, the second drug to be licensed in the UK specifically for Alzheimer's disease, was launched in 1998. It is taken twice daily, starting with a low dose of 3 mg/day and increasing to between 6 and 12 mg/day. It has a dual action, inhibiting both AChE and butyrylcholinesterase (BChE). It must be used with caution in cases of renal impairment, mild or moderate hepatic impairment, sick sinus syndrome, conduction abnormalities, or gastric or duodenal ulcers and in patients with a history of asthma or obstructive pulmonary disease. The three systematic reviews (discussed above) found rivastigmine to improve cognition (measured using the ADAS-cog rather than the MMSE) and to benefit quality of life (at the high dose) compared with placebo. The data on quality of life are derived from the study by Corey-Bloom et al (1998), which involved 699 patients with mild to moderate probable Alzheimer's disease treated for 26 weeks. Quality of life, measured using the Progressive Deterioration Scale, was significantly improved compared with placebo. The percentage of patients seen to benefit globally was approximately 40%, compared with 20% on placebo. Side effects are similar to those of donepezil, with the addition of fatigue, headaches and abdominal pain.

Metrifonate

Metrifonate is a drug that has been used for the treatment of schistosomiasis and has yet to be licensed in the UK or the USA for Alzheimer's disease, although several studies have shown benefit. Becker et al (1996), at the Southern Illinois University School of Medicine, were the first to report an advantage for metrifonate over placebo in a small double-blind randomized trial, initially of 3 months duration and then of 6 months duration (Becker et al 1998). Three large trials, one of 480 patients (treated for 12 weeks) (Cummings et al 1998), one of 264 (treated for 26 weeks) (Raskind et al 1999) and one of 605 patients (treated for 24 weeks) (Dubois et al 1999) have all reported slowing of cognitive decline. The last-mentioned study also reported behavioural improvement (mainly in apathy), psychiatric improvement (in hallucinations), improvement in functioning and, in a separate publication, reductions in carer stress (Shikiar et al 2000). Adverse effects were predominantly mild in intensity, and no hepatotoxicity was observed. A caution against the use of metrifonate is that it can induce muscle weakness that can affect respiration.

Xanomeline

The muscarinic M_1 receptor is abundant in areas of the brain concerned with learning but, unlike the nicotinic receptor, it is not affected in Alzheimer's disease. Nevertheless, muscarinic agonists may have beneficial effects on cognition. Xanomeline is a second-generation muscarinic receptor agonist with a structure similar to that of arecoline. Bodick et al (1997) conducted a large, double-blind, randomized placebo-controlled 6-month trial of xanomeline in 343 patients with Alzheimer's disease. Positive effects on behaviour, mood and cognition were noted. A substantial proportion of patients were unable to tolerate the drug, owing to gastrointestinal side effects, sweating and syncope. A new patch form of the drug is being developed.

Physostigmine

Physostigmine was the first AChE inhibitor, investigated under double-blind conditions, as early as 1979. It is widely used in the diagnosis of myasthenia gravis, but its advantage in that use (i.e. its short half-life) is a disadvantage in chronic diseases. Its use is also limited by a narrow therapeutic index and frequent side effects. Nevertheless, the long-acting form was trialed in 1111 patients with mild to moderate Alzheimer's disease (Thal et al 1997). In an unusual study design after a 2 week washout period, patients with initial improvement ($n = 366$) were randomized to receive either placebo or their best dose of physostigmine in a 6-week double-blind trial. After 6 weeks there was a small improvement in cognition, but not in function, in initial responders but not in initial non-responders. Nausea and vomiting occurred in 50% of patients, limiting the value of the drug.

OTHER DRUGS THAT INFLUENCE COGNITION

Memantine

Memantine is a non-competitive N-methyl-D-aspartate (NMDA) receptor antagonist which acts selectively (at therapeutic doses) on brain NMDA receptors. It was launched in November 2002 by Lundbeck for the treatment of moderate to severe Alzheimer's disease on the basis of one double-blind RCT in comparison with placebo in 252 patients with severe dementia (median MMSE score 7.9) over 28 weeks (Reisberg et al 2003). Results showed modest benefits in cognition, function and carer burden. In an open 24-week extension, patients switched from placebo to memantine appeared to make superior gains to those on memantine all along. An earlier study of the drug in 166 patients with severe Alzheimer's disease and vascular dementia was also positive in both subgroups. One significant attraction of the drug is the paucity of adverse effects, which include dizziness, headache and tiredness in about 2% of patients. There is a theoretical risk of hallucinations or confusion (recorded in 2% of phase III patients) and this is more likely if the drug is combined with ketamine or dextromethorphan. The question of whether memantine should be added to the regimens of patients with moderate or severe Alzheimer's disease who are taking AChE inhibitors has recently been addressed. In a 24-week RCT, 400 patients were randomized to memantine or placebo augmentation of donepezil. There was a significant benefit in cognition and function in the memantine–donepezil group (Farlow et al 2003).

Others

Some studies suggest that the selective-type monoamine oxidase inhibitor (MAOI) selegiline has cognitive and behavioural benefits in Alzheimer's disease, especially in combination with tacrine. However, results were inconsistent (Birks & Flicker 1998). Acetyl-L-carnitine has been investigated in several conditions that feature cognitive impairment. The definitive study in Alzheimer's disease was a multicentre, double-blind RCT comparing 1 year of acetyl-L-carnitine with placebo treatment (Thal et al 1996). At the trial endpoint, there were no statistical differences between 431 patients, although in early-onset cases there was a trend for benefit with active drug, whereas in late-onset cases there was a trend for hazard with active drug (Thal et al 2000). There is some evidence that oestrogens can prevent the development of Alzheimer's disease (Clinical Pointer 56.1). So far the therapeutic effects of oestrogen have been disappointing (Mulnard et al 2000). One small, placebo-controlled RCT of 15 patients with symptoms of aggression in dementia found beneficial effects of conjugated oestrogens on behaviour (Kyomen et al 1999).

Clinical Pointer 56.1

Oestrogens and cognition

Oestrogens in the form of hormone replacement therapy (HRT) appear to be beneficial in preventing age-associated memory impairment. The effects of HRT may depend on the type of therapeutic intervention used, although this is not well studied. Epidemiological studies suggest that HRT protects against the development of clinically diagnosed Alzheimer's disease. A large-scale prospective study funded by the US National Institute of Health is under way.

Three recent controlled experimental studies using HRT showed no appreciable effects of HRT in preventing further cognitive decline in women who already have Alzheimer's disease, but one very small study did find an effect. Larger studies are desperately needed. The duration of treatment seems to play an important role, with beneficial effects declining—and even reversing—with longer treatment in women with Alzheimer's disease.

Further reading *Hogervorst E, Williams J, Budge M et al 2000 The nature of the effect of female gonadal hormone replacement therapy on cognitive function in post-menopausal women: a meta-analysis. Neuroscience 101:485–512*
LeBlanc ES, Janowsky J, Chan BKS et al 2001 Hormone replacement therapy and cognition: systematic review and meta-analysis. JAMA 285:1489–1499
Paganini Hill A, Henderson VW 1996 Estrogen replacement therapy and risk of Alzheimer disease. Archives of Internal Medicine 156:2213–2217
van Amelsvoort T, Compton J, Murphy D 2001 In vivo assessment of the effects of estrogen on human brain. Trends in Endocrinology and Metabolism 12:273–276

TREATMENT OF THE NEUROPSYCHIATRIC COMPLICATIONS OF ALZHEIMER'S DISEASE

Depression and antidepressants

Patients with dementia are sensitive to the anticholinergic, antiadrenergic and antihistaminergic side effects inherent in tricyclic antidepressants. Several RCTs support the safe and efficacious use of the selective serotonin reuptake inhibitors to treat depression in Alzheimer's disease (Nyth & Gonfries 1990, Olafsson et al 1992, Volicer et al 1994). Of the few modest-sized older antidepressant trials in Alzheimer's disease, one study with imipramine (Reifler et al 1989) and one study with maprotiline (Fuchs et al 1993) have not shown an advantage over placebo. On the other hand, Nyth et al (1992) found an advantage of citalopram over placebo in a double-blind, multicentre RCT of 149 patients with a diagnosis of dementia with and without depression. Of note, both depressive symptoms and cognitive symptoms showed some improvement with citalopram compared with placebo, although side effects were more commonly reported than in comparable studies of primary depression.

Trazadone is commonly prescribed for patients with dementia, and sometimes for behavioural problems alone. One small trial supports the view that it may be more effective than haloperidol for agitation, but patients are prone to develop postural hypotension and excess sedation (Sultzer et al 1997). One recent attempt to replicate these results in 149 patients with Alzheimer's disease was probably underpowered, owing to its four-arm design and 38% drop-out rate. Thirty-four per cent of patients with agitation improved, but there was no difference between haloperidol, trazodone, behavioural management techniques and placebo (Teri et al 2000). Several open-label studies report success with methylphenidate, MAOIs and ECT.

Mood stabilizers

There has been one modest-sized, double-blind RCT of carbamazepine in the treatment of the agitation and aggression of dementia (Tariot et al 1998). The study was relatively small (51 subjects) and relatively brief (6 weeks). After assessment using the crude Clinician's Global Clinical Impression, 77% of patients improved on carbamazepine compared with 21% on placebo. There was also good response on the Overt Aggression Scale.

Three RCTs of sodium valproate have been reported. Sival et al (2000) enrolled 42 patients with dementia (Alzheimer's disease and vascular dementia) in an 8-week study of fixed-dose sodium valproate (480 mg/day) versus placebo. There was a non-significant trend for improvement in aggression, the lack of statistical significance perhaps being due to the inadequate power of the study. In a similarly powered study, Porsteinsson et al (2001) assessed the value of variable dose divalproex semi-sodium (mean 826 mg/day) in agitated demented patients. There was a marked response in 40% of the divalproex group and 10% on placebo at 6 weeks, a finding of borderline significance given the group size of 56 patients. One study has shown divalproex to be effective in the treatment of agitation in patients with dementia and mania (Tariot et al 2001).

Lithium may be effective in some patients, but it is more difficult in practice, owing to the need for blood monitoring.

Psychosis, behavioural disturbance and antipsychotics

In the dementias, behavioural problems such as agitation, aggression and insomnia, as well as anxiety and psychosis, are often treated with typical antipsychotics. In reviewing these studies it is difficult to separate those that examined patients who were agitated but not aggressive from those that rated aggression in a meaningful way.

A meta-analysis of a handful of small clinical trials supports the clinical observation that these drugs can be useful in the treatment of behavioural disturbance when prescribed with care (Lanctut et al 1998). Only two trials involving more than 70 patients have been published. Devanand et al (1998) compared haloperidol with placebo in 71 patients with Alzheimer's disease, who were treated for 6 weeks. At doses above 2 mg/day (but not under 1 mg/day), psychosis, agitation and aggression improved in more than half of patients. In the second study, Nygaard et al (1994) treated 73 patients with dementia with various doses of zuclopenthixol using an unusual study design without a placebo group. Patients were randomized to fixed daily doses of 2, 4 or 6 mg zuclopenthixol or to a daily dose that could be increased from 4 to 20 mg. Improvements were seen with all but the lowest doses, and outcome was not correlated with serum drug levels.

Antipsychotics are liable to cause severe side effects, including extrapyramidal side effects in at least one-fifth of elderly patients. Such side effects are probably exacerbated by a biological predisposi-

---

Clinical Pointer 56.2

Non-pharmacological treatment of non-cognitive symptoms of dementia

Patients with dementia, rather like children, are often unable to express discomfort or distress verbally, and resort to behavioural means of doing so. Before pharmacological treatment for behavioural symptoms are considered, all potential exogenous factors should be identified and, if possible, modified. Such external factors may include change of environment or reference person, confrontation with carers, or too much or too little external stimuli. There is often a breakdown in communication as patients fail to understand complex, quickly spoken instructions. Written statements that can be carried by the patient are often helpful. Intercurrent illnesses and adverse effects of medication used for other purposes should be considered as well. The family is most often the first line of defence in the management of such behaviours, and therefore considerable effort should be given to helping the family understand and manage the patient. Video tapes of family members may help. Behaviour diaries can help document the difficulties, and an 'ABC' model is easy for people to understand (antecedents–behaviour–consequences).

As the patient deteriorates, increasing control of the environment is necessary and, moreover, helps the patient's sense of stability. Principles of environmental intervention in dementia include: provision of a safe environment, reducing over-stimulation but introducing a regular activity programme, using positive aspects of the natural environment (e.g. sunlight, gardens) and using reminders or cues whenever possible. An hour-by-hour schedule may be necessary, with particular emphasis on toileting, bathing, hygiene, sleep and eating. Wandering is a common behavioural problem in dementia and one that is rarely appropriately treated pharmacologically. Safely identifying and returning patients, giving verbal and visual instruction, distraction, using overlearned routines or locking doors are sensible alternatives. Pharmacological treatment can be used as a supplement when these measures are unsuccessful.

Further reading   Ballard C, O'Brien J, James I et al 2001 Dementia: management of behavioural and psychological symptoms. Oxford University Press, Oxford
Cohen-Mansfield J 2000 Nonpharmacologic interventions for inappropriate behaviors in dementia: a review, summary, and critique. American Journal of Geriatric Psychiatry 9:361–381
Doody RS, Steven JC, Beck C et al 2001 Practice parameter: management of dementia (an evidence-based review). Neurology 56:1154–1166

Clinical Pointer 56.3

Future developments in the treatment of Alzheimer's disease

One promising idea is to use neuroprotective agents. Given the early success of the NMDA antagonist memantine, newer NMDA agents are under investigation (e.g. L-701252 and WIIN-63480–2). A second neuroprotective option are the nerve growth factor enhancers. One example is Neotrofin (AIT-082), which is under intense study. However, the most aggressive treatments for Alzheimer's disease will surely attempt to prevent the accumulation of the biological substrates of dementia. Therein lies a problem, because the exact biological factors that are instrumental in the progression of the disease are not known. Plaques and tangles are the most likely candidates, but in reality it is only after they are actually prevented in vivo that we will discover whether or not they are innocent bystanders. The enzymes responsible for phosphorylation of tau include protein kinase I and II and glycogen synthase kinase 3 (GSK-3). This is of note because lithium and insulin both inhibit GSK-3 and may have occult clinical benefits that are yet to be demonstrated.

There are various options that may prevent synthesis of amyloid in the brain. Inhibitors of β-site amyloid precursor protein cleaving enzyme (BACE) and β/γ-secretases, such as Calpeptin or MG-132, may prevent synthesis of β-amyloid. Oestrogens may also have a similar action, and specific CNS-acting oestrogen agonists have been developed. The presence of complement in amyloid plaques and an excess of microglia suggests that anti-inflammatory drugs are worth examining, and hence the interest in cyclo-oxygenase 1, cyclo-oxygenase 2 and/or leukotriene inhibitors, such as GR-253035 and Celecoxib. This could also be the mechanism of action of propentofylline. Indeed, some existing non-steroidal anti-inflammatory drugs (NSAIDs) (including ibuprofen and indomethacin) reduce brain β-amyloid and in large surveys have been associated with a reduced risk of developing Alzheimer's disease, but there is a big question of whether they are effective if started after diagnosis of Alzheimer's disease has been made. This is exactly the hypothesis of the large US ADAPT study (Martin et al 2002).

Much excitement surrounds the development of an ingenious way to clear amyloid plaques immunologically. From animal models, passive peripheral immunization against β-amyloid helps clear pre-existing plaques in mature transgenic animals, with possible direct benefits in cognitive function. Unfortunately, recent phase II trials of AN-1792 in humans were abandoned by Elan Pharmaceuticals after 15% of patients developed encephalitis. Further developments in this field are sure to follow.

Further reading   Emilien G, Beyreuther K, Masters CL et al 2000 Prospects for pharmacological intervention in Alzheimer's disease. Archives of Neurology 57:454–459

Martin BK, Meinert CL, Breitner JCS 2002 Double placebo design in a prevention trial for Alzheimer's disease. Controlled Clinical Trials 23:93–99

Schenk D 2002 Amyloid-beta immunotherapy for Alzheimer's disease: the end of the beginning. National Reviews in Neuroscience 3:824–828

tion to hypotension, parkinsonism, constipation and urinary retention, the inability to complain about treatment-emergent problems and the likelihood of polypharmacy. As a result, dose-related side effects can appear even at low doses. There is also evidence that conventional antipsychotics may worsen cognitive function in patients with dementia (McShane et al 1997).

For these reasons, there is considerable interest in atypical antipsychotics. At least three atypical antipsychotics have been studied in placebo-controlled trials involving the treatment of behavioural disturbance. Both risperidone (De Deyn et al 1999, Katz et al 1999) and olanzapine (Street et al 1999, 2000) appear to be effective and well-tolerated treatments in this regard. In a large study coordinated by the University of Pennsylvania, 625 patients with Alzheimer's disease, vascular dementia or mixed dementia and significant psychotic or behavioural symptoms were randomly assigned to placebo or low-dose risperidone for 12 weeks (Katz et al 1999). Significantly greater reductions using the Behavioural Pathology in Alzheimer's Disease Rating Scale occurred in the patients receiving risperidone 1 mg/day or 2 mg/day than in the patients receiving placebo and with the 1 mg dose was associated with the least extrapyramidal side effects. Approximately 33% in the placebo group improved, compared with 50% on 2 mg risperidone. Improvement in aggression was independent of improvement in psychosis.

In a second study, from De Dyen et al (1999), risperidone was compared with placebo and haloperidol in a three-arm trial. In a 13-week, double-blind study, 344 patients with dementia were randomly assigned to receive placebo or flexible doses (0.5–4 mg/day) of risperidone (mean dose 1.1 mg/day) or haloperidol (mean dose 1.2 mg/day).

Reductions in the BEHAVE-Alzheimer's disease total score were significantly greater with risperidone than with placebo at 12 weeks, although the effect was modest. There were also significantly greater reductions in the BEHAVE-Alzheimer's disease aggressiveness score with risperidone than haloperidol at 12 weeks. The severity of extrapyramidal side effects with risperidone did not differ significantly from that of placebo and was less than that with haloperidol.

In a 6-week study with open-label extension, Street et al (2000) conducted a multicentre, double-blind, placebo-controlled study of 206 elderly US nursing home residents with Alzheimer's disease who exhibited psychotic or behavioural symptoms. Low-dose olanzapine produced significant improvement compared with placebo on the Neuropsychiatric Inventory and the Occupational Disruptiveness Score (reflecting the impact on the carer). Post hoc analysis also illustrated improvement in anxiety items (Mintzer et al 2001). Somnolence was significantly more common among patients receiving olanzapine (occurring in a quarter of patients), although no significant cognitive impairment or extrapyramidal symptoms occurred. Olanzapine appears to be advantageous only at low doses (5 and 10 mg) and, although generally reasonably tolerated, side effects require special monitoring in patients with dementia, who are less likely to complain (Street et al 2000). Finally the new partial dopamine agonist Aripiprazole has been trialed in 208 moderate-severe Alzheimer patients experiencing psychotic symptoms. There was a significant benefit at 10 weeks, although results in the placebo group were surprisingly good (De Dyen et al 2003).

In acutely agitated patients there is an issue with the most appropriate route of administration of medication. It is therefore of interest that Meehan et al (2001) on behalf of Eli Lilly, have conducted a randomized trial of rapid-acting intramuscular olanzapine to treat agitated inpatients with dementia ($n = 205$) compared with a placebo injection ($n = 67$). They found that 2 hours after the initial injection, improvements were seen on the Posture and Negative Symptom Scale (PANSS) Excited Component subscale and the Cohen–Mansfield Agitation Inventory. This benefit was maintained for 24 hours. There were no reported problems of extrapyramidal side effects, orthostasis or QT prolongation.

Despite these possible benefits of atypical antipsychotics, there are still pharmacological differences between them (Table 56.1). Anticholinergic action is strongest for olanzapine and clozapine (partial agonists) and relatively weak for quetiapine, risperidone and ziprasidone. Thus, there is the possibility that olanzapine may not be the best choice in patients with Alzheimer's disease. To address this, one small study from Eli Lilly randomized 43 patients with Alzheimer's to olanzapine 5, 10 or 15 mg or placebo (Kennedy et al 2001). The authors reported that the 5 mg dose had no deleterious cognitive or behavioural effects.

Acetylcholinesterase inhibitors

Studies are progressively being completed that report favourable behavioural outcomes using AChE inhibitors. As mentioned above, in open-label

Table 56.1 Pharmacological differences between antipsychotic drugs

Drug	Dopamine D$_2$	Dopamine D$_1$	Serotonin 5HT$_2$	α$_1$-Adrenergic	α$_2$-Adrenergic	Histamine H$_1$	Muscarinic M$_1$
Chlorpromazine	✓	✓		✓		✓✓	✓✓
Haloperidol	✓✓			✓		✓	
Thioridazine	✓	✓				✓	✓✓
Clozapine	✓	✓	✓	✓	✓	✓✓	✓✓
Olanzapine	✓	✓	✓	✓		✓✓	✓✓
Risperidone	✓✓	✓	✓✓	✓✓	✓	✓	
Sertindole*	✓	✓	✓✓	✓✓			
Quetiapine	✓			✓		✓✓	
Ziprasidone*	✓		✓✓	✓		✓	

✓, Moderate level of receptor binding; ✓✓, high level of receptor binding
*Not currently available in the UK (2003)

Clinical Pointer 56.4

The importance of insight in neuropsychiatry

Insight has an important role in every neurological and psychiatric disorder. 'Insight' refers to a person's awareness of not only his or her current symptoms, but also the disorder, its treatment and its influences. Awareness of symptoms is important because it determines help-seeking behaviour, not just on first presentation but also on subsequent occasions (relapse prevention). Awareness of the disorder is important in terms of planning for the future in the case of recurrent or degenerative conditions and using available support when in remission. Insight into treatment will have a dominant effect on compliance and thus on outcome. The same is true regarding an awareness of modifying variables such as social stressors in alcoholism.

Diseases that affect cognition are likely to affect insight. Alzheimer's disease is a classic example, although this association has also been shown in schizophrenia. Insight is good in the early stages of the disease, but this predisposes to greater depressed mood and is inversely correlated with agitation (which is often present in the later stages). Neurological disorders of awareness (neglect and anosognosia) appear to have a distinct neuronal mechanism and are discussed in Section I of this book.

Further reading *Harwood DG, Sultzer DL, Wheatley MV 2000 Impaired insight in Alzheimer disease: association with cognitive deficits, psychiatric symptoms, and behavioural disturbances. Neuropsychiatry, Neuropsychology and Behavioural Neurology 13:83–88*

Clinical Pointer 56.5

Detention of patients who lack capacity

Doctors have a duty of care to act in a person's best interests, particularly when that person is unable to state his or her own wishes. However, there is also requirement to respect a person's wishes, and sometimes this causes conflict over the treatment of physical disorders when a patient with capacity refuses treatment. In the UK, a relative has no legal right to consent on a patient's behalf. The Mental Health Act (1983) does not take into account capacity, but it does require that the Act should be used only if absolutely necessary. In 1997 the Court of Appeal ruled that it was unlawful to admit an autistic adult to a psychiatric hospital on an informal basis when the patient lacked the capacity but did not object. The implication was that any person incapable of consenting to informal admission could only lawfully be admitted under the statutory Mental Health Act. This was overturned by the House of Lords who decided the Mental Health Act could be used but did not have to be used. In the new Department of Health document, Reforming the Mental Health Act (2000), new guidelines are suggested: 'It is essential to ensure that the best interests of these patients are properly considered and protected and this can only be achieved through independent scrutiny. New legislation will place a duty on the clinical supervisor responsible for the care and treatment of a patient with long-term mental incapacity to refer the care plan to a member of the expert panel for a second opinion when the care and treatment for a mental disorder continues for longer than 28 days.'

Further reading *Jones R 2002 Mental Health Act manual, 8th edn. Sweet and Maxwell, London*

studies tacrine and metrifonate, and in RCTs donepezil, galantamine and rivastigmine improve non-cognitive symptoms. As of March 2003, only a handful of RCTs have been published. One modestly sized study showed a favourable effect of donepezil measured by the Neuropsychiatric Inventory (Feldman et al 2001), whereas another did not (Tariot et al 2001). Two larger studies have shown beneficial effects for galantamine over placebo (Kaufer et al 2002). Interestingly the magnitude of the effect may be greater than the effect on cognition alone. From pooled metrifonate studies using the Neuropsychiatric Inventory, 60% of patients did not deteriorate further and 40% of patients improved significantly (Cummings et al 2001). From open-label data on rivastigmine, the areas that showed most improvement were night-time wandering, hallucinations, apathy, motor symptoms, irritability and aggression.

Other drugs

Beta blockers (e.g. propranolol) and benzodiazepines can be effective in controlling overaroused behaviour in dementia (Schneider & Sobin 1992).

They must be used with caution because of their side effects at higher doses. Small doses of benzodiazepines can also cause disinhibition, exacerbating the underlying problem. Benzodiazepines can also impair cognitive performance and therefore should be avoided except for very short periods or where the benefits outweigh the disadvantages.

SUMMARY

The management of the neuropsychiatric complications of Alzheimer's disease can be summarized as follows:

- A trial of an AChE inhibitor should be considered, particularly for those with co-existing behavioural symptoms and those with early dementia. However, in patients who do not benefit by 6 months, medication should be discontinued.
- Donezepil or memantine (or a combination of the two) should be considered for moderate to severe Alzheimer's disease.
- Screen for depression at all stages and consider newer antidepressants as first-line treatment. (Be prepared to use non-cognitive indicators of depression.)
- Take a holistic view in assessing and managing behavioural disturbance – no medication may be necessary (see Clinical Pointer 56.2). In those with persistent symptoms an atypical antipsychotic is preferred; carbamazepine divalproex and low-dose benzodiazepines are alternatives.
- Do not accept withdrawal and social isolation as a normal variant. Screen for apathy and treat accordingly.
- Treat distressing psychotic symptoms with atypical antipsychotics as first-line treatment – olanzapine and risperidone have a reasonable evidence base.
- Take time to educate and advise patients and relatives about driving, genetic risks, prognosis, treatment alternatives and available sources of help.

REFERENCES AND FURTHER READING

Becker RE, Colliver JA, Markwell SJ et al 1996 Double-blind, placebo-controlled study of metrifonate, an acetylcholinesterase inhibitor, for Alzheimer disease. Alzheimer's Disease and Associated Disorders 10:124–131

Becker RE, Colliver JA, Markwell SJ et al 1998 Effects of metrifonate on cognitive decline in Alzheimer disease: a double-blind, placebo-controlled, 6-month study. Alzheimer's Disease and Associated Disorders 12:54–57

Birks J, Flicker L 1998 The efficacy and safety of selegiline for the symptomatic treatment of Alzheimer's disease. A systematic review of the evidence. Cochrane Review, issue 3. Oxford, Update Software

Birks JS, Melzer D 1998 Donepezil for mild and moderate Alzheimer's disease (Cochrane Review). The Cochrane Library, issue 1. Oxford, Update Software

Bodick NC, Offen WW, Lewy AI et al 1997 Effects of xanomeline, a selective muscarinic receptor agonist on cognitive function and behavioural symptoms in Alzheimer's disease. Archives of Neurology 54:465–473

Burback D, Molnar FJ, St John P et al 1999 Key methodological features of randomized controlled trials of Alzheimer's disease therapy. Minimal clinically important difference, sample size and trial duration. Dementia and Geriatric Cognitive Disorders 10:534–540

Corey-Bloom J, Anand R, Veach J 1998 A randomized trial evaluating the efficacy and safety of ENA 713 (rivastigmine tartrate): a new acetylcholinesterase inhibitor, in patients with mild to moderately severe Alzheimer's disease. International Journal of Geriatric Psychopharmacology 1:55–65

Cummings JL, Askin-Edgar S 2000 Evidence for psychotropic effects of acetylcholinesterase inhibitors. CNS Drugs 13:385–395

Cummings JL, Cyrus PA, Bieber F et al 1998 Metrifonate treatment of the cognitive deficits of Alzheimer's disease. Metrifonate Study Group. Neurology 50:1214–1221

Cummings JL, Nadel A, Masterman D et al 2001 Efficacy of metrifonate in improving the psychiatric and behavioural disturbances of patients with Alzheimer's disease. Journal of Geriatric Psychiatry and Neurology 14:101–108

De Deyn PP, Rabheru K, Rasmussen A et al 1999 A randomized trial of risperidone, placebo, and haloperidol for behavioural symptoms of dementia. Neurology 53:946–955

De Deyn PP, Jeste DV, Auby P et al 2003 Aripiprazole for psychosis of Alzheimer's disease. Presented at the 156th American Psychiatric Association Annual Meeting, San Francisco, CA, 17–22 May

Devanand DP, Marder K, Michaels K et al 1998 A randomized, placebo-controlled, dose-comparison of haloperidol for psychosis and disruptive behaviours in Alzheimer's disease. American Journal of Psychiatry 155:1512–1520

Doody RS, Geldmacher DS, Gordon B et al 2001 Open-label, multicenter, phase 3 extension study of the safety and efficacy of donepezil in patients with Alzheimer disease. Archives of Neurology 58:427–433

Dubois B, McKeith I, Orgogozo J M et al 1999 A multicentre, randomized, double-blind, placebo-controlled study to evaluate the efficacy, tolerability and safety of two doses of metrifonate in patients with mild-to-moderate Alzheimer's disease: the MALT study. International Journal of Geriatric Psychiatry 14:973–982

Farlow MR, Tariot PN, Grossberg GT et al 2003 Memantine/donepezil dual therapy is superior to placebo/donepezil therapy for treatment of moderate-to-severe Alzheimer's disease. Presented at the 55th Annual Meeting of the American Academy of Neurology, Hawaii, 29 March to 5 April

Feldman H, Gauthier S, Hecker J et al and the Donepezil MSAD Study Investigators Group 2001 A 24-week, randomized, double-blind study of donepezil in moderate to severe Alzheimer's disease. Neurology 57:613–620

Fitzgerald MJT, Folan-Curran J 2001 Clinical neuroanatomy and related neuroscience, 4th edn. Saunders, Philadelphia

Fuchs A, Hehnke U, Erhart C et al 1993 Video rating analysis of effect of maprotiline in patients with dementia and depression. Pharmacopsychiatry 26:37–41

Gauthier S, Feldman H, Hecker J et al 2003 Donepezil shows significant benefits in global function, cognition, ADL and behavior in patients with severe Alzheimer's disease. Presented at the 55th Annual Meeting of the American Academy of Neurology, Hawaii, 29 March to 5 April

Greenberg SM, Tennis MK, Brown LB et al 2000 Donepezil therapy in clinical practice: a randomized crossover study. Archives of Neurology 57:94–99

Han L, Cole M, Bellavance F et al 2000 Tracking cognitive decline in Alzheimer's disease using the Mini-Mental State Examination: a meta-analysis. International Psychogeriatrics 12:231–247

Katz IR, Jeste DV, Mintzer JE et al 1999 Comparison of risperidone and placebo for psychosis and behavioural disturbances associated with dementia: a randomized, double-blind trial. Risperidone Study Group. Journal of Clinical Psychiatry 60:107–115

Kaufer DI, Cummings JL, Christine D 1996 Effect of tacrine on behavioural symptoms in Alzheimer's disease: an open-label study. Journal of Geriatric Psychiatry and Neurology 9:1–6

Kaufer D, Lilienfeld S, Schwalen S et al 2002 Beneficial effects of galantamine on patient behaviour and caregiver distress in Alzheimer's disease and dementia associated with cerebrovascular disease. Journal of Neurology 249(suppl 1):130

Kennedy J, Basson B, Street J et al 2001 The effects of olanzapine on Alzheimer's disease assessment scale scores in patients with mild to moderate Alzheimer's disease with psychosis and behavioural disturbances. Biological Psychiatry 49:378

Knapp MJ, Knapman DS, Soloman PR et al 1994 A 30-week randomized controlled trial of high dose tacrine in patients with Alzheimer's disease. JAMA 271:985–991

Kopman D, Schneider L, Davis K et al 1996 Long term tacrine (Cognex) treatment: effects on nursing home placement and mortality. Neurology 47:166–177

Kyomen HH, Satlin A, Hennen J et al 1999 Estrogen therapy and aggressive behavior in elderly patients with moderate-to-severe dementia: results from a short-term, randomized, double-blind trial. American Journal of Geriatric Psychiatry 7:339–348

Lanctot KL, Best TS, Mittmann N et al 1998 Efficacy and safety of neuroleptics in behavioural disorders associated with dementia. Journal of Clinical Psychiatry 59:550–561

Livingston G, Katona C 2000 How useful are cholinesterase inhibitors in the treatment of Alzheimer's disease? A number needed to treat analysis. International Journal of Geriatric Psychiatry 15:203–207

McKeith I, Truyen L, Lilienfeld S et al 2003 The long-term treatment response in patients with moderate-to-severe Alzheimer's disease: galantamine vs donepezil. Presented at the 55th Annual Meeting of the American Academy of Neurology, Hawaii, 29 March to 5 April

McShane R, Keene J, Gedling K et al 1997 Do neuroleptic drugs hasten cognitive decline in dementia? Prospective study with necropsy follow-up. BMJ 7076:266–270

Maelicke A, Samochocki M, Jostock R et al 2001 Allosteric sensitization of nicotinic receptors by galantamine, a new treatment strategy for Alzheimer's disease. Biological Psychiatry 493:279–288

Mastey V, Wimo A, Winblad B et al 2001 Donepezil reduces the time caregivers spend providing care: results of a one-year, double-blind randomized trial in patients with mild to moderate Alzheimer's disease. Journal of the American Geriatric Society 49:P16

Meehan K, Wang H, David S et al 2001 Intramuscular olanzapine: efficacy and safety in acutely agitated patients with dementia. Seventh World Journal of Biological Psychiatry Abstracts 2(suppl 1):11

Mintzer JE, Street JS, Clark WS et al 2001 Olanzapine in the treatment of anxiety in patients with Alzheimer's disease. Biological Psychiatry 49:379

Mohs R, Doody R, Morris J et al for the '312' Study Group 2001 A 1-year, placebo-controlled preservation of functional survival study of donepezil in AD patients. Neurology 57:481–488

Mulnard RA, Cotman CW, Kawas C et al 2000 Estrogen replacement therapy for treatment of mild to moderate Alzheimer disease: a randomized controlled trial. Alzheimer's Disease Cooperative Study. JAMA 283:1007–1015

Nordberg A, Svensson AL 1998 Cholinesterase inhibitors in the treatment of Alzheimer's disease: a comparison of tolerability and pharmacology. Drug Safety 19:465–480

Nordberg A, Hellstrom-Lindahl E, Lee M et al 2002 Chronic nicotine treatment reduces beta-amyloidosis in the brain of a mouse model of Alzheimer's disease (APPsw). Journal of Neurochemistry 81:655–658

Nygaard HA, Bakke K, Brudvik E et al 1994 Dosing of neuroleptics in elderly demented patients with aggressive and agitated behaviour: a double-blind study with zuclopenthixol. Current Medical Research and Opinions 13:222–232

Nyth AL, Gonfries CG 1990 The clinical efficacy of citalopram in treatment of emotional disturbances in dementia disorders. A Nordic multicentre study. British Journal of Psychiatry 157:894–901

Nyth AL, Gottfries CG, Lyby K et al 1992 A controlled multicenter clinical study of citalopram and placebo in elderly depressed patients with and without concomitant dementia. Acta Psychiatrica Scandinavica 86:138–145

Olafsson K, Jorgensen S, Jensen HV et al 1992 Fluvoxamine in the treatment of demented elderly patients: a double blind, placebo-controlled study. Acta Psychiatrica Scandinavica 85:453–456

Porsteinsson AP, Tariot PN, Erb R 2001 Placebo-controlled study of divalproex sodium for agitation in dementia. American Journal of Geriatric Psychiatry 9:58–66

Raskind MA, Sadowsky CH, Sigmund WR et al 1997 Effects of tacrine on language, praxis and noncognitive behavioural problems in Alzheimer's disease. Archives of Neurology 54:836–840

Raskind MA, Cyrus PA, Ruzicka BB et al 1999 The effects of metrifonate on the cognitive, behavioural, and functional performance of Alzheimer's disease patients. Metrifonate Study Group. Journal of Clinical Psychiatry 60:318–325

Raskind MA, Peskind ER, Wessel T et al 2000 Galantamine in AD. A 6-month randomized, placebo-controlled trial with a 6-month extension. Neurology 54:2261–2268

Reifler BV, Teri L, Raskind M et al 1989 Double-blind trial of imipramine in Alzheimer's disease patients with and without depression. American Journal of Psychiatry 146:45–49

Reisberg B, Doody R, Stöffler A et al 2003 Memantine in moderate-to-severe Alzheimer's disease. New England Journal of Medicine 348:1333–1341

Schneider LS, Sobin PB 1992 Non-neuroleptic treatment of behavioural symptoms and agitation in Alzheimer's disease and other dementia. Psychopharmacology Bulletin 28:71–79

Shikiar R, Shakespeare A, Sagnier PP et al 2000 The impact of metrifonate therapy on caregivers of patients with Alzheimer's disease: results from the MALT clinical trial. Metrifonate in Alzheimer's Disease Trial. Journal of the American Geriatric Society 48:268–274

Sival RC, Haffmans PMJ, Jansen PAF et al 2002 Sodium valproate in the treatment of aggressive behavior in patients with dementia – a randomized placebo controlled clinical trial. International Journal of Geriatric Psychiatry 17:579–585

Smith F, Talwalker S, Gracon S et al 1996 The use of survival analysis techniques in evaluating the effect of long-term tacrine (Cognex) treatment on nursing home placement and mortality in patients with Alzheimer's disease. Biopharmaceutical Statistics 6:395–409

Street JS, Clark WS, Mitan S et al 1999 Olanzapine in the treatment of psychiatric disturbances associated with Alzheimer's disease. Neurology 52:396–397

Street JS, Clark WS, Gannon KS et al 2000 Olanzapine treatment of psychotic and behavioural symptoms in patients with Alzheimer disease in nursing care facilities: a double-blind, randomized, placebo-controlled trial. Archives of General Psychiatry 57:968–976

Sultzer DL, Gray KF, Gunnay I et al 1997 A double-blind comparison of trazadone and haloperidol for treatment of agitation inpatients with dementia. American Journal of Geriatric Psychiatry 5:60–69

Summers WK, Majovski LV, Marsh GM et al 1986 Oral tetrahydroaminoacridine in long term treatment of senile dementia, Alzheimer type. New England Journal of Medicine 315:1241–1245

Tariot PN, Erb R, Podgorski CA et al 1998 Efficacy and tolerability of carbamazepine for agitation and aggression in dementia. American Journal of Psychiatry 155:54–61

Tariot PN, Solomon PR, Morris J et al 2000 A 5-month, randomised, placebo-controlled trial of galantamine in AD. Neurology 54:2269–2276

Tariot PN, Schneider LS, Mintzer JE et al 2001a Safety and tolerability of divalproex sodium in the treatment of signs and symptoms of mania in elderly patients with dementia: results of a double-blind, placebo-controlled trial. Current Therapy, Research and Clinical Experiments 62:51–67

Tariot PN, Cummings JL, Katz IR et al 2001b A randomized, double-blind, placebo-controlled study of the efficacy and safety of donepezil in patients with Alzheimer's disease in the nursing home setting. Journal of the American Geriatrics Society 49:1590–1599

Teri L, Logsdon RG, Peskind E et al 2000 Treatment of agitation in AD. A randomized, placebo-controlled clinical trial. Neurology 55:1271–1278

Thal LJ, Carta A, Clarke WR et al 1996 A 1-year multicenter placebo-controlled study of acetyl-L-carnitine in patients with Alzheimer's disease. Neurology 47:705–711

Thal L J, Schwartz G, Sano M et al 1997 A multicenter double-blind study of controlled-release physostigmine for the treatment of symptoms secondary to Alzheimer's disease. Physostigmine Study Group. Neurology 47:1389–1395

Thal LJ, Calvani M, Amato A et al 2000 A 1-year controlled trial of acetyl-L-carnitine in early-onset AD. Neurology 55:805–810

Volicer L, Rheaume Y, Cyr D 1994 Treatment of depression in advanced Alzheimer's disease using sertraline. Journal of Geriatric Psychiatry and Neurology 7:227–229

Weinstock M 1999 Selectivity of cholinesterase inhibition: clinical implications for the treatment of Alzheimer's disease. CNS Drugs 12:307–323

Wilcock GK, Lilienfeld S, Gaens E 2000 Efficacy and safety of galantamine in patients with mild to moderate Alzheimer's disease: multicentre randomised controlled trial. British Medical Journal 321:1445–1449

Winblad B, Brodaty H, Gauthier S et al 2001a Pharmacotherapy of Alzheimer's disease: is there a need to redefine treatment success? International Journal of Geriatric Psychiatry 16:653–666

Winblad B, Engedal K, Soininen H et al and the Donepezil Nordic Study Group 2001b A 1-year, randomized placebo-controlled study of donepezil in patients with mild to moderate AD. Neurology 57:489–495

Wolfson C, Moride Y, Perrault A et al 2000 Drug treatments for Alzheimer's disease. I. A comparative analysis of clinical trials. Canadian Coordinating Office of Health Technology Assessment (CCOHTA), Ottawa

57

Treatment in Patients with Lewy Body Dementia

TREATMENT OF COGNITIVE IMPAIRMENT IN LEWY BODY DEMENTIA

One of the most troublesome symptoms in Lewy body dementia (LBD) is fluctuating dementia, although this is actually present in only one-third of patients, whereas specific fluctuations of memory or orientation or function are present in 85% of patients (Londos et al 2000). One of the most useful strategies is to attempt to exclude any extraneous organic disease that when superimposed on Alzheimer's disease might mimic LBD. Patients with dementia are more likely to develop delirium (acute-on-chronic global cognitive impairment), and this may easily be mistaken for LBD. Patients with LBD may be particularly sensitive to the anti-dopaminergic effects of psychotropic medication. In McKeith's case series, 80% had side effects with conventional antipsychotics compared with 30% of patients with Alzheimer's disease, although a subsequent series showed a narrower differential of 48% and 36%, respectively (McKeith et al 1992, Londos et al 2000). The most common drug-induced adverse effects include confusion, hypotension and extrapyramidal side effects (EPSE). Early evidence suggests that atypical antipsychotics are preferable.

A small, placebo-controlled double-blind trial involving 29 patients with LBD showed improvements in psychosis and cognition (2.5 points on the Mini-Mental State Examination) without worsening of EPSE after 6 weeks of olanzapine (Kennedy et al 2001). Furthermore, acetylcholinesterase inhibitors may be as effective in LBD as in Alzheimer's disease, or perhaps even more so.

TREATMENT OF THE NEUROPSYCHIATRIC COMPLICATIONS OF LEWY BODY DEMENTIA

Neuropsychiatric complications are such an inherent part of LBD that treatments aimed at improving cognition are likely to benefit psychiatric complications as well. One of the best demonstrations of this is the multicentre study by McKeith et al (2000), in which 120 patients with LBD from the UK, Spain and Italy were randomized to rivastigmine 12 mg/day or placebo for 20 weeks. Assessment by means of the Neuropsychiatric Inventory was made at baseline and again at 12, 20 and 23 weeks. Computerized cognitive assessment and neuropsychological tests were also used. Patients taking rivastigmine were significantly less apathetic and anxious and had fewer delusions and hallucinations while on treatment than did controls. In the computerized cognitive assessment system and the neuropsychological tests, treated patients were significantly faster and better than those on placebo, particularly in tasks with a substantial attentional component. However, 3 weeks after discontinuation of rivastigmine most cognitive benefits were lost. Further studies of acetylcholinesterase inhibitors in LBD are awaited with great interest.

In most cases, symptomatic treatment of psychotic symptoms, agitation, behavioural disturbance or mood disturbance is also required. Without specific evidence to the contrary, the principles of treatment from studies of Alzheimer's disease can also be applied to LBD. The exception to this may be psychotic symptoms (see below).

Psychosis and antipsychotics

Psychotic symptoms in LBD often require treatment, but many clinicians are naturally cautious in view of the purported sensitivity of these patients to antipsychotics. Sensitivity to antipsychotics is certainly not limited to LBD, and it has yet to be definitively established whether it is any more severe than is seen in Parkinson's dementia or HIV dementia. In any case, possible sensitivity should not prevent the appropriate treatment of psychotic symptoms, although a very slow titration of the antipsychotic agent is indicated. Almost certainly, atypical antipsychotics are the drugs of choice.

Parkinsonian symptoms

Parkinsonian symptoms may be troublesome in LBD. The first step is to exclude a possible iatrogenic cause, by reviewing recent psychotropic medication. Although systematic evidence is lacking, it may be possible to treat parkinsonian symptoms with a mild dopaminergic agent, such as amantadine, or the antispasmodic agent baclofen.

SUMMARY

The management of the neuropsychiatric complications of LBD can be summarized as follows:

- in patients with psychosis, parkinsonism and dementia, atypical antipsychotics are preferred first-line treatment – one small randomized controlled trial (RCT) supports olanzapine, but other antipsychotic drugs may be more or less effective
- acetylcholinesterase inhibitors should be considered – one RCT supports rivastigmine, but benefits will be lost on discontinuation
- low doses of typical antipsychotics can be used with caution; note that antipsychotic sensitivity is not seen in every patient, and low doses can be used with close monitoring
- consider amantadine or dopamine agonists for troublesome motor symptoms, but beware of exacerbating psychosis or sleep disturbance.

REFERENCES AND FURTHER READING

Kennedy JS, Clark WS, Sanger TM 2001 Reduction of psychotic symptoms by olanzapine in patients with possible Lewy body dementia. Journal of Neuropsychiatry and Clinical Neurosciences 13:138

Londos E, Passant U, Brun A et al 2000 Clinical Lewy body dementia and the impact of vascular components. International Journal of Geriatric Psychiatry 15:40–49

McKeith IG, Fairbairn A, Perry R et al 1992 Neuroleptic sensitivity in patients with senile dementia of Lewy body type. British Medical Journal 305:673–678

McKeith I, Del Ser T, Spano P et al 2000 Efficacy of rivastigmine in dementia with Lewy bodies: a randomised, double-blind, placebo-controlled international study. Lancet 356:2031–2036

58

Treatment in Patients with HIV and AIDS Dementia

OVERVIEW OF NEUROLOGICAL TREATMENTS OF HIV AND AIDS

The clinical management of HIV-infected patients continues to improve rapidly. The first antiretroviral agent, zidovudine (AZT), was introduced in 1987. Three classes of antiretrovirals now exist (Box 58.1). Nucleoside and non-nucleoside reverse transcriptase inhibitors work by preventing reverse transcriptase from binding to the RNA chain. Protease inhibitors prevent maturation of HIV virions by blocking the action of the protease enzyme late in the life cycle of the virus. These are known collectively as highly active antiretroviral therapy (HAART). Approximately 80–90% of patients who are compliant with antiretroviral treatment achieve undetectable viral levels. A concern is that drug resistance may be increasing. Future developments may include drugs that prevent the virus from entering the immune system.

PRE-TEST COUNSELLING

Counselling is really no more than a frank discussion aimed at improving coping and adjustment to a difficult decision (Box 58.2). HIV counselling is for both prevention and support. People have very different levels of knowledge about HIV and AIDS, and hence their expectations of counselling will differ. A few people attend for HIV testing without any significant history of exposure but with an irrational fear that they may have been infected. At the other end of the spectrum, some people with repeated high-risk behaviour refuse to consider testing, usually because they they are afraid of the implications of being HIV-positive.

TREATMENT IN HIV AND AIDS

The goal of treatment is to help the body's natural defences reduce viral load to 'undetectable levels' (<20 virions/mm^3) for as long as possible. Combinations of antiretroviral drugs are often used, and at high doses, for theoretical maximum efficacy. In patients who have developed AIDS dementia there is even greater impetus to slow down the rate of viral replication. Therefore, a combination of a nucleoside and non-nucleoside reverse transcriptase inhibitors together with a protease inhibitor is often used. One important question is when to start treatment and whether early treatment of the primary

---

Box 58.1 Antiretroviral medications*

Nucleoside analogue reverse transcriptase inhibitors
Abacavir
Didanosine
Lamivudine[†]
Stavudine[†]
Zalcitabine
Zidovudine[†]

Non-nucleoside analogue reverse transcriptase inhibitors
Delavirdine
Efavirenz[†]
Nevirapine[†]

Protease inhibitors
Amprenavir
Indinavir[†]
Lopinavir
Nelfinavir
Ritonavir
Saquinavir

*All drugs are licensed in the UK, except delavirdine, amprenavir and lopinavir
[†]Drugs that achieve good CNS penetration

HIV infection (usually indicated by the acute sero-conversion syndrome) makes a difference to long-term outcome. So far, studies have failed to show any effect on long-term prognosis, despite early suppression of plasma viral load. There is also the risk of toxicity, drug interactions, adverse effects (including lipodystrophy) and the risk of developing drug resistance. These are the reasons given by the British HIV Association to delay treatment in cases of asymptomatic HIV until the CD4$^+$ cell count is within the range 200–350 cells/ml. Once treatment has begun, strict adherence to the protocol is necessary to ensure effectiveness. Symptomatic treatment with antibiotics and a variety of other medications are used as necessary. Up-to-date evidence-based guidelines for conventional treatment of HIV and AIDS has been published in the UK (BHIVA 2001) and the USA (US Department of Health and Human Services 2001).

TREATMENT OF THE NEUROPSYCHIATRIC COMPLICATIONS OF HIV AND AIDS

Cognition

Three main syndromes of cognitive impairment exist in patients with HIV–HIV dementia, HIV-related cognitive impairment and HIV-related delirium. One underpowered randomized controlled trial (RCT) of drug treatment in HIV delirium exists (see Ch. 46), and there are only a handful of studies concerned with HIV dementia or HIV-related cognitive impairment that falls short of dementia.

HIV-related cognitive impairment

Treatment with the antiviral zidovudine has been tested in several placebo-controlled trials. In the first study, Schmitt et al (1988) studied the neurological performance of subjects during the licensing trial for zidovudine. Significant improvement in performance on multiple tests was documented within weeks of initiating therapy. The same positive effect was found in children given intravenous zidovudine (Pizzo et al 1988) and in a separate study of didanosine (Butler et al 1991). Advantages are likely to be modest or weak and to diminish with time (Llorente et al 2001). Zidovudine is not well tolerated by all patients. Furthermore, certain antiviral agents do not adequately penetrate the CNS, including didanosine and zalcitabine (see Box 58.1). Several nucleoside reverse transcriptase inhibitors can cause psychiatric complications such as delirium, anxiety and insomnia. One interesting lead comes from the DANA consortium study of selegiline in HIV. In this limited study (selegiline versus thioctic acid versus placebo, with nine patients in each arm), those taking selegiline showed modest improvements (DANA Consortium 1998).

AIDS dementia

As HIV dementia is a clinical diagnosis, every effort must be made to rule out any other candidate dementias. In patients with HIV infection, this particularly includes untreated secondary infections and vitamin deficiencies. The AIDS Clinical Trial Groups study (ACTG005) compared high doses of zidovudine with placebo in those with HIV dementia, over 32 weeks of treatment. The study was ended prematurely because zidovudine was efficacious for treatment of HIV and also improved neuropsychological function, although benefits plateau (Sidtis et al 1993). The benefit of zidovudine is clearest at the high dose of 2000 mg/day, which may be difficult for patients to tolerate. Approximately 50–60% of patients show neurological or cognitive response, and there are accompanying improvements in immune or viral markers (such as CSF viral load and β_2-microglobulin); however, it is not clear if these can be used as predictors of response. Patients with a history of intravenous drug abuse have less likelihood of response than do those without.

Abacavir is a new reverse transcriptase inhibitor that is metabolized intracellularly to a T-deoxyguanosine nucleoside analogue that competitively inhibits HIV reverse transcriptase and terminates proviral DNA chain extension. A large double-blind RCT failed to demonstrate significant benefit over placebo in AIDS dementia when abacavir was added to existing antiretrovirals (Brew 1999).

Two studies of novel treatments for HIV dementia have recently been published. Peptide T (D-ala-

---

Box 58.2 Aspects of HIV pre-test counselling

- The basics of seroconversion
- High-risk activities and risk reduction
- Who to tell about a result
- Treatment options
- Confidentiality

Clinical Pointer 58.1

Psychosocial predictors of HIV progression

A wide range of biological and immunological factors moderate the effects of HIV infection. Surprisingly to some, psychological and social factors also may have a significant influence. It is widely accepted that measures of severe psychological distress (e.g. depression) can suppress immune function. One possible mechanism is the immunosuppressive actions of induced hypercortisolaemia.

The relationship between depression and immune status has been examined in patients with HIV. In a prospective cohort study over 66 months, Burack et al (1993) studied 277 HIV-positive men. Twenty per cent were found to be depressed. Although depression was associated with a decline in CD4$^+$ cell count, in a larger 8-year study of 1809 HIV-seropositive homosexual men without AIDS, no such relationship was apparent. In neither study did depression influence clinical outcome, although two subsequent studies have refuted this. Mayne et al (1996) found that depression adversely affected mortality in a 7-year follow-up study of 402 HIV-positive sufferers. In the HIV Epidemiologic Research Study, Ickovics et al (2001) examined 765 HIV-seropositive women aged 16–55 years. Chronic depressive symptoms were also associated with significantly greater decline in CD4$^+$ cell counts, although this may have reflected a secondary effect of illness severity rather than a direct effect of depression. Moreover, in multivariate analyses controlling for clinical findings, treatment and other factors, women with chronic depressive symptoms were twice as likely to die as women with limited or no depressive symptoms.

As many people with HIV infection also experience bereavement of loved ones, the impact of depression could be mediated by grief, or vice versa. This was examined by Kemeny et al (1994). Interestingly, the adverse effect of depression on outcome was present only in the non-bereaved subjects. Faster progression to AIDS may also be associated with coping by means of denial, higher serum cortisol, and lower satisfaction with social support (Leserman et al 2000).

Further reading *Balbin EG, Ironson GH, Solomon G F 1999 Stress and coping: the psychoneuroimmunology of HIV/AIDS. Baillière's Clinical Endocrinology and Metabolism 13:615–633*
Burack JH, Barrett DC, Stall RD et al 1993 Depressive symptoms and CD4 lymphocyte decline among HIV-infected men. JAMA 270:2568–2573
Ickovics JR, Hamburger ME, Vlahov D et al 2001 Mortality, CD4 cell count decline, and depressive symptoms among HIV-seropositive women: longitudinal analysis from the HIV Epidemiology Research Study JAMA 285:1466–1474
Kemeny ME, Weiner H, Taylor S et al 1994 Repeated bereavement, depressed mood, and immune parameters in HIV-seropositive and seronegative gay men Health Psychology 13:14–24
Leserman J, Petitto JM, Golden RN et al 2000 Impact of stressful life events, depression, social support, coping, and cortisol on progression to AIDS. American Journal of Psychiatry 157:1221–1228
Lyketsos CG, Hoover DR, Guccione M et al 1993 Depressive symptoms as predictors of medical outcomes in HIV-infection JAMA 270:2563–2567
Mayne TJ, Vittinghoff E, Chesney M A et al 1996 Depressive affect and survival among gay and bisexual men infected with HIV. Archives of Internal Medicine 156:2233–2238

peptide T-amide) has been reported to block the binding of gp120 to brain tissue and to protect neurones from the in vitro toxic effects of gp120. Heseltine et al (1998) at the University of Chicago conducted a three-site, double-blind, placebo-controlled trial of peptide T given intranasally for 6 months. Participants were 23 HIV-seropositive patients with evidence of cognitive deficits on a screening test battery. There was no statistically significant difference between the peptide T group and the placebo group on deficit scores, but after adjusting for CD4$^+$ cell count between treatment arms analyses suggested a trend towards a greater improvement in the peptide T group. Shifitto et al (1999) published a study involving lexipafant, a platelet-activating factor antagonist in HIV demen-

tia. The rationale is that there is evidence that a variety of inflammatory mediators, including platelet-activating factor, may contribute to neuronal injury in HIV infection. In a randomized, double blind, placebo-controlled trial of lexipafant, 30 patients with cognitive impairment were enrolled. A trend towards greater improvement was seen in neuropsychological performance, especially verbal memory, in the lexipafant treatment group.

Psychosis and antipsychotics

The two main issues in prescribing antipsychotics to patients with early HIV infection are drug–drug interactions and side effects. Clozapine may be relatively contraindicated with zidovudine, since each can cause bone marrow suppression, and in any case iatrogenic neutropenia in HIV patients should be avoided, for obvious reasons. In late stages of symptomatic HIV infection, extrapyramidal sensitivity to antipsychotics necessitates a low starting dose and careful titration of chosen drugs. This may arise because of a predilection of HIV for dopaminergic neurones of the basal ganglia (see Ch. 26). For this reason, atypical antipsychotics are usually preferred. Case reports of seizures following antipsychotic treatment have been published, and therefore it is wise to consider this when starting drugs that alter the seizure threshold. Risperidone and olanzapine have been used successfully in HIV-positive patients according to open-label studies and clinical experience. Amisulpride has not been examined but has a low rate of seizures, extrapyramidal side effects and blood dyscrasias. Caution should still be exercised. In practice, this means using low doses, titrating slowing and discontinuing slowly.

Depression, fatigue and antidepressants

Patients with HIV infection are often sensitive to psychotropic medication. The frequency of adverse effects, particularly with tricyclics, is often higher than is seen in primary depression. Symptomatic patients with HIV infection are also more sensitive to anticholinergic and antidopaminergic effects than are asymptomatic patients and healthy controls (see above). The side-effect profile alone may guide antidepressant choice (Elliot et al 1998). In terms of efficacy, several RCTs have examined the effect of antidepressants in HIV infection. In a 6-week study of imipramine versus placebo, Rabkin & Harrison (1994) examined 97 people with HIV (with or without AIDS) and depression. Imipramine was more effective than placebo and there was no evidence that imipramine adversely affected CD4$^+$ cell counts. Mauri et al (1994) conducted a double-blind study of fluvoxamine versus placebo in 26 HIV-positive patients with depression. There was a significant advantage of fluvoxamine over placebo at the end of the 8-week trial. Fernandez et al (1995), from Houston, Texas, presented results of a small randomized trial of methylphenidate versus desipramine in HIV-related depression. Both treatments were found to be equally effective. Elliot et al (1998) compared placebo, paroxetine (up to 40 mg/day) and imipramine (up to 200 mg/day) in a 12-week three-arm study in 75 HIV-positive patients

(45% of whom had AIDS). Of note, only 45% completed the 12 week trial, with imipramine being responsible for twice as many drop-outs as paroxetine. Both active drugs were more effective than placebo. In another RCT, from Rabkin et al (1999), 87 HIV-seropositive patients (50% with AIDS) with major depression or dysthymia completed 8 weeks of treatment of fluoxetine versus placebo and had the option of a 4-month extension. In completor analysis there was a significant benefit for fluoxetine (74% responded to fluoxetine and 47% to placebo). In a third RCT in this area, from the New York State Psychiatric Institute, Wagner & Rabkin (2000) studied the effect of dextroamphetamine on 22 men with DSM-IV depressive disorder featuring debilitating fatigue. In the 2-week study, eight of 11 patients assigned to dextroamphetamine reported significant improvement in mood and energy, compared with three of 12 placebo patients.

Markowitz et al (1995, 1998) examined cognitive and pharmacological intervention in a rather complex four-arm study of 101 HIV-positive men with depression. Interventions were cognitive–behavioural therapy, interpersonal therapy, supportive therapy, and supportive therapy plus imipramine for 16 weeks. The authors reported that last-observation-carried-forward analysis and completer analysis showed that depression scores decreased, with greater improvement noted with interpersonal psychotherapy and supportive psychotherapy with imipramine. Zisook et al (1998) studied 47 HIV-positive males with DSM-III major depressive disorder. The intervention was fluoxetine plus group psychotherapy versus placebo plus group psychotherapy for 7 weeks. After a 1-week placebo run-in, patients were randomized, and 25 were administered fluoxetine and 22 were given placebo. At 7 weeks, there was greater benefit in those who had received group therapy plus fluoxetine.

The use of psychostimulants is supported by one open trial and one placebo-controlled trial. Methylphenidate or dextroamphetamine may be effective for depression in HIV. Stimulants are sometimes given to improve fatigue symptoms (along with the cannabinoid dronabinol, the steroids oxandrolone and megestrol acetate, and the growth hormone somatotropin, all of which are approved by the Food and Drug Administration in the USA). Breitbart et al (1999) conducted a randomized RCT of methylphenidate and pemoline for fatigue in HIV. Both were superior to placebo, with a stronger effect of methylphenidate. Improvement in fatigue also improved symptoms of depression. Two groups have reported positive benefits of testosterone in depressed patients with HIV (Grinspoon et al 2000, Rabkin et al 2000). This observation related to the finding that symptoms of hypogonadism overlap with depression and that testosterone may be lower in depressed subjects than non-depressed HIV subjects. However, a third group has recently reported a negative result (Seidman et al 2001). Thus a larger scale RCT is required before an informed decision about the effects of psychostimulants on mood can be made.

Finally, one group performed an RCT to examine the use of simple relaxation therapies for depression in 81 outpatients with HIV. Interventions were guided imagery and relaxation therapy versus usual care. No significant effect on depression scores was found (Eller 1995). The possibility of drug interactions should be considered in those taking SSRIs, refazedone, trazedone, buproprion or tricyclic antidepressants along with antiretrovirals (see Ch. 64).

Mood stabilizers

Mood stabilizers should be used with caution in patients with HIV infection. Patients with AIDS are sensitive to lithium and can present with signs of toxicity, particularly tremor, ataxia and diarrhoea, even when lithium levels are in the therapeutic range. This may be related to the tendency to unstable fluid status and diarrhoea. Lithium is contraindicated for patients with HIV-related neuropathy and HIV-associated nephropathy, and has a particular interaction with indinavir. Carbamazepine can cause bone marrow suppression, and therefore is not commonly used (although this can be monitored); it also is an enzyme inducer, possibly reducing antiviral levels. Sodium valproate is probably the safest mainstream choice, although it does inhibit glucuronyl transferase, which can lead to elevated zidovudine concentrations. The use of lamotrigine and topiramate requires further investigation in patients with secondary mania, mainly from the perspective of tolerability.

SUMMARY

The management of the neuropsychiatric complications of HIV infection can be summarized as follows:

- investigate patients presenting with delirium for CNS involvement and offer symptomatic treatment
- rule out secondary complications in those with suspected AIDS dementia, including CNS infections, vitamin deficiencies and side-effects of medication
- document baseline cognitive performance in all patients with AIDS
- consider acetylcholinesterase inhibitors for cognitive impairment (one small RCT supports rivastigmine)
- atypical antipsychotics are recommended for psychosis and agitation, and amisulpride may be the drug of choice
- newer antidepressants are the preferred treatment for depression, but methylphenidate is an alternative, particularly where fatigue co-exists
- in mania, sodium valproate or divalproex are the drugs of choice, but carbamazepine is an alternative; all can cause drug interactions
- beware of drug–drug interactions in those taking antiretrovirals
- multidisciplinary, continued care is essential.

REFERENCES AND FURTHER READING

BHIVA Writing Committee on behalf of the BHIVA Executive Committee 2001 British HIV Association (BHIVA) guidelines for the treatment of HIV-infected adults with antiretroviral therapy. HIV Medicine 2:276–313

Breitbart WS, Rosenfeld B, Kaim M et al 1999 Psychostimulants for fatigue in the HIV$^+$ patients: preliminary findings of a placebo-controlled trial of methylphenidate vs pemoline. Psychosomatics 40:160–161

Brew BJ 1999 AIDS dementia complex. Neurologic Clinics 17:861–881

Butler KM, Husson RN, Balis FM et al 1991 Dideoxyinosine in children with symptomatic human immunodeficiency virus infection. New England Journal of Medicine 324:137–144

DANA Consortium on the Therapy of HIV Dementia Related Cognitive Disorders 1998 A randomized, double-blind, placebo-controlled trial of deprenyl and thioctic acid in human immunodeficiency virus-associated cognitive impairment. Neurology 50:645–651

Eller L 1995 Effects of two cognitive–behavioral interventions in immunity and symptoms in persons with HIV. Annals of Behavioral Medicine 17:339–348

Elliott AJ, Uldall KK, Bergam K et al 1998 Randomized, placebo-controlled trial of paroxetine versus imipramine in depressed HIV-positive outpatients. American Journal of Psychiatry 155:367–372

Fernandez F, Levy JK, Samley HR et al 1995 Effects of methylphenidate in HIV-related depression: a comparative trial with desipramine. International Journal of Psychiatry in Medicine 25:53–67

Grinspoon S, Corcoran C, Stanley T et al 2000 Effects of hypogonadism and testosterone administration on depression indices in HIV-infected men. Journal of Clinical Endocrinology and Metabolism 85:60–65

Heseltine PNR, Goodkin K, Atkinson JH et al 1998 Randomized double-blind placebo-controlled trial of peptide T for HIV-associated cognitive impairment. Archives of Neurology 55:41–51

Llorente AM, Gorp WGV, Stern MJ et al 2001 Long-term effects of high-dose zidovudine treatment on neuropsychological performance in mildly symptomatic HIV-positive patients: results of a randomized, double-blind. Placebo-controlled investigation. Journal of the International Neuropsychology Society 7:27–32

Markowitz JC, Klerman GL, Clougherty KF et al 1995 Individual psychotherapies for depressed HIV-positive patients. American Journal of Psychiatry 152:1504–1509

Markowitz JC, Peterkin J, Goggin KJ et al 1998 Treatment of depressive symptoms in human immunodeficiency virus-positive patients. Archives of General Psychiatry 55:452–457

Mauri MC, Ferrara A, Fabiano L et al 1994 A double blind study on fluvoxamine vs. placebo in depressed HIV positive patients: short-term and perspective results. Integrative Psychiatry 10:199–201

Pizzo PA, Eddy J, Falloon J et al 1988 Effect of continuous intravenous infusion of zidovudine (AZT) in children with symptomatic HIV infection. New England Journal of Medicine 319:889–896

Rabkin JG, Rabkin R, Harrison W et al 1994 Effect of imipramine on mood and enumerative measures of immune status in depressed patients with HIV illness. American Journal of Psychiatry 151:516–523

Rabkin JG, Wagner GJ, Rabkin R 1999 Fluoxetine treatment for depression in patients with HIV and AIDS: a randomized, placebo-controlled trial. American Journal of Psychiatry 156:101–107

Rabkin JG, Wagner GJ, Rabkin R 2000 A double-blind, placebo-controlled trial of testosterone therapy for HIV-positive men with hypogonadal symptoms. Archives of General Psychiatry 57:141–147

Schifitto G, Sacktor N, Marder K et al 1999 Randomized trial of the platelet-activating factor antagonist lexipafant in HIV-associated cognitive impairment. Neurology 53:391–396

Schmitt FA, Bigley JW, McKinnis R et al The AZT Collaborative Working Group 1988 Neuropsychological outcome of zidovudine (AZT) treatment of patients with AIDS and AIDS-related complex. New England Journal of Medicine 319:1573–1578

Seidman SN, Spatz E, Rizzo C et al 2001 Testosterone replacement therapy for hypogonadal men with major depressive disorder: a randomized, placebo-controlled clinical trial. Journal of Clinical Psychiatry 62:406–412

Sidtis JJ, Gatsonis C, Price RW et al for the AIDS Clinical Trials Group 1993 Zidovudine treatment of the AIDS dementia complex: results of a placebo-controlled trial. Annals of Neurology 33:343–349

US Department of Health and Human Services 2001 The HIV/AIDS Treatment Information Service (ATIS). http://hivatis.org/trtgdlns.html

Wagner G J, Rabkin R 2000 Effects of dextroamphetamine on depression and fatigue in men with HIV: a double-blind, placebo-controlled trial. Journal of Clinical Psychiatry 61:436–440

Zisook S, Peterkin J, Goggin KJ et al 1998 Treatment of major depression in HIV-seropositive men. Journal of Clinical Psychiatry 59:217–224

59

Treatment in Patients with CNS Tumours

NEUROLOGICAL TREATMENTS FOR CNS TUMOURS

Although the goal of intervention is to alleviate symptoms and modify the disease course, in the short-term patients undergoing treatment for CNS tumours may suffer an exacerbation of their neuropsychiatric problems. Disentangling these from the baseline deficits may not be straightforward. Patients undergoing treatment for intracranial tumours have a high frequency of baseline symptoms, including fatigue, motor difficulties, drowsiness, communication difficulties and headache. Superimposed are the adverse effects of chemotherapy or radiotherapy (or both) and the effects of steroids or other symptomatic treatments.

Chemotherapy

The main problem with cytotoxic agents is their effect on normal tissue. The antimetabolite methotrexate and the plant alkaloid cisplatin are among the most neurotoxic (Table 59.1). Methotrexate administration has been associated with the later development of dementia with leukoencephalopathy. Cisplatin has been observed to cause delirium, more commonly after intra-arterial infusion with symptoms of seizures, focal cortical signs including cortical blindness and cognitive impairment. Immunotherapy can have neu-

ropsychiatric complications. Interleukin-2 can cause cerebral oedema, delirium and, rarely, leukoencephalopathy. β-Interferons can cause delirium and dementia associated with parkinsonism. For a review see DeAngelis et al (2001).

Radiation therapy

The effect of radiotherapy on the CNS is a complex topic, well beyond the scope of this chapter. The neuropsychiatric complications are usually discussed in terms of encephalopathy (delirium) and diffuse tissue necrosis (dementia). Acute delirium occurs if an excessive dose of radiation is administered in one sitting. Pretreatment with corticosteroids may help prevent this. The onset may be within hours or delayed for days or weeks. Breakdown of white matter is the putative mechanism. Months or years after cessation of radiotherapy, focal or diffuse coagulative necrosis in white matter, sometimes accompanied by cerebral atrophy, has been observed. Varying degrees of cognitive impairment is one consequence of this. A minority of patients appear to suffer serious adverse cognitive effects, although the mean effect may be appreciable. Surma-aho et al (2001) compared 28 patients who had undergone postoperative irradiation after surgery for low-grade glioma with 23 who had not. The group that had undergone postoperative irradiation had poorer cognitive performance, a difference that was not accounted for by histological diagnosis or the location or size of the tumour. Leukoencephalopathy was more severe in the group that had received postoperative irradiation than in the group that had not, and it correlated with poor memory performances only in the postoperative radiotherapy group.

TREATMENT OF THE NEUROPSYCHIATRIC COMPLICATIONS OF CNS TUMOURS

This area is desperately under-researched. There have been no randomized controlled trials, but there has been one open-label study that is of particular interest. Meyers et al (1998) asked 30 patients with primary brain tumours to undertake neuropsychological assessment before and during treatment with methylphenidate. Activities of daily living and

Table 59.1 Neuropsychiatric effects of chemotherapeutic and related agents

Drug name	Delirium	Dementia	Visual loss	Ataxia	Aseptic meningitis	Seizures	Peripheral neuropathy
Hormonal agents							
Prednisolone	✓	✓					
Tamoxifen	✓		✓				
Plant alkaloids							
Vincristine	✓			✓		✓	✓
Etoposide	✓					✓	✓
Antimetabolites							
Methotrexate	✓	✓			✓	✓	
5-Fluorouracil				✓			
Cytarabine		✓		✓	✓		✓
Alkylating agents							
Cyclophosphamide							
Cisplatin	✓		✓			✓	✓
Chlorambucil							
Carmustine		✓				✓	
Other							
Interleukin	✓						
Interferons	✓	✓					
Cyclosporin	✓			✓		✓	

Adapted from DeAngelis et al (2001)

MRI results were also documented. Significant improvements in cognitive function were observed on a 10 mg twice-daily dose. Functional improvements included improved gait, increased stamina and better motivation to perform activities. Adverse effects were minimal. Gains in cognitive function were seen in half of the subjects.

SUMMARY

The management of the neuropsychiatric complications of CNS tumours can be summarized as follows:

- Evaluate the patient's understanding of the illness: is the patient underestimating the prognosis, and does the patient understand the treatment options?
- Assess the patient's adjustment to the life-threatening condition – has he or she responded with fighting spirit, denial or dysphoria or giving up?

- Assess the biological effects of the tumour on higher function.
- Review the site and size of the lesion.
- Assess the level of support and ascertain whether the family has come to terms with the changes in mood or personality and the prognosis.
- Offer a multidisciplinary approach to ongoing care.

REFERENCES AND FURTHER READING

DeAngelis LM, Delattre JY, Posner JB 2001 Neurological complications of chemotherapy and radiation therapy. In: Aminoff MJ (ed) Neurology and general medicine, 3rd edn. Churchill Livingstone, Edinburgh, p 347–358

Surma-aho O, Niemelä M, Vilkki J et al 2001 Adverse long-term effects of brain radiotherapy in adult low-grade glioma patients. Neurology 56:1285–1290

Meyers CA, Weitzner MA, Valentine AD et al 1998 Methylphenidate therapy improves cognition, mood, and function of brain tumor patients. Journal of Clinical Oncology 16:2522–2527

60

Treatment in Patients with Motor Neurone Disease (Amyotrophic Lateral Sclerosis)

NEUROLOGICAL TREATMENTS FOR MOTOR NEURONE DISEASE

Riluzole is a sodium channel blocker that inhibits the release of glutamate. In a comparatively large trial published in 1994, Bensimon et al reported a prospective, double blind, placebo-controlled study in 155 outpatients with motor neurone disease (MND). After 12 months, more patients with bulbar-onset disease (but not other types) were alive after taking riluzole. The deterioration of muscle strength was slightly slower in the riluzole group than in the placebo group. About one-third of patients in the riluzole group withdrew from the study because of adverse reactions (asthenia and spasticity). Since that time, three other randomized controlled trials (RCTs) have been published and reviewed (National Institute for Clinical Excellence 2001).

At the present time very limited evidence supports a positive effect on quality of life, extended time to mechanical ventilation, or prevention of functional deterioration. Nevertheless, in the UK the National Institute for Clinical Excellence (NICE) has recommended that riluzole should be made available in the NHS for patients with MND. In the real world, the effect will be a prolongation of life for 2–6 months, which will arguably be hardly noticeable to most patients, who will still be suffering the same symptoms. Accordingly, patients' perspective on riluzole is mixed. Many people do not wish to have treatment to extend life once physically very unwell. Indeed, Ganzini et al (1998) reported that over half of a sample of 100 patients with MND said they would consider assisted suicide in these circumstances.

TREATMENT OF THE NEUROPSYCHIATRIC COMPLICATIONS OF MOTOR NEURONE DISEASE

There have been no RCTs (or any other studies) in this area.

SUMMARY

The management of the neuropsychiatric complications of MND can be summarized as follows:

- Elucidate the patient's understanding of MND and ascertain whether the patient understands the prognosis, treatment options and level of support available.
- Assess the patient's adjustment to the life-threatening condition – has he or she responded with fighting spirit, denial or dysphoria or by giving up?
- Screen for the presence of cognitive impairment, apathy, depression and suicidal thoughts.
- Assess the level of support.
- Ascertain how well the family has come to terms with the illness.
- Offer a multidisciplinary approach to the treatment of neuropsychiatric complications.

Clinical Pointer 60.1

Assisted suicide and euthanasia in terminal neurological illnesses

This is a very emotive topic for doctors, who are naturally uncomfortable with the concept of avoidable accelerated death. Attitudes of doctors, patients and carers have been surveyed extensively, but results are highly dependent on the way sensitive questions are asked (Emanuel 2002). One large survey of primary care physicians in Northern Ireland found that 70% of GPs believe that passive euthanasia is ethically acceptable and that 50% would be prepared to condone it (McGlade et al 2000). Furthermore, 30% had received requests from patients for assisted euthanasia (physician-assisted suicide) in the preceding 5 years.

Whatever the attitudes of doctors, the feelings of patients and carers must be taken into account. One of the most comprehensive surveys of attitudes examined 1341 HIV-infected sufferers in 11 European countries (Andraghetti et al 2001). Seventy-eight per cent of the patients were in favour of legalizing euthanasia in the case of severe physical suffering and 47% in order to alleviate severe psychological suffering. Importantly, half of the people living with HIV-infection or AIDS reported that the option of euthanasia would reduce their current anxiety about the future. Ganzini et al (1998) in Portland, Oregon, asked 100 patients and carers with MND about assisted suicide after the 'Oregon Death with Dignity Act' legalized physician-assisted suicide in 1997. Over 56% of sufferers said they would consider euthanasia, and this was more likely in men with a higher level of education but a low level of religious beliefs with more hopelessness and lower quality of life. However, it is important to remember that patients' attitudes are not fixed. One survey found that within the space of a year, half of those supporting euthanasia had changed their minds, but an equal number of dissenters had also changed. Ultimately, there will always be divided opinion on this topic, with sticking points being how to decide when a terminal illness is really terminal, when to accept the patient's view as final, what to do in case of conflict with carers, and how much to be involved in ending life. A final point to consider is that patients with high rates of depression are much more likely to request euthanasia, and thus depression should be considered and treated before such a decision is taken to be final.

Further reading *Andraghetti R, Foran S, Colebunders R et al 2001 Euthanasia: from the perspective of HIV infected persons in Europe. HIV Medicine 2:3–10*
Emanuel EJ 2002 Euthanasia and physician-assisted suicide. A review of the empirical data from the United States. Archives of Internal Medicine 162:142–152
Emanuel EJ, Fairclough DL, Emanuel LL 2000 Attitudes and desires related to euthanasia and physician-assisted suicide among terminally ill patients and their caregivers. JAMA 284:2460–2468
Ganzini L, Johnston WS, McFarland BH et al 1998 Attitudes of patients with amyotrophic lateral sclerosis and their care givers toward assisted suicide. New England Journal of Medicine 339:967–973
McGlade KJ, Slaney L, Bunting BP et al 2000 Voluntary euthanasia in Northern Ireland: general practitioners' beliefs, experiences, and actions. British Journal of General Practice 50:794–797

REFERENCES AND FURTHER READING

Bensimon G, Lacomblez L, Meininger V et al 1994 A controlled trial of riluzole in amyotrophic lateral sclerosis. New England Journal of Medicine 330:585–591

Ganzini L, Johnson WS, McFarland BH et al 1998 Attitudes of patients with amyotrophic lateral sclerosis and their care givers toward assisted suicide. New England Journal of Medicine 339:967–973

National Institute for Clinical Excellence 2001 Guidance on the use of riluzole (Rilutek) for the treatment of motor neurone disease. Technology Appraisal Guidance No. 20

61

Treatment in Patients with Sleep Disorders

NARCOLEPSY

If the disability is mild, no pharmacological treatment is necessary. Behavioural treatment, particularly a schedule of short naps several times a day, can be very successful. Sufferers who schedule brief naps report improved alertness for up to 2 hours subsequently (Guilleminault & Brooks 2001). There is often an interaction with meals (which could be an effect of hypocretin), and thus dietary manipulation can be useful. Advice and support regarding work, hobbies and driving is usually required. Patients should be encouraged to lead as active a life as possible. Often their own fears are more than sufficient in answering concerns about safety.

If medication is required, stimulants are usually the drugs of choice. Alternatives are amphetamine, methamphetamine, dextroamphetamine, methylphenidate and pemoline (for a review, see Littner et al 2001). Modafinil, a benzohydrylsulfinyl acetamide derivative, is being evaluated as a safer alternative to stimulants. The mechanism of action of modafinil remains to be defined, but it appears to have a low abuse potential. In a 6-week randomized controlled trial of 75 narcoleptic patients, Broughton et al (1997) compared modafinil with placebo. Modafinil significantly increased the mean sleep latency and reduced the number of daytime sleep episodes. There were no effects on nocturnal sleep. This was followed by two larger multicentre studies by the US Modafinil in Narcolepsy Multicenter Study Group. In the first study, 283 people with narcolepsy received modafinil or placebo for 9 weeks (Mitler et al 1998). Modafinil significantly reduced all measures of sleepiness and was associated with significant improvements in level of illness. Medication-related adverse experiences were few, dose-dependent and mostly rated as mild to moderate. Mild headache was the most common adverse effect. Modafinil demonstrated an excellent safety profile for up to 40 weeks of open-label treatment, and efficacy was maintained, suggesting that tolerance is unlikely to develop with long-term use. In the second study, an 8-week treatment discontinuation phase was included to evaluate the effects of withdrawal on patients who had been receiving modafinil (Becker et al 2000). A total of 240 patients received modafinil in the discontinuation phase. Previous results were replicated, and during treatment discontinuation patients did not experience an amphetamine-like withdrawal syndrome. Unfortunately, modafinil does not seem to work well for cataplexy and response may be inferior in those previously treated with amphetamines. Tricyclic antidepressants, selective serotonin reuptake inhibitors (SSRIs) and γ-hydroxybutyrate (GHB) can be used to treat catalepsy as well as sleep paralysis.

SLEEP APNOEA

Sleep apnoea is a difficult condition to treat successfully. Treatments include positional alterations, intraoral devices and surgical procedures aimed at improving the flow of air. Continuous positive air-

---

Box 61.1 Sleep hygiene recommendations

- Create sleep–wake habits
- Use the bedroom for sleep and the living room for wake periods exclusively
- Avoid stimulants such as caffeine
- Moderate alcohol and food consumption
- Take regular exercise in the day
- Do something relaxing
- Get up if not sleeping within 20 minutes
- Maintain comfortable sleeping conditions (mattress, sheets)
- Avoid daytime sleeping

way pressure therapy has become the treatment of choice for obstructive sleep apnoea, with accumulating evidence suggesting benefit in both the apnoea–hypopnoea and diurnal tiredness when compared with a suitable sham control (Loredo et al 1999). However, non-compliance is the largest problem and it may be ineffective in people without daytime sleepiness; this is still unclear (Barbe et al 2001). Pharmacological strategies have been disappointing, including the use of modafinil in sleep apnoea (Grunstein et al 2001).

CHRONIC INSOMNIA

Beyond modulation of environmental factors (including diet, exercise and substance abuse), education and behavioural techniques, more specialized approaches include relaxation therapies, cognitive–behavioural treatment for insomnia and drug treatment. Ironically, much of the difficulty surrounding the pharmacological management of chronic insomnia involves how to stop medication rather than how to start it. The following principles apply. Prescribing medication for the shortest possible period (usually less than 4 weeks), gradually discontinuing medication and being alert for rebound insomnia following discontinuation. Self-medication strategies (alcohol and over-the-counter agents) are only minimally effective in inducing sleep, but detract from sustained quality of sleep, often at the expense of daytime performance. A number of groups have undertaken meta-analyses of pharmacotherapy and behavioural therapy for chronic insomnia, with broadly similar conclusions (Smith et al 2002). Both modalities improve sleep latency and interruption of sleep, although non-pharmacological treatments may have more enduring effects. Mirtazepine, nefazadone, trazadone and paroxetine are often used to treat depression with associated insomnia in preference to older sedating tricyclic antidepressants. However, data to support their use in primary insomnia are currently scarce.

Box 61.2 Drugs that can cause insomnia

- Alcohol
- Amphetamines
- Anticholinergics
- Beta blockers
- Caffeine
- Cimetidine
- Cytotoxics
- Monoamine oxidase inhibitors
- Methyldopa
- Reserpine
- Selective serotonin reuptake inhibitors
- Sympathomimetics

Clinical Pointer 61.1

Basic approach to patients with uncomplicated sleep problems

A sleep history is most useful when corroborated by a sleeping partner. A partner is better placed to report bruxism, snoring, apnoea, abnormal movements or somnambulism. A sleep history should include the nature of the sleep problem, sleeping environment, sleep hygiene, dietary habits, and a systematic medical and psychiatric enquiry. A family history may reveal hereditary narcolepsy or periodic limb movement disorder. A 2-week sleep diary is recommended for most patients. Mental state examination should help eliminate the common psychiatric causes of poor sleep, including psychophysiological insomnia, depression and primary anxiety disorder. Somatic symptoms such as restless legs, myoclonus and breathing problems may highlight a medical cause for disturbed sleep.

Hypersomnia is often investigated using the Multiple Sleep Latency Test. Here the subject is enticed to sleep in a darkened room in 20-minute periods across 2-hour intervals. An average sleep latency of less than 5 minutes is abnormal. Other specific sleep investigations include video sleep recording and polysomnography.

Treatment always begins with a review of sleep hygiene. Psychological treatments for sleep disorder are effective and well tolerated. These usually involve cognitive–behavioural therapy. Medication should be used with caution, since hypnotics are liable to be effective in the short term and may be associated with dependency. The hypnotics zopiclone and zolpidem do not cause REM suppression or rebound or significant dependency, but they have a short half-life that can cause mid-insomnia. Alcohol and caffeinated drinks should be gradually reduced. Good sleep habits should gradually return.

Further reading Antonio Culebras 1999 Sleep disorders and neurological disease. Marcel Dekker, New York
Seyone C, Shapiro C 1995 Long-term therapy of insomnia. In: Ancil RJ, Lader MH (eds) Pharmacological management of chronic psychiatric disorders. Baillière's Clinical Psychiatry 1:605–637

SUMMARY

The management of sleep disorders can be summarized as follows:

- elucidate factors contributing to disrupted sleep (e.g. stimulants, lifestyle, sleeping conditions, work, stress)
- screen for any unusual sleep disorders
- screen for depression, anxiety, mania and substance abuse
- recommend a sleep diary
- provide information about good sleep hygiene
- consider specialist investigations or referral if problems persist.

REFERENCES AND FURTHER READING

Barbe F, Mayoralas L R, Duran J et al 2001 Treatment with continuous positive airway pressure is not effective in patients with sleep apnea but no daytime sleepiness: a randomized, controlled trial. Annals of Internal Medicine 134:1015–1023

Becker PM, Jamieson AO, Jewel CE et al 2000 Randomized trial of modafinil as a treatment for the excessive daytime somnolence of narcolepsy. Neurology 54:1166–1175

Broughton RJ, Fleming JAE, George CFP et al 1997 Randomized, double-blind, placebo-controlled crossover trial of modafinil in the treatment of excessive daytime sleepiness in narcolepsy. Neurology 49:444–451

Grunstein RR, Hedner J, Grote L 2001 Treatment options for sleep apnoea. Drugs 61:237–251

Guilleminault C, Brooks SN 2001 Excessive daytime sleepiness. A challenge for the practising neurologist. Brain 124:1482–1491

Littner M, Johnson SF, McCall WV et al 2001 Practice parameters for the treatment of narcolepsy: an update for 2000. Sleep 24:451–466

Loredo JS, Ancoli-Israel S, Dimsdale JE 1999 Effect of continuous positive airway pressure vs placebo continuous positive airway pressure on sleep quality in obstructive sleep apnea. Chest 116:1545–1549

Mitler MM, Guilleminault C, Harsh JR et al 1998 Randomized trial of modafinil for the treatment of pathological somnolence in narcolepsy. Annals of Neurology 43:88–97

Smith MT, Perlis ML, Park A et al 2002 Comparative meta-analysis of pharmacotherapy and behavior therapy for persistent insomnia. American Journal of Psychiatry 159:5–11

62

Management of Carer Stress

Carer stress is reciprocally related to patient well-being. Chronic debilitating illnesses affect both the patient and their carers. As an example, 90% of stroke survivors are able to return home after the acute hospitalization. This is compounded by the fact that at least half of all patients with brain injury are suddenly unable or unwilling to leave the home and lose previous sources of support outside the family. It should be of no surprise that significant distress is present in more than half of carers of these patients. Equally, three-quarters of patients with dementia are cared for at home by carers. Most often this is a close family member who, statistically, is more likely to be female. The burden felt by carers of dementia sufferers is equal to that experienced by the relatives of stroke victims, and in both cases it is strongly related to the psychiatric and behavioural complications in the patient (Draper et al 1992).

It is hard to imagine the frustration that looking after a disabled family member creates. Such persistent stress takes its toll in the form of distress, depression, anxiety and a decline in the physical health and social function of the carer. Several studies have found that predictors of carer stress include severe disability or neuropsychiatric disturbance in the patient, an uncertain prognosis, absence of family or professional support (for the carer), poor carer coping skills and poor carer physical health (Han & Haley 1999). The psychiatric and behavioural problems of patients with dementia impact on carers more powerfully than impaired cognition alone. In addition, individual psychiatric symptoms influence carers differently in different stages of dementia (Kaufer et al 2002).

Management of carer stress sensibly involves additional help where available. This can come in a variety of forms, from residential care, to home nursing assistance, to delivered meals. Interventions generally need to be ongoing. For example, respite care is widely accepted for dementia, but beneficial effects quickly wear off, and so regular repetition is needed. Local or national support groups are often the best source of information for carers. Provision of appropriate information from an early stage is likely to minimize the difficulty that the patient and relatives have in coming to terms with a new diagnosis. Questions of driving, medication, prognosis and legal status are commonly raised. Effective treatment of the underlying condition has a role in reducing carer stress, with studies in Alzheimer's disease showing that galantamine (and other effective treatments) reduce the time required in assisting with activities of daily living.

STUDIES OF INTERVENTIONS DIRECTED AT CARERS

Many studies have examined whether specific interventions may improve coping abilities or well-being in carers of patients with Alzheimer's disease, but few have looked at other conditions. Studies have employed education, support, training and counselling as the main interventions, and have often included a mixture of approaches. In an excellent

Clinical Pointer 62.1

A multidisciplinary approach to neuropsychiatric treatment

The multidisciplinary approach aims to use skills from different professionals to maximize patient care. Several groups have reported success using a multidisciplinary intervention for patients with memory complaints. The memory clinic team usually comprises a neurologist, a psychologist and a psychiatrist. Unless an individual has expertise in all areas, this core team would be an advantage in assessing inpatients and outpatients with neuropsychiatric complaints. Additional members of the team might also include an occupational therapist to assess the patient's activities of daily living skills, a social worker to examine the patient's social needs and living conditions, and a community psychiatric nurse to observe the patient's symptoms and drug responses outside of the clinic or ward. It is a mistake to think that medical staff are the only professionals capable of delivering quality care. Several studies have shown that non-medical staff are, with appropriate training and supervision, perfectly capable of accurate diagnoses and competent treatment of many common conditions (Collighan et al 1993, Sakr et al 1999). However, some diagnoses are more difficult than others and hence require structured supervision. The strengths of the multidisciplinary team are often in degree of engagement and rapport, detailed monitoring, and the supervision and feedback structure.

The team also has an important educational and supportive role for both the patient and their relatives. The multidisciplinary team share information in each of their specialized areas with the team leader (usually the consultant), in order that the optimum care package is coordinated and kept under review. Thus, the overall package of care focuses on all aspects of the patient's needs, whether it be medical, psychological or social.

Further reading   Collighan G, Macdonald A, Herzberg J et al 1993 Evaluation of the multidisciplinary approach to psychiatric diagnosis in elderly people. BMJ 306:821–824
Sakr M, Angus J, Perrin J et al 1999 Care of minor injuries by emergency nurse practitioners or junior doctors: a randomized controlled trial. Lancet 354:1321–1326
Sorensen L, Foldspang A, Gulmann NC et al 2001 Assessment of dementia in nursing home residents by nurses and assistants: criteria validity and determinants. International Journal of Geriatric Psychiatry 16:615–621

review Green & Brodaty (2002) appraised 35 of the more stringent articles in the dementia field. The following randomized controlled trials (RCTs) involving more than 100 subjects have been conducted using a multifaceted intervention strategy to gain maximum possible benefit.

Zarit et al (1987) provided eight sessions of counselling and support for 145 carers of dementia in comparison with 39 waiting list controls. There was a reduction in carer stress in the active arms (more so in those who received counselling than support), but no effect on nursing home placement. Mittelman et al (1996) conducted an RCT to determine the long-term effectiveness of six sessions of support and counselling for 206 families coping with Alzheimer's disease sufferers in the community. The intervention group took longer than the control group in admitting relatives to nursing home care (by 329 days) and ultimately reduced the nursing home placement rate by one-third. Not surprisingly, the effect was mostly seen in people with mild to moderate dementia. Teri et al (1997) in Seattle examined interventions for carers of Alzheimer's disease patients who were also depressed. They asked 72 patient–carer dyads to consent to randomization to behavioural therapy (emphasizing either carer problem solving or patient pleasant events) compared with usual care and waiting list alone. Carers who received behavioural therapy showed significant improvement in depressive symptoms, while carers in the two other conditions did not. Benefits were maintained at the 6-month follow-up. Brodaty et al (1997) reported 8-year outcome data on an ongoing RCT involving 96 people less than 80 years old with mild to moderate dementia and their cohabiting carers. All patients received a 10-day structured memory retraining and activity programme, but carers received either a structured, residential 10-day training programme with booster sessions or 10 days' respite and booster sessions. Effects were modest, but demonstrable. At 8 years, the nursing home admission rate was 79% in the training group versus 90% in the respite group. There was also a small effect on survival. Eloniemi-Sulkava et al (1999) used a comprehensive programme (with two refresher courses) in 53 relatives of dementia patients and 47 controls. There was an effect in delaying time to institutionalization, but not on the rate of institutionalization or mortality at 2 years.

In stroke, only two studies were identified. Mant et al (2000) examined 323 patients and 267 carers in a single-blind RCT to assess the impact of family support on stroke patients and their carers. Patients with acute stroke were assigned to family support or normal care within 6 weeks of stroke. After 6 months, the carer's knowledge about stroke, social activities and quality of life was better in the family support group, although no beneficial effect to the patients was demonstrated. In the second study, carers of stroke patients from four regions of The Netherlands were assigned in blocks to a control group, a group programme or individual home visits (Van den Heuvel et al 2000). In the short term both interventions contributed significantly to an increase in confidence of knowledge about patient care and confidence in seeking social support. There were no significant differences between group support and individual support.

SUMMARY

The management of carer stress can be summarized as follows:

- listen to the carer's issues and problems – additional help, information or respite may be necessary
- explain to carers that they are not alone and not constantly indispensable – feeling isolated and without options predicts depression
- screen for depression, adjustment disorder and complicated grief
- recommend support group(s)
- recommend further sources of information – patients and carers are entitled to know as much about the index condition as they wish, but they often do not know where best to look
- consider referral for psychological treatment, if problems are refractory – carers' mental health needs should not be overlooked
- consider setting up a comprehensive support

programme for carers locally – this is likely to bring benefits to both patients and carers.·

REFERENCES AND FURTHER READING

Brodaty H, Gresham M, Luscombe G 1997 The Prince Henry Hospital dementia caregivers' training programme. International Journal of Geriatric Psychiatry 12:183–192

Draper BM, Poulos CJ, Cole AMD et al 1992 A comparison of caregivers for elderly stroke and dementia victims. Journal of the American Geriatric Society 40:896–901

Eloniemi-Sulkava U, Sivenius J, Sulkava R 1999 Support program for demented patients and their carers: the role of dementia family care coordinator is crucial. In: Iqbal K, Swaab DF, Winblad B et al (eds) Alzheimer's disease and related disorders. Wiley, New York, p 795–802

Green A, Brodaty H 2002 Care-giver interventions. In: Qizilbash N, Schneider LS, Chui H et al (eds) Evidence-based dementia practice. Blackwell, Oxford, p 764–794

Han B, Haley WE 1999 Family caregiving for patients with stroke: review and analysis. Stroke 30:1478–1485

Kaufer DI, Lingler JA, Ketchel PJ et al 2002 cognitive and neuropsychiatric symptoms in Alzheimer's disease: differential relationship to global functioning and caregiver distress. Presented at the American Academy of Neurology 54th Annual Meeting, Denver, 13–20 April

Mant J, Carter J, Wade DT et al 2000 Family support for stroke: a randomised controlled trial. Lancet 356:808–813

Mittelman MS, Ferris SH, Shulman E et al 1996 A family intervention to delay nursing home placement of patients with Alzheimer disease: a randomized controlled trial. JAMA 276:1725–1731

Teri L, Logsdon RG, Uomoto J et al 1997 Behavioral treatment of depression in dementia patients: a controlled clinical trial. Journal of Gerontology, Series B 52:159–166

Van den Heuvel ETP, de Witte LP, Nooyen-Haazen I et al 2000 Short-term effects of a group support program and an individual support program for caregivers of stroke patients. Patient Education and Counseling 40:109–120

Zarit SH, Anthony CR, Boutselus M 1987 Interventions with care givers of dementia patients: comparison of two approaches. Psychology and Aging 2:225–232

63

Issues relating to Prescribing Psychotropic Drugs in Pregnancy

Psychotropic prescribing in pregnancy is a huge topic and could justify a textbook in itself. The issues include the following. Does the neuropsychiatric disease or its treatment harm fertility? Are there genetic or parenting issues? Does pregnancy influence the psychiatric manifestations? Are psychotropic drugs safe during breast feeding? Are psychotropic drugs safe in pregnancy? If drug safety is not certain, what is the threshold for treatment? I will concentrate on the last two issues.

DRUG SAFETY DURING PREGNANCY

It is important to consider possible teratogenicity in women of childbearing age as about half of pregnancies are unplanned. Some studies estimate that one-third of pregnant women take psychotropic medication during the pregnancy. This area has been comprehensively reviewed (Austin & Mitchell 2000, Ward et al 2000). Estimates of risk for drugs used during pregnancy are derived largely from case reports or retrospective cohort epidemiological stud-ies because prospective, randomized studies are considered unethical.

Depression and antidepressants

Antidepressants are essentially safe during pregnancy, the most common adverse effects being withdrawal reactions following delivery and dose-related (anticholinergic effects) side effects due to the slow metabolism of the foetus. The US Food and Drug Administration advises that there is evidence of risk with amitriptyline and nortriptyline, but their use is acceptable when indicated. Antidepressants are similarly safe in breast-feeding, with on average less than 0.5% of the agent being passed to the neonate.

Psychosis and antipsychotics

There are few data to suggest antipsychotics are unsafe in pregnancy and accumulating evidence to suggest that they are safe. Exceptions are prochlorperazine, loxapine and clozapine, which should be avoided. Breast-feeding may be problematic because of hyperprolactinaemia, although sulpiride is only passed to the neonate at 1% of the mother's levels.

Anxiety and anxiolytics

Benzodiazepines appear to increase the relative risk of cleft palate and lip with first-trimester exposure (especially to alprazolam) from 0.06% to 0.7% (Altshuler et al 1996). Exposure to benzodiazepines in the third trimester may lead to hypotonicity in the child at birth.

Antiepileptic drugs and mood stabilizers

Congenital malformations and other poor neonatal outcomes are three times more common in women who have been maintained on antiepileptic drugs (AEDs) during pregnancy. Lithium is a problem because it crosses the placenta and causes Epstein's anomaly in about 1 in 1000 cases when taken from weeks 2 to 6 of pregnancy. It should be used only if essential and then only with foetal echocardiography. After delivery, lithium is passed to the neonate in breast-feeding at one-third the maternal level. Sodium valproate and carbamazepine are associated with foetal abnormalities, including spina bifida in

1% of cases. Valproate may have a greater toxicity profile than carbamazepine, especially at high doses (over 1 g/day); however, it is tolerated while breast-feeding. This may be reflected in a higher rate of learning disabilities in children of mothers on valproate (Adab et al 2001). Other AEDs associated with increased risk include phenobarbitone, phenytoin, tiagabine, topiramate and vigabatrin. Folic acid is recommended for women with epilepsy who are pregnant. Overall, the rate of foetal malformations is 2% for the general population and 6% for patients on one AED, but 20% for patients on three AEDs.

THRESHOLD FOR TREATMENT DURING PREGNANCY

Like all prescribing situations, prescribing during pregnancy is a balance of risks versus benefits. Discontinuing medication increases the likelihood of relapse, suicidal thoughts, poor self-care or nutrition, and poor antenatal clinic compliance. There is also the consideration of the effect of maternal illness on the child, both prenatally and after birth.

Predictably, accurate risks concerning newer drugs are not known. A guiding principle is to avoid drugs wherever possible in pregnancy, particularly in the first trimester. The first trimester is the time when medication is most likely to cause malformations of the foetus. Ideally, medication should be stopped before trying to conceive, unless there are clear predictors of poor outcome. Drug treatment should be interrupted during labour.

SUMMARY

The issues to consider when prescribing during pregnancy can be summarized as follows:

- consider the balance of risk versus benefits and inform the patient of these
- beware of mood disorders during and after pregnancy
- try to avoid medication during the first trimester
- use only necessary medication during the second and third trimesters, but the consequences of not treating should be considered equally seriously
- avoid sedative medication during labour
- advise on breast-feeding and familial risks
- restart medication, where indicated, after the pregnancy.

REFERENCES AND FURTHER READING

Adab N, Jacoby A, Smith D et al 2001 Additional educational needs in children born to mothers with epilepsy. Journal of Neurology, Neurosurgery and Psychiatry 70:15–21

Altshuler LL, Cohen L, Szuba MP et al 1996 Pharmacologic management of psychiatric illness during pregnancy: dilemmas and guidelines. American Journal of Psychiatry 153:592–606

Austin MP, Mitchell P 2000 Psychotropic medications in pregnant and breast-feeding women: a review of the literature and treatment guidelines. Australian and New Zealand Journal of Psychiatry 34(suppl S):A4

Ward RM, Bates BA, McCarver DG et al 2000 Use of psychoactive medication during pregnancy and possible effects on the fetus and newborn. Pediatrics 105:880–887

64

Psychotropic Drug Interactions

There are many reasons why concomitant prescribing of multiple drugs should be avoided where ever possible. Polypharmacy is associated with poor compliance, administration errors and an increased risk of adverse effects. Drug–drug interactions can lead to greatly altered pharmacological effects. Only a brief summary is possible here. The reader is referred elsewhere for further detail (Stockley 1999). The two main types of drug interactions are pharmacokinetic and pharmacodynamic. Pharmacokinetic interactions occur when one medication affects the plasma concentration of another medica-tion by altering its absorption, distribution, metabolism or elimination. The most common type of interaction involves induction or inhibition of the cytochrome p450 system. Pharmacodynamic interactions occur when one drug affects the therapeutic target or receptor of the other drug. Drug interactions are subject to great individual differences, being modified by genetic factors, ageing, pregnancy and disease states.

PHARMACODYNAMIC INTERACTIONS

As with pharmacokinetic interactions, pharmacodynamic interactions can be beneficial. This is the principle underlying augmentation treatment strategies. When prescribing for patients with brain injury, extra care should be taken to avoid additive adverse effects. Common examples include:

- sedation, when using tricyclic antidepressants, antipsychotics, older antiepileptic drugs together, or in combination with hypnotics or benzodiazepines
- anticholinergic symptoms, when using any combination of tricyclic antidepressants, antipsychotics or antimuscarinics
- hypotension, when using several tricyclic antidepressants, antipsychotics or beta blockers
- haematological or electrolyte abnormalities when using lithium, clozapine or carbamazepine.

PHARMACOKINETIC INTERACTIONS

Most drugs are predominantly metabolized by the liver and excreted by the kidney. The cytochrome p450 enzymes, located in the smooth endoplasmic reticulum, are responsible for this metabolism. These enzymes can be inhibited, causing a rise in the plasma level of the substrate, or induced, causing a fall in concentration. In general, induction takes longer than inhibition. Several drugs are not metabolised by the liver. This can be used to good effect in patients with hepatic impairment (see Clinical Pointer 54.1). However, these drugs may accumulate by other means. For example, lamotrigine is metabolized by the conjugating enzyme uridine diphosphate glucuronosyltransferase (UGT). This enzyme may be inhibited by sertraline, risking

---

Box 64.1 Drugs with serious P450 interaction potential

- Calcium channel blockers
- Cisapride
- Cyclosporine
- Flecainide
- Haloperidol
- Lovastatin
- Phenytoin
- Propafenone
- Protease inhibitors
- Simvastatin
- Theophylline
- Tricyclic antidepressants
- Triazolam/alprazolam
- Warfarin

Table 64.1 Psychotropic drug interactions

P450 enzyme	Substrates: psychotropic	Substrates: non-psychotropic	Inducers: psychotropic	Inducers: non-psychotropic	Inhibitors: psychotropic	Inhibitors: non-psychotropic
CYP1A2	*Antidepressants* Amitriptyline* Clomipramine* Desipramine* Imipramine* *Antipsychotics* Clozapine* Olanzapine* Chlorpromazine* Haloperidol* Trazodone *Benzodiazepines* Chlordiazepoxide Diazepam	Cyclobenzaprine Naproxen Propranolol Riluzole Theophylline*		Smoking	Fluvoxamine	*Antibiotics* Ciprofloxacin Clarithromycin Erythromycin Levofloxacin Norfloxacin *Other* Cimetidine Grapefruit juice Ketoconazole
CYP2C9	*Antidepressants* Fluoxetine Sertraline *Benzodiazepines* Diazepam	NSAIDs Oral hypoglycaemics Angiotensin II antagonists Fluvastatin Naproxen Phenytoin* Tamoxifen Tolbutamide Warfarin*	Barbiturates	Prednisone Rifampicin	Fluoxetine Fluvoxamine	Amiodarone Chloramphenicol Fluconazole Omeprazole
CYP2C19	*Barbiturates* Diazepam Phenobarbitone *Antidepressants* Moclobemide Venlafaxine Citalopram Amitriptyline* Imipramine* Clomipramine*	Omeprazole Lansoprazole Cyclophosphamide Progesterone	Barbiturates	Rifampicin	Fluoxetine Fluvoxamine	Fluconazole Omeprazole

	Substrates		Inducers	Inhibitors
CYP2D6	*Antipsychotics* Risperidone* Clozapine Olanzapine Thioridazine* Chlorpromazine* Haloperidol *Antidepressants* Venlafaxine Antipsychotics Mirtazapine SSRIs *Other* Donepezil	Beta blockers *Analgesics* Codeine Dextromethorphan *Antiarrhythmics* Flecainide* Propafenone Ondansetron Tamoxifen Tramadol	Barbiturates	Paroxetine Fluoxetine Haloperidol Fluphenazine Methanol Amiodarone, Propafenone Quinidine

CYP3A4	*Mood stabilizers*
	Carbamazepine*
	Ethosuximide*
	
	Antipsychotics
	Clozapine
	Pimozide
	Quetiapine
	Ziprasidone
	
	Antidepressants
	Nefazodone
	Citalopram
	Desipramine*
	Buspirone
	Trazodone
	Venlafaxine
	
	Other
	Benzodiazepines
	Methadone
	Donepezil
		Cytotoxics
		Macrolide antibiotics
		Quinidine anti-
		  arrhythmics
		Cyclosporin
		Antiviral protease
		  inhibitors
		Cisapride
		Antihistamines
		Calcium channel
		  blockers
		HMG COA reductase
		  inhibitors (not
		  parvastatin)
		Tamoxifen
		Vincristine
			Barbiturates
			Phenytoin
			Carbamazepine
			St. John's Wort
			
			HIV antivirals
			Efavirenz
			Efavirenz
			Nevirapine
			
			Other
			Barbiturates
			Glucocorticoids
			Modafinil
			Phenobarbital
			Phenytoin
			Pioglitazone
			Rifampicin
			St. John's Wort
			Troglitazone
				Fluvoxamine
				Nefazodone
				
				Amiodarone
				
				Antibiotics
				Clarithromycin
				Erythromycin
				Metronidazole
				Norfloxacin
				Troleandomycin
				
				Antifungals
				Fluconazole
				Ketoconazole
				Itraconazole
				
				Calcium channel
				antagonists
				Verapamil
				Diltiazem

*Drugs of low therapeutic index

lamotrigine toxicity. Knowledge of the effects of drugs at each isoenzyme can help predict and prevent adverse drug–drug interactions.

CYP1A2

The 1A2 enzyme is inhibited by fluvoxamine, leading to raised blood levels of tricyclic antidepressants and antipsychotics, including clozapine and olanzapine. Conversely, smoking lowers the concentration the these drugs.

CYP2C9

Warfarin and phenytoin are primarily metabolized via CYP2C9, although CYP2C19 may also play a small role. Cimetidine is a weak inhibitor of CYP2C9, as are fluoxetine and fluvoxamine.

CYP2D6

Many antidepressants are metabolized by CYP2D6. The SSRIs inhibit this enzyme, leading to elevated levels of tricyclics, olanzapine, clozapine and risperidone if prescribed concomitantly. The order of potency, with the strongest inhibitor first, is paroxetine > fluoxetine > sertraline (high dose) > fluvoxamine > nefazodone > venlafaxine.

CYP3A

CYP3A accounts for one-third of the P450 enzymes in the liver and is the most important enzyme. The selective serotonin reuptake inhibitors (SSRIs) are weak inhibitors compared with ketoconazole and nefazodone. Nefazodone inhibits the CYP3A4 enzyme, leading to increases in antihistamines, carbamazepine and atypical antipsychotics. In vitro, the rank potency of inhibition is: nefazodone > fluvoxamine/norfluoxetine > fluoxetine > sertraline/desmethylsertraline > paroxetine > venlafaxine. Several clinically important cardiac events have been reported in patients receiving fluoxetine or fluvoxamine with terfenadine or astemizole. AEDs commonly induce drug metabolism, leading to possible reductions in the concentration of tricyclic antidepressants and oral contraceptives.

CYP2E1

The substrate of this enzyme is ethanol, and CYP2E1 is induced by ethanol and inhibited by disulfiram (a feature of the antabuse reaction). It is worth noting that a non-drinker who overdoses with alcohol and tricyclic antidepressants will triple the peak concentration of the tricyclic. Although regular drinkers can induce CYP isoenzymes, and thereby lower tricyclic plasma concentrations, alcoholic cirrhosis tends to increase levels of tricyclics.

SUMMARY

Psychotropic drug interactions can be summarized as follows:

- nicotine and alcohol are cytochrome P450 enzyme inducers, leading to lower substrate levels (including clozapine and tricyclic antidepressants)
- carbamazepine and phenytoin induce the 3A4 enzyme, leading to lower substrate levels (including tricyclic antidepressants and oral contraceptives)
- nefazodone can inhibit the 3A4 enzyme, leading to higher substrate levels (including clozapine, pimozide and antihistamines)
- fluoxetine and fluvoxamine inhibit the 2C9 enzyme, increasing the levels of warfarin and phenytoin
- paroxetine and fluoxetine inhibit the 2D6 enzyme, increasing the levels of risperidone, clozapine, olanzapine and tricyclics
- expect considerable inter-individual variation.

REFERENCES AND FURTHER READING

Stockley IH 1999 Drug interactions: a source book of adverse interactions, their mechanisms, clinical importance and management, 5th edn. Pharmaceutical Press, London

65

Driving and Neuro-psychiatric Conditions

BACKGROUND

Cognitive impairment and daytime tiredness are as important in their contribution to road traffic accidents as drink driving. Yet these factors are overlooked both in research and in practice. In a wider context, medical illness is the cause of fatal road traffic accidents in about one in five cases where the victim is over 65 years old. Related to this, 41% of those aged over 70 years (nearly 1 million people) hold a driving licence. Advice given to patients is patchy. A third of patients will return to driving after traumatic brain injury, but less than 20% receive advice about driving (Hawley 2001). At least a half of such patients report some sort of driving problem when asked.

NEUROPSYCHIATRIC FACTORS AFFECTING DRIVING COMPETENCE

Normal ageing adversely effects driving skills, causing an increase in accidents in those aged over 60 years (when corrected for the reduced number of miles driven). However, this deterioration is not uniform and is difficult to predict. Ultimately, only direct tests of performance reveal an individual's competence or otherwise. This is exactly the same when the cause of suspected impaired driving ability is a neuropsychiatric disorder. Few conditions automatically exclude an individual from driving for a long period. Factors that impair driving ability include motor and coordination problems, sensory difficulties and disorders of consciousness. Common cognitive domains that impair driving include attention, executive capacity and processing speed. In addition, abnormalities in insight, impulsivity, psychosis, mood and even personality exert a more complex influence on driving. Medication has a serious part to play in driving competence. Users of benzodiazepines or tricyclic antidepressants are about 50% more likely than non-users to be involved in a crash.

Table 65.1 Odds ratios for the causes of serious vehicle accidents

Cause	Odds ratio
Overtaking	5.6
Non-use of seat belts	4.0
Age >80 years	2.3
Changing lanes	2.1
Disobeying traffic signs	1.7
Snowy weather	1.6
Male gender	1.4

Adapted from Zhang et al (2000)

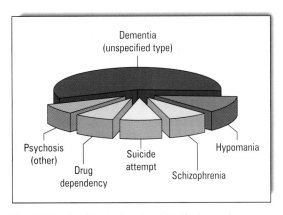

Fig. 65.1 Psychiatric disorders identified on police reports as the cause of 250 road traffic accidents. Data from Harris (2000)

405

MANAGEMENT OF THE DRIVER WITH A NEUROPSYCHIATRIC DISORDER

Management of drivers with a neuropsychiatric disorder can be divided into advice, testing, prevention of dangerous driving and alternatives to driving. As noted above, many conditions do not automatically exclude an individual from driving, and therefore some judgement is required before correct advice can be given. It is important to assess areas that are likely to impact directly on driving performance rather than penalizing someone on the basis of their age or disease history alone. Where only slight difficulty in driving is present, advice to restrict driving to the day, in good weather and on familiar routes is sensible. There is some benefit of driving accompanied rather than alone. Testing fitness to drive is an extremely valuable resource, where available. In the UK there is a network of regional mobility centres that can provide off-road testing. Certain driving instructors offer specialist advice for people with disabilities and can test on the road, where appropriate.

When doctors assess patients who are unfit to drive there is a balance to make between confidentiality and protection. In most countries it is the licence holder's legal responsibility to notify regulatory authorities such as the Driver and Vehicle Licensing Agency (DVLA) in the first instance. This is an obvious weakness in the system, as many risky drivers are either unwilling or unable to recognize their limitations. The doctor's responsibility is particularly important in these circumstances (Box 65.2). A clinician can act as a patient's advocate, as the DVLA will often consider the merits of individual cases.

There should be some planning for alternative methods of transportation when driving ceases. It is worth reminding patients that it is more economical to use taxis than a car when less than 4000 miles are covered in a year.

REGULATIONS

In Europe, driving regulations vary by country. In the UK, the DLVA maintains a series of rather complex recommendations. Details are available online. The DVLA's aim is to remove licences from anyone at more than 20% chance of having an accident.

The guidelines produced by the DVLA for psychiatry are:

> All psychiatric conditions which are relapsing, recurrent, or progressive, and which may make the driver a source of danger, must be notified to DVLA and medical enquiry will ensue....A licence is issued subject to medical review in 1, 2 or 3 years. It is the way in which the disorder manifests itself in behaviour and

---

Box 65.1   DLVA guidelines on psychotropic drugs

- Driving while unfit through drugs prescribed or illicit is an offence and may lead to prosecution.
- All CNS active drugs can impair alertness, concentration and driving performance. This is particularly so within the first month of starting or increasing the dose. It is important to cease driving during this time if adversely affected.
- Benzodiazepines are most dangerous, and are over-represented in drivers involved in road traffic accidents.
- Drugs having anticholinergic side effects should be avoided in drivers. These include tricyclic antidepressants and phenothiazines. Antihistamine effects of some antidepressants may cause drowsiness and care must be taken.
- Selective serotonin reuptake inhibitors, monoamine oxidase inhibitors and noradrenaline (norepinephrine) reuptake inhibitors have fewer side effects and are safer. However, some patients have idiosyncratic responses, and should be advised accordingly.
- Long-acting depot neuroleptics and the newer antipsychotic drugs can impair driving, but sedation usually diminishes after approximately 3 months. Parkinsonian side effects can be dangerous. Drivers on these drugs should be carefully assessed clinically. A formal driving assessment may be required.
- The interaction of all CNS active drugs with alcohol will increase impairment and affect driving ability.
- Drivers with psychiatric illnesses are usually safer when well and on regular psychotropic medication than when they are ill. Inadequate treatment or lack of compliance may render the driver impaired by both illness and medication.
- Prescribers should be aware of the epileptogenic potential of psychotropic drugs.
- Doctors who fail to advise their patients of the dangers of side effects of medication may have serious medicolegal difficulties should an accident occur.

Box 65.2   GMC guidelines concerning disclosure of information about patients to the DVLA (September 2000)

- The DVLA is legally responsible for deciding if a person is medically unfit to drive. The Agency needs to know when driving-licence holders have a condition which may now, or in the future, affect their safety as a driver.
- Therefore, where patients have such conditions you should:
  - Make sure that patients understand that the condition may impair their ability to drive. If a patient is incapable of understanding this advice, for example because of dementia, you should inform the DVLA immediately.
  - Explain to patients that they have a legal duty to inform the DVLA about the condition.
- If patients refuse to accept the diagnosis or the effect of the condition on their ability to drive, you can suggest that the patients seek a second opinion, and make appropriate arrangements for the patients to do so. You should advise patients not to drive until the second opinion has been obtained.
- If patients continue to drive when they are not fit to do so, you should make every reasonable effort to persuade them to stop. This may include telling their next of kin.
- If you do not manage to persuade patients to stop driving, or you are given or find evidence that a patient is continuing to drive contrary to advice, you should disclose relevant medical information immediately, in confidence, to the medical adviser at the DVLA.
- Before giving information to the DVLA you should try to inform the patient of your decision to do so. Once the DVLA has been informed, you should also write to the patient, to confirm that a disclosure has been made.

Clinical Pointer 65.1

Cognitively impaired and fit to drive?

Neuropsychological testing shows a weak ability to predict driving errors. Overlearned skills (procedural memory) are likely to be resistant to deterioration in early dementia and thus people may perform better in automatic situations (e.g. the emergency stop) than ones requiring some thought (e.g. pulling away from a junction with poor visibility). The association between dementia and driving competence is very difficult to study because for any individual person a crash is a relatively rare event. Retrospective studies relying on recall are likely to be flawed for obvious reasons. Raw statistics suggest that as many as half of elderly drivers killed in road traffic accidents have actual or incipient Alzheimer's disease. Prospective studies have problems with consent and information reporting. For these reasons, studies of accident frequency among drivers with Alzheimer's disease have yielded conflicting results about risk. Driving simulator work attempts to solve these problems. In high-risk scenarios, patients with early dementia are approximately twice as likely to experience 'close calls', and predictors of poor performance include visuospatial impairment and reduction in the useful field of view. This level of risk is similar to that posed by young drivers or driving whilst intoxicated. The effects of other neuropsychiatric disorders that influence cognition require further study. One important caveat is that many people with deteriorating performance limit the amount they drive, so that the actual risk is lower than predicted from individual performance tests.

Further reading   Dubinsky RM, Stein AC, Lyons K 2000 Practice parameter: risk of driving and Alzheimer's disease (an evidence-based review) – Report of the Quality Standards Subcommittee of the American Academy of Neurology. Neurology 54:2205–2211

Johansson K, Bogdanovic N, Kalimo H et al 1997 Alzheimer's disease and apolipoprotein E epsilon 4 allele in older drivers who died in automobile accidents. Lancet 349:1143–1144

Rizzo M, Dingus T 1996 Driving in neurological disease. Neurologist 2:150–160

psychomotor function appropriate to safe driving which is relevant, the diagnosis is not necessarily important."

The guidelines produced by the DVLA for neurology are:

There is no single or simple marker for assessment of impaired cognitive function although the ability to manage day to day living satisfactorily is a possible yardstick of cognitive competence ... mild cognitive

disability may be compatible with safe driving and individual assessment will be required. Impairment of cognitive functioning is not usually compatible with the driving of these vehicles.

Regarding epilepsy, the DLVA states:

Epileptic attacks are the most frequent medical cause of collapse at the wheel. A person who has suffered an epileptic attack whilst awake must refrain from driving for one year from the date of the attack *before a driving licence may be issued. A person who has suffered an attack whilst asleep must also refrain from driving for one year from the date of the attack, unless they have had an attack whilst asleep more than three years ago and have not had any awake attacks since that asleep attack.*

SUMMARY

The issue of driving and neuropsychiatric disorders can be summarized as follows:

- take cognitive impairment and daytime sleepiness seriously and ask you patients to do the same
- advise patients not to drive when acutely unwell, intoxicated or on sedative medication
- assess the risks in those who continue to drive despite advice not to
- involve regulatory authorities where necessary
- try to follow local guidelines

- be prepared to advise patients when to recommence driving
- consider alternative transport arrangements for patients advised not to drive
- consider the risk of unsafe driving over the next year, as this is the minimum period for which a licence can be issued in the UK

REFERENCES AND FURTHER READING

Harris M 2000 Psychiatric conditions with relevance to fitness to drive. Advances in Psychiatric Treatment 6:261–269

Hawley CA 2001 Return to driving after head injury. Journal of Neurology, Neurosurgery and Psychiatry 70:761–766

Zhang J, Lindsay J, Clarke K et al 2000 Factors affecting the severity of motor vehicle traffic crashes involving elderly drivers in Ontario. Accident Analysis and Prevention 32:117–125

66

Treatment of Medically Unexplained Symptoms

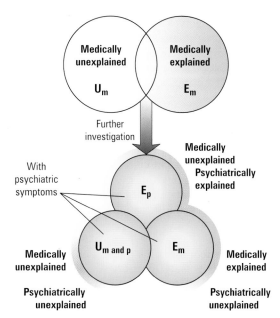

Fig. 66.1 Classification of medically unexplained symptoms. Every branch of medicine has its share of presentations that do not fit the conventional medical model of the day. In some cases this is due to inadequacy in medical science, as only arrogance could suggest that current diagnostic tests are flawless (E_m). After thorough investigation some cases are better accounted for by psychological or psychiatric factors (E_p). Such patients consider themselves to be severely ill, and they tend to suffer over many years as multiple health professionals attempt to fit their symptoms into a medical model. Finally, a small proportion of cases remain unexplained, yet these patients still require support and strategies to manage disability.

Understanding symptoms and signs not accounted for by known medical diseases is an important part of all clinical specialties.

Between a third and a half of all patients presenting to secondary care physicians have a medically unexplained disorder. How common are medically unexplained symptoms in neurology? In a Scottish study of 300 newly referred neurological outpatients, neurologists rated over half of all presentations as not completely explained by organic disease (Carson et al 2000). Such patients are often imprecisely labelled as having 'psychogenic' or 'non-organic' illnesses, and they may present with a wide variety of complaints, including seizures, chronic pain, movement disorder, aphonia, erectile dysfunction, memory impairment, disturbed vision and weakness.

CLASSIFICATION OF MEDICALLY UNEXPLAINED SYMPTOMS

On closer examination, medically unexplained disorders encompass three very different presentations (Fig. 66.1). The first category are those patients who are labelled as having medically unexplained symptoms but whose underlying physical disease has not been diagnosed by current tests. These are cases of diagnostic error or diagnostic delay. An average diagnostic delay of over 1 year is seen in several neurological disorders, including Parkinson's disease (Vieregge et al 1994), motor neurone disease (Househam & Swash 2000), idiopathic generalized epilepsy (Cachera et al 2000), Wilson's disease (Miranda et al 1995) and Alzheimer's disease (Cattel et al 2000). It is worth remembering that certain presentations that are now thought to reflect neurological disease were considered psychogenic at the turn of the century. These included migraine, Tourette's syndrome and trigeminal neuralgia.

The second category are those patients whose disorders are better accounted for by the way people deal with distress than by a medical illness. This is the category of somatoform disorder (sometimes confusingly referred to as 'somatization' in Europe).

The third category, rarely mentioned in the literature, are those patients whose symptoms are not satisfactorily explained by either medical or psychological influences (Hamilton et al 1996). These could be viewed as examples of diagnostic failure or uncertainty.

Deciding which of these categories applies to a given presentation can be problematic. It is often better to acknowledge that both a biological and a psychological explanation of the presentation is applicable. Medical uncertainty at the time of initial presentation is not prima facie evidence of a psychological explanation. Premature use of labels such as 'dissociative', 'hysterical' and 'supratentorial' can lead to diagnostic error. A classic case series from Elliot Slater found that 60% of patients diagnosed with hysteria at the National Hospital for Nervous Diseases in London developed evidence of organic pathology, although to what extent this pathology was causative was not addressed (Slater & Glithero 1965). One should note that more recent case series suggest that this may have been an overestimate (Crimlisk et al 1998, Moene et al 2000). Naturally, the opposite situation can occur. Patients with medically explained symptoms may on further investigation and observation turn out to have symptoms that are better described by psychological factors. An example is patients who are initially thought to have epilepsy but, on further testing, have pseudo-seizures. These examples lie on opposite ends of a spectrum. In between are the majority of presentations in neuropsychiatry, in which both medical and psychological factors interact.

A clinician who uses only a dichotomous model of 'either medically explained or psychologically explained' would poorly categorize the majority of presentations. One reason for this is that many people have both a psychiatric and a neurological disorder (Raja 1995). A second reason is that psychological factors are important in most cases, even when the biological basis of the disorder is known. For example, the way in which a disease manifests itself is highly dependent on the individual patient's personality structure (coping style, resilience, outlook and so on). It is common rather than uncommon for distress to be expressed in emotional, behavioural or somatic terms. In addition, psychological variables determine the burden of disease that the patient perceives or, to put it more simply, the amount of distress a person suffers (see Clinical Pointers 30.1 and 58.1).

THE SPECIAL CASE OF SOMATOFORM DISORDER

The term 'somatoform disorder' attempts to bring together several quite different presentations, including body dysmorphic disorder, conversion disorder (also known as dissociative disorder or hysteria), hypochondriasis, somatoform pain disorder and somatization disorder. What is it that unites these syndromes?

Many people have difficulty expressing distress verbally and instead use a language of behaviour and physical complaints. In addition, certain aspects of the sick role, such as freedom from responsibilities and care from health professionals, can be reinforcing. Over a period of time this can lead to recurrent somatic complaints that have no primary pathological basis. However, patients with somatoform disorder consider themselves to be severely ill, often more so than the ratings of patients with chronic medical conditions.

Distress may also be expressed in other ways in patients with somatoform disorder. About half have either comorbid depression or anxiety disorders. A similar proportion have a personality disorder, although some authorities argue that somatization is itself a form of personality disorder. When assessing a patient with a somatoform disorder, it is often difficult to understand why the patient expresses distress in this way. Unfortunately, such patients are often dismissed as intentionally fabricating symptoms (malingering). Several studies have shown that very few patients intentionally set out to deceive medical staff with invented symptoms. The origin of somatoform disorder is complex, but it is probably related to learning from others in their formative years how distress is expressed. Consistent with this, families of patients with somatoform disorder have higher rates of physical and sexual abuse and more medical illnesses than control families. Ultimately, ignoring this problem may prove costly because, without modification, medically unexplained symptoms are extremely disabling and a burden to the individual patient and to the health service. As an example, one study of non-organic abnormal movements showed that symptoms persisted in 90% of patients 3 years after the initial assessment (Feinstein et al 2001). Poor outcome was associated with long duration of symptoms, insidious onset of abnormal movements and psychiatric comorbidity.

Clinical Pointer 66.1

Recognizing 'psychogenic' neurological symptoms

Recognizing and managing presentations that are not explained by known organic diseases is one of the most difficult problems in neurology. Movement disorders, amnesia, weakness, sensory symptoms, aphonia and seizures are just some of the presentations that can have a psychological basis. Only rarely is there a diagnostic test that can disprove the medical model during life. That said, simultaneous EEG and videotaping of pseudoseizures (see Clinical Pointer 18.2), an optokinetic drum test in conversion blindness, cortical evoked potentials for auditory and visual deficits, and examination of personal memory in dissociative memory loss can be useful. Such specialist tests may not be necessary if a clinician makes a thorough clinical assessment of the patient.

Context

The best starting place is usually the context in which the patient presents. A person with multiple investigations without satisfactory cause raises suspicions about abnormal illness behaviour. A past psychiatric history (particularly featuring depression, repeated self-harm or substance abuse) and a personal history of abuse or neglect in childhood, medical illnesses in the family or absence of appropriate role models all increase the probability of a psychosomatic explanation. If complaints are severe but the injury or insult is minor, or if compensation has been mentioned, another question mark is raised. It is important to emphasize that these pointers in the history are not by any means foolproof in isolation. The whole picture should always be considered in difficult cases.

Mental state and physical examination

The next step is to examine the patient in detail. Do not overlook the neurological examination, since 'medically explained' is as likely as 'medically unexplained' at this stage. Engage the patient in a non-threatening dialogue and try to understand the patient's perspective. This will give valuable clues as to why the patient is presenting at this moment. What does the patient understand by his or her complaints? What does the patient think has caused them? What would relieve these symptoms? Has stress played a role? What are the recent events in the patient's life?

Clinical clues of a non-organic presentation from the physical examination include bizarre or unusual signs incongruous with the medical model, severe or inconsistent fatigue, and remissions paralleling psychosocial events. In patients with non-organic tremor, tapping with the unaffected limb tends to recruit the frequency of movement in the affected limb – a phenomenon known as 'entrainment'. In patients with non-organic paresis, the examiner places a hand under the patient's contralateral heel while the patient attempts to raise the affected limb. The patient with true organic weakness will exert downward pressure on the contralateral heel.

Longitudinal observation

In many ways observation over time is the most valuable form of investigation. Symptoms or signs that that are paroxysmal or that vary with observation or periods of leave are suspicious. Inconsistencies when the patient is visited or is accompanied by family and friends are also a valuable indication of psychological factors. Occasionally, patients may refuse a second opinion or refuse videotaping, although this could have many non-sinister explanations. If a diagnosis cannot be made after a period of observation, symptomatic treatment may help to elucidate the underlying cause. An alternative is the abreaction technique, whereby a drug with disinhibiting properties is used to elucidate underlying drives.

If psychological factors are discovered, do not fall into the trap of assuming there are no organic factors at work or of assuming that the patient has created the condition intentionally.

Further reading   Halligan P, Bass C, Marshall JC 2001 Contemporary approaches to the study of hysteria. Oxford University Press, Oxford
Landau ME 2001 Conversion disorders. eMedicine Journal 2:11

TREATMENT OF SOMATOFORM AND RELATED DISORDERS

Unlike other types of treatment in neurology, the treatment of neurologically unexplained symptoms cannot be reduced to something that can be easily administered to the patient. Rather it is more concerned with the doctor's approach to and ongoing interactions with that person. In many cases, the doctor will discover the patient with somatoform disorder is wary of medical professionals and can cite a long list of past problems. It is vital to acknowledge that their disabling symptoms are being taken seriously and that you, as the patient's doctor, have the same goal as the patient – the resolution of these problems. Because extensive series of tests performed to date have not helped to locate the problem, further testing is likely to maintain rather than reduce anxiety. Continuing to search for a pathological abnormality that is not present reinforces the idea that one may be present.

Many patients and doctors lack an adequate understanding of the interaction between psychological stress and somatic symptoms. Instead of further investigations, one should begin to look for factors in the person's background that help shape how he or she deals with distress. Consistency and appropriate boundaries are essential to continuing treatment. The person should agree to participate in a treatment programme. This involves not presenting to other healthcare professionals. Where a family is involved, the family should not encourage maladaptive behaviour and should reward improvements in functioning. Progress can be slow and difficult and there is a temptation for the patient to slip back into the old, natural somatizing style. Thus, specific behavioural treatment can be used to good effect. The patient's natural reaction is to increasingly limit activities and personal contact on account of physical complaints. A behavioural programme gradually encourages activity in a graded manner (see Clinical Pointer 52.1). Evidence supports the use of cognitive therapy in somatization. This includes challenging negative assumptions and automatic thoughts, avoiding catastrophic thinking, and examining the evidence for and against health assumptions. Two recent systematic reviews both show the effectiveness of cognitive–behavioural therapy for medically unexplained symptoms in many, but not all, cases (Kroenke & Swindle 2000, Nezu et al 2001). About half of the individual studies reviewed showed functional or psychological improvements following cognitive–behavioural therapy. Yet some patients remain significantly disabled by somatoform disorders despite treatment. In such cases, one option is to use a model of 'living with disability'. The message here is that a cure is unlikely but quality of life can still be improved, even in the face of continuing symptoms. We must not forget that the presence of psychiatric symptoms requires recognition and treatment in itself.

Several variants of somatoform disorder may require a slightly different approach. Cognitive–behavioural therapy appears to be effective in the specific somatoform disorders of chronic fatigue, irritable bowel syndrome and chronic pain as well as

in multiple somatization disorder (Briquet's syndrome). In the dissociative disorder, there is a specific symptom or sign, such as weakness, aphonia or memory loss, that does not conform to the pathophysiology of the nervous system but does conform to the patient's understanding of disease. It typically occurs in a setting of stress and produces considerable dysfunction. Although the diagnosis is a clinical one, occasionally specific tests or investigations can be helpful (e.g. simultaneous EEG and videotaping of pseudoseizures) (see Clinical Pointer 18.2). Once the diagnosis is made, the duration of symptoms is usually brief and the outcome good. Gentle exploration about current stressors and social supports should be addressed.

In resistant cases, a problem-solving approach or hypnosis may be helpful. In neuropsychiatry, dissociative or psychogenic amnesia has special significance because memory loss is at the root of many conditions. DSM-IV further defines five types of dissociative amnesia, but the validity of these has not been tested. Again, dissociative amnesia is difficult to diagnose because some aspects of memory loss may be quite plausible. In order to demonstrate a dissociative rather than an organic amnesia one must show that the memory loss is of a type or severity that should not normally occur. (Ask the subject to remember 10 items. After 5 minutes offer each true item along with a false item in 10 pairs. By chance alone a person in the most severe cases of anterograde amnesia, should score roughly 5 correct answers. Subjects with dissociative amnesia may score 0 correct items.) One also might observe inconsistencies on repeated testing. Emotional incongruity (Janet (1920) described a lack of concern about physical symptoms or la bélle indifference in association with dissociative disorder) or emotional distress may be pointers towards possible underlying psychological factors, but these are not robust associations (see anosodiaphoria in Ch. 14). Minor fluctuations in symptom severity, changes in the ability of a person to cope with symptoms, and variation in symptoms with changes in perceived stress or support should not be regarded as pointers towards a non-organic disorder. Several questionnaires to detect non-organic amnesia have been developed.

SUMMARY

The management of medically unexplained symptoms can be summarized as follows:

Clinical Pointer 66.2

The importance of a healthy lifestyle in neuropsychiatry

Physical activity and physical fitness reduce the likelihood of cardiovascular disease and, to a lesser extent, stroke. Weight loss in obese people is associated with modest reductions in blood pressure. A body mass index above 30 kg/m² is linked with a two-fold increase in the likelihood of stroke, but this effect may be confined to men. Eating a healthy diet reduces blood pressure and also reduces the risk of cardiovascular and cerebrovascular disease. This may be via an effect on cholesterol or other lipids, since cholesterol is associated with an increased risk of vascular disease in a dose–response relationship. Advice on diet can reduce cholesterol levels in the long term and in turn reduce cardiovascular mortality. Smoking is associated with a roughly two-fold increase in the risk of myocardial infarction and stroke, with the effect being strongest in the middle-aged. Stopping smoking gradually eliminates these risks but it does not appear to influence blood pressure.

Of interest, weight loss is a predictor of poor prognosis in most neurodegenerative diseases, although the effect of weight alteration per se on outcome is unknown. Often the weight loss seems beyond expectations given calorie intake, and conceivably nutritional compromise could influence cognitive decline. There is also accumulating evidence that physical exercise can protect against age-related cognitive decline. There is some evidence that an unhealthy diet is a risk factor for Alzheimer's disease. One trial showed a benefit of treatment with high-dose vitamin E in delaying the cognitive decline in those recently diagnosed. Cross-sectional evidence suggested that cholesterol reduction using statins protected against later dementia. However, the prospective (PROSPER) study, which enrolled 5804 high-risk individuals to 40 mg/day pravastatin or placebo for an average of 3 years, showed no appreciable effect on stroke or cognitive function. A second large study (The Heart Protection Study) demonstrated a reduction in stroke, but no benefit on cognition.

Further reading   González-Gross M, Marcos A, Pietrzik K 2001 Nutrition and cognitive impairment in the elderly. British Journal of Nutrition 86:313–321

Laurin D, Verreault R, Lindsay J et al 2001 Physical activity and risk of cognitive impairment and dementia in elderly persons. Archives of Neurology 58:498–504

Rexrode KM, Hennekens CH, Willett WC et al 1997 A prospective study of body mass index, weight change, and risk of stroke in women. JAMA 277:1539–1545

Shepherd J, Blauw GJ, Murphy MB et al 2002 Pravastatin in elderly individuals at risk of vascular disease (PROSPER): a randomized controlled trial. Lancet 360:1623–1630

- examine the published evidence with caution – research in this area is beset by difficulties because of the minefield of poorly defined terms and the absence of standardized case definitions
- do not assume that 'medically unexplained' is necessarily 'psychologically explained' – a combination of neurological and psychological factors is more likely
- consider the context, the patient's mental state and physical examination, and longitudinal observation in evaluating suspected somatoform disorder
- take every patient's complaints seriously – engaging with rather than dismissing the patient (and his or her symptoms) is one of the most important steps
- consider referral for cognitive–behavioural therapy
- treat any co-existing psychiatric symptoms
- be wary of accusing any patient of intentionally fabricating symptoms.

REFERENCES AND FURTHER READING

Cachera C, Baulac M, Fagnani F et al 2000 Epilepsies and time to diagnosis. Revue Neurologique 156:481–490

Carson AJ, Ringbauer B, Stone J et al 2000 Do medically unexplained symptoms matter? A prospective cohort study of 300 new referrals to neurology outpatient clinics. Journal of Neurology, Neurosurgery and Psychiatry 68:207–210

Cattel C, Gambassi G, Sgadari A et al 2000 Correlates of delayed referral for the diagnosis of dementia in an outpatient population. Journals of Gerontology Series A – Biological Sciences and Medical Sciences 55:M98–M102

Crimlisk HL, Bhatia K, Cope H et al 1998 Slater revisited: 6 year follow up study of patients with medically unexplained motor symptoms. British Medical Journal 316:582–586

Feinstein A, Stergiopoulos V, Fine J et al 2001 Psychiatric outcome in patients with a psychogenic movement disorder. Neuropsychiatry, Neuropsychology and Behavioral Neurology 14:169–176

Hamilton J, Campos R, Creed F 1996 Anxiety, depression and management of medically unexplained symptoms in medical clinics. Journal of the Royal College of Physicians, London 30:18–20

Househam E, Swash M 2000 Diagnostic delay in amyotrophic lateral sclerosis: what scope for improvement? Journal of the Neurological Sciences 180:76–81

Janet P 1920 The major symptoms of hysteria. Macmillan, New York

Kroenke K, Swindle R 2000 Cognitive–behavioral therapy for somatization and symptom syndromes: a critical review of controlled clinical trials. Psychotherapy and Psychosomatics 69:205–215

Miranda M, Brinck P, Roessler JL et al 1995 Wilson's disease: report of 16 patients. Revista Medica de Chile 123:1098–1107

Moene FC, Landberg EH, Hoogduin KAL et al 2000 Organic syndromes diagnosed as conversion disorder: identification and frequency in a study of 85 patients. Journal of Psychosomatic Research 49:7–12

Nezu AM, Nezu CM, Lombardo ER 2001 Cognitive–behavior therapy for medically unexplained symptoms: a critical review of the treatment literature. Behavioral Therapy 32:537–583

Raja M 1995 Neurological diagnoses in psychiatric patients: the uncertain boundaries between neurology and psychiatry. Italian Journal of Neurological Sciences 16:153–158

Slater E, Glithero E 1965 A follow up of patients diagnosed as suffering from 'hysteria'. Journal of Psychosomatic Research 9:9–13

Vieregge P, Kortke D, Meyerbornsen C 1994 Medical and social care in elderly parkinsonian patients. Zeitschrift fur Gerontologie 27:260–269

Weatherall J, Ledingham JGG, Warrell DA (eds) 1995 Oxford textbook of medicine, 3rd edn. Oxford University Press, Oxford

Pathogenesis of Neuro-psychiatric Presentations

67

Why and How Neurological Disease Causes Psychiatric Symptoms

Not many neurological diseases escape without psychiatric or behavioural complications (see Table I.1). Possible exceptions are neurological diseases that are limited to peripheral nerves and muscle. From this it is safe to conclude that damage to the brain, whether that be from tumour, ischaemia, infection or degenerative disease, causes changes in thinking, emotions and behaviour. By inference, it must therefore be that the physiological basis for thinking, emotions and behaviour is seated in the brain and that these mechanisms are specifically disrupted by CNS lesions. Keen readers will not be happy with this level of explanation and will demand a more precise explanation for the pathophysiology of every symptom or syndrome. Fortunately, we can learn more about the physiological basis of mood, psychosis, cognition and behaviour by closely observing the relationship between specific neurological lesions and specific neuropsychiatric complications. These associations are discussed in the following chapters. It is logical to divide the aetiology of a complication into risk factors, pathogenetic factors and main pathological findings. Risk factors are remote influences that are neither necessary nor sufficient in themselves. Pathogenesis is the direct mechanism by which a complication arises. Pathological findings are associated structural changes, either macroscopic or microscopic. Several examples are illustrated in Figure 67.1.

However, a word of caution. In order to study this relationship scientifically, we must not fall into the trap of assuming that the measurable neurological insult (e.g. haemorrhage) is an adequate explanatory variable in determining outcome (e.g. depression). The measurable insult is, in most cases, a marker of a more fundamental disease process associated with other neurobiological consquences, of which we may be totally unaware. The neurological disease also causes an array of psychosocial changes that have a major contribution to the ultimate complications.

That said, an equally serious error in logic is to assume that because the complication is in the psychiatric domain then the cause cannot be organic, and, worse, must be volitional. An excellent example is the description of postconcussional symptoms as psychogenic. In the majority of cases, such symptoms are no more invented or desired by the patient than are the cognitive deficits of Alzheimer's disease.

For most psychiatric complications of neurological disease the explanation of how they occurred is complex. Furthermore, the explanation will vary from one individual to the next. A combination of interdependent direct and indirect mechanisms are likely to co-exist. The wider perspective here is that the boundaries of psychiatry and neurology overlap. Neurological symptoms are those based on damage to neurones and related systems. Psychiatric symp-

> **Box 67.1 The ten most prevalent neurological diagnoses**
>
> - Migraine
> - Tension headache
> - Alzheimer's disease
> - Active epilepsy
> - Essential tremor
> - Chronic fatigue syndrome
> - Multiple sclerosis
> - Parkinson's disease
> - Cluster headache
> - Neurofibromatosis
>
> Data from Warlow (2001)

Risk factors		Primary pathology		Pathogenesis		Disease		Complications	
Exercise Genetic factors Hyperlipidaemia Hypertension Medical illness Smoking		Atheroma Emboli		Hypoxia		*Cerebrovascular accident*		Falls High mortality rate Incontinence Memory loss	→ **Aetiology of ischaemic stroke**

Risk factors		Primary pathology		Pathogenesis		Disease		Complications	
Alcohol consumption Nutritional compromise Liver disease Medical illness		Neuronal loss Synaptic degeneration		Direct neurotoxity		*Dementia*		Disintegration of personality Loss of function Self-neglect Social isolation Unemployment	→ **Aetiology of alcohol-induced dementia**

Risk factors		Primary pathology		Pathogenesis		Disease		Complications	
Blood transfusion HIV exposure Immunosuppression Unsafe sex		HIV in CNS		Metabolic dysregulation		*Delirium*		Agitation Hallucinations High mortality rate Poor compliance	→ **Aetiology of HIV-related delirium**

Risk factors		Primary pathology		Pathogenesis		Disease		Complications	
Disability and handicap Genetic factors Medication Parkinson's disease Stressful life events		? Basal ganglia disease		? Psychological mechanisms ? Stress hormone dysregulation		*Depression*		Parasuicide Poor compliance Self-neglect Social isolation	→ **Aetiology of depression in Parkinson's disease**

Fig. 67.1 Examples of the different components of aetiology. ?, Possible association.

toms concern dysfunctional levels of distress, whether or not neuronal damage is the precipitating factor.

REFERENCES AND FURTHER READING

Donaghy M, Compston A, Rossor M et al 2001 Clinical diagnosis. In: Donaghy M (ed) Brain diseases of the nervous system, 11th edn. Oxford University Press, Oxford, p 2–59

Warlow CP 2001 The frequency of neurological disease. In: Donaghy M (ed) Brain diseases of the nervous system, 11th edn. Oxford University Press, Oxford

68

Modifying Variables that Influence Neuro-psychiatric Complications

Psychological, environmental and therapeutic factors can powerfully influence the impact of a disease on the sufferer as well as the extent of further complications. Historically, there has been a tendency to overlook these influences in favour of biological factors. This has led to the simplification of a complex relationship between a disease and its manifestations into a wholly clinicoanatomical model.

LIMITATIONS OF THE CLINICOANATOMICAL MODEL

The majority of published work has concentrated on the clinicoanatomical relationships of neurological disease and psychiatric complications. This is not surprising because neurologists and pathologists have spent hundreds of years defining the anatomical basis of neurological diseases (see Appendix I). The limitations of a simple clinicoanatomical model of complex brain function were recognized by the brilliant Russian neurologist AR Luria, who proposed the concept of functional systems. On critical analysis, a purely anatomical model of psychopathology begins to break down on a number of fronts. First, not all neurological diseases have a simply described gross anatomical basis (consider transient global amnesia, infectious CNS disease or Tourette's syndrome). Secondly, an apparently neat anatomical lesion frequently affects diffuse areas and related systems such as neurotransmitters, neuromodulators, neuropeptides, the autonomic nervous system and gene expression. Any of these may be more important in the genesis of the complication in question. Thirdly, the anatomical lesion tends to be fairly static, with modest resolution with time, whereas the psychiatric and behavioural complications can vary enormously. Fourthly, therapeutic evidence offers greater support for a biochemical or neuroendocrine model of many psychiatric prob-

Table 68.1 Generic quality of life instruments

Instrument	No. of items	Completion time	Domains rated				
			Physical	Emotional	Social	Cognitive	Communication
Nottingham Health Profile	45	10 min	✓	✓	✓	✗	✗
Sickness Impact Profile	136	30 min	✓	✓	✓	✗	✓
36-Item Short-Form Health Survey	36	5 min	✓	✓	✓	✗	✗
Farmer Quality of Life Index	41	20 min	✓	✓	✓	✗	✗
EuroQoL	5	2 min	✓	✓	✗	✗	✗
Functional Status Questionnaire	34	15 min	✓	✓	✓	✗	✗
Quality of Life-Index MS-Version	72	45 min	✓	✓	✓	✗	✗

Box 68.1 Modifying variables that influence the extent of neuropsychiatric complications

Neurological modifying variables
Concomitant neurological Illness
Family neurological history (genetic and non-genetic)
Lesion evolution
Lesion location
Lesion size
Lesion type
Previous brain pathology
Stage of development of the brain

Psychosocial modifying variables
Concomitant life events (stressors)
Concomitant psychiatric illness
Family psychiatric history (genetic and non-genetic)
Family, carer and peer expectations
Previous psychiatric Illness
Resources (financial, housing, information)
Sufferer's perception, understanding and outlook
Support (social and professional)

Therapeutic variables
Compliance with intervention
Intervention timing (early versus late)
Intervention type and duration
Therapeutic relationship
Therapist factors (skill, time, personality)

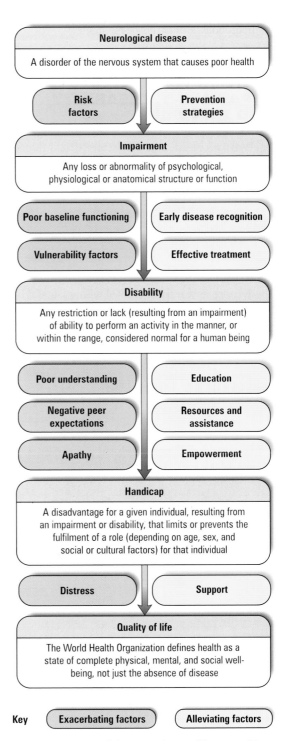

Fig. 68.1 Impact of disease and its modifying variables.

lems. Fifthly, evidence from primary psychiatric disorders emphasizes the importance of modifying variables upon the manifestation of these disorders.

With all this in mind, we must acknowledge the limitations of a purely anatomical model of neuropsychiatric disease. Moreover, we should acknowledge the limitations of any single-factor model in just about every medical or psychiatric disease.

LIMITATIONS OF THE MEDICAL MODEL

Throughout this book, I have put forward various descriptions of the medical model in order to further our understanding of neuropsychiatric disease. In some circumstances even the most comprehensive medical model may fail to explain fully the presentation and course of certain complications. In terms of understanding causation, presentations such as normal grief, acute stress disorders and several personality traits are probably not clarified by a classical medical approach. In terms of treatments,

421

the role of the family, peer-group support, self-help techniques and alternative medicine can be extremely valuable to patients, but often lie beyond the traditional boundaries of medicine.

FACTORS THAT INFLUENCE IMPAIRMENT, DISABILITY AND HANDICAP

One way of considering the factors that influence the impact of a disease in more detail is the model of impairment, disability and handicap proposed by the World Health Organization:

- impairment is the primary medical dysfunction
- disability is a reduced ability to perform daily activities
- handicap is the resultant disadvantage due to reduced participation in society.

These concepts are closely linked with quality of life (Fig. 68.1); in other words, the global well-being of the person. Many factors interact with a disease to increase or decrease its impact. Many factors interact with a disease to increase or decrease its impact (Box 68.1). The degree of neurological impairment may be influenced while the disease is in evolution. This may be a long window of opportunity in some diseases, such as Parkinson's disease, or a relatively short period, for example in subarachnoid haemorrhage. The degree of disability arising from a given impairment is particularly influenced by environmental factors. With sufficient resources, individuals with a given impairment can reduce their daily restrictions to a minimum. Psychological factors are heavily involved in the relationship between disability and handicap. These are in turn modified by support and encouragement from friends, family and health professionals. Psychiatric factors are one of the most important influences on health-related quality of life, although many other factors also have an influence (see Ch. 82). Treatments can work at all these levels. Treatments may modify the evolution of the disease influencing impairment, may provide a way of managing the impairment to reduce disability, may improve participation and reduce distress and therefore improve quality of life.

69

The Origin of Cognitive Impairment

WHAT AREA OF THE BRAIN IS RESPONSIBLE FOR MEMORY?

Learning, storage and recall (condensed into the term 'memory') is not one process but several brilliantly integrated processes. New information is not randomly acquired, but filtered according to importance. Consider the example of 'traumatic remembrance' in post-traumatic stress disorder. These are memories acquired during emotionally laden events that become indelibly stamped upon the brain, much to the distress of the sufferer. By contrast, in everyday life the majority of information does not reach conscious awareness, and even the information that does is discarded within a few seconds. This is the ruthless efficiency of working memory. Conditions that influence working memory are predominantly those that affect attention and concentration (e.g. delirium). Patients with frontal lobe lesions, for example after head injury, have been observed to have significant problems with working memory. This aspect of memory does not appear to be well localized; nevertheless, working memory involves specific parts of the brain. For example, the supramarginal gyrus is involved in verbal working memory, whereas the dorsolateral prefrontal cortex and the posterior association cortex are involved in spatial working memory. Furthermore, GABAergic and cholinergic input from the medial septum of the diagonal band of Broca to the hippocampus are important for spatial working memory.

Attempts to pin down short-term and long-term memory to one anatomical area have been unsuccessful. In Korsakoff's syndrome, lesions to the mammillary bodies, anterior nucleus of the thalamus and dorsomedial nucleus of the thalamus cause similar or identical profound deficits in new learning (Visser et al 1999). Such lesions do not always differentiate amnesic from non-amnesic alcoholics (see Ch. 35).

Dense amnesia can result from rupture of an anterior communicating artery aneurysm, which causes damage to the basal forebrain (diagonal band of Broca, septal nucleus and medial septum, nucleus basalis of Meynert and anterior hypothalamus) (Rajaram 1997). This area is rich in cholinergic projections that are also widely disrupted in Alzheimer's disease. Indeed, white matter hyperintensities in acetylcholinergic pathways correlate with the degree of executive and visuospatial attentional deficits in Alzheimer's disease (Swartz & Black 2002). Various neuropsychiatric conditions highlight the importance of the prefrontal cortex in memory (Fletcher & Henson 2001). For example, in cognitive impairment caused by cerebrovascular disease, deficits in episodic memory correlate with PET hypoperfusion in the left dorsolateral prefrontal cortex and the right orbital prefrontal cortex (Reed et al 2000). In multiple sclerosis lesions to the periventricular area have been linked with memory impairments (Izquierdo et al 1991), but not all studies agree and many unmeasured microscopic lesions may exert a more powerful influence than a single macroscopic lesion (Rovaris et al 1998). Persistent deficits in verbal episodic memory are greater following closed head injury than spinal cord injury. The severity of the head injury is associated with bilateral atrophy of the fornix and hippocampal formation (Bigler et al 1996, Tate & Bigler 2000). Trauma to the frontal lobes also influences subsequent learning performance (Di Stefano et al 2000). In epilepsy, several studies conclusively show that the medial temporal lobes are linked with memory performance (Lencz et al 1992). The hippocampi are damaged by recurrent seizures and, in turn, predispose to further seizures, a vicious feedback loop.

Thus, apparently disparate areas are concerned with memory, and yet damage to the medial temporal lobe structures and diencephalon produce similar deficits in new learning. These deficits are characterized by rapid rates of forgetting of new information, with episodic memory affected more than semantic memory. Patients with frontal lobe damage are often described as having retrieval problems because they fail to recall information that they recognize on prompting. They also have problems assessing their own deficits (*meta-memory deficits*). The neuroanatomy of memory is clearly more complex than it first appears. One attractive explanation is that the transmission of filtered working information into short-term memory involves two closely integrated anatomical circuits (D'Esposito 2000). The well-known Papez circuit has the hippocampus as its core component. On the basis of PET scans, it has been suggested that the rostral hippocampus is activated during episodic memory encoding, whereas the caudal hippocampus is activated during retrieval (Lepage et al 1998). The hippocampus projects via the fornices to the mammillary bodies and basal forebrain. The mammillary bodies are in communication with the anterior nucleus of the thalamus via the mammillothalamic tract, which in turn projects to the posterior and anterior cingulate cortex. The circuit is completed by connection back to the hippocampus. The hippocampus is adjacent to the entorhinal temporal cortex, which is increasingly thought to have a major role in episodic (particularly visual recognition) memory. The entorhinal cortex receives vast projections from the orbit-frontal cortex, cingulate cortex, parahippocampal gyrus and superior temporal gyrus, all of which interface with the hippocampus. The entorhinal cortex acts as a routing system for information from the cortex concerned with memory. It may be the entorhinal cortex that is the first to be affected in Alzheimer's disease. Furthermore, the entorhinal cortex shows an annual rate of atrophy of 15% in Alzheimer's disease, compared with 5% for the hippocampus (Schuff et al 2002). The less well-known amygdala circuit projects from the amygdala (mainly from the lateral nucleus) to the dorsomedial nucleus of the thalamus and, in turn, via reciprocal connections to the prefrontal cortex (Fig. 69.1).

This still leaves unaddressed the physiological mechanism underlying long-term memory storage. In every diffuse brain disease, long-term memories are left relatively unscathed despite the accumulation of other neuropsychiatric symptoms. This is consistent with the neural network theory of long-term memory, in which memory is a function of synaptic plasticity rather than a categorical effect of the neurones themselves. Hopfield (1982) showed that interconnected networks of model neurones can form associative memories based on the strength of synaptic connections, modified by prior activity. Individual neurones are not linked with one particular memory but are involved in many memory pathways. This model fits neatly the clinical findings in Alzheimer's disease. Of all the candidate markers of cognitive decline, the strongest association found to date is with synapse density (meas-

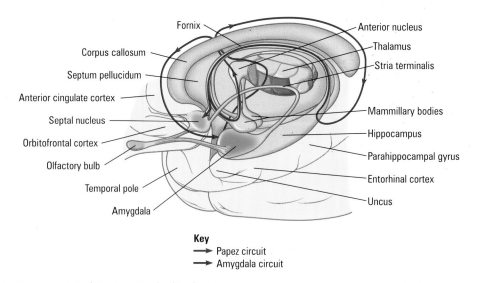

Fig. 69.1 Neuroanatomical structures involved in short-term memory.

ured by synaptophysin immunoreactivity) in the hippocampus (Sze et al 1997).

WHAT IS THE MECHANISM OF DELIRIUM?

Although many of the fundamental causes of delirium are well known, the mechanism by which environmental and metabolic insults result in temporary brain dysfunction are not well understood. Clues come from the study of the metabolic correlates of hepatic encephalopathy, hypoxic encephalopathy, hypercapnic encephalopathy, hypoglycaemic encephalopathy and uraemic encephalopathy (Pulsinelli & Cooper 1989). From the common factors in the many diverse causes, it must be concluded that the mechanism involves disruption of neuronal activity that is sufficiently subtle for consciousness not to be completely lost and for deficits to be able to reverse completely. The degree of slowing on EEG parallels the degree of brain dysfunction clinically. This is likely to be an adaptive change to reduce demands for tissue ATP. Furthermore, in the early stages of delirium, EEG activity correlates with decreases in cerebral blood flow (although in later stages regulation of cerebral blood flow breaks down) (Ingvar 1971).

Studies of the mechanism of status epilepticus may also help shed light on the mechanism of delirium. A seizure is a defined brain event that disturbs homeostasis and produces increasing severity of dysfunction. In the early phase of the convulsion, cerebral blood flow is increased (to compensate for the massive increase in metabolic demands from the discharging neurones) and there is a systemic attempt to maintain cerebral glucose supply with a stress hormone response (glucolysis and gluconeogenesis) together with autonomic hyperactivity. As the seizure continues past 30 minutes, with rising lactic acidosis, cerebral blood flow falls, causing a mismatch between neuronal supply and demand for oxygen and glucose. This metabolic perspective on brain dysfunction may well apply to delirium, although in this case the driving force is not necessarily increased neuronal activity. Neurones require a constant supply of oxygen and glucose to manufacture high-energy organic phosphates such as phosphocreatine and ATP in mitochondria. Even subtle mismatches between supply (e.g. in hypoglycaemia, hypoxia, artificial ventilation) and demand (e.g. in hypoglycaemia seizures, fever, systemic illness) may cause temporarily inadequate oxidative metabolism, leading to reduced cellular levels of ATP and reductions in dependent membrane ion pumps. In turn, this leads to suppression of neuronal function and abnormal neurotransmitter release (Brown 1999). The secondary effects of reduced cholinergic function, excess release of dopamine, noradrenaline (norepinephrine) and glutamate, and changes in serotonergic and GABA activity may underlie the different symptoms and clinical presentations of delirium.

Table 69.1 Summary of cognitive deficits in common neurological disorders

Disorder	Patients affected (%)	
	Mild to moderate deficits	Dementia
AIDS (late stage)*	80	25
Alcoholism (chronic)	80	15
Alzheimer's disease	100	100
CNS tumour*	50	10
Epilepsy	Unknown	Rare
Huntington's disease	40	Unknown
Lewy body dementia	100	100
Motor neurone disease	30	5–10
Multiple sclerosis*	50	5
Normal control	5	2
Parkinson's disease	80	30
Subarachnoid haemorrhage*	35	Unknown
Severe head injury*	≥50	3
Stroke*	50	30

*Highly dependent on subtypes, duration and/or regional effects

HOW MUCH DOES TREATMENT MODIFY THE COURSE OF A PROGRESSIVE DISEASE?

The natural history of Alzheimer's disease is discussed in Chapter 40, but let us now consider this from an integrated point of view. In the early *at-risk* stage a person carries a predisposition to develop the disease in later life. A classic example of such a predisposition can be seen with the carriers of the Huntington gene, who are certain to develop the condition at a later date (the disorder has 100% penetrance). All clinical, neuropsychological and neurobiological markers are likely to be normal at this stage. In the late *presymptomatic at-risk* stage, the underlying pathology of the disease begins to accumulate in the CNS, although all but the most sensitive investigations would prove negative and no clinical features are apparent. An example is found in patients at risk of Parkinson's disease who happen to die years before developing clinical symptoms. Neuropathological investigation shows early changes in the substantia nigra. PET studies confirm a rate of cell loss and plasma membrane dopamine transporter loss of about 10% per year in Parkinson's disease (compared to 1% in controls) and it is thought that the disease process takes at least 5 years to reach a critical threshold for causing symptoms. Another example is people at risk of Huntington's disease who show subtle cognitive deficits before clinical onset, in proportion to the number of trinucleotide repeats (Jason et al 1997). Gradually the pathology has an impact on cognition and other neuropsychiatric domains. The patient enters the *preclinical stage*. Deficits are subtle and firm diagnosis is usually impossible. As the disease progresses the patient crosses an arbitrary threshold for diagnosis and the *early clinical stage* is reached. Even at this point with positive clinical and investigative evidence of disease, a diagnosis may be difficult and may be delayed until more evidence of deterioration is obtained. The disease continues to develop, often at an accelerating pace, and function is progressively affected, initially for complex tasks and then for simple tasks.

With a strongly progressive condition such as Alzheimer's disease, the likelihood of a treatment having a powerful effect on the course is small and is further reduced with time as the biology of the condition marches on. Patients may achieve a temporary plateau in progression together with improvements in specific areas. However, after a treatment is withdrawn patients typically deteriorate back to their projected level. In a weakly progressive condition, such as chronic alcohol poisoning (surprisingly, alcohol is a low-potency drug), early treatment should restore function to near-premorbid levels in the absence of continued drinking. Some conditions may begin with a relatively benign profile and gradually become more severe with time. Examples include bipolar affective disorder and multiple sclerosis. In these conditions, the effect of treatment delay on outcome is being tested. The question being asked is, does time spent unwell (as opposed to time spent with an illness effectively treated) in itself influence long-term outcome? The design of one study in multiple sclerosis enabled the effect of early intervention to be examined. In the PRISMS study, patients were randomized to receive one of two doses of interferon-β-1a or placebo for 2 years. Both groups then continued to take interferon in a blind 2-year extension (PRISMS Study Group 2001). Those who had begun treatment early and continued for 4 years had less deterioration in disability and MRI measures, although only those on a high dose (44 µg three times weekly) actually improved over 4 years. The same question has been asked in patients with epilepsy – that is, does early treatment alter the long-term course of the condition? This has been studied using animal models of kindling, but rarely in humans. One exception comes from Musicco et al (1997). In a multicentre, randomized but non-blinded trial involving 419 patients, those with a first tonic–clonic seizure were randomized to immediate treatment with carbamazepine, phenytoin, phenobarbital or sodium valproate or to delayed treatment (beginning only after another seizure). Twenty-four per cent of patients randomized to immediate treatment and 42% of those randomized to delayed treatment experienced a seizure recurrence during follow-up. At 2 years, 68% of the early group had had no seizures, whereas 60% of the delayed group had not experienced any further seizures. This difference was not statistically significant, but whether it is clinically insignificant is a more difficult question to answer. In Parkinson's disease, clinicians have wondered whether treatment slows progression and reduces mortality. Naturalistic examination before and after the introduction of levodopa in the UK seems to suggest reduced mortality for up to 5 years, followed by a 'catch-up effect' where the overall mortality rises towards previous levels (Clarke 1995). A population-based study in Italy highlights a modest effect of levodopa on survival over an 8-year period (Morgante et al 2000). However, one 10-year follow-up study could not demonstrate an effect of early treatment upon mortality (Hely et al 1999).

SHOULD TREATMENTS THAT ARREST RATHER THAN REVERSE DETERIORATION BE GIVEN?

If treatments for progressive diseases such as Alzheimer's disease cause the course of the disease

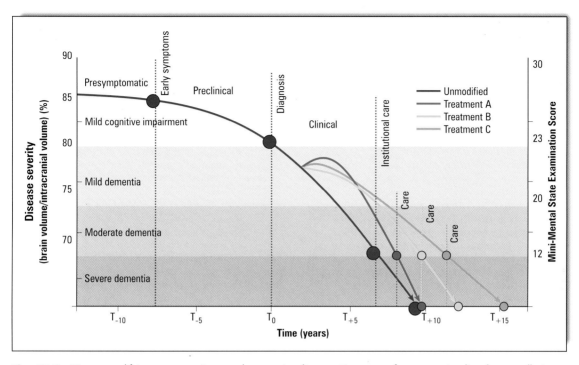

Fig. 69.2 Disease-modifying treatments in neurodegenerative diseases. Treatment of a progressive disorder may alleviate current symptoms and signs, but when treatment is stopped those symptoms and signs return. This is symptomatic treatment. Alternatively, treatment may prevent further deterioration and restore acquired deficits. In this example, treatment is altering the natural course of the disease. In most neurological conditions it is usually accepted that once damage to the CNS has occurred the damage is essentially irreversible. However, there may be a critical period in which early treatment can arrest or reverse decline. It is important to consider the effect of the treatment on each stage of the disease (i.e. the phase associated with good quality of life and that without good quality of life).

to arrest but not to reverse, how does this influence the decision to treat? In patients with good function at baseline, the promise of not losing that function is ample reason to justify treatment. However, in patients with very poor function at baseline, the preservation of the associated poor quality of life is not a desirable outcome. There is a caveat in that in the real world response to treatment is variable, such that one subgroup will show a relatively good response whereas another subgroup will show little or no response (see Fig. 69.2). In the trials in Alzheimer's disease to date, about 50% of patients do not deteriorate over 1 year (compared with one-third on placebo), but 30% show some improvement (compared with 20% on placebo) and 20% show a greater than 7-point improvement on the ADAS-cog (compared with none on placebo). Perhaps unexpectedly, patients who are severely cognitively impaired are more likely to show cognitive and behavioural benefits. It is exactly because of

these behavioural benefits that treatment may be justified even without palpable benefits upon cognition.

Most progressive conditions eventually 'overtake' the effect of treatment, such that several years down the line patients given treatment are no better off than patients not given treatment, although owing to the short length of clinical trials this has not been conclusively demonstrated in Alzheimer's disease. The disease course has been altered, but only modestly so and for a temporary period. In these examples, the treatment is buying X years without deterioration from baseline, Y years of cognitive benefit over placebo and Z years of behavioural benefit over placebo. This X–Y–Z formula is complex, and to many purchasers the superficial cost–benefit ratio is too large to justify treatment. However, to most sufferers any cost is justifiable if the benefit is appreciable or even possible.

REFERENCES AND FURTHER READING

Bigler ED, Johnson SC, Anderson CV et al 1996 Traumatic brain injury and memory: the role of hippocampal atrophy. Neuropsychology 10:333–342

Brown TM 1999 Basic mechanisms in the pathogenesis of delirium. In: Stoudemire A, Fogel BS, Greenberg DB (eds) Psychiatric care of the medical patient, 2nd edn. Oxford University Press, Oxford, p 571–579

Clarke CE 1995 Does levodopa therapy delay death in Parkinson's disease? A review of the evidence. Movement Disorders 10:250–256

D'Esposito M 2000 Neurobehavioural syndromes. In: Coffey CE, Cummings JL (eds) Textbook of neuropsychiatry, 2nd edn. American Psychiatric Press, Washington, DC

Di Stefano G, Bachevalier J, Levin HS et al 2000 Volume of focal brain lesions and hippocampal formation in relation to memory function after closed head injury in children. Journal of Neurology, Neurosurgery and Psychiatry 69:210–216

Fawcett JW, Rosser AE, Dunnett SB 2001 Brain damage, brain repair. Oxford University Press, Oxford

Fletcher PC, Henson RNA 2001 Frontal lobes and human memory: insights from functional neuroimaging. Brain 124:849–881

Hely MA, Morris JGL, Traficante R et al 1999 The Sydney multicentre study of Parkinson's disease: progression and mortality at 10 years. Journal of Neurology, Neurosurgery and Psychiatry 67:300–307

Hopfield JJ 1982 Neural networks and physical systems with emergent collective computational abilities. Proceedings of the National Academy of Sciences USA 79:2554–2558

Ingvar DH 1971 Cerebral blood flow and metabolism related to EEG and cerebral function. Acta Anaesthiologica Scandinavica 45:110–114

Izquierdo G, Campoy F, Mir J et al 1991 Memory and learning disturbances in multiple sclerosis: MRI lesions and neuropsychological correlation. European Journal of Radiology 13:220–224

Jason GW, Suchowersky O, Pajurkova EM et al 1997 Cognitive manifestations of Huntington disease in relation to genetic structure and clinical onset. Archives of Neurology 54:1081–1088

Lencz T, Mccarthy G, Bronen RA et al 1992 Quantitative magnetic resonance imaging in temporal lobe epilepsy: relationship to neuropathology and neuropsychological

function. Annals of Neurology 31:629–637

Lepage M, Habib R, Tulving E 1998 Hippocampal PET activation of memory encoding and retrieval: the HIPER model. Hippocampus 8:313–322

Morgante L, Salemi G, Meneghini F et al 2000 Parkinson disease survival: a population-based study. Archives of Neurology 57:507–512

Musicco M, Beghi E, Solari A et al 1997 Treatment of first tonic–clonic seizure does not improve the prognosis of epilepsy. Neurology 49:991–998

PRISMS Study Group and University of British Columbia MS/MRI Analysis Group 2001 PRISMS-4: long term efficacy of interferon-β-1a in relapsing MS. Neurology 56:1628–1636

Pulsinelli WA, Cooper AJL 1989 Metabolic encephalopathies and coma. In: Siegel G, Agranoff B, Albers RW et al (eds) Basic neurochemistry: molecular, cellular, and medical aspects, 4th edn. Raven Press, New York, p 765–791

Rajaram S 1997 Basal forebrain amnesia. Neurocase 3:405–415

Reed BR, Eberling JL, Mungas D et al 2000 Memory failure has different mechanisms in subcortical stroke and Alzheimer's disease. Annals of Neurology 48:275–284

Rovaris M, Filippi M, Falautano M et al 1998 Relation between MR abnormalities and patterns of cognitive impairment in multiple sclerosis. Neurology 50:1601–1608

Schuff N, Du AT, Chui H et al 2002 Differences between hippocampus and entorhinal cortex atrophy in normal aging and dementia. Presented at the 32nd Annual Meeting of the Society of Neuroscience, Orlando, FL, 2–7 November

Swartz RH, Black SE 2002 Are there strategic cognitive effects from diffuse white matter hyperintensities? The role of damage to cortical acetylcholine pathways. Presented at the 32nd Annual Meeting of the Society of Neuroscience, Orlando, FL, 2–7 November

Sze CI, Troncoso JC, Kawas C et al 1997 Loss of the presynaptic vesicle protein synaptophysin in hippocampus correlates with cognitive decline in Alzheimer's disease. Journal of Neuropathology and Experimental Neurology 56:933–944

Tate DF, Bigler ED 2000 Fornix and hippocampal atrophy in traumatic brain injury. Learning & Memory 7:442–446

Visser PJ, Krabbendam L, Verhey FRJ et al 1999 Brain correlates of memory dysfunction in alcoholic Korsakoff's syndrome. Journal of Neurology, Neurosurgery and Psychiatry 67:774–778

70

The Origin of Depression

IS DEPRESSION IN NEUROLOGICAL DISEASE ENDOGENOUS OR REACTIVE?

After many years of debate about the classification of depression, most authorities acknowledge that primary depression is often both endogenous and reactive. To be more accurate, there are some important environmental factors that contribute to the onset, severity and duration of an episode, but there are also biological factors that can explain some of the variance. The complex balance between the two will depend on the quality of the measures used and the population under study. This argument should not be confused with the question of whether the depression is volitional (*malingering*) or genuine. Pure factitious disorder is very uncommon, occurring in less than 0.3% of routine cases, and has little to do with whether the symptoms are psychiatric or physical (Bauer & Boegner 1996). The same question is asked repeatedly in neuropsychiatry: 'Is depression following stroke biological or psychological in origin?' This question becomes harder to answer the more it is examined. First, every patient is different, and therefore is the question restricted to those with a typical presentation, all cases or this particular case? Second, when a possible aetiological factor is identified, how do we know it is definitely a causative factor?

Authors frequently suggest that if the severity of depression (whether after stroke or after onset of Parkinson's disease) is tightly correlated with the degree of neurological impairment then a reactive

aetiology is confirmed. This is a logical error, as a significant neurological impairment implies a significant brain lesion and hence an equally likely biological contribution. Another strand of evidence is the relation to physical disease markers, in particular those that are caused by the original disease and that are not an epiphenomenon of the mood disorder. Comparisons of patients with secondary depression and healthy age-matched controls are of little use here, because any finding may be secondary to depression itself. A comparison needs to be made with primary depression. A change in neurotransmitter concentration in Huntington's disease or Parkinson's disease, or an elevation of the hypothalamopituitary–adrenal (HPA) axis function after stroke are examples of biological factors that could influence the development of depression. However, as it has not been possible to study these in a prospective way, their actual role remains speculative. A handful of studies have measured multiple risk factors for depression in high-risk neuropsychiatric patients. Andersen et al (1995) looked at 285 stroke patients, of whom 41% developed depression in the first year. Factors that predicted post-stroke depression were cognitive impairment, a history of previous stroke or depression, female gender, living alone and social distress. Anatomical factors were not contributory. One interpretation is that measurable biological factors (e.g. anatomical change) are unimportant, while another is that our measures are inadequate markers of brain dysfunction. In summary, depression in the context of neurological disease is a complex disorder with psychological and biological influences. The brain injury is usually the causative event, but the moderating factors vary enormously between individuals and in most cases cannot be reduced to one category alone.

WHAT UNIQUE FACTORS ARE INVOLVED IN THE PATHOGENESIS OF DEPRESSION IN NEUROLOGICAL DISEASE?

There are many reasons why the rate of depression is higher than expected in patients with CNS disease, but are specific biological factors involved? Most biological theories that have been applied to primary depression have also been applied to secondary depression. Serotonergic dysfunction is the most widely purported mechanism of primary affective disorder. Serotonergic function has also been examined in the depression of Parkinson's disease (Mayeux et al 1988). Mayeux et al (1984) found significantly lower concentrations of 5-hydroxyindoleacetic acid in the CSF of depressed versus non-depressed patients with Parkinson's disease. Unfortunately, this study did not include a control group of patients with primary depression, and this finding has not been consistently replicated (Kuhn et al 1996).

In Alzheimer's disease, Lopez et al (1997) found an association between deep white matter lesions and psychological aspects of depression. Post-mortem studies have suggested that there is more extensive

neuronal loss in the locus ceruleus and raphe nuclei in depressed compared with non-depressed patients with Alzheimer's disease (Zweig et al 1988). This may also be reflected by lower neurotransmitter levels in the cortex (Zubenko et al 1990). Change in the locus ceruleus in depressed patients was not found in a small study in Huntington's disease (Zweig et al 1992).

In multiple sclerosis, Sabatini et al (1996) studied 10 non-depressed and 10 depressed patients matched for age, sex and functional disability. No differences between the two groups were seen on MRI, but there were differences in perfusion asymmetries in the limbic cortex. Bakshi et al (2000) compared dif-

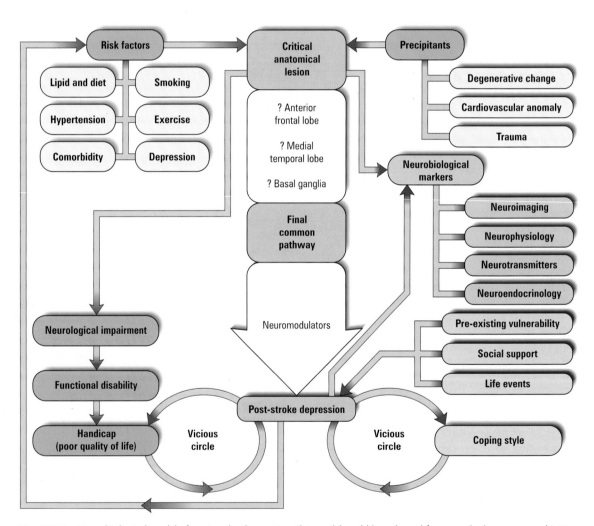

Fig. 70.1 Neurobiological model of post-stroke depression. This model could be adapted for several other neuropsychiatric complications. The presence of feed-forward or feedback loops acts as a significant maintaining factor in many conditions.

Table 70.1 Neurobiological correlates of post-stroke depression

Association with depression	Positive studies	Negative studies	Original observation	Recognized in primary depression	Comments
Anatomical factors					
Left hemisphere lesion	7	7	Gainotti (1972)	No	Confounders likely
Anterior lesion	10	3	Robinson et al (1984)	No	Publication bias likely
Subcortical lesion	6	1	Robinson et al (1988)	Yes	Publication bias likely
Temporal hypoperfusion	3	1	Mayberg et al (1991)	Yes	Functional neuroimaging
Ventricular enlargement	2	0	Starkstein et al (1988)	Yes	Not systematically studied
Neurophysiological factors					
Reduced REM latency	1	0	Kapen & Greiffenstein (1989)	Yes	Isolated report
Increased theta activity	1	0	Giaquinto et al (1994)	Yes	Isolated report
Neurotransmitter factors					
Low serotonin function	1	1	Bryer et al (1992)	Yes	Not systematically studied
Low NA function	2	0	Meyer et al (1974)	Yes	Not systematically studied
Neuroendocrinological factors					
DST non-suppression	8	4	Ross & Rush (1981)	Yes	Well replicated
Blunted thyrotropin-releasing hormone test	1	1	Dam et al (1994)	Yes	Not systematically studied
Blunted GH responses	1	0	Barry & Dinan (1990)	Yes	Isolated report

DST, dexamethasone suppression test; GH, growth hormone; NA, noradrenaline

ferences in 19 depressed and 29 non-depressed multiple sclerosis patients who were matched for severity of disability. A number of hypodense regions seen on T1-weighted MRI were linked with the presence of depression. These included changes in the superior frontal, parietal and temporal lobes. There were also less specific findings of ventricular enlargement and cortical atrophy. In a similar study, Berg et al (2000) used the DSM-IV criteria to compare 31 depressed and 47 non-depressed multiple sclerosis patients. They again found lesions in the right parietal and right frontal lobes, but it was an excess of temporal lobe lesions that most clearly differentiated depressed from non-depressed patients. Most recently, Zorzon et al (2001) conducted an assessment of 95 patients with definite multiple sclerosis (18 of whom were depressed), 97 patients suffering from chronic rheumatoid diseases and 110 healthy subjects. On MRI, both the severity of depressive symptoms and a diagnosis of major depression were weakly correlated with right frontal lesion load, total temporal brain volume, right hemisphere brain volume and the degree of disability in the patients.

Studies in multiple sclerosis that highlight the temporal lobe (among other regions) as potentially important in the pathogenesis of depression should be compared with studies in epilepsy. Several studies have documented higher depression scores in patients with temporal lobe epilepsy than other types of epilepsy (Lambert & Robertson 1999). Piazzini & Canger (2001) went further and rated depression in 106 patients with temporal lobe epilepsy, 44 with frontal lobe epilepsy and 70 with generalized epilepsy. Depression scores were highest in the patients with left temporal lobe epilepsy. Furthermore, it may be hippocampal damage that is particularly relevant (Quiske et al 2000).

The disorder that it is most often hoped will reveal secrets about the biological basis of depression is stroke. In patients with stroke a variety of biological and psychological mechanisms could mediate the influence of stroke on later depression (Fig. 70.1). The best studied are anatomical factors and neuroendocrine factors. The literature concerning the anatomical basis of post-stroke depression is large, but flawed in a number of ways (Aben et al 2001). One criticism is that clinical confounding variables, such as aphasia and anosognosia, will influence depression and its recognition and lead to artefactual reasons why depression is associated with particular brain areas. The second major criticism is that, while the anatomical lesion of stroke occurs quickly and resolves slowly, post-stroke depression appears gradually and then waxes and wanes. The third criticism is that there is a substantial publication bias – there has been only one methodologically sound review of the literature (Carson et al 2000). The conclusion of this review was that there is no particular association between lesion location and post-stroke depression (Fig. 70.2).

Neuroendocrine dysfunction is a consistent finding in a subgroup of patients with moderate or severe depression. The dexamethasone suppression test has been most commonly used as a marker of HPA axis function in primary and secondary depressions. In Parkinson's disease, Kostic et al (1990) found a 75% rate of non-suppression in depressed patients with Parkinson's disease, compared to 28% in non-depressed patients with Parkinson's disease. Frochtengarten et al (1987) found lower rates of 14% and 0%, respectively. Cerebrovascular insult elevates the HPA axis function acutely, due in part to local release of the regulating hormone corticotropin-releasing hormone from damaged tissue. Usually this HPA overdrive corrects within weeks. However, in patients with severe stroke, post-stroke delirium, post-stroke depression and post-stroke cognitive impairment this HPA overdrive is prolonged (Mitchell 1997). Considerable evidence suggests that this biological finding may be more than a marker of poor outcome (Sapolsky 1992). The ultimate test of this kind of biological finding is whether it can lead to diagnostic therapeutic advances in the field.

Changes seen on functional imaging, such as hypofrontality, have been robustly demonstrated in primary depression and documented in Parkinson's disease (Mayberg et al 1990), Huntington's disease (Mayberg et al 1992) and temporal lobe epilepsy (Bromfield et al 1992). Unfortunately, these studies tell us almost nothing about the biological basis of depression, because these findings are impossible to disprove as state-related phenomena of low mood. That is, these changes could occur as a consequence of depression itself and be unrelated to the cause. At the very least, repeat testing is required upon remission (a protocol that is used in primary but not sec-

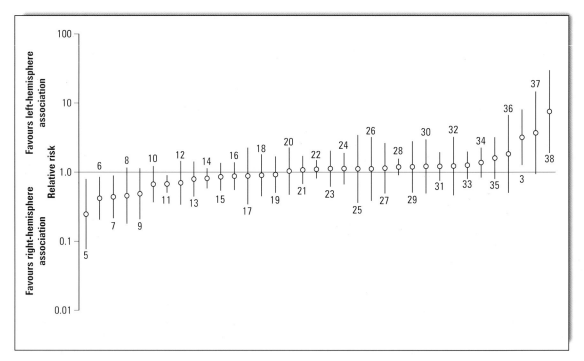

Fig. 70.2 Study-specific relative risks (log scale) for association of depression with left-hemisphere stroke. For studies in which assessment of depression was done at more than one time point (6, 9 and 20) the earliest assessment is shown. Error bars are 95% confidence intervals. Data from Carson et al (2000).

ondary depression). Of slightly more interest are the associations between atrophy of the basal ganglia and the degree of depression in Huntington's disease (De La Monte et al 1988), Parkinson's disease (Taylor et al 1986) and, possibly, idiopathic basal ganglia calcification (Trautner et al 1988).

CAN DEPRESSION BE DIAGNOSED RELIABLY IN PHYSICAL ILLNESS?

There are three closely related issues here:

- Is depression overdiagnosed because of contamination from disease-related somatic complaints?
- Is the syndrome of depression itself phenotypically different in the context of neurological disease?
- Is depression under-recognized because of the difficulty of assessing mood in patients with neurological disabilities?

It is often stated that the physical symptoms of neurological illness will prejudice the diagnosis of depression. In stroke, for example, a high frequency of somatic symptoms occurs in non-depressed patients (e.g. the rate of fatigue is twice that seen in age-matched controls). On most occasions, detailed questioning will reveal whether physical symptoms such as insomnia are a direct effect of stroke or a consequence of low mood. Certain somatic symptoms may be specific indicators of depression. For example, Randolph et al (2000) examined the intercorrelations of somatic symptoms with disability and low mood in multiple sclerosis. Disinterest in sex (not strictly a somatic symptom) was associated with depression, but not with fatigue or disability. Most somatic symptoms were contributed to by both depression and fatigue. Kalichman et al (2000) investigated the effect of somatic symptoms in HIV on the validity of the Beck Depression Inventory and the Centers for Epidemiological Studies Depression Scale (both self-report scales). Removing somatic subsets of depression symptoms improved the clinical utility of the scales, but at the possible cost of reduced sensitivity. Furthermore, it is not clear what effect the skill or experience of the investigator would have in detecting depression. Another disorder that poses particular difficulty is Parkinson's disease. There are strong parallels between the somatic symptoms of severe depression and the typical motor symptoms of Parkinson's disease (Table

70.2). The diagnosis of severe (melancholic) depression requires extra care in Parkinson's disease, because symptoms of anergia (lethargy), psychomotor retardation (bradykinesia) and sleep disturbance are essential features of both conditions. Despite this, the use of other somatic symptoms, the psychological and emotional features of depression and an exploration of the course will enable the careful clinician to make an accurate assessment. For this to occur, the use of clinician-reported scales rather than self-reported scales is recommended. Authors that have examined the use of conventional depression rating scales in Parkinson's disease have suggested that slightly higher cut-off scores are advisable (Leentjens et al 2000). The same situation of confounders is often seen in cases of head injury, where sleep disturbance, loss of libido and poor concentration are not useful in isolation, but in the context of other indicators of low mood do have diagnostic significance (Jorge et al 1993). In Alzheimer's disease many fundamental symptoms are similar to those with primary depression. This creates two problems: difficulty distinguishing early Alzheimer's disease from depression-related cognitive impairment; and difficulty spotting subtle depressions in Alzheimer's disease (Emery & Oxman 1992). This is made more hazardous by the fact that depression may be a risk factor for later dementia and a prodromal symptom of early dementia (see Clinical Pointer 40.3). If diagnosis remains uncertain, treatment of the suspected depression is indicated with later assessment. Depressive pseudodementia does not occur when the episode is in remission. Thus there appears to be little need to change the diagnostic criteria for depression in most neurological diseases without clear evidence that depression is being systematically overdiagnosed compared with a robust gold standard.

The second issue is whether depression itself presents differently in certain neurological illnesses. Studies to date have shown relatively subtle differences between primary and secondary depressions. Where there were differences these usually represent contamination from the underlying somatic symptoms of the disease itself (see above). Suggestions of phenomenological differences have been discussed in each chapter of this book, and need not be repeated here. However, on close examination, there may be psychological differences such as frequent worries about the future of the illness, difficulty coming to terms with disability and

Table 70.2 Similarities in presentation between primary depression, Parkinson's disease and Alzheimer's disease

Clinical feature	Depression	Parkinson's disease	Alzheimer's disease
Psychological features			
Loss of interest	+ + +	+	+ + +
Poor motivation	+ + +	+	+ +
Indecisiveness	+ + +	+	+ + +
Guilt	+ + +	0	0
Loss of self-esteem	+ + +	+	0
Suicidality	+ + +	+	0
Anxiety	+ + +	+ + +	+
Somatic features			
Reduced energy	+ + +	+ +	0
Disturbed appetite	+ + +	0	+ +
Fatigue	+ + +	+ +	+
Sleep disturbance	+ + +	+ +	+ + +
Mental state features			
Psychomotor retardation	+ +	+ + +	+
Psychomotor agitation	+ +	0	+ + +
Poverty of speech and thought	+ +	+	+ + +
Reduced blink rate	+	+ + +	0
Stooped posture	+ +	+ + +	+
Psychosis	+ +	+	+ + +
Cognitive features			
Poor concentration	+ + +	+ +	+ + +
Frontal/executive deficits	+	+ +	+ + +
Dementia or pseudodementia	+	+ +	+ + +

0, Not a characteristic feature; +, recognized feature; ++, common feature; +++, characteristic feature

loss, and often blame for being unwell or handicapped by the medical illness. Of course, these are important issues to explore in every patient with a chronic illness.

The third issue concerns the underdetection of depression. There is no doubt that depression is not diagnosed reliably in the general hospital setting, but neither is depression diagnosed reliably in the community. However, are there specific issues that lead to the under-recognition of depression in neurological patients? For example, visual–analogue or observer-rated scales can be valuable in patients who have severe communication or intellectual problems, and several have been specifically developed for patients with neurological disease. That said, scales and diagnostic schedules that purport to improve on the detection of depression should not be accepted without clear evidence concerning their sensitivity and specificity compared with conventional measures. This has rarely been tested. In an exceptional study, Nicholl et al (2001) examined the

relative sensitivity and specificity of eight mood scales in 98 multiple sclerosis patients. They found that the General Health Questionnaire GHQ-28 and GHQ-12 scales detected about twice as many cases as the Hospital Anxiety and Depression (HAD) scale, with the Beck Anxiety and Depression Scales performing at an intermediate level.

In summary, the diagnosis of depression does not rely on one or two non-specific somatic symptoms, and the worries about overdiagnosis have largely been overstated. Multiple somatic symptoms associated with core psychological features of depression still have validity for diagnosis and severity ratings (Stein et al 1996). To look at this another way, depression is rarely systematically overdiagnosed by clinicians, but it is frequently underdiagnosed. Core features of low mood (tearfulness, loss of interest/motivation, loss of enjoyment) accompanied by psychological features (pessimistic view of the future, self-blame or guilt, loss of confidence and low self-esteem) and somatic complaints are valid in cases of secondary depression, but some effort may be required to elicit these features in patients with apathy, dysphasia or cognitive impairment.

REFERENCES AND FURTHER READING

Aben I, Verhey F, Honig A et al 2001 Research into the specificity of depression after stroke: a review on an unresolved issue. Progress in Neuropsychopharmacology and Biological Psychiatry 25:671–689

Andersen G, Vestergaad K, Ingemann-Nielsen M et al 1995 Risk factors for post-stroke depression. Acta Psychiatrica Scandinavica 92:193–198

Bakshi R, Czarnecki D, Shaikh ZA et al 2000 Brain MRI lesions and atrophy are related to depression in multiple sclerosis. Neuroreport 11:1153–1158

Barry S, Dinan TG 1990 Alpha-2 adrenergic receptor function in post-stroke depression. Psychological Medicine 20:305–309

Bauer M, Boegner F 1996 Neurological syndromes in factitious disorder. Journal of Nervous and Mental Disease 184:281–288

Berg D, Supprian T, Thomae J et al 2000 Lesion pattern in patients with multiple sclerosis and depression. Multiple Sclerosis 6:156–162

Bromfield EB, Altshuler L, Leiderman DB et al 1992 Cerebral metabolism and depression in patients with complex partial seizures. Archives of Neurology 49:617–623

Bryer JB, Starkstein SE, Votypka V et al 1992 Reduction of CSF monoamine metabolites in poststroke depression: a preliminary report. Journal of Neuropsychiatry and Clinical Neuroscience 4:440–442

Carson AJ, MacHale S, Allen K et al 2000 Depression after stroke and lesion location: a systematic review. Lancet 356:122–126

Dam H, Pedersen HE, Dige-Petersen H et al 1994 Neuroendocrine tests in depressive stroke patients. Progress in Neuropsychopharmacology & Biological Psychiatry 18:1005–1013

De La Monte SM, Vonsattel JP, Richardson EP 1988 Morphometric demonstration of atrophic changes in the cerebral cortex, white matter and neostriatum in Huntington's disease. Journal of Neuropathology and Experimental Neurology 47:516–525

Emery VO, Oxman TE 1992 Update on the dementia spectrum of depression. American Journal of Psychiatry 149:305–317

Frochtengarten ML, Villares JCB, Maluf E et al 1987 Depressive symptoms and the dexamethasone suppression test in Parkinsonian patients. Biological Psychiatry 22:386–389

Gainotti G 1972 Emotional behaviour and hemispheric side of the lesion. Cortex 8:41–55

Giaquinto S, Cobianchi A, Macera F et al 1994 EEG recordings in the course of recovery from stroke. Stroke 25:2204–2209

Jorge RE, Robinson RG, Arndt SV 1993 Are there symptoms which are specific for a depressed mood in patients with traumatic brain injury? Journal of Nervous and Mental Disorders 181:91–99

Kalichman SC, Rompa D, Cage M 2000 Distinguishing between overlapping somatic symptoms of depression and HIV disease in people living with HIV-AIDS. Journal of Nervous and Mental Disorders 188:662–670

Kapen S, Greiffenstein M 1989 Stroke and depression: the cholinergic sleep induction test. In: Horne J (ed) Sleep '88. Gustav Fischer, New York, p 238–240

Kostic VS, Sternic NC, Bumbasirevic LB et al 1990 Dexamethasone suppression test in patients with Parkinson's disease. Movement Disorders 5:23–26

Kuhn W, Muller T, Gerlach M et al 1996 Depression in Parkinson's disease: biogenic amines in the CSF of 'de-novo' patients. Archives of Neurology 54:982–986

Lambert MV, Robertson MM 1999 Depression in epilepsy: etiology, phenomenology, and treatment. Epilepsia 40(suppl 10):S21–S47

Leentjens AFG, Verhey FRJ, Lousberg R et al 2000 The validity of the Hamilton and Montgomery–Asberg depression rating scales as screening and diagnostic tools for depression in Parkinson's disease. International Journal of Geriatric Psychiatry 15:644–649

Lopez OL, Becker JT, Reynolds I et al 1997 Psychiatric correlates of MR deep white matter lesions in probable Alzheimer's disease. Journal of Neuropsychiatry and Clinical Neuroscience 9:246–250

Mayberg HS, Starkstein SE, Sadzot B et al 1990 Selective hypometabolism in the inferior frontal-lobe in depressed patients with Parkinson's disease. Annals of Neurology 28:57–64

Mayberg HS, Starkstein SE, Morris PL et al 1991 Remote cortical hypometabolism following focal basal ganglia injury: relationship to secondary changes in mood. Neurology 41(suppl 1):266

Mayberg HS, Starkstein SE, Peyser CE et al 1992 Paralimbic frontal lobe hypometabolism in depression associated with Huntington's disease. Neurology 42:1791–1797

Mayeux R, Stern Y, Cote L et al 1984 Altered serotonin metabolism in depressed patients with Parkinson's disease. Neurology 34:642–646

Mayeux R, Stern Y, Sano M et al 1988 The relationship of serotonin to depression in Parkinson's disease. Movement Disorders 3:237–244

Meyer JS, Welch KMA, Okamoto S et al 1974 Disordered neurotransmitter function: demonstration by measurement of norepinephrine and 5-hydroxydopamine in CSF of patients with recent cerebral infarction. Brain 97:655–664

Mitchell AJ 1997 Clinical implications of post-stroke hypothalamo-pituitary adrenal axis dysregulation: a critical review. Journal of Stroke and Cerebrovascular Disorders 6:377–388

Nicholl CR, Lincoln NB, Francis VM et al 2001 Assessment of emotional problems in people with multiple sclerosis.

Clinical Rehabilitation 15:657–668

Piazzini A, Canger R 2001 Depression and anxiety in patients with epilepsy. Epilepsia 42(supp 1):29–31

Quiske A, Helmstaedter C, Lux S et al 2000 Depression in patients with temporal lobe epilepsy is related to mesial temporal sclerosis. Epilepsy Research 39:121–125

Randolph JJ, Arnett PA, Higginson CI et al 2000 Neurovegetative symptoms in multiple sclerosis: relationship to depressed mood, fatigue and physical disability. Archives of Clinical Neuropsychology 15:387–398

Robinson RG, Kubos KG, Starr LB 1984 Mood disorders in stroke patients: importance of location of lesion. Brain 107:81–93

Robinson RG, Boston JD, Starkstein SE et al 1988 Comparison of mania and depression after brain injury: causal factors. American Journal of Psychiatry 145:172–178

Ross ED, Rush AJ 1981 Diagnosis and neuroanatomical correlates of depression in brain damaged patients: implications for a neurology of depression. Archives of General Psychiatry 38:1344–1354

Sabatini U, Pozzilli C, Pantano P et al 1996 Involvement of the limbic system in multiple sclerosis patients with depressive disorders. Biological Psychiatry 39:970–975

Sapolsky RM 1992 Stress, the aging brain, and the mechanisms of neuron death. MIT Press, Cambridge, MA

Starkstein SE, Robinson RG, Price TR 1988 Comparison of patients with and without post-stroke major depression matched for size and location of lesion. Archives of General Psychiatry 45:247–252

Stein PN, Sliwinski MJ, Gordon WA et al 1996 Discriminative properties of somatic and nonsomatic symptoms for post stroke depression. Clinical Neurologist 10:141–148

Taylor AE, Sain-Cyr JA, Land AE et al 1986 Parkinson's disease and depression: a critical re-evaluation. Brain 109:279–292

Trautner RJ, Cummings JL, Read SL et al 1988 Idiopathic basal ganglia calcification and organic mood disorder. American Journal of Psychiatry 145:350–353

Zorzon M, de Masi R, Nasuelli D et al 2001 Depression and anxiety in multiple sclerosis. A clinical and MRI study in 95 subjects. Journal of Neurology 248:416–421

Zubenko GS, Moosy J, Kopp U 1990 Neurochemical correlates of major depression in primary dementia. Archives of Neurology 47:209–214

Zweig RM, Ross CA, Hedreen JC et al 1988 The neuropathology of aminergic nuclei in Alzheimer's disease. Annals of Neurology 24:233–242

Zweig RM, Ross CA, Hedreen JC et al 1992 Locus coeruleus involvement in Huntington's disease. Archives of Neurology 49:152–156

71

The Origin of Anxiety

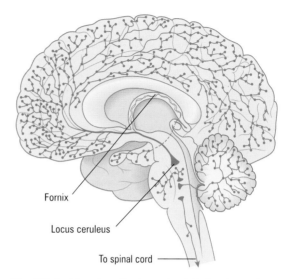

Fig. 71.1 Noradrenaline (norepinephrine) pathways in the brain. After Baynes & Dominiczak (2000).

Fornix

Locus ceruleus

To spinal cord

Anxiety disorders are in danger of becoming the lost diagnosis in neuropsychiatry. Few investigators have asked patients with neurological disorders whether they have suffered anxiety problems, let alone examined the cause or course of this distressing condition. This is perplexing when one considers that anxiety disorders compete with depression as the most common psychiatric diagnosis, being present in up to 30.5% of women and 19.2% of men over a lifetime (Kessler et al 1994). Phobias are seen in 9% of the general population, and generalized anxiety disorder and panic disorder in about 3%.

Of the few biological studies of secondary anxiety disorder, Kurlan et al (1989) noted increased susceptibility to yohimbine-induced panic attacks in Parkinson's disease. Yohimbine is an α_2 antagonist that increases noradrenaline (norepinephrine) firing. Patients with Parkinson's disease are thought to have a loss of inhibitory mesencephalic dopamine projections to the locus ceruleus, resulting in high levels noradrenaline (norepinephrine) relative to dopamine in the locus ceruleus, and perhaps oversensitivity. Serotonin has an important role in anxiety and depression. Abnormalities in the serotonin reuptake transporter and its gene have been documented in primary depression. In Parkinson's disease there is degeneration of serotonergic neurones and loss of the serotonin transporter. In an interesting study concerning the genetics of anxiety in Parkinson's disease, Menza et al (1999) found that patients who carried the short allele of the serotonin transporter gene had higher anxiety scores than those who did not. This has also been shown in rela-

tion to depression scores (Mossner et al 2001), suggesting a common biological mechanism of anxiety and depression in Parkinson's disease.

Many lessons for the biological basis of secondary anxiety can be gleaned from the study of patients with temporal lobe epilepsy. Although anxiety disorder can occur in many forms, patients' ictal fear is among the most interesting. Intraoperative electrical stimulation implicates the amygdala, locus ceruleus and, to a lesser extent, the hippocampus in the generation of the acute fear response (Halgren et al 1978). The amygdala is a key component of the primitive brain's defence system, which includes threat analysis, complex conditioning (e.g. avoidance) and generation of basic emotions (possibly via the septohippocampal system). Stimuli that activate the amygdala are those that produce a high level of physiological arousal. As a structure, the amygdala receives high-level sensory information from the cortex and low-grade but affectively labelled sensory information from the thalamus. The response from the amygdala is output to the medial hypothalamus (including the paraventricular nucleus) and periaqueductal grey matter if simple autonomic, neuroendocrine and motor responses are required, and output to the cortex and basal ganglia if a more flexible response is required. Serotonergic neurones of the raphe nuclei have an inhibitory effect on the amygdala, locus ceruleus and periaqueductal grey matter.

Box 71.1 The ten most frequent neurological causes of secondary anxiety

- Delirium
- Head injury
- Stroke
- Alzheimer's disease
- Mixed dementia
- Vascular dementia
- Lewy body disease
- Parkinson's disease
- Multiple sclerosis
- Epilepsy

In vivo MRI has also shown that patients with ictal fear have smaller amygdala volumes than do temporal lobe epilepsy patients without fear (Cendes et al 1994). In two fascinating reports, Abraham & Duffy (1991) and Jabourian et al (1992) both reported an extremely high rate of EEG abnormalities (on 24-hour EEG monitoring) in patients with panic disorder. In fact, they found about four times the rate of EEG abnormalities compared with the rate in depressed patients. This has been replicated with routine EEG studies and in drug-free subjects, with the conclusion that up to one-third of patients with panic disorder have EEG abnormalities, and of these approximately 60% will have MRI evidence of structural anomalies, particularly in the hippocampal area (Bystritsky et al 1999, Dantendorfer et al 1996). This overlooked association has important implications for the investigation and treatment of anxiety disorder.

REFERENCES AND FURTHER READING

Abraham HD, Duffy FH 1991 Computed EEG abnormalities in panic disorder with and without premorbid drug abuse. Biological Psychiatry 29:687–690

Baynes J, Dominiczak M 2000 Medical biochemistry. Mosby, St. Louis

Bystritsky A, Leuchter AF, Vapnik T 1999 EEG abnormalities in non-medicated panic disorder. Journal of Nervous and Mental Disorders 187:13–114

Cendes F, Andermann F, Gloor P et al 1994 Relationship between atrophy of the amygdala and ictal fear in temporal-lobe epilepsy. Brain 117:739–746

Dantendorfer K, Prayer D, Kramer J et al 1996 High frequency of EEG and MRI brain abnormalities in panic disorder. Psychiatry Research – Neuroimaging 68:41–53

Halgren E, Walter RD, Cherlow DG et al 1978 Mental phenomena evoked by electrical stimulation of the human hippocampal formation and amygdala. Brain 101:83–117

Jabourian AP, Erlich M, Desvignes C et al 1992 Panic-attacks and 24 hours EEG by out-patients. Annales Medico-Psychologiques 150:240–245

Kessler RC, McGonagle KA, Zhao S et al 1994 Lifetime and 12-month prevalence of DSM-III-R psychiatric disorders in the United States. Results from the National Comorbidity Survey. Archives of General Psychiatry 51:8–19

Kurlan R, Lichter D, Schiffer RB 1989 Panic/anxiety in Parkinson's disease: yohimbine challenge. Neurology 39:421

Menza MA, Palermo B, DiPaola R et al 1999 Depression and anxiety in Parkinson's disease: possible effect of genetic variation in the serotonin transporter. Journal of Geriatric Psychiatry and Neurology 12:49–52

Mossner R, Henneberg A, Schmitt A et al 2001 Allelic variation of serotonin transporter expression is associated with depression in Parkinson's disease. Molecular Psychiatry 6:350–352

72

The Origin of Mania

The lifetime risk of primary mania is about 1%. Bipolar affective disorder is one of the most strongly genetic of all psychiatric disorders, yet in the vast majority of cases other factors are involved. Several studies highlight that people who present with mania for the first time in late life have more than a 50% chance of the episode being caused by a comorbid neurological illness (Van Gerpen et al 1999). This is the disorder known as secondary mania.

In secondary mania, the contribution of genetic factors is considerably less than in primary mania but is still present. In an important neuroimaging study, Fujikawa et al (1995) examined 20 patients with late-onset mania, 20 age- and sex-matched patients who developed mania while younger than 50, and 20 patients with late-onset major depression. The incidence of silent cerebral infarctions was 65.0% in patients with late-onset mania, 55% in those with late-onset depression and 25% in those with early-onset mania. Patients with late-onset mania also have higher cholesterol levels and more vascular risk factors than comparable patients with early-onset mania (Cassidy & Carroll 2002). Many other conditions, including neurodevelopmental and neurodegenerative conditions, predispose to secondary mania (Box 72.1).

One important difference between primary mania and secondary mania is that sufferers of secondary mania are more likely to experience unipolar mania or hypomania rather than the typical mix of both highs and lows seen in patients with primary bipolar affective disorder. The clinical features of primary and secondary manias have not been found to be sufficiently different from each other to allow a diagnosis on this basis alone. Nevertheless, cognitive impairment does appear to be more common in secondary mania than primary mania.

CLINICOANATOMICAL MECHANISMS OF MANIA

One of the earliest models of secondary mania came from Welt (1888), who suggested that orbitofrontal lesions may produce mania by disinhibition. This popular theory has been revisited over the years, but it is neither a complete nor an accurate explanation. Patients with orbital surface damage often display labile, incongruous or euphoric mood. This affect state may have an empty, childlike quality sometimes referred to as 'moria.' There may be accompanying hyperactivity of thought, action and biological drives (e.g. hypersexuality, hyperphagia, insomnia, sleep–wake dysregulation). Where behavioural features are present but the condition is not driven by

---

Box 72.1 Neurological causes of secondary mania

Cerebrovascular disease

Head injury

Cerebral tumours

Multiple sclerosis

Temporal lobe epilepsy

Movement disorders:
- Huntington's disease
- neuroacanthocytosis
- Sydenham's chorea
- Wilson's disease

CNS infections:
- AIDS
- Creutzfeldt–Jakob disease
- Lyme disease
- neurosyphilis
- prion disease
- viral encephalitis

Neurodevelopmental disorders:
- adrenoleukodystrophy
- fragile X syndrome
- tuberous sclerosis
- Kleine–Levin syndrome

Adapted from Mendez (2000)

euphoric or irritable mood, the disorder may be conceptualized as pseudomania (i.e. a behavioural phenocopy of mania). This link between frontal disinhibition and euphoria is consistent with the observation that elated Alzheimer patients have more frontal hypoperfusion and executive deficits than do non-euphoric patients with Alzheimer's disease (Lebert et al 1994). One issue when reviewing the literature is that many authors do not specify the duration of symptoms. For this reason, the syndrome of mania may be confused with emotionalism and the subsyndromal bipolar disorders. Starkstein & Robinson (1997) have suggested that various syndromes of disinhibition may exist. These include motor disinhibition from disconnection of the ventromedial prefrontal cortex, instinctive disinhibition from orbitofrontal lesions, cognitive and sensory disinhibition from the basotemporal cortex, and emotional disinhibition from paleocortical–paralimibc disconnections. The clinical support for these proposed syndromes is currently poor. Case series of patients who have sustained head injury or focal cerebrovascular lesions suggest an association between mania and right-sided lesions (Braun et al 1999). This applies to cortical areas (orbitofrontal and basotemporal) as well as subcortical areas (including the thalamus, hypothalamus, caudate and surrounding the third ventricle) (Cummings & Mendez 1984, Leibson 2000, Starkstein et al 1991). Structural lesions producing mania are said by some authors to involve the basotemporal region, the parathalamic structures and the inferior medial frontal lobe. However, as with many clinicoanatomical associations in neuropsychiatry these findings are neither sensitive nor specific enough to be used reliably in a clinical setting.

REFERENCES AND FURTHER READING

Braun CM, Larocque C, Daigneault S et al 1999 Mania, pseudomania, depression and pseudodepression resulting from focal unilateral cortical lesions. Neuropsychiatry, Neuropsychology and Behavioral Neurology 12:35–51

Cassidy F, Carroll BJ 2002 Vascular risk factors in late onset mania. Psychological Medicine 32:359–362

Cummings JL, Mendez MF 1984 Secondary mania with focal cerebrovascular lesions. American Journal of Psychiatry 141:1084–1087

Fujikawa T, Yamawaki S, Touhouda Y 1995 Silent cerebral infarctions in patients with late-onset mania. Stroke 26:946–949

Lebert F, Pasquier F, Danel T et al 1994 Psychiatric, neuropsychologic, and SPECT evidence of elated mood in dementia of Alzheimer type. Neuropsychiatry, Neuropsychology and Behavioral Neurology 7:299–302

Leibson E 2000 Anosognosia and mania associated with right thalamic haemorrhage. Journal of Neurology, Neurosurgery and Psychiatry 68:107–108

Mendez MF 2000 Mania in neurologic disorders. Current Psychiatry Reports 2:440–445

Starkstein SE, Robinson RG 1997 Mechanism of disinhibition after brain lesions. Journal of Nervous and Mental Disorders 185:108–114

Starkstein SE, Federoff P, Berthier ML et al 1991 Manic–depressive and pure manic states after brain lesions. Biological Psychiatry 29:149–158

Van Gerpen MW, Johnson JE, Winstead DK 1999 Mania in the geriatric patient population: a review of the literature. American Journal of Geriatric Psychiatry 7:188–202

Welt L 1888 Uber Charakterveränderungen der Menschen infolge von Läsionen des Stirnhirm. Deutsch Archiv fur Klinische Medizinische 42:339–390

73

The Origin of Apathy

Apathy is a complex symptom that can occur in a variety of medical and psychiatric conditions. In addition to loss of motivation or volition (hence the term *amotivational syndrome*), patients (and their relatives) often complain of loss of emotional interest for positive and negative events (a condition described by Habib as *athymhormia*) (Habib 2000). There is a strong overlap with depression. About one-third of depressed patients also have apathy, and because depression is a very common condition, this mixed disorder accounts for two-thirds of all cases of apathy. In other words, only one-third of people with apathy have pure apathy. Certain neuropsychiatric conditions, such as the degenerative dementias, Parkinson's disease, traumatic brain

injury and stroke, feature apathy about as commonly as primary depression – these tend to be conditions in which insight is impaired. If one compares patients who have Alzheimer's disease and depression with patients who have pure depression, apathy is commoner in the depressed Alzheimer's disease sufferers. This shows that apathy is not a product of depression alone.

In medicine, the amotivational syndrome presents a particular problem with recognition. Such patients do not ask for help or 'cause a fuss', and hence are much more likely to be overlooked on busy wards. In addition, clinicians are simply not good at helping patients who at face value appear unwilling to help themselves, even though this condition is no more deserved by the patient than any other symptom or sign. Furthermore, amotivational syndromes are notoriously difficult to treat, requiring considerable persistence by the patient and carers alike (see Clinical Pointer 52.1).

CLINICOANATOMICAL MECHANISMS

As with depression, it is difficult to pin down where motivation resides in the brain. This is, in part, because motivation is not a pure neurological function but a complex interaction of consciousness, awareness, arousal, perception, emotion and interaction with the environment (see Fig. 73.1). Disruption in any of these areas can impair motivation. It is still interesting to ask that, if one excludes

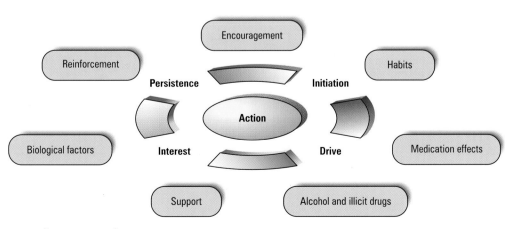

Fig. 73.1 Influences on apathy.

Box 73.1 Neuropsychiatric causes of apathy

Acquired brain injury
Any degenerative dementia
Cerebrovascular disease
Encephalitis
Head injury
Herpes simplex encephalitis
HIV encephalopathy
Huntington's disease
Hydrocephalus
Lewy body disease
Motor neurone disease
Multiple sclerosis
Parkinson's disease
Parkinsonian syndromes
Prion disease
Wilson's disease

Drug induced
Alcohol
Cannabis
Chronic stimulant use
Heavy metal poisoning
Typical antipsychotics

patients with emotional and cognitive deficits, what newly acquired lesions occur in patients with post-stroke or post-head injury apathy? Case series suggest that the orbitofrontal and mesial frontal cortex, the basal ganglia, the internal capsule and the thalamus are involved. Bilateral lesions are usually implicated, but occasionally unilateral lesions of the caudate, globus pallidus and thalamus are responsible. One small study in brain-injured patients found that patients with right hemisphere lesions and subcortical lesions were most likely to suffer apathy. Unfortunately, these anatomical associations are not sufficiently precise to be diagnostically useful (Andersson et al 1999). In Alzheimer's disease, functional imaging has demonstrated an association between apathy and right cingulate hypoperfusion (Benoit et al 1999). The same association with (bilateral) anterior cingulate dysfunction has been replicated in patients with 'organic brain syndrome' with and without dementia (Migneco et al 2001). In frontotemporal dementia there may be an association with hypometabolism in the prefrontal cortex (Diehl et al 2002).

Of course it is an error to consider the physiology and pathophysiology of motivation in purely anatomical terms. Cognitive correlates of apathy have been studied in HIV and post-head injury. The biochemical foundations of motivation are quite well described, but beyond the scope of this book. In animal models, considerable evidence supports a prominent role for mesocortical dopamine from the ventral tegmental area in arousal, drive and novelty-seeking behaviour (Tzschentke 2001). This may be of relevance to the negative syndrome of schizophrenia, depression and the reward systems in addictions. It also provides a scientific foundation for the treatment of apathy with dopamine-enhancing drugs.

REFERENCES AND FURTHER READING

Andersson S, Krogstad JM, Finset A 1999 Apathy and depressed mood in acquired brain damage: relationship to lesion localization and psychophysiological reactivity. Psychological Medicine 29:447–456

Benoit M, Dygai I, Migneco O et al 1999 Behavioral and psychological symptoms in Alzheimer's disease: relation between apathy and regional cerebral perfusion. Dementia and Geriatric Cognitive Disorders 10:511–517

Diehl J, Grimmer T, Drzezga A et al 2002 Association of apathy with cerebral glucose metabolism in frontotemporal dementia. Presented at 8th International Conference on Alzheimer's Disease and Related Disorders, Stockholm, 20–25 July

Habib M 2000 Disorder of motivation. In: Bogousslavsky J, Cummings JL (eds) Behaviour and mood disorders in focal brain lesions. Cambridge University Press, Cambridge, p 261–284

Migneco O, Benoit M, Koulibaly PM et al 2001 Perfusion brain SPECT and statistical parametric mapping analysis indicate that apathy is a cingulate syndrome: a study in Alzheimer's disease and non-demented patients. Neuroimage 13:896–902

Tzschentke TM 2001 Pharmacology and behavioral pharmacology of the mesocortical dopamine system. Progress in Neurobiology 63:241–320

74

The Origin of Aggression

Inappropriate aggression and irritability are increasingly recognized as valid symptoms of brain injury. As with all complex behaviours, both organic brain injury or psychological factors may be to blame. Aggression is a behaviour associated with the emotion of anger, with the goal of attack. Violence implies an actual assault. Irritability is an emotion associated with frustration – that is, a failure to attain goals as planned. Disinhibition is the tendency to think, feel or act without the required evaluation. It may be described using the terms 'poor judgement', 'emotional lability' and 'impulsivity'. Frustration combined with disinhibition or dysphoria can add up to severe outbursts when perceived failure occurs, a response sometimes labelled as the *catastrophic reaction* in patients with stroke, dementia and head injury (see also Ch. 2). There is a strong sociocultural component to aggression, and men are consistently more likely to commit aggressive acts. There is no doubt that psychiatric disorders increase the relative risk of violence, although the actual risk of violence remains low (Swanson et al 1990). For example, a number of studies suggest that the relative risk of violence in sufferers with schizophrenia is between 5- and 10-fold that in aged-matched controls. Within this group alcohol has a powerful effect. In one study, alcoholic men with schizophrenia were 25 times more likely to commit a violent crime than mentally healthy men, and 3.6 times more likely where alcohol was not involved (Rasanen et al 1998).

An interest in the biological origins of aggression in humans stems from studies of violent offenders, who, more often than not, have antisocial personality disorder. Such patients have an increased rate of *minimal brain dysfunction* (i.e. subtle brain damage acquired very early in life and possibly perinatally). If seen when they are children, such patients could attract a diagnosis of attention deficit hyperactivity disorder (ADHD), a disorder that overlaps with conduct disorder. In adult life, violent offenders have a higher rate of EEG abnormalities, perhaps as a reflection of early life insults. They also have abnormalities in serotonergic function that may be more highly correlated with impulsivity than aggression (Dolan et al 2002).

That is not to say that aggression is entirely biologically determined. People who are violent for psychological or cultural reasons tend to be more impulsive and more easily aroused and to have high novelty-seeking traits. They also have lower problem-solving capabilities.

NEUROPSYCHIATRIC CONDITIONS AND AGGRESSION

Traumatic brain injury is one of the most common conditions associated with aggression in the literature, but statistically delirium and dementia are far more common causes. In head injury this occurs on an almost universal background of frustration at the very common deficits in attention and processing speed. These force the patient to try harder in order to achieve the same result (McAllister et al 2001). Patients who sustain a head injury to the orbital surface of the frontal lobes (and perhaps the ventromedial frontal lobes and anterior temporal lobes) are

---

Box 74.1   The ten most common neuropsychiatric causes of aggression*

- Alcohol
- Illicit drug use
- Delirium
- Dementia
- Normal frustration
- Head injury
- Frontal lobe stroke
- Frontal tumour
- Iatrogenic disinhibition
- Delusions (any cause)

*Excluding personality disorder

more likely to lash out impulsively at people around them following minor provocation (Grafman et al 1996). Characteristically this is without planning and, although the patient is aware of his or her actions, the normal degree of remorse is usually absent. These patients are sometimes described as having *acquired sociopathy*. Very rarely, patients with hypothalamic lesions may have similar outbursts, again precipitated by no obvious cause, except perhaps irritability through hunger or poor sleep. These observations have led to the formulation of an organic aggressive syndrome (see Box 74.2), although it must be said that the validity of this is unknown.

In children the significance of minimal brain dysfunction is often debated (see Clinical Pointer 19.1).

Elliott (1982) reported neurological findings in 286 patients with a history of recurrent attacks of uncontrollable rage, many dating from early childhood. Objective evidence of developmental or acquired brain defects was found in 94%. The most common abnormality was minimal brain dysfunction, found in 41%.

Stroke is now recognized as a cause of outbursts of anger, a symptom that relatives find particularly distressing. In this context, anger can occur spontaneously but is more likely to be an overreaction to minor provocation. This has been called an 'inability to control anger or aggression after stroke' (Kim et al 2002). There is a significant overlap with the inability to control crying (emotionalism). Occasionally, stroke patients who suffer a lesion to the orbitofrontal or right hemisphere lose their understanding of emotional events and empathy – a feature that has parallels with 'aquired sociopathy' (Eslinger et al 2002).

Epilepsy is often quoted as a cause of aggression, but in reality this is very rare. When it does occur, it is usually is a post-ictal phenomenon during a period of confusion, when a person acts instinctively and after which he or she has little or no memory of the events. This is similar to the violence that can

---

Box 74.2 The organic aggressive syndrome

- Reactive – only small triggers necessary
- Non-reflective – no planning beforehand
- Non-purposeful – no clear goal
- Explosive – sudden onset
- Periodic – episodes are brief
- Ego-dystonic – no explanation given

Modified from Yudofsky et al (1990)

Clinical Pointer 74.1

Assessing and managing the risk of acute violence in patients

The first principle is that prevention is better than cure. Therefore try to predict who is likely to become aggressive using early warning signs (such as shouting, threats, agitation, distress, restlessness, disinhibition and alcohol abuse) and offer to help, reassure or distract the person. Be as calming as possible (i.e. use de-escalation techniques).

The risk of violence can be divided into four types of factors:

- demographic factors (e.g. male sex, young, low social class)
- predisposing factors (e.g. a history of violence, prison, psychiatric illness or antisocial personality disorder; being a victim of violence; having disinhibition, a history of substance use or unpleasant symptoms such as akathisia)
- precipitating factors (e.g. current adversity, feeling under threat, conflict with others (including staff))
- perpetuating factors (e.g. repetition of previously adverse circumstances, social isolation).

Once violence has started to occur it should be contained for the safety of the patient and staff. If you are not equipped or able to deal with the problem on your own, immediately ask for help. Once the patient can be safely approached make a clear verbal statement for the violence to cease. If this is ineffective remove the violent patient from the provoking situation or restrain the patient using the least force possible. Where violence has occurred in response to mental illness sedating medication is usually necessary to prevent recurrence. This is usually administered using the route that produces the fastest and most predictable effect (i.e. intravenous rapid tranquillization). Intravenous injection of benzodiazepines is routinely used in anaesthesia and general medicine and is a safe procedure when monitored. Rapid onset allows the sedative effect to be titrated with the dose administered. Duration of action is a matter of hours, and therefore combination with a high-potency antipsychotic is often recommended. Very occasionally the patient may need to be in an appropriate seclusion area; however, this requires careful supervision. Analysis of the violent incident is also recommended to discover any avoidable factors. If there appears to be repeated aggressive behaviour, consider the use of a psychiatric intensive care facility, where available.

occur in the context of delirium after head injury.

Occasionally, CNS tumours are associated with aggression. Much more frequently there is irritability with verbal outbursts directed towards carers. In some case series an association with temporal lobe and anterior hypothalamic tumours has been suggested.

Obviously, alcohol and drugs (e.g. phencyclidine, anabolic steroids) are prime causes of aggressive behaviour, either in the intoxication or withdrawal phase, and this is usually due to disinhibition, increased arousal and paranoid ideas. A widely quoted figure is that 50% of men arrested for violent crime are intoxicated.

Aggression and violence occurring in the course of delirium and dementia are major problem areas for staff in hospitals and residential homes. Patients with delirium often respond to repeated reassurance, but many patients with dementia do not. Enlisting the assistance of family members may help, but medication is often needed.

Violence can occur in the context of REM and non-REM sleep disorders. Assault is well documented but poorly understood in the context of somnambulism.

CLINICOANATOMICAL AND OTHER MECHANISMS OF AGGRESSION

There is a genetic basis underlying aggression and antisocial behaviour, most clearly illustrated in studies of monozygotic twins reared apart (Rhee & Waldman 1997). The hereditary effect is more powerful in children than in adults (Grove et al 1990). It is of interest that male carriers of the Huntington gene have an increased prevalence of criminal behaviour (Jensen et al 1998).

Both human and animal studies show a convergence of interest in the diencephalon and amygdala. In animals, septal lesions and stimulation of the posterior lateral hypothalamus may produce *sham rage*. Bard (1928) described sham rage as a response observed in decorticate animals without conscious experience. Septal stimulation results in an additional syndrome of self-stimulation (described by Olds in 1958). Conversely, stimulation of the ventromedial hypothalamus may produce a defensive posture. The amygdala is involved in matching the environmental stimuli with appropriate emotional and behavioural responses. Lesions generally result in placidity along with a failure to filter signals for food or sexual partners appropriately. In humans, other centres, such as the subcortical grey matter, prefrontal cortex, hippocampus and anterior cingulate gyrus are thought to modulate aggressive responses. In the Vietnam Head Injury Study, aggression was associated with ventromedial frontal lobe lesions but not lesion size or the presence of seizures (Grafman et al 1996).

Neurotransmitter alterations have been much investigated in animals and humans models of violence, but are beyond the scope of this discussion.

In Alzheimer's disease and other dementias, the biological basis of aggression is most often assumed to result from disinhibition. Clinical predictors of

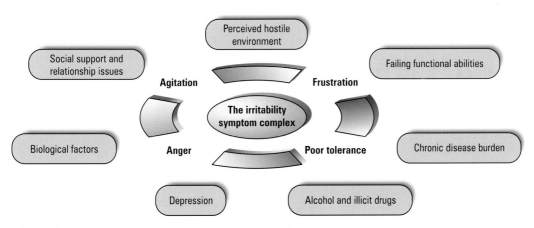

Fig. 74.1 Influences on the irritability–aggression symptom complex.

agitation in Alzheimer's disease include male sex, degree of cognitive impairment (and impaired communication skills) and the presence of delusions (Eutace et al 2000). In early functional neuroimaging studies, agitation and disinhibition scores in Alzheimer's disease has been correlated with hypometabolism in the frontal and temporal lobes (but this could simply be an effect of severity) (Sultzer et al 1995). Hirono et al (2000) also demonstrated that patients with aggression had hypoperfusion in the left anterior temporal cortex. One recent innovative study from the same group sought to examine the neuropathological correlates of behavioural changes in 31 patients with Alzheimer's disease examined at autopsy. Behavioural changes were assessed using the Neuropsychiatric Inventory. Neurofibrillary tangles in the left orbitofrontal cortex correlated with agitation scores and aberrant motor behaviour. Neurofibrillary tangles in the left anterior cingulate correlated highly with agitation and apathy (Tekin et al 2001).

Some patients experience recurrent aggressive episodes 'beyond their control' associated with some regret. If this is a change from baseline, the term *episodic dyscontrol syndrome* (or intermittent explosive disorder) has been used (Bach-y-Rita 1971). It has no clear identifiable basis in most patients, but a subgroup have paroxysmal EEG abnormalities (temporal lobe sharp waves or spikes in particular). One study of patients with temporal lobe epilepsy found a greater frequency of either left-sided or bilateral EEG and MRI abnormalities, along with a lower than expected IQ and more frequent mood problems in those with aggression than in those without. However, the same study found no differences in the hippocampus or amygdala volumes (Van Elst et al 2000).

REFERENCES AND FURTHER READING

Bach-y-Rita G, Lion JR, Climent CE et al 1971 Episodic dyscontrol: a study of 130 violent patients. American Journal of Psychiatry 127:1473–1478

Bard P 1928 A diencephalic mechanism for the expression of rage with special reference to the sympathetic nervous system. American Journal of Physiology 84:490–515

Dolan M, Deakin WJF, Roberts N et al 2002 Serotonergic and cognitive impairment in impulsive aggressive personality disordered offenders: are there implications for treatment? Psychological Medicine 32:105–117

Elliott F 1982 Neurological findings in adult minimal brain dysfunction and the dyscontrol syndrome. Journal of Nervous and Mental Disorders 170:680–687

Eslinger PJ, Parkinson K, Shomay SG 2002 Empathy and social–emotional factors in recovery from stroke. Current Opinion in Neurology 15:91–97

Eutace A, Greene E, Ni Bhriain S et al 2000 Determinants of agitation in Alzheimer's disease: clinical, functional and neuropsychological correlates. Presented at the International Psychogeriatrics' Association Annual Meeting. Newcastle upon Tyne, 4–7 April

Grafman J, Schwab K, Warden D et al 1996 Frontal lobe injuries, violence, and aggression: a report of the Vietnam Head Injury Study. Neurology 46:1231–1238

Grove WM, Eckert ED, Heston L et al 1990 Heritability of substance abuse and antisocial behavior: a study of monozygotic twins reared apart. Biological Psychiatry 27:1293–1304

Hirono N, Mega MS, Dinov ID et al 2000 Left frontotemporal hypoperfusion is associated with aggression in patients with dementia. Archives of Neurology 57:861–866

Jensen P, Fenger K, Bolwig TG et al 1998 Crime in Huntington's disease: a study of registered offences among patients, relatives, and controls. Journal of Neurology, Neurosurgery and Psychiatry 65:467–471

Kim JS, Choi S, Kwon SU et al 2002 Inability to control anger or aggression after stroke. Neurology 58:1106–1108

McAllister TW, Sparling MB, Flashman LA et al 2001 Differential working memory load affects mild traumatic brain injury. Neuroimage 14:1004–1012

Olds J 1958 Self-stimulation of the brain. Science 127:315–324

Rasanen P, Tiihonen J, Isohanni M et al 1998 Schizophrenia, alcohol abuse, and violent behavior: a 26-year follow-up study of an unselected birth cohort. Schizophrenia Bulletin 24:437–441

Rhee SH, Waldman ID 1997 A meta-analysis of twin and adoption studies examining antisocial behavior. Behavior and Genetics 27:603–603

Sultzer DL, Mahler ME, Mandelkern MA et al 1995 The relationship between psychiatric symptoms and regional cortical metabolism in Alzheimer's disease. Journal of Neuropsychology and Clinical Neuroscience 7:476–484

Swanson JW, Holzer CE, Ganju VK et al 1990 Violence and psychiatric-disorder in the community: evidence from the epidemiologic catchment-area surveys. Hospital and Community Psychiatry 41:761–770

Tekin S, Mega MS, Masterman DM et al 2001 Orbitofrontal and anterior cingulate cortex neurofibrillary tangle burden is associated with agitation in Alzheimer's disease. Annals of Neurology 49:355–361

Van Elst LT, Woermann FG, Lemieux L et al 2000 Affective aggression in patients with temporal lobe epilepsy: a quantitative MRI study of the amygdala. Brain 123:234–243

Yudofsky SC, Silver JM, Hales RE 1990 Pharmacologic management of aggression in the elderly. Journal of Clinical Psychiatry 51(suppl 10):22–28

75

The Origin of Emotionalism

Psychiatrists have long recognized sudden swings of mood, which occur rapidly and inappropriately in patients with mixed affective disorder, mania and post-partum psychosis. Similarly, neurologists have recognized the condition of pseudobulbar palsy in stroke, motor neurone disease and multiple sclerosis affecting the frontal lobe (Wilson 1924). The defining features are that the mood state is intense, occurring with little (but not necessarily no) stimulus, resulting in laughing or, more often, crying that may be socially inappropriate. In pure emotionalism, the majority of patients recognize their condition as inappropriate and find it deeply embarrassing. This condition is descriptively called *pathological crying* or *pathological laughing*. Recently, clinicians have begun to recognize that there is a continuum of abnormal emotionalism, just as there is a continuum of abnormal low mood (McGrath 2000). In mild to moderately severe cases the emotionalism is precipitated by relevant stimuli and the intensity of the reaction is understandable and not overwhelming. In severe cases, there are no relevant stimuli and the emotional reaction is in itself distressing to the patient. If all types of emotionalism are included in the definition, then emotionalism may occur in as many as one-third of patients with stroke or severe head injury. If a pure syndrome is required then the rate is nearer to 5–10%. Emotionalism has been described in stroke, multiple sclerosis, dementia and Parkinson's disease (Box 75.1). Poeck (1985) attempted to delineate the characteristics of pathological laughing or crying, based on the following features:

- response is triggered by non-specific stimuli
- lack of a relationship between affective change and observed expression
- absence of a change in mood lasting beyond the episode of emotionalism
- absence of voluntary control of facial expression.

This definition has abnormal motor expression of mood at its core. House et al (1989) examined the prevalence of emotionalism in 128 patients who had suffered a first ever stroke. Emotionalism was reported by 15% of patients at 1 month post-stroke, 21% at 6 months and 11% at 12 months. Only two patients described problems with pathological laughing. In stroke patients, the syndromes of emotionalism and depression frequently co-exist, with about 50% of patients with emotionalism also suffering syndromal depression (with an even greater overlap with depressive symptoms). In patients with mixed emotionalism and depression there is often irritability, anger and anxiety, as well (Calvert et al 1998).

CLINICOANATOMICAL MECHANISMS

Emotionalism has been associated with lesions of corticobulbar (or supranuclear) pathways in many cases, but not all (Poeck 1985). Morris et al (1993) noted a relationship between the proximity of the lesion to the frontal and temporal poles and the

---

Box 75.1 Neuropsychiatric diseases featuring emotionalism

- AIDS dementia
- Alzheimer's disease
- Frontotemporal dementia
- Head injury
- Huntington's disease
- Lewy body dementia
- Multiple sclerosis
- Neurosyphilis
- Neurotoxicity
- Normal-pressure hydrocephalus
- Parkinson's disease
- Stroke
- Vascular dementia
- Wilson's disease

presence of emotionalism. House et al (1989) found that patients with emotionalism tended to have larger lesions and that when intrahemispheric variations were examined there was an association between left anterior lesions and the presence of emotionalism. Andersen et al (1993) noted that patients with pathological crying had frequent involvement of the subcortical structures. In McGrath's examination of 82 severely brain-injured patients, independent variables that predicted emotionalism were female sex and focal damage to the right cerebral hemisphere (McGrath 2000). In Alzheimer's disease, provisional evidence suggests greater asymmetry on SPECT scanning in patients with emotionalism (Lebert et al 1994). Emotionalism has been studied in patients with Parkinson's disease. In one study there was no association between emotionalism and cognitive impairment or depression (Madely et al 1992). Rarely, patients with epilepsy may suffer paroxysmal laughter, known as *gelastic epilepsy*. Irritative lesions in the orbitofrontal and temporal lobes as well as subcortical areas appear to be responsible (Striano 1999).

The mechanisms underlying emotionalism are informed by studies of the closely related phenomenon of the *catastrophic reaction*. In one study the catastrophic reaction occurred in about 5% of stroke patients, usually those with left hemisphere lesions (Carota et al 2001). Specific areas implicated were the temporal cortex and insula, the frontal opercular and parietal cortex along with the cingulate gyrus, and the thalamic nuclei. Two-thirds of patients were reclassified as having emotionalism within 3 months of their diagnosis of catastrophic reaction. The boundaries of these two overlapping syndromes has yet to be delineated.

REFERENCES AND FURTHER READING

Andersen G, Vestergaard K, Riis J 1993 Citalopram for post-stroke pathological crying. Lancet 342:837–839

Calvert T, Knapp P, House A 1998 Psychological associations with emotionalism after stroke. Journal of Neurology, Neurosurgery and Psychiatry 65:928–929

Carota A, Rossetti AO, Karapanayiotides T et al 2001 Catastrophic reaction in acute stroke: a reflex behavior in aphasic patients. Neurology 57:1902–1905

House A, Dennis M, Molyneux A et al 1989 Emotionalism after stroke. British Medical Journal 298:991–994

Lebert F, Pasquier F, Steinling M et al 1994 Affective disorders related to SPECT patterns in Alzheimer's disease: a study of emotionalism. International Journal of Geriatric Psychiatry 9:327–329

Madely P, Biggins CA, Boyd JL et al 1992 Emotionalism and Parkinson's disease. Irish Journal of Psychological Medicine 9:24–25

McGrath J 2000 A study of emotionalism in patients undergoing rehabilitation following severe acquired brain injury. Behavioural Neurology 12:201–207

Morris PLP, Robinson RG, Raphael B 1993 Emotional lability after stroke. Australian and New Zealand Journal of Psychiatry 27:601–605

Poeck K 1985 Pathological laughter and crying. In: Fredricks JAM (ed) Handbook of clinical neurology. Vol 1: Clinical neuropsychology. Elsevier Science, Amsterdam, p 219–225

Striano S 1999 Gelastic epilepsy. Epilepsia 40:294–302

Wilson SAK 1924 Some problems in neurology. II. Pathological laughing and crying. Journal of Neurology and Psychopathology 4:299–333

76

The Origin of Psychosis

HALLUCINATIONS

There are common themes that underlie the presence of psychosis in different neuropsychiatric disorders. Studies in Parkinson's disease have helped to clarify that there is not one single cause of psychosis but several causes (see Fig. 21.4). Whether these causes share a common pathophysiological mechanism is another question. The mechanisms that underlie mild transient hallucinations occurring in clear consciousness have recently been shown to involve reduced visual acuity, and this in turn may result from reduced dopamine content in the retina in sufferers of Parkinson's disease (Holroyd et al 2001). This mechanism is also operational in Alzheimer's disease (Ballard 2001, Holroyd & Keller 1995) and in patients with macular degeneration (Holroyd et al 1994). There is also an association between visual agnosia and visual hallucinations in vascular dementia and between poor visual attention, defective visual perception and visual hallucinations in Lewy body dementia (Ballard 2001). For example, Mori et al (2000) found that on tasks of visual perception (the object size discrimination, form discrimination, overlapping figure identification, and visual counting tasks), patients with probable Lewy body dementia scored significantly lower than patients with Alzheimer's disease. There may also be a parallel deficit in auditory comprehension in elderly patients prone to auditory hallucinations – a phenomenon recognized in Alzheimer's disease (Lopez et al 1991). (Patients with acquired peripheral deafness often experience auditory hallucinations in clear consciousness.) These findings

have an implication for conditions in nursing homes, since ambient lighting can affect visual acuity and subsequent visual hallucinations (Murgatroyd & Prettyman 2001). Severe hallucinations are also heavily influenced by deficits in cognition. This mechanism is involved in the genesis of hallucinations in Alzheimer's disease, macular degeneration and Parkinson's disease (Holroyd & Keller 1995, Holroyd et al 1994, 2001). A role of specific pathology in the limbic and temporal areas has been suggested (see delusions, below). Late-onset, well-formed visual hallucinations were associated with increased numbers of Lewy bodies in the basolateral amygdaloid nucleus in cognitively impaired Parkinson's patients (Harding et al 2002), whereas early-onset hallucinations in both Parkinson's dementia and Lewy body dementia were related to greater Lewy body density in the temporal cortices, parahippocampi and amygdala (Harding et al 2002). Destruction of the limbic and temporal areas may cause loss of visual cortical inhibition.

From this we can deduce that one circumstance in which hallucinations and illusions occur is when the accuracy of information processing is decreased and, furthermore, an ambiguous stimulus is pre-

---

Box 76.1 Neuropsychiatric diseases that feature psychosis

Disorders of early life
Adrenoleukodystrophy
CNS trauma
Metachromatic leukodystrophy
Multiple sclerosis
Temporal lobe epilepsy

Disorders of later life
CNS tumours
Delirium
Dementias:
● AIDS dementia
● Alzheimer's disease
● Lewy body disease
● vascular dementia
Movement disorders:
● Fahr's syndrome
● Huntington's disease
● Parkinson's disease
● Wilson's disease
Prion disease
Occult microvascular CNS disease
Stroke

sented. This is most clearly demonstrated in delirium when the patient describes florid but transient visual hallucinations, often with features that parallel the patient's prevailing emotional tone. The effect of established sensory deficits are important, since these alter clarity of the perception. In the Charles Bonnet syndrome, sensory deprivation is associated with typically visual hallucinations without delusions or loss of insight (see Ch. 2). The syndrome is considered not to represent psychiatric illness, despite the hallucinations causing distress in about one-quarter of patients (Teunisse et al 1996). Studies of hallucinatory experiences in patients with epilepsy have found that irritative lesions in the temporal lobe, insula or opercular areas produce complex hallucinations in several sensory modalities. Irritative lesions in the occipital lobe produce simple (or elementary) visual hallucinations such as flashes and lines. Illusions, dysmorphopsia and dymegalopsia have been associated with non-dominant seizures in some patients.

DELUSIONS

Studies of psychosis in patients with recent stroke are contaminated by the effect of dementia and delirium. A single stroke leading to a defined psychotic episode (or syndrome) is a rare phenomenon. Psychotic symptoms occur in less than 10% of stroke patients at 1 year (Verdelho et al 2002). There are case reports of patients with temporoparietal lesions resulting in delusions and hallucinations, but more common is the delusion-like syndrome of anosognosia (denial of disability) that typically follows a parietal lesion. Temporal lobe involvement is also seen in adults and children who have psychosis associated with CNS tumours (Malamud 1967), and in adults who have psychosis associated with head injury (Achte et al 1969). In the case of CNS tumours, the effect of co-existent seizure disorder must be accounted for. Pure delusions (such as in the Capgras misidentification syndrome) and pure visual hallucinations may be slightly more common in patients with right-sided lesions. (Capgras & Lachaux (1923) described a female patient with the delusion that members of her family had all been gradually replaced by doubles and that all her surroundings and all her acquaintances were doubles.)

Perhaps the most important model of psychosis is temporal lobe epilepsy. The relationship between temporal lobe epilepsy and interictal psychosis

became accepted after the description given by Flor-Henry in 1969. An attractive hypothesis is that the medial temporal lobe is central to the production of delusions and hallucinations, this being supported by the frequent observation that patients with schizophrenia have temporal lobe damage (Arnold 1997). In patients with established temporal lobe epilepsy and psychosis (with either delusions or hallucinations), implanted subcortical electrode studies have demonstrated spike and wave activity in the amygdala, hippocampus and septal areas, which are not seen in patients without psychosis. Patients with first-episode schizophrenia have reduced hippocampal volumes compared with healthy controls, as do patients with both left- and right-focused temporal lobe epilepsy (Barr et al 1997). Patients with schizophrenia may have more atrophy on the left than the right side, as do patients with left-sided temporal lobe epilepsy and psychotic patients with temporal lobe epilepsy (Maier et al 2000). Yet an excess of hippocampal atrophy or mesial temporal sclerosis in temporal lobe epilepsy patients with psychosis versus temporal lobe epilepsy patients without psychosis has not been found in all neuroimaging studies (Marsh et al 2001, Sachdev 1998). Furthermore, the analogy between temporal lobe epilepsy and schizophrenia is limited by the fact that temporal lobe epilepsy is usually a localized, unilateral disorder of the brain (i.e. bitemporal foci are rare), whereas schizophrenia is not. The link between temporal damage and psychosis in epilepsy could still be valid if there was some special significance of when in life the lesion was acquired, or perhaps differences either outside the hippocampus or even at the microscopic level. One possibility is that involvement of the temporal neocortex rather than the hippocampus is the critical factor (Kanemoto et al 1996, Marsh et al 2001).

Research involving degenerative disorders offers the advantage of pathological samples. In a landmark study in Alzheimer's disease, Förstl et al (1994) from the Institute of Psychiatry, London, examined the neuropathological characteristics of 56 patients with Alzheimer's disease in relation to psychosis. Thirteen had hallucinations and 22 had delusions. Psychotic patients had lower neurone counts in the dorsal raphe nucleus, although a more specific association was found between higher neurofibrillary tangle count in the parahippocampal gyrus and paranoid delusions. An association between lower neurone counts in the CA-1 field of the hippocampus and the presence of delusional misidentification was also documented. In a larger study, Farber et al (2000) found a 2.3-fold greater density of neocortical neurofibrillary tangles in Alzheimer's disease patients with psychosis versus patients without psychosis, but no difference in senile plaques or subcortical tangles. Another group found the same results and refined the association of tangle pathology and psychosis to the cingulate gyrus, superior temporal gyrus and nucleus accumbens (Cairns et al 2000). However, at least one publication has failed to confirm these findings (Sweet et al 2000). Several groups have used functional neuroimaging to document regional metabolic correlates of psychosis in Alzheimer's disease. Associations with the frontal lobe (Sultzer et al 1995), dorsolateral frontal, left anterior cingulate and dorsolateral parietal cortex have been recorded (Mega et al 2000). It would seem that in Alzheimer's disease at least, pathology in areas of the brain responsible for the integration of current experiences with existing memories can lead to misinterpretations and then delusions.

From a biochemical perspective, psychosis in amphetamine abusers highlights the importance of dopamine excess. In Parkinson's disease, dopaminergic agents may also cause psychosis. Presumably, it is dopamine excess in the frontal and limbic areas that is important to the generation of complex psychotic experiences (Engelien et al 2001). Reviews of the neurochemical basis of psychosis are available elsewhere.

Several conclusions are warranted from this body of work. First, it is a mistake to assume that all cases of 'organic' psychosis are the same. Not only are there several important types of psychosis associated with neurological disease (e.g. psychosis in delirium, psychosis in dementia, pure visual hallucinations, pure delusions), but most, perhaps all, of these types of organic psychosis are distinct from the psychosis seen in schizophrenia. Schizophrenia is a complex disorder, which may not be one single disease, and is distinguished by recognizable changes in function, cognition and personality. A greater understanding of the biological basis of psychosis will only provide one part of the puzzle that is the aetiology of schizophrenia. Reductions in clarity of perception or alterations in processing ability lead to errors in stimulus identification and hence misinterpretations and hallucinations. By the same token, increasing difficulty in understanding the complex motives of others leads to suspiciousness and delusions. This is particularly the case when one's own database of the world (i.e. memory) is eroded.

REFERENCES AND FURTHER READING

Achte KA, Hillbom E, Aaalberg V 1969 Psychoses following war brain injuries. Annals of Clinical Psychiatry 45:1–18

Arnold SE 1997 The medial temporal lobe in schizophrenia. Journal of Neuropsychiatry and Clinical Neuroscience 9:460–470

Ballard C 2001 Visual hallucinations in dementia. Journal of Neurology, Neurosurgery and Psychiatry 71:139

Barr WB, Ashtari M, Bilder RM et al 1997 Brain morphometric comparison of first-episode schizophrenia and temporal lobe epilepsy. British Journal of Psychiatry 170:515–519

Cairns NJ, Murray A, Holmes C et al 2000 Neuropathological correlates of psychotic symptoms in Alzheimer's disease. Brain Pathology 10:515

Capgras J, Lachaux J 1923 L'illusion des 'sosies' dans un délire systématisé chronique. Bulletin de Société Clinique de Médecine Mentale 11:6–16

Engelien A, Stern E, Silbersweig D 2001 Functional neuroimaging of human central auditory processing in normal subjects and patients with neurological and neuropsychiatric disorders. Journal of Clinical and Experimental Neuropsychology 23:94–120

Farber NB, Rubin EH, Newcomer JW et al 2000 Increased neocortical neurofibrillary tangle density in subjects with Alzheimer disease and psychosis. Archives of General Psychiatry 57:1165–1173

Flor-Henry P 1969 Psychosis and temporal lobe epilepsy. Epilepsia 10:363–365

Förstl H, Burns A, Levy R et al 1994 Neuropathological correlates of psychotic phenomena in confirmed Alzheimer's disease. British Journal of Psychiatry 165:53–59

Harding AJ, Broe GA, Halliday GM 2002 Visual hallucinations in Lewy body disease relate to Lewy bodies in the temporal lobe. Brain 125:391–403

Holroyd S, Keller AS 1995 A study of visual hallucinations in Alzheimer's disease. American Journal of Geriatric Psychiatry 3:198–205

Holroyd S, Rabins PV, Finkelstein D et al 1994 Visual hallucination in patients with macular degeneration. American Journal of Psychiatry 149:1701–106

Holroyd S, Currie L, Wooten GF 2001 Prospective study of hallucinations and delusions in Parkinson's disease. Journal of Neurology, Neurosurgery and Psychiatry 70:734–738

Kanemoto K, Takeuchi J, Kawasaki J et al 1996 Characteristics of temporal lobe epilepsy with mesial temporal sclerosis, with special reference to psychotic episodes. Neurology 47:1199–1203

Lopez OL, Becker JT, Brenner RP et al 1991 Alzheimer's disease with delusions and hallucinations: neuropsychological and electroencephalic correlates. Neurology 41:906–912

Maier M, Mellers J, Toone B et al 2000 Schizophrenia, temporal lobe epilepsy and psychosis: an in vivo magnetic resonance spectroscopy and imaging study of the hippocampus/amygdala complex. Psychological Medicine 30:571–581

Malamud N 1967 Psychiatric disorders with intracranial tumours of limbic system. Archives of Neurology 17:113–123

Marsh L, Sullivana EV, Morrell M et al 2001 Structural brain abnormalities in patients with schizophrenia, epilepsy, and epilepsy with chronic interictal psychosis. Psychiatry Research – Neuroimaging 108:1–15

Mega MS, Lee L, Dinov ID et al 2000 Cerebral correlates of psychotic symptoms in Alzheimer's disease. Journal of Neurology, Neurosurgery and Psychiatry 69:167–171

Mori E, Shimomura T, Fujimori M et al 2000 Visuoperceptual impairment in dementia with Lewy bodies. Archives of Neurology 57:489–493

Murgatroyd C, Prettyman R 2001 An investigation of visual hallucinosis and visual sensory status in dementia. International Journal of Geriatric Psychiatry 16:709–713

Sachdev P 1998 Schizophrenia-like psychosis and epilepsy: the status of the association. American Journal of Psychiatry 155:325–336

Sultzer DL, Mahler ME, Mandelkern MA et al 1995 The relationship between psychiatric symptoms and regional cortical metabolism in Alzheimer's disease. Journal of Neuropsychiatry and Clinical Neuroscience 7:476–484

Sweet RA, Hamilton RL, Lopez SL et al 2000 Psychotic symptoms in Alzheimer's disease are not associated with more severe neuropathologic features. International Psychogeriatrics 12:547–558

Teunisse RJ, Cruysberg JR, Hoefnagels WH et al 1996 Visual hallucinations in psychologically normal people: Charles Bonnet's syndrome. Lancet 347:794–797

Verdelho A, Hénon H, Lebert F et al 2002 Psychotic symptoms after stroke: a 3-year follow up study. Journal of Neurology 249(suppl 1):184

77

The Origin of Personality Change

Neurodegenerative disease, particularly dementia, has personality change at its core. Personality alterations may be the first sign of illness, manifest only to close family members, as subtle changes, long before clinical diagnosis is made. Early in Alzheimer's disease patients become disengaged and lose interest and confidence in hobbies. In studies that have used the Blessed Dementia Scale, passivity was the most common behavioural change reported by carers. Patients may become increasingly moody or irritable as their abilities are inexplicably eroded. Sufferers prefer to stay at home rather than face increasingly awkward social encounters. As the condition progresses, there is less and less regard for social conventions. Frontotemporal dementias are particularly likely to cause impairments in judgement, inhibition and empathy in advance of clear cognitive changes. Lesions of the frontal lobes (after head injury or in tumours or frontal vascular dementia) can produce a similar picture, emphasizing the importance of the frontal cortex in regulating higher social functions. The alterations in behaviour following head injury are reasonably well described. Organic personality change is seen in the majority of those with severe head injury, but in less than 10% of those with mild head injury (Max et al 2001). Characteristic traits are disinhibition and apathy and, in severe cases, antisocial, obsessive–compulsive, borderline, avoidant, paranoid or narcissistic personality disorder (Hibbard et al 2000).These kinds of personality change can occur after most

causes of brain injury, including stroke (Golden et al 2002). Contrary to many expectations, such personality changes are dynamic during the first 2 years after injury and become more stable with time (Malia et al 1995). Individuals with the apathy of Huntington's disease are sometimes described as having a personality characterized by a lack of initiative, impersistence and disinterest. Personality is affected early, probably preclinically, in many sufferers of Parkinson's disease. Compared with matched medical controls with rheumatological problems, Parkinson's disease patients have fewer novelty-seeking traits (Menza et al 1993). There is a continuing debate about whether personality is altered in a predictable way in chronic sufferers of epilepsy (Devinsky & Najjar 1999). Yet, why is it that the characteristics of 'sticky thoughts', religiosity, expressiveness, irritability and hypergraphia have been described? Irritability is the most easily explained, since this is a non-specific feature of living with stress. Hypergraphia and religiosity could be related to temporal lobe involvement and 'sticky thoughts' could be a reflection of cognitive impairment. It is very likely that these subtle personality alterations are a rather crude description of the secondary effects that one would more accurately describe as mood disorder, psychosis, behavioural change and cognitive disturbance. Personality change has also been described in other neuropsychiatric disorders, including Wilson's disease and multiple sclerosis (Dhossche & Shevitz 1999).

It is interesting to ask whether there are *behavioural phenotypes* associated with specific brain lesions. One study recently reported an association with personality change in multiple sclerosis and frontal lobe neuropsychological impairment (Benedict et al 2001). The placidity and compulsive exploration of environmental stimuli that is seen in bilateral tem-

---

Box 77.1 The ten most frequent neuropsychiatric causes of personality change

- Alcohol
- Illicit drug use
- Alzheimer's disease
- Stroke
- Vascular dementia
- Head injury
- Parkinson's disease
- Lewy body dementia
- Frontotemporal dementia
- Cerebral tumour

poral lobe lesions has already been mentioned (see Ch. 13). Placidity is also a description attached to patients who have undergone frontal lobotomy (leukotomy). Some reports suggest that patients with lesions in Wernicke's area are suspicious, demanding and irritable. However, it is difficult to disentangle these reports from what one would anticipate given significant communication difficulties. Contrastingly, non-dominant hemisphere lesions might interfere with the expression of emotions (alexithymia) and social interactivity (autistic spectrum disorder). Do characteristic behavioural phenotypes occur in specific neurodevelopmental disorders? A strong case was made by William Nyhan during an address to the American Pediatric Association in 1971 (Nyhan 1972). He suggested that persistent self-injurious behaviour was a hallmark of Lesch–Nyhan disease. In this X-linked recessive disease, a deficiency in the enzyme hypoxanthine phosphoribosyltransferase (HPRT) causes an accumulation of uric acid peripherally and hypoxanthine centrally. The result is cognitive impairment, developmental delay and motor abnormalities (choreoathetosis, dystonia, spasticity and hyperreflexia) emerging in the first few years of life. Strikingly, 90% also have self-biting or other destructive behaviours that he or she is unable to resist. The pathophysiology of this complication is not yet understood.

The work to date on acquired personality change reveals that personality alterations do not arise de novo but are part of a constellation of changes that include the effects of brain lesions on cognition, mood and behaviour. In the majority of cases, it is simplistic to define a single disease-related personality syndrome, in just the same way it would be to say that all suffers of Parkinson's disease develop a particular type of depression. Furthermore, in addition to organic explanations of personality alteration in neuropsychiatric disease, psychosocial factors such as uncertainty about the future, difficulty coming to terms with loss, perceived support, the reactions of others and ongoing stressors no doubt play an extremely important role.

Table 77.1 DSM-IV defined change in personality traits

Type	Predominant feature
Labile	Affective lability
Disinhibited	Poor impulse control
Aggressive	Aggression
Apathetic	Apathy and indifference
Paranoid	Suspiciousness and paranoid ideation
Combined	More than one feature is present

REFERENCES AND FURTHER READING

Benedict RHB, Priore RL, Miller C et al 2001 Personality disorder in multiple sclerosis correlates with cognitive impairment. Journal of Neuropsychiatry and Clinical Neuroscience 13:70–76

Devinsky O, Najjar S 1999 Evidence against the existence of a temporal lobe epilepsy personality syndrome. Neurology 53(suppl 2): S13–S25

Dhossche DM, Shevitz SA 1999 Assessment and importance of personality disorders in medical patients: an update. Southern Medical Journal 92:546–556

Golden ZL, Seldon J, Greene L et al 2002 National differential impact of alternate etiologies of brain injury or personality change. Archives of Clinical Neuropsychology 17:715–867

Hibbard MR, Bogdany J, Uysal S et al 2000 Axis II psychopathology in individuals with traumatic brain injury. Brain Injury 14:45–61

Malia K, Powell G, Torode S 1995 Personality and psychosocial function after brain injury. Brain Injury 9:697–712

Max JE, Robertson BAM, Lansing AE 2001 The phenomenology of personality change due to traumatic brain injury in children and adolescents. Journal of Neuropsychiatry and Clinical Neuroscience 13:161–170

Menza MA, Golbe LI, Cody RA et al 1993 Dopamine-related personality-traits in Parkinson's disease. Neurology 43:505–508

Nyhan WL 1972 Behavioral phenotypes in organic genetic disease. Pediatric Research 6:1–9

78

The Origin of Suicide

Suicide is the most unfavourable outcome of any illness. Medical illnesses are very distressing and, in essence, difficult to live with. A high proportion of patients with acute medical illness report that 'life is not worth living' (Shah et al 2000). Alcohol dependence or abuse is a strong predictor of suicide in its own right, although it is also linked with depression (Berglund & Ojehagen 1998). At least 50% of suicide victims have evidence of depression, and 40% have evidence of alcohol problems during life (Henriksson et al 1993). In case–control studies, medical illness is often reported as a risk factor associated with suicide. This is particularly the case in suicides in the elderly, who often do not present with attempted suicide before successfully taking their lives (Carney et al 1994). It is then pertinent to ask how the presence of physical disease influences the frequency of adequate treatment for depression, and also to ask what particular medical disorders confer the highest suicide risk.

The relationship between physical illness and antidepressant treatment has been studied in a large epidemiological study of almost 8000 people older than 55 years (Egberts et al 1997). One would anticipate that the presence of a major medical disease would be associated with increased rates and treatment of depression. The authors did indeed detect an association between osteoarthritis and stroke and initiation of antidepressants, but no such link with many other medical diseases such as myocardial infarction, rheumatoid arthritis and Parkinson's disease. It should be remembered that, although there is an association between impaired function and suicide, the relationship between medical illness and suicide is likely to be played out through depression for the most part. Depression causes physical symptoms and physical symptoms cause depression (Hotopf et al 1998). The take-home message is that depression is the most important risk factor for suicide in all groups, not least of which is because it is treatable.

SUICIDE IN SPECIFIC NEUROPSYCHIATRIC DISORDERS

Discovering the actual suicide rate in specific diseases is more difficult than it would first appear. Suicide is a rare outcome, which means that prospective studies are very time-consuming. Examination of case registers of all patients in a large area with a condition for rates of suicide is usually more productive. Rates are usually compared with those found in the background population, adjusted for age and sex. This is the standardized mortality ratio (SMR). Comparison with other

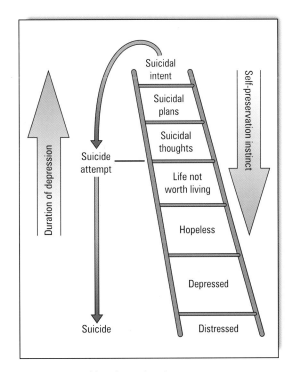

Fig. 78.1 Ladder of suicide risk.

groups of patients, matching for degree of disability, are also of great interest.

As a reference point, a number of studies have examined suicide rates in patients with cancer. Clearly, the stage and type of cancer will have an influence. In large studies, the relative risk of suicide in cancer patients is marginally raised at about twice the risk in the general population (Storm et al 1992). In a recent large study from Japan, Tanaka et al (1999) followed 23,979 cancer patients for up to 16 years. Suicide risk was significantly increased within the first 5 years after cancer diagnosis (relative risk for males, 1.62; for females, 2.13), but not after 5 years. Patients in their fifties with remote metastasis at their initial diagnosis and genital organ involvement had a significantly higher suicide risk within 5 years.

In multiple sclerosis, one large study of over 5000 patients on the Danish MS Register documented an SMR of 3.12 in men and 2.12 in women who had an onset of multiple sclerosis before the age of 40 years (Stenager et al 1992). Risk was highest within the first 5 years. The risk of suicide was not increased in patients with an onset after 40 years of age.

In epilepsy, a long-term follow-up of 2000 patients treated with antiepileptic drugs was published by White et al (1997). The age- and sex-adjusted SMR was 5.4. A more recent study of nearly 800 patients suggested a lower SMR of 2.1, but the rate was much higher in patients with a congenital neurological disorder. Deaths were not due to epilepsy per se.

In stroke patients, Stenager et al (1998) examined suicide rates in a large cohort of 37,869 patients over 17 years. In patients aged over 60 years (the largest group), relative risk was modestly raised at between 1.5 and 2. In those below 60 years of age the relative risk was 13 in women and 6 in men.

In Parkinson's disease, Stenager et al (1994) published the results of a 20-year follow-up of 485 patients. The risk of suicide was not affected in women; in men it appeared to be slightly lower than in the general population. The results of this study await replication.

Two large epidemiological studies have looked at suicide rates in head injury (Achté et al 1971, Teasdale & Engberg 2001). Teasdale & Engberg (2001) examined 145,000 patients who had suffered a head injury in adult life between 1979 and 1993 and looked at suicides up to 1994. About 10% of subjects had died from natural causes, but accidents accounted for 1.4% of deaths and suicides for 0.62%. Comparing rates with the general population the SMRs were about three-fold. The presence of contusions or intracerebral haemorrhage, female sex and substance abuse increased the relative risk of suicide. There was no particular 'high-risk' period following the injury.

Finally, studies in HIV infection have found greatly elevated relative risks of suicide compared with the general population, with figures of 36-fold, 21-fold and 7.4-fold having been reported. However, rates differ widely depending on the methodology used

---

Clinical Pointer 78.1

Assessing suicide risk

Assessing suicide risk is a dynamic process with limited evidence for success in prevention of future suicides. The predicted risk may be elevated 10-fold in an individual patient, but even so that patient is still unlikely to commit suicide. In other words, the problem of false positives is legion. The most practical epidemiological (policy) method is to use predictive factors that themselves require intervention (e.g. the presence of depression). However, on an individual basis, consider how close a person has come to overcoming his or her natural self-preservation instincts. The longer someone is distressed or depressed the more natural barriers will be overcome (see Fig. 78.1). The risk of completed suicide is increased by the following factors:

- demographic factors (male sex, middle aged, divorced, single, bereaved, low social class, low income, unemployed)
- psychiatric history (previous attempts, any psychiatric history, non-compliance, recently discharged from hospital)
- current features (depression, hopelessness, psychosis, command hallucinations, akathisia, isolation from staff)
- suicidal thoughts (death wish, suicidal plans, suicidal intent)
- recent attempted suicide (with concealment, intent to die, serious attempt, accidental discovery, carrying out final acts).

Further reading   Hawton K, Van Heeringen K (eds) 2000 The international handbook of suicide and attempted suicide. Wiley, Chichester

Box 78.1 Suicide markers in various groups

Suicidal thoughts, 12-month prevalence
25–33% of acutely physically unwell elderly
13–17% of the elderly
2.5–5% of the general adult population
80% of depressed patients

Suicide attempts, 12-month prevalence
0.3% of the elderly
1% of the general adult population
3% of depressed patients

Actual suicide, 12-month prevalence
10 per 100,000 of population
100 per 100,000 of depressed patients

and, in particular, on the demographic factors and other risk factors of HIV sufferers. Dannenberg et al (1996) looked at suicide rates through the National Death Index, using 4147 HIV-positive military service applicants, who were disqualified from Military Service. Suicide rates were two-fold higher than the general population adjusted for age, race and sex. Recently, a study has examined suicidal thoughts in four groups (HIV-seropositive, HIV-seronegative, hepatitis C virus-seropositive, hepatitis C virus-seronegative) of injecting drug users (Grassi et al 2001). One-third of patients in all the groups had suicidal ideation, with no significant differences between groups.

ATTEMPTED SUICIDE IN NEUROPSYCHIATRIC DISORDERS

Physical comorbidity is seen in a substantial proportion of people attending A&E departments with *deliberate self-harm*. Some estimates suggest 50% of self-harmers have either acute, chronic or relapsing–remitting medical illnesses (De Leo et al 1999). Furthermore, 22% of people in this study rated their medical disease as a major factor in their suicide attempt. About a quarter of these patients had neurological disease. Rates of self-harm have rarely been adequately documented in any specific medical diseases. Further self-harm is not synonymous with attempted suicide, but includes a mixture of motivations and methods. One study of 130 patients with epilepsy found an elevated rate of self-poisoning, at seven times higher than expected in the population (Mackay 1979).

REFERENCES AND FURTHER READING

Achté KA, Lönnqvist J, Hillborm E 1971 Suicides following brain injuries. Acta Psychiatrica Scandinavica (suppl 225):1–94

Berglund M, Ojehagen A 1998 The influence of alcohol drinking and alcohol use disorders on psychiatric disorders and suicidal behavior. Alcohol Clinical and Experimental Research 22(suppl S):333S–345S

Carney SS, Rich CL, Burke PA et al 1994 Suicide over 60: the San Diego Study. Journal of the American Geriatrics Society 42:174–180

Dannenberg AL, McNeil JG, Brundage JF et al 1996 Suicide and HIV infection: mortality follow-up of 4147 HIV-seropositive military service applicants. Journal of the American Medical Association 276:1743–1746

De Leo D, Scocco P, Marietta P et al 1999 Physical illness and parasuicide: evidence from the European Parasuicide Study Interview Schedule (EPSIS/WHO-EURO). International Journal of Psychiatry and Medicine 29:149–163

Egberts ACG, Leufkens HGM, Hofman A et al 1997 Incidence of antidepressant drug use in older adults and association with chronic diseases: the Rotterdam Study. International Clinical Psychopharmacology 12:217–223

Grassi L, Mondardini D, Pavanati M et al 2001 Suicide probability and psychological morbidity secondary to HIV infection: a control study of HIV-seropositive, hepatitis C virus (HCV)-seropositive and HIV/HCV-seronegative injecting drug users. Journal of Affective Disorders 64:195–202

Henriksson MM, Aro HM, Marttunen MJ 1993 Mental disorders and comorbidity in suicide. American Journal of Psychiatry 150:935–940

Hotopf M, Mayou R, Wadsworth M et al 1998 Temporal relationship between physical symptoms and psychiatric disorder: results from a national birth cohort. British Journal of Psychiatry 173:255–261

Lhatoo SD, Johnson AL, Goodridge DM et al 2001 Mortality in epilepsy in the first 11 to 14 years after diagnosis: multivariate analysis of a long-term, prospective, population-based cohort. Annals of Neurology 49:336–344

Mackay A 1979 Self-poisoning: a complication of epilepsy. British Journal of Psychiatry 134:277–282

Shah A, Hoxey K, Mayadunne V 2000 Suicidal ideation in the acutely medically in elderly inpatients: prevalence, correlates and longitudinal stability. International Journal of Geriatric Psychiatry 15:162–169

Stenager EN, Stenager E, Koch-Henrikson N et al 1992 Suicide and multiple sclerosis: an epidemiological investigation. Journal of Neurology, Neurosurgery and Psychiatry 55:542–545

Stenager EN, Madsen C, Stenager E et al 1998 Suicide in patients with stroke: epidemiological study. British Medical Journal 316:1206

Stenager EN, Wermuth L, Stenager E et al 1994 Suicide in patients with Parkinson's disease – an epidemiologic study. Acta Psychiatrica Scandinavica 90:70–72

Storm HH, Christensen C, Jensen OM 1992 Suicide, violent death and cancer. Cancer 69:1507–1512

Tanaka H, Tsukuma H, Masaoka T et al 1999 Suicide risk among cancer patients: experience at one medical center in Japan, 1978–1994. Japanese Journal of Cancer Research 90:812–817

Teasdale TW, Engberg AW 2001 Suicide after traumatic brain injury: a population study. Journal of Neurology, Neurosurgery and Psychiatry 71:436–440

White SJ, McLean AEM, Howland C 1979 Anticonvulsant drugs and cancer. Lancet ii:458–461

79

The Origin of Obsessive– Compulsive Symptoms

Our knowledge of the link between obsessional thoughts or compulsive behaviours and neurological disease took a significant step forward with the observations made of sufferers of encephalitis lethargica. Encephalitis lethargica is not the only neurological disease to feature an unexpectedly high rate of obsessive–compulsive disorder (OCD) (Box 79.1). Such disorders may provide clues to the aetiology or pathogenesis of idiopathic OCD.

Symptoms of OCD in secondary disorders do not seem particularly different from symptoms of primary OCD, with the possible exception of a higher rate of cognitive abnormalities in the former conditions (Berthier et al 1996, 2001). OCD may result from head injury (including birth trauma), frontal lobe tumours and temporal lobe epilepsy. However, in most conditions OCD is a fairly rare complication and is therefore difficult to study. Brain regions associated with post-head injury OCD are the frontal cortex and basal ganglia (Berthier et al 2001). In addition, OCD is seen in up to 70% of patients with Tourette's syndrome and in approximately one-quarter of first-degree relatives. This may suggest a common pathology that can be genetically inherited. One group of conditions of great potential in elucidating the mechanisms of OCD are the paediatric autoimmune neuropsychiatric disorders associated with streptococcal infections (PANDAS). Perhaps as many as 50% of children who develop streptococcal-related autoimmune disease develop obsessional symptoms. In the OCD subtype of the PANDAS syndrome, volumes of the caudate, putamen and globus pallidus, but not of the thalamus or total cerebrum, are larger than in matched controls (Giedd et al 2000). Acquired damage to the caudate nucleus or basal ganglia caused by degenerative or acquired lesions is a common theme in patients with secondary obsessional symptoms (see Table I.1) and could represent an anatomical final common pathway. The basal ganglia are of particular importance in OCD, as evidenced by the overlap with movement disorders such as Sydenham's chorea, Tourette's syndrome and post-encephalitic Parkinson's disease. OCD can result from isolated focal lesions of the basal ganglia, although such lesions are usually bilateral (Laplane et al 1989). In addition to lesions of the basal ganglia, disease of the frontal lobe has also been linked with OCD. Some studies report that 60% of those with fronto-temporal dementia have some degree of compulsive behaviour. Furthermore, this has been correlated with the degree of temporal atrophy and the degree of caudate atrophy (Rosso et al 2001).

Box 79.1 Conditions that feature obsessions and compulsions

Neurological disorders
Carbon monoxide poisoning
Epilepsy
Huntington's disease
Ischaemic stroke of the caudate
Ischaemic stroke of the globus pallidus
Lesch–Nyhan syndrome
Manganese poisoning
PANDAS syndrome
Parkinson's disease
Pick's disease
Post-encephalitis
Progressive supranuclear palsy
Sydenham's chorea
Tourette's syndrome

Psychiatric disorders
Anankastic personality disorder
Anxiety disorder
Autism
Depression
Eating disorders
Use of dopamine agonists
Use of stimulants

Tumours of the medial frontal and orbitofrontal surface are occasionally thought to cause obsessional symptoms without other evident pathology.

MECHANISMS OF OBSESSIONS AND COMPULSIONS

One theoretical model of OCD is that an imbalance in the frontal–subcortical motor loops is responsible for the generation of symptoms. The involvement of these circuits in Parkinson's disease and Huntington's disease has been discussed (see Figs 51.2 and 52.1). In OCD it is suggested that repetitive compulsive actions arise from excess activity in the direct motor pathway relative to the indirect pathway. This produces activation of the ventral nucleus of the thalamus, which reinforces the motor signals of the supplementary motor area of the frontal lobe. This model is essentially the opposite of that proposed in Parkinson's disease.

Why should this dysregulation in the two motor circuits arise in the first place? Conceivably this could be due to neurotransmitter changes or even to functional changes in the cortex itself. The orbitofrontal circuit has a role in activating the direct loop, whereas the dorsolateral circuit tends to activate the indirect loop. Functional imaging studies in primary OCD show that the orbitofrontal cortex is overactive – a finding that would be consistent with

the proposed model. Very few studies have attempted to study functional correlates in secondary OCD, and the results of these are, as yet, uncertain (Hugo et al 1999).

REFERENCES AND FURTHER READING

Berthier ML, Kulisevsky J, Gironell A et al 1996 Obsessive–compulsive disorder associated with brain lesions: clinical phenomenology, cognitive function, and anatomic correlates. Neurology 47:353–361

Berthier ML, Kulisevsky J, Gironell A et al 2001 Obsessive–compulsive disorder and traumatic brain injury: behavioral, cognitive, and neuroimaging findings. Neuropsychiatry, Neuropsychology and Behavioral Neurology 14:23–31

Giedd JN, Rapoport JL, Garvey MA et al 2000 MRI assessment of children with obsessive–compulsive disorder or tics associated with streptococcal infection. American Journal of Psychiatry 157:281–283

Hugo F, van Heerden B, Zungu-Dirwayi N et al 1999 Functional brain imaging in obsessive–compulsive disorder secondary to neurological lesions. Depression and Anxiety 10:129–136

Laplane D, Levasseur M, Pilloni B et al 1989 Obsessive–compulsive and behavioural changes with bilateral basal ganglia lesions. Brain 112:649–725

Rosso SM, Roks G, Stevens M et al 2001 Complex compulsive behaviour in the temporal variant of frontotemporal dementia. Journal of Neurology 248:965–970

80

Neurobiology of Appetite and Weight

The basic biological drives to sleep, eat and reproduce are ancient in evolutionary terms and therefore their control centres must be located in ancient parts of the brain. The diencephalon, or more specifically the hypothalamus, is the most plausible candidate, as it regulates the pituitary gland and, in addition, controls thirst and thermal regulation. In 1954, Bauer described the characteristics of 60 people with hypothalamic disease – 70% had endocrine consequences (hypogonadism, precocious puberty, diabetes insipidus), 30% had hyperphagia or obesity, 25% had anorexia, 30% had hypersomnolence and 20% had problems with temperature regulation. It is perhaps surprising, given the fundamental nature of appetite, sleep and libido, that these areas are not better protected from insults. Good evidence from many medical conditions demonstrates that these functions are peculiarly sensitive to non-specific disruption. One clue as to why this sensitivity exists lies in the fact that these areas receive major feedback following the success of the organism in the environment. A dominant, successful chimpanzee will expect to feed first, mate regularly and sleep well. Conversely, a chimp lower in the social hierarchy would not receive these advantages; therefore, low sex drive and poor appetite is adaptive in this situation. In our world, these functions are disrupted by human stressors (e.g. work hassles, marital disharmony, medical illness) and usually return when the hassles remit.

EATING AND APPETITE

An old notion, arising from animal studies in the 1950s, is that the biological control of appetite is seated exclusively in the hypothalamus and that lesions of the ventral medial nucleus of the basal hypothalamus result in obesity, whereas lesions to the lateral hypothalamus produce anorexia. However, ventral medial lesions cause parasympathetic overarousal and a secondary anabolic state, and lateral hypothalamic lesions cause a general apathetic state. Thus, it is an oversimplification to reduce the control of eating to signals in the hypothalamus. As with disturbances in cognition, disturbances in eating can result from lesions to several interlinked areas. Central to this is the *nucleus of the tractus solitarius*, which receives inputs from the periphery (with short, medium and long feedback from the mouth, stomach and gut) and from the area postrema, which keeps track of plasma osmolality. Satiety (inhibition of food intake) appears to be mediated, in part, by oxytocin neurones originating in the parvocellular division of the paraventricular nucleus of the hypothalamus. Peripherally, the release of cholecystokinin (CCK) informs the brain when food has been detected in the gut. Serotonin, oestradiol and glucagon suppress feeding and stressors that increase CRF increase oxytocin and reduce appetite. The 'set-point' for feeding is closely associated with the peripheral amount of body fat. High blood glucose levels stimulate insulin, which acts directly on the hypothalamus to reduce the hormone neuropeptide Y (NPY). NPY is the most powerful appetite stimulant. Low levels of NPY reduce the inhibition of oxytocin. Adipose cells secrete leptin, particularly in the anabolic state, and this acts on the arcuate nucleus of the hypothalamus and in the caudal dorsal raphe and median raphe nuclei to inhibit NPY release and increase the release of coticotropin releasing hormone, which, with melanocortin, is an appetite suppressor. Central serotonergic receptors, particularly the serotonin-2c receptor, may be the target of the leptin signal (or the two may be separate systems, with serotonin being part of an integrated network for short-acting satiety signals and leptin acting as a hormonal dictator of long-term (tonic) energy reserves) (Halford & Bundell 2000, Nonogaki et al 1998). Adrenaline (epinephrine) increases thermogenesis and lipolysis, leading to increased energy expenditure and decreased fat stores. It is likely that β-3 adrenergic receptors mediate these responses (Fig. 80.1).

An understanding of the physiology of hunger and feeding is not synonymous with an understanding of obesity or anorexia. The majority of neurobiological changes observed in those who are over- or underweight appear to be compensatory mechanisms.

Appetite in neuropsychiatry

Appetite and eating can be disturbed in several neuropsychiatric conditions. Shortly after severe closed head injury, the majority of patients are unable to manage the task of feeding independently. Also, they tend to have a high metabolic rate. In late Alzheimer's disease, spontaneous feeding reduces with disease severity. Swallowing can also be disrupted. For these reasons, there is sometimes the dilemma whether to use forced feeding via percutaneous endoscopic gastrostomy. Usually little is to be gained from this intervention. Low body weight and low body fat is a recognized complication of

Parkinson's disease and progressive supranuclear palsy. Patients with progressive supranuclear palsy may have worse dysphagia and dysarthria than patients with Parkinson's disease (Jankovic et al 1992), although the mechanisms are not entirely clear. It is not clear what the underlying mechanisms are in these diseases. Weight loss is seen in Huntington's disease, probably due to a combination of persistent movements and inadequate intake. One study found that sedentary energy expenditure, but not total free-living energy expenditure, is higher in patients than controls because patients with Huntington's disease engage in less voluntary physical activity (Pratley et al 2000).

Lessons for the neurobiology of anorexia

The biology of anorexia nervosa is the same as the biology of long-term starvation (Müller & Locatelli

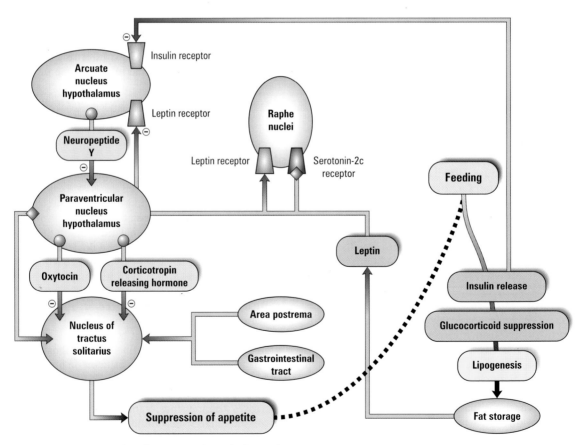

Fig. 80.1 Overview of mechanisms regulating body weight.

1992). Studies report no robust biological differences between these conditions (except where the omission of certain foods causes specific consequences). This is not surprising, since the nutritionally challenged body does not know whether calories are being withheld or are unavailable. In both enforced starvation and anorexia nervosa there are massive hormonal attempts to maintain blood glucose at an appropriate level. The immediate effects are reductions in leptin and increases in NPY to stimulate appetite, although appetite usually diminishes with time. Centrally, the hypothalamic–pituitary–adrenal axis is overactive, in an attempt to maintain plasma glucose via gluconeogenesis. The other main catabolic hormone, growth hormone, is also elevated. Conversely, the hypothalamic–pituitary–gonadal axis is underactive, a necessary adaptive function to conserve energy during starvation. Low activity of the hypothalamic–pituitary–thyroid axis has the advantage of reducing the basal metabolic rate. In terms of actual plasma glucose, basal levels may be normal or low, but there is instability, with a tendency to impaired glucose tolerance tests and increased sensitivity to insulin (there is a reduced growth hormone response to insulin-induced hypoglycaemia). Anorexic patients perform poorly on tests of pituitary reserve, with blunted corticotropin-releasing factor, thyrotropin-releasing hormone and gonadotropin-releasing hormone induced responses. Water deprivation may elicit subnormal increases in vasopressin. The longer these endocrine changes persist, the more likely they are to result in undesirable secondary changes, including hypogonadism (causing hyposexuality and amenohrroea) and a slow metabolism (causing bradycardia, hypothermia and constipation). Hypercortisolaemia may contribute to osteoporosis, immunosuppression and sleep disturbance. Studies now demonstrate that patients with anorexia nervosa have changes in neuroanatomy and neuropsychology. These studies have recruited only small numbers of patients to date. Typical findings on neuroimaging include ventricular enlargement, cortical atrophy, pituitary atrophy and, possibly, adrenal hypertrophy. Global hypometabolism has been shown on functional imaging. Changes in cognition, although recognized, are not yet well characterized. All the above changes are thought to be state dependent and, given time and adequate nutrition, revert back to normal levels.

Anorexia of old age

Ageing is associated with changes in eating habits, which are most likely adaptive in response to reduced calorie requirements. There is a diminished desire to eat and reduced hunger and a slowing of gastric emptying. More worrying are changes in appetite or eating habits that are maladaptive. This is commonly seen in the context of medical and psychiatric illnesses in elderly people with a vulnerable baseline nutritional state. The effect of a new illness is to disturb appetite and, in some diseases, increase calorie requirements. The most obvious example is loss of weight and appetite in cancer (cancer cachexia). Refusal to eat while unwell may have a critical influence on prognosis, although it is more often than not (perhaps falsely) considered to be an unalterable secondary consequence (Davis & Dickerson 2000).

REFERENCES AND FURTHER READING

Bauer HG 1954 Endocrine and other manifestations of hypothalamic disease: a survey of 60 cases, with autopsies. Journal of Clinical Endocrinology and Metabolism 14:13–31

Davis MP, Dickerson D 2000 Cachexia and anorexia: cancer's covert killer. Supportive Care in Cancer 8:180–187

Halford JCG, Blundell JE 2000 Separate systems for serotonin and leptin in appetite control. Annals of Medicine 32:222–232

Jankovic J, Wooten M, Vanderlinden C et al 1992 Low body-weight in Parkinson's disease. Southern Medical Journal 85:351–354

Nonogaki K, Strack AM, Dallman MF et al 1998 Leptin-independent hyperphagia and type 2 diabetes in mice with a mutated serotonin 5-HT2C receptor gene. Nature Medicine 4:1152–1156

Müller EE, Locatelli V 1992 Undernutrition and pituitary function: relevance to the pathophysiology of some neuroendocrine alterations of anorexia nervosa. Journal of Endocrinology 132:327–329

Pratley RE, Salbe AD, Ravussin E, Caviness JN 2000 Higher sedentary energy expenditure in patients with Huntington's disease. Annals of Neurology 47:64–70

Rang HP 1999 Pharmacology. Churchill Livingstone, Edinburgh

Swaab DF, Purba JS, Hofman MA 1995 Alterations in the hypothalamic paraventricular nucleus and its oxytocin neurons (putative satiety cells) in Praeder–Willi syndrome: a study of 5 cases. Journal of Clinical Endocrinology and Metabolism 80:573–579

81

Stress Biology as an Integrative Concept

It should be obvious from the preceding discussion that there is no 'master theory' that unites all of neuropsychiatry or even the major presentations. There is increasing understanding about the causes of delirium and many dementias. There are also reasonable explanations about the pathogenesis of depression, apathy, anxiety, anger, memory deficits, delusions and hallucinations. It is important to recognize that each presentation may have a different mechanism in different circumstances (e.g. the origin of mild cognitive impairment in multiple sclerosis and mild cognitive impairment in Parkinson's disease differ). Yet part of the pathophysiology may be common. This is the elusive *final common pathway* that could ultimately shed light on primary psychiatric illnesses that also feature these symptoms and signs. Several such pathways have been mentioned already and only you, the reader, can answer how convincing these integrative theories are. However, I feel that one system is worth revisiting, as it tries particularly hard to unite social experiences with neurobiology and neuropsychiatric complications.

Clinical Pointer 81.1

The role of stress (life events) in the onset of neuropsychiatric disease

In general medicine, a surprising finding in recent years has been that the onset of several biological illnesses is often heralded by stressful life events. This has been seen in myocardial infarction, Cushing's disease, hyperprolactinaemia, diabetes, rheumatoid arthritis, asthma and Graves' disease. It is important to remember that these are not crisis events in the hours or days before disease onset, but rather a build up of stressful life events over the preceding months. Some work has drawn a similar conclusion in neuropsychiatric conditions, most notably in stroke where it may be long-term threatening events that are significant. In dementia, preceding stressful life events are important, but easier to understand. Here it is the social disruptiveness of the event rather than the threat or neuroendocrine consequence of the event that is likely to be the crucial factor. Stress has been examined in Tourette's syndrome, with generally consistent findings that stress worsens tics whereas reduced stress (including relaxation) diminishes tics. Stressful life events have been found to increase the odds of HIV progression, but it was not as clear if they influence AIDS progression (if at all) (Bablin et al 1999).

Life events also have a role in prognosis and ongoing quality of life, although this requires much closer study. There are several reasons why the association of life events and disease onset might not be causative: life events may reflect a subtle preclinical manifestation of the disease; or life events may not be recalled accurately after a disease has developed (the so-called 'search after meaning', i.e. an attempt to find factors that explain why this has happened). That said, one should keep an open mind about the link between stressors and disease, given what we already know from the huge field of psychoneuroendocrinology.

Further reading   *Balbin EG, Ironson GH, Solomon GF 1999 Stress and coping: the psychoneuroimmunology of HIV/AIDS. Baillière's Clinical Endocrinal Metabolism 13:615–633*
Biondi M, Picardi A 1999 Psychological stress and neuroendocrine function in humans: the last two decades of research. Psychotherapy and Psychosomatics 68:114–150
Orrell M, Bebbington P 1995 Life events and senile dementia. 1. Admission, deterioration and social-environment change. Psychological Medicine 25:373–386
Schneck MJ 1997 Is psychological stress a risk factor for cerebrovascular disease? Neuroepidemiology 164:174–179

THE HYPOTHALAMIC–PITUITARY–ADRENAL AXIS IN NEUROPSYCHIATRY

In 1936, Hans Selye introduced the world to the concept of non-specific biological stress responses in the *general adaption syndrome*. Although Selye discussed only glucocorticoids in the initial alarm phase, adrenaline (epinephrine) and noradrenaline (norepinephrine) are hormonal effectors of acute stress, while the hypothalamic–pituitary–adrenal (HPA) axis is better viewed as the hormonal mediator of chronic stress. These three hormones (glucocorticoids, adrenaline and noradrenaline) form part of three interrelated systems: the sympathoneural (or sympathetic nervous) system (the main effector of which is noradrenaline), the adrenomedullary hormonal system (which produces adrenaline) and the HPA system (which relies on cortisol). The physiological role of glucocorticoids is complex, involving an integrated catabolic response. This breaks down and redistributes fat, protein and mineral stores to satisfy the potential demands of a continuing threat. Unfortunately, a prolonged catabolic response becomes increasingly hazardous as the unwanted effects of sleep disturbance, osteoporosis, appetite suppression, anergia, hyperglycaemia, hypertension and immunosuppression result from hypercortisolaemia. The HPA axis is a dynamic hormonal system, which is usually tightly controlled, with a periodicity that can be measured in hours, days or months. Hypothalamic corticotropin releasing hormone and vasopressin are centrally active neuropeptides with an important neurotransmitter-like role and also act as secretagogues for adrenocorticotropic hormone (ACTH), which is produced by the anterior pituitary. ACTH stimulates the production of cortisol and other steroid hormones, such as dehydroepiandrosterone from the adrenal gland. Cortisol acts on glucocorticoid receptors, including those in the hippocampus that regulate the HPA axis via negative feedback.

The HPA axis theory of neuropsychiatric disorders is based on the following observations:

- the HPA axis is dysregulated in several psychiatric and neuropsychiatric disorders
- the dysregulation correlates (to a variable degree) with hippocampal atrophy, mood disturbance and cognitive impairment
- the origins of HPA dysregulation include early life adversity, recent life stressors and other individual differences

- some patients at high risk of psychiatric disorders also have a moderately disturbed HPA axis function
- endogenous and exogenous medical causes of HPA axis activity feature high rates of psychiatric disturbance
- normalization of peripheral endogenous glucocorticoids appears to be beneficial in the treatment of mood disorders
- established antidepressants actually reduce HPA activity in healthy controls, a possible novel antidepressant mechanism.

In healthy controls, treatment with medium to high doses of cortisol produces reversible decreases in verbal declarative memory without effects on nonverbal memory, sustained or selective attention, or executive function (Newcomer et al 1999). Acute cortisone administration impairs retrieval of long-term declarative memory (de Quervain et al 2000). Clinically, patients on long-term steroids have explicit memory deficits (Keenan et al 1996).

In normal ageing, studies demonstrate that aged humans with prolonged cortisol elevations show reduced hippocampal volume (of the order of 10–20%) and deficits in hippocampus-dependent memory tasks compared with normal-cortisol controls. Moreover, the degree of hippocampal atrophy correlates with basal and sustained cortisol levels (Lupien et al 1998).

In alcoholism, a reduction in hippocampal volume is well described, but this appears to be proportional to total brain atrophy (Agartz et al 1999). The HPA axis is abnormally hyperactive during withdrawal, but normalizes thereafter (Hundt et al 2001). Corticotropin-releasing hormone may have a role in addiction (Sarnyai et al 2001), but to date it has not been shown to play a role in cocaine abuse (Jacobsen et al 2001).

The HPA changes that follow stroke are reasonably well characterized. Plasma cortisol concentrations are high within hours of a stroke (typically over 800 nmol/l or 30 μg/dl), with lower mean concentrations thereafter (Murros et al 1993). This is a picture also seen in patients with any acute critical illness. Astrom et al (1993) administered the dexamethasone suppression test to 70 patients at 1 week, 3 months and 3 years post-stroke. Although there was a high rate of attrition, non-suppression was evident in about one-quarter of patients and showed an association with post-stroke depression. Animal work has not proven that post-stroke HPA axis activation has a strong clinicoanatomical basis (i.e. stress hormone activation can be induced by diffuse brain injury). Clinical correlations of stroke-related HPA activation include the severity of the stroke, delirium, cognitive impairment and depression. Uski et al (2000) performed lumbar punctures 3–6 months after surgery in 17 patients who experienced good outcomes after aneurysmal subarachnoid haemorrhage. Patients with cognitive impairment after aneurysmal subarachnoid haemorrhage exhibited higher CSF concentrations of endorphins, corticotropin-releasing factor, and δ-sleep-inducing peptide than did those with normal capacity (Uski et al 2000).

In Parkinson's disease, a small post-mortem study of hypothalamic corticotropin-releasing hormone neurones did not find an increased number of neurones expressing corticotropin-releasing hormone in depressed ($n = 6$) or non-depressed patients ($n = 6$) with Parkinson's disease (Hoogendijk et al 1998).

In Huntington's disease the HPA axis is overactive, as evidenced by higher basal cortisol and ACTH levels than in controls and a blunted ACTH response (with normal cortisol response) to corticotropin-releasing hormone (Heuser et al 1991). Dehydroepiandrosterone concentrations are also lower in Huntington's disease than in age-matched controls (Leblhuber et al 1995).

In systemic lupus erythematosus, low levels of dehydroepiandrosterone sulphate are associated with poor memory in subjects who do not have CNS involvement (Kozora et al 2001).

HPA axis activity in multiple sclerosis has been investigated using the comparatively sensitive combined dexamethasone–corticotropin-releasing-hormone test (Bergh et al 1999). The degree of hyperactivity was moderate in patients with relapsing–remitting multiple sclerosis ($n = 38$), intermediate in patients with the secondary progressive form of the disease ($n = 16$) and marked in patients with primary progressive multiple sclerosis ($n = 6$). There was also a correlation with the degree of neurological impairment (including cognition), but there was no correlation between HPA activity and depression. This finding has been replicated. On pathological examination, in comparison with control subjects there were elevated levels of corticotropin-releasing hormone immunoreactivity in the paraventricular nucleus of the hypothalamus (Purba et al 1995). Normalization of HPA axis overactivity occurs with antidepressant augmentation of steroid treatment, but not with steroid treatment alone (Bergh et al

2001). A correlation with abnormalities seen on MRI of the brain suggests that critical areas of inflammation are the cause (Wei & Lightman 1997).

In Alzheimer's disease, a large series of studies has established modest increases in HPA axis activity. However, similar results are also seen in vascular dementia and elderly patients with depression, so the test cannot be used diagnostically. There are also no differences between young-onset and senile-onset cases (Bernardi et al 2000, Gottfries et al 1994). Of more interest is what the HPA axis hyperactivity is due to, and whether it has any clinical significance. To answer this, it is necessary to examine the levels of corticotropin-releasing hormone in central sites. Extrahypothalamic corticotropin-releasing hormone is reduced in Alzheimer's disease, which is consistent with widespread tissue loss. Hypothalamic corticotropin-releasing hormone mRNA (but not corticotropin-releasing hormone neuronal counts) is increased compared with controls (Raadsheer et al 1995). In addition, hypothalamic (but again, not extrahypothalamic) vasopressin appears to be either elevated or unchanged in Alzheimer's disease, depending on the study (Lucassen et al 1997). This is consistent with central overdrive of the HPA axis in dementia (i.e. it is not a result of pituitary–adrenal hyper-responsivity). One attractive hypothesis is that elevated levels of corticotropin-releasing hormone and arginine vasopressin are caused by impaired glucocorticoid feedback from damaged neurones in the hippocampus (a primary site of pathology in Alzheimer's disease). The first study to report glucocorticoid receptor and mineralocorticoid receptor mRNA levels in individual hippocampal neurones of patients with Alzheimer's disease found that the distribution and intensity were similar to those in controls (although there was a significantly lower expression in the CA1 subfield) (Seckl et al 1993). A second study found higher levels of hippocampal glucocorticoid mRNA in patients with Alzheimer's disease than in controls (Wetzel et al 1995). However, this could simply have been a compensating response secondary to general neuronal loss in the hippocampus.

CLINICAL CORRELATIONS

Most, but not all, groups have found that high levels of cortisol are inversely correlated with the degree of cognitive impairment in Alzheimer's disease (Murialdo et al 2001). That said, the strength of this

Table 81.1 Association between the HPA axis function and clinical variables in neuropsychiatric disorders

Patient group	HPA axis function	Cognition deficits	Depressed mood	Medial temporal damage
Alzheimer's disease	Overactive	✓ (correlated with HPA activity)	✓ (correlated with HPA activity)	✓ (weakly correlated with HPA activity)
Bipolar depression	Overactive	✓	✓ (correlated with HPA activity)	✓ (small samples)
Cushing's disease	Overactive	✓ (correlated with HPA activity)	✓ (correlated with HPA activity)	✓ (correlated with HPA activity)
Head injury	Overactive (acutely)	✓	✓	✓
Huntington's disease	Overactive	✓	✓ (correlated with HPA activity)	0
Korsakoff's syndrome/ alcoholism	Overactive (in withdrawal)	✓	✓	✓ (correlated with HPA activity)
Multiple sclerosis	Overactive (in severe illness)	✓	✓	0
Normal ageing	Overactive (in oldest old)	✓ (mild) (correlated with HPA activity)	✓ (variable)	✓ (correlated with HPA activity)
Parkinson's disease	Normal	✓	✓	0
Post-traumatic stress disorder	Underactive peripherally	✓	✓	✓ (correlated with cognition)
Schizophrenia	Near normal	✓	✓	✓
Stroke	Overactive (acutely)	✓ (correlated with HPA activity)	✓ (correlated with HPA activity)	0
Temporal lobe epilepsy	Overactive (acutely)	✓	✓	✓
Unipolar depression	Overactive	✓ (weakly correlated with HPA activity)	✓ (correlated with HPA activity)	✓ (correlated with HPA activity)

✓, Significant correlations have been reported, but the strength of the association varies

0, no association

correlation is, at best, modest (Gottfries et al 1994). This has led to a rise in popularity of the *glucocorticoid cascade hypothesis* as applied to Alzheimer's disease. Sapolsky et al (1986) proposed the glucocorticoid cascade hypothesis, which can be summarized as the theory that hippocampal cell loss results in hypercortisolism, which in turn leads to hypercortisolaemia. This acts as a co-factor in further hippocampal degeneration and thus creates a feedforward loop. Against this hypothesis, longitudinal studies to date have not shown a deterioration in HPA axis function with worsening dementia, as predicted by the model (Swanwick et al 1998). In favour of the hypothesis, using MRI, Deleon et al (1988) demonstrated a correlation between the 2-hour plasma cortisol response to the glucose tolerance test and both cognitive status and hippocampal size. In addition, Polleri and colleagues at the University of Genoa examined the HPA axis and brain activity in 14 patients with Alzheimer's disease and 12 controls (Murialdo et al 2000). Hippocampal SPECT data correlated directly with mean dehydroepiandrosterone sulphate levels and inversely with cortisol/dehydroepiandrosterone sulphate ratios. Using a large sample from Melbourne, O'Brien et al (1996) observed a relationship between post-dexamethasone cortisol levels and both MRI hippocampal atrophy and minor mood symptoms. A fourth study found a correlation between high salivary cortisol, low Mini-Mental State Examination scores and cortical atrophy (Monti et al 2000). It will be interesting to see whether the same association exists in people with mild cognitive impairment (Wolf et al 2002).

In summary, hippocampal lesions, particularly in the CA1 and CA3 subfields, are well recognized as producing a variety of cognitive deficits in animals and humans. Although the short-term glucocorticoid response is adaptive, prolonged exposure to glucocorticoids is neurotoxic (probably via the action of excitatory amino acids on N-methyl-D-aspartate receptors) to apical dendrites of the CA3 region of the hippocampus, causing an abnormality of structure or function. The degree of hypercortisolaemia has been correlated with either in vivo measures of hippocampal atrophy or cognitive impairment in normal ageing, Cushing's disease, post-traumatic stress disorder, stroke, Korsakoff's syndrome, depression, Huntington's disease and Alzheimer's disease (Axelson et al 1993, Emsley et al 1994, Starkman et al 1992). Steroid-related apoptosis is commonly seen in the hippocampi of depressed patients, but only to a relatively minor degree, and therefore its clinical significance is not yet known (Lucassen et al 2001). These data alone do not answer the question of cause or effect. Hippocampal atrophy, from whatever cause, would be expected to produce HPA overdrive because hippocampal glucocorticoid receptors are an important source of negative feedback in the axis. To improve the theory, what is needed are good studies that monitor the integrity of the hippocampus (and higher function) during a protracted course of treatment with exogenous steroids.

REFERENCES AND FURTHER READING

Agartz I, Momenan R, Rawlings RR et al 1999 Hippocampal volume in patients with alcohol dependence. Archives of General Psychiatry 56:356–363

Astrom M, Olsson T, Asplund K 1993 Different linkage of depression to hypercortisolism early versus late after stroke. A three year longitudinal study. Stroke 24:52–57

Axelson DA, Doraiswamy PM, McDonald WM et al 1993 Hypercortisolaemia and hippocampal changes in depressives. Psychiatric Research 47:163–173

Bergh FT, Kumpfel T, Trenkwalder C et al 1999 Dysregulation of the hypothalamo–pituitary–adrenal axis is related to the clinical course of MS. Neurology 53:772–777

Bergh FT, Kumpfel T, Grasser A et al 2001 Combined treatment with corticosteroids and moclobemide favors normalization of hypothalamo–pituitary–adrenal axis dysregulation in relapsing–remitting multiple sclerosis: a randomized, double blind trial. Journal of Clinical Endocrinology and Metabolism 86:1610–1615

Bernardi F, Lanzone A, Cento RM et al 2000 Allopregnanolone and dehydroepiandrosterone response to corticotropin-releasing factor in patients suffering from Alzheimer's disease and vascular dementia. European Journal of Endocrinology 142:466–471

Deleon MJ, Mcrae T, Tsai JR et al 1988 Abnormal cortisol response in Alzheimer's disease linked to hippocampal atrophy. Lancet ii:391–392

de Quervain DJF, Roozendaal B, Nitsch RM et al 2000 Acute cortisone administration impairs retrieval of long-term declarative memory in humans. Nature Neuroscience 3:313–314

Emsley RA, Roberts MC, Albers C et al 1994 Endocrine function in alcoholic Korsakoff's syndrome. Alcohol and Alcoholism 29:187–191

Gottfries CG, Balldin J, Blennow K et al 1994 Regulation of the hypothalamo–pituitary–adrenal axis in dementia disorders. Annals of the New York Academy of Sciences 739:336–343

Heuser IJE, Chase TN, Mouradian MM 1991 The limbic hypothalamic–pituitary–adrenal axis in Huntington's disease. Biological Psychiatry 30:943–952

Hoogendijk WJG, Purba JS, Hofman MA et al 1998 Depression in Parkinson's disease is not accompanied by more corticotropin-releasing hormone expressing neurons in the hypothalamic paraventricular nucleus. Biological Psychiatry 43:913–917

Hundt W, Zimmermann U, Pottig M et al 2001 The combined dexamethasone-suppression/CRH-stimulation test in alcoholics during and after acute withdrawal. Alcohol Clinical and Experimental Research 25:687–691

Jacobsen LK, Giedd JN, Kreek MJ et al 2001 Quantitative medial temporal lobe brain morphology and hypothalamic–pituitary–adrenal axis function in cocaine dependence: a preliminary report. Drug and Alcohol Dependency 62:49–56

Keenan PA, Jacobson MW, Soleymani RM et al 1996 The effect on memory of chronic prednisone treatment in patients with systemic disease. Neurology 47:1396–1402

Kozora E, Laudenslager M, Lemieux A et al 2001 Inflammatory and hormonal measures predict neuropsychological functioning in systemic lupus erythematosus and rheumatoid arthritis patients. Journal of the International Neuropsychological Society 7:745–754

Leblhuber F, Peichl M, Neubauer C et al 1995 Serum dehydroepiandrosterone and cortisol measurements in Huntington's chorea. Journal of Neurological Science 132:76–79

Lucassen PJ, VanHeerikhuize JJ, Guldenaar SEF et al 1997 Unchanged amounts of vasopressin mRNA in the supraoptic and paraventricular nucleus during aging and in Alzheimer's disease. Journal of Neuroendocrinology 94:297–305

Lucassen PJ, Muller MB, Holsboer F et al 2001 Hippocampal apoptosis in major depression is a minor event and absent from subareas at risk for glucocorticoid overexposure. American Journal of Pathology 158:453–468

Lupien SJ, de Leon M, de Santi S et al 1998 Cortisol levels during human aging predict hippocampal atrophy and memory deficits. Nature Neuroscience 1:69–73

Monti MS, Giubilei F, Tisei P et al 2000 Alzheimer's dementia and circadian rhythm of cortisol: clinical and neuroradiological aspects. Giornale di Neuropsicofarmacologia 22:163–169

Murialdo G, Nobili F, Rollero A et al 2000 Hippocampal perfusion and pituitary–adrenal axis in Alzheimer's disease. Neuropsychobiology 42:51–57

Murialdo G, Barreca A, Nobili F et al 2001 Relationships between cortisol, dehydroepiandrosterone sulphate and insulin-like growth factor-I system in dementia. Journal of Endocrinological Investigation 24:139–146

Murros K, Fogelholm R, Kettunen S et al 1993 Serum cortisol and outcome of ischemic brain infarction. Journal of Neurological Science 116:12–17

Newcomer JW, Selke G, Melson AK et al 1999 Decreased memory performance in healthy humans induced by stress-level cortisol treatment. Archives of General Psychiatry 56:527–533

O'Brien JT, Ames D, Schweitzer I et al 1996 Clinical and magnetic resonance imaging correlates of hypothalamic–pituitary–adrenal axis function in depression and Alzheimer's disease. British Journal of Psychiatry 168:679–687

Purba JS, Raadsheer FC, Hofman MA et al 1995 Increased number of corticotropin-releasing hormone expressing neurons in the hypothalamic paraventricular nucleus of patients with multiple sclerosis. Neuroendocrinology 62:62–70

Raadsheer FC, Vanheerikhuize JJ, Lucassen PJ et al 1995 Corticotropin-releasing hormone messenger-RNA levels in the paraventricular nucleus of patients with Alzheimer's disease and depression. American Journal of Psychiatry 152:1372–1376

Sapolsky RM, Krey LC, McKewan BS 1986 The neuroendocrinology of stress and aging: the glucocorticoid cascade hypothesis. Endocrine Reviews 7:284–301

Sarnyai Z, Shaham Y, Heinrichs SC 2001 The role of corticotropin-releasing factor in drug addiction. Pharmacological Reviews 53:209–243

Seckl JR, French KL, O'Donnell D et al 1993 Glucocorticoid receptor gene expression is unaltered in hippocampal neurons in Alzheimer's disease. Molecular Brain Research 18:239–245

Selye H 1936 A syndrome produced by diverse noxious agents. Nature 138:32

Starkman MN, Gebarski SS, Berent SA et al 1992 Hippocampal formation volume, memory dysfunction and cortisol levels in patients with Cushing's syndrome. Biological Psychiatry 32:756–765

Swanwick GRJ, Kirby M, Bruce I et al 1998 Hypothalamic–pituitary–adrenal axis dysfunction in Alzheimer's disease: lack of association between longitudinal and cross-sectional findings. American Journal of Psychiatry 155:286–289

Uski TK, Lilja A, Saveland H et al 2000 Cognitive functioning and cerebrospinal fluid concentrations of neuropeptides for patients with good neurological outcomes after aneurysmal subarachnoid hemorrhage. Neurosurgery 47:812–818

Wei T, Lightman SL 1997 The neuroendocrine axis in patients with multiple sclerosis. Brain 120:1067–1076

Wetzel DM, Bohn MC, Kazee AM et al 1995 Glucocorticoid receptor messenger RNA in Alzheimer's diseased hippocampus. Brain Research 679:72–81

Wolf OT, Convit A, Thorn E et al 2002 Salivary cortisol day profiles in the elderly with mild cognitive impairment. Psychoendocrinology 27:777–789

Epilogue

82

Maxims of Neuro- psychiatry Revisited

Having examined most of the important neuropsychiatric conditions individually, Let us re-examine the maxims of neuropsychiatry presented at the beginning of this book (see Box I.1), this time looking at the supporting evidence.

Any significant brain lesion can cause diverse neuropsychiatric complications

There is considerable heterogeneity in the presentation of disease. One disease will affect different people in different ways. There may be common strands, such as the predominantly subcortical pathology of Parkinson's disease, but there will also be important differences. These individual differences tend to be lost in the summated results published in large studies, but are very important for clinicians treating individual patients. Even when the pathology is well localized (e.g. in a caudate infarct) the neurological and psychiatric complications can be diverse (e.g. as in depression, apathy, cognitive impairment). Why is this? Every area of the brain is directly (and indirectly) interconnected, and therefore a change in function in one area influences the

function in other areas. The take-home message is that clinicians should be vigilant for the unexpected, and should not automatically dismiss unusual symptoms or signs as non-organic or psychosomatic.

Predicting which neuropsychiatric complication(s) will develop after brain injury is difficult

The clinicoanatomical basis of many neurological symptoms and signs is reasonably well localized. In contrast, psychiatric symptoms are generally poorly localized. Despite much research, studies have failed to find a convincing anatomical basis for mood, psychosis or behaviour. There is a haphazard and hence incalculable element to all presentations. It is not possible to look at an MRI scan of a patient with newly diagnosed multiple sclerosis or an EEG of a patient with epilepsy and discern exactly which symptoms will be present. Similarly, it is difficult to review the environmental and personality variables and conclude what complications will develop. Usually no single biological or psychosocial variable is necessary, sufficient and exclusively associated with any one neuropsychiatric complication. Multiple risk factors interact in a complex way that defies expression mathematically (see Ch. 68). At best, while assessing presenting symptoms and signs we use ancillary information to make an informed judgement about the most likely diagnosis.

Psychological symptoms may manifest before neurological symptoms of neurological disease

In a number of neuropsychiatric conditions, psychological, behavioural and mood symptoms occur before the onset of neurological symptoms. For example, in Parkinson's disease, studies suggest that about one-third of patients have depressive or anxiety symptoms (or both) before motor symptoms (Henderson et al 1992). In particular, anxiety disorders have been recognized up to 20 years before the onset of Parkinson's disease (Shiba et al 2000). Psychological symptoms are known regularly to manifest before neurological symptoms in Huntington's disease, CNS tumours, Alzheimer's disease, vascular dementia and, less commonly, multiple sclerosis, systemic lupus erythematosus, HIV infection and Wilson's disease (Bachoud-Levi et al 2001, Dening & Berrios 1989, Mintz 1994, Schiffer et al 1983, Steinlin et al 1995).

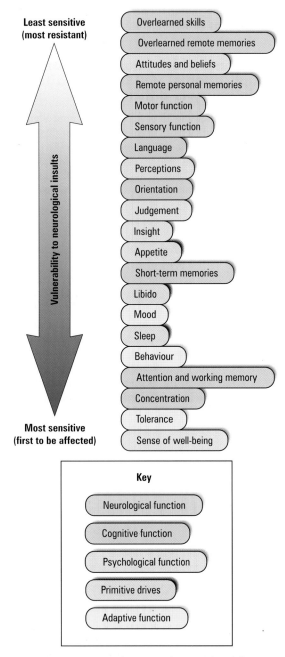

Least sensitive
(most resistant)

Vulnerability to neurological insults

Overlearned skills

Overlearned remote memories

Attitudes and beliefs

Remote personal memories

Motor function

Sensory function

Language

Perceptions

Orientation

Judgement

Insight

Appetite

Short-term memories

Libido

Mood

Sleep

Behaviour

Attention and working memory

Concentration

Tolerance

Sense of well-being

Most sensitive
(first to be affected)

Key

Neurological function

Cognitive function

Psychological function

Primitive drives

Adaptive function

Fig. 82.1 Overview of neuropsychiatric vulnerability. Certain higher functions are very vulnerable to dysfunction. Clinically, these areas are often the first to be lost in the presence of neuropsychiatric disease and the last to return. Others are extremely stable and hence will only become eroded by a severe disorder. The exact order of loss of function will depend on disease- and host-related variables.

What could be the explanation for these observations? In the case of Alzheimer's disease, depression in late life is a risk factor for later dementia (see Clinical Pointer 40.3). In addition, patients with subtle subjective memory complaints are likely to develop dysphoria, and possibly depression, before the cognitive problems become severe enough to warrant a medical opinion. In other words, the patient begins to suffer as a result of perceived deficits before he or she seeks medical help. This explanation falls short of explaining the early presentation with other neuropsychiatric complaints, such as anxiety, psychosis and cognitive impairment, that are seen in several conditions. Another intriguing possibility is that neurobiological changes associated with early degenerative disease cause psychological changes before the point of diagnosis.

Should we be surprised that in neuropsychiatric disorders, mental symptoms may present before physical symptoms? Most conditions begin gradually, and hence it may be vulnerable higher functions that are most easily disrupted by the early stages of CNS disease and these alert the patient or their relatives to a problem. Overlearned primitive skills are most resistant to degradation and are only affected in the most severe conditions (Fig. 82.1).

The relationship between neuropsychiatric complication(s) and health-related disability is not simple

Researchers have been struggling for.years to understand the determinants of disability in the common neurological disorders. Most studies have not accounted for the influence of psychiatric, psychological and social variables. Studies that use objective measures of disability tend to show a weaker relationship with psychiatric outcome than do studies that use measures rated by patients themselves (Griffin et al 1998, Schrag et al 2001). For example, Gilchrist & Creed (1994) found that depression and cognitive deficits in multiple sclerosis were not associated with duration of disease, physical impairments, disability or handicap. However, a larger study did link subjective disability ratings with depressive symptoms (Chwastiak et al 2002). Other studies have found little or no relationship between physical disability in multiple sclerosis and severity of cognitive deficits. In Alzheimer's disease, the decline in function is an integral part of the disease that is secondarily influenced by medical and psychiatric comorbidity (Espiritu et al 2001, Rapoport et al 2001, Thomas 2001). In an elegant study, Artero et al (2001) examined neuropsychiatric predictors of decline in disability over a 3-year period in patients with mild cognitive impairment. Decline in visuospatial performance on cognitive tests was the most significant predictor of decline in ability to dress, bathe, use the telephone or retain mobility. Decline in attention also reduced the capability of independent toileting, and a decline in language was associated with poor telephone use. Memory impairment alone did not have a large effect. Patient-rated disability and handicap are major determinants of quality of life and are also affiliated with hopelessness and suicide.

Most neuropsychiatric complications go unrecognized and untreated

Many studies show that at least half of all psychiatric problems of patients on medical wards go unrecognized. Similarly, about 50% of organic disease also goes unrecognized by psychiatrists (Dening & Berrios 1989). In the community, primary care physicians appear to overlook dementia in the majority of cases (Callahan et al 1995). In hospitals, delirium is identified by nursing staff in less than one in three cases. Risk factors for non-recognition are hypoactive presentations, old age, visual impairment and co-existing dementia (Inouye et al 2001). Indeed, when dementia is also present, delirium is overlooked 90% of the time.

There are two outstanding studies in this area. Wancata et al (2000) looked at the recognition of psychiatric disorders on medical hospital wards and assessed case recognition by asking physicians themselves rather than relying on medical notes. A total of 187 of 505 inpatients had a psychiatric disorder. Physicians managed to pick up 54% of these cases, although their accuracy varied by diagnosis. Balestrieri et al (2002) detected depression in 195 of 1039 medical or surgical inpatients. General hospital physicians correctly identified one-third of these cases and began antidepressant treatment in about one-third of this group. In other words, 17 out of 195 depressed patients were prescribed antidepressants. Other studies with similar findings show that this is not an anomaly (Hansen et al 2001). Three recent studies show low rates of detection and/or investigation for alcohol problems in medical inpa-

tients, psychiatric inpatients and patients in general practice (Hansen et al 2000, Rumpf et al 2001, Schneekloth et al 2001). Few case-recognition studies have been conducted specifically in neurological patients. In a prospective evaluation of 101 patients with Parkinson's disease, Shulman et al (2002) found that neurologists picked up 35% of cases of depression, 42% of cases of anxiety, 25% of cases of fatigue and 60% of cases of sleep disturbance. Clinicians have also been found to overlook depression in stroke (Pohjasvaara et al 2001), epilepsy (Wiegartz et al 1999), multiple sclerosis (Minden et al 1989) and dementia (Margallo-Lana et al 2001). The solution to this problem is not easy. What is known is that improving clinicians' communication style and increasing consultation times improves detection rates (Fallowfield et al 2001).

Treatment of secondary psychiatric complications is similar to treatment of primary psychiatric disorders

There is little evidence to suggest that mood disorder or psychotic disorder caused by organic brain disease requires qualitatively different treatment to a primary mood or psychotic disorder on account of efficacy. However, the course of recovery will not necessarily be the same in both types of presentation. In neurological disease, the prognosis will be largely determined by the underlying condition. Thus, if psychosis occurs following steroid treatment for multiple sclerosis, the psychosis will tend to resolve quickly once the steroid treatment is reduced. This emphasizes the importance of treating the underlying condition as well as the neuropsychiatric complication.

Does the organic condition determine which specific treatment to use? Much of the choice of a particular drug is determined by likely side effects. Patients with organic brain disease, particularly Parkinson's disease, Lewy body dementia, HIV-related disease and Huntington's disease, are particularly sensitive to the antidopaminergic, antiadrenergic and antihistaminic effects of medication. Thus, the percentage of patients who are unable to tolerate medication (particularly older receptor non-specific agents) may approach 50% (Elliot et al 1998). Drug–drug interactions may also be important (see Ch. 64). ECT should also be used with caution because of the increased frequency of ECT-induced delirium (Moellentine et al 1998). It is therefore more important to treat all neuropsychiatric conditions with care than to withhold vital treatment for fear of potential side effects.

Neuropsychiatric complications affect neurological recovery and mortality

Neurological recovery is not a purely physical process. The effect of motivation, cooperation, goal setting and support should not be underemphasized. Neuropsychiatric illness acts as a barrier to rehabilitation and in some cases accelerates mortality. This effect has been seen in most chronic medical diseases where this relationship has been studied. For example, post-stroke depression is a major influence on rehabilitation recovery and long-term mortality (Morris et al 1993) (see Ch. 47). The same relationship is recognized in head injury (Satz et al 1998), Parkinson's disease (Hughes 2000) and possibly HIV progression to AIDS (Lesserman et al 2002). Psychosis has also been linked with mortality in several neuropsychiatric diseases including Parkinson's disease (Goetz & Stebbins 1995). Although the mechanism could be an epiphenomenon of severity of disease, it could also represent an overlap with delirium. In Alzheimer's disease psychotic symptoms predict institutionalization but not survival, perhaps because psychotic symptoms tend to occur in the middle rather than the late stages of the disease.

Neurobiological markers are the same in primary and secondary psychiatric disorders

Studies have found that in some patients with depression and Parkinson's disease there is a decrease in CSF 5-hydroxyindole acetic acid compared with non-depressed patients with Parkinson's disease (Mayeux et al 1984). However, this finding is also seen in primary depression. In two PET series from different groups, Mayberg et al (1992) compared depressed patients with Parkinson's disease, Huntington's disease and caudate stroke with patients suffering primary depression. Depressed patients, independently of group, had frontal and temporal cortex hypometabolism. Ring et al (1994) replicated this finding in depressed and non-depressed patients with Parkinson's disease. The depressed patients had bilateral reductions in prefrontal cortex blood flow.

In depression following stroke, several studies have shown an association between non-suppression after the dexamethasone suppression test and the presence of depression (Astrom et al 1993). This change is recognized in primary depression, so what useful information does this reveal and therefore what additional information does it convey? Without being too negative, this association might be of interest if the biological marker is in fact driven by the underlying physical condition and precedes the development of depression. Conceivably, it could be important if the biological marker is driven by the underlying condition and occurs before the onset of mood symptoms. In other words, the biological finding moves from an epiphenomenon to one that may be involved in pathogenesis.

Neuropsychiatric complications arise from a combination of organic and non-organic factors

Neuropsychiatric disorders are complex in their aetiology, manifestations and treatment. More than in any other branch of medicine there are considerable individual differences between sufferers of the same condition. This leads to problems with initial recognition, problems with differential diagnosis and the repeated question of whether the condition is organic or psychological in origin. Consider two examples of this dichotomy. In a patient with post-stroke dementia, it may be clear that the recent infarct has caused the cognitive impairment, but many psychosocial factors will determine the extent of the disability and handicap that the person endures. In a patient with dissociative pseudo-seizures, a psychological explanation may be the best-fitting model, but an associated seizure disorder is always a possibility and could co-exist with a diagnosis of pseudoseizures. If a clinician believes that all conditions are either entirely organic or entirely psychosomatic in origin there is the danger of missing psychological distress, which in itself adversely effects compliance, rehabilitation outcome and perhaps mortality. At the same time, there is the danger of missing organic factors in patients presenting with psychiatric symptoms. If, on the other hand, a clinician behaves as if there is likely to be both a psychological component and an organic component to every presentation, these problems are rare. The relative weight of psychological, social, psychiatric and organic factors will vary

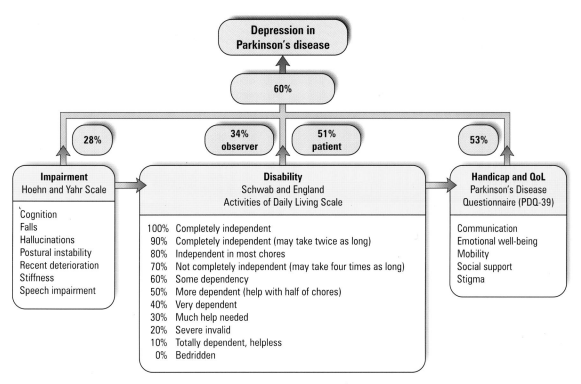

Fig. 82.2 Predictors of depression in Parkinson's disease. Schrag et al (2001) studied the predictors of depression (and quality of life) in Parkinson's disease. As predicted, neurological impairment was modestly related to depression. Observer-rated disability was also a rather poor indicator. Patient-related disability and handicap were strongly correlated with severity of depression in Parkinson's disease. Adapted from Schrag et al (2001).

in every case, but these may be difficult or impossible to calculate with accuracy.

Neuropsychiatric complications dramatically affect quality of life

'Quality of life' refers to the positive aspects of daily living that healthy people normally take for granted. It includes adequate level of interest and motivation (vitality), ability to carry out essential tasks (e.g. washing, dressing, eating, sleeping) and the option to engage in self-directed hobbies, work and relationships. Many of these are captured in the Short Form with 36 Items (SF-36), a widely used quality of life scale (see Table 68.1). Stavem et al (2000) administered the SF-36 questionnaire to 397 patients with epilepsy, 785 with angina pectoris, 1030 with rheumatoid arthritis, 117 with asthma and 221 with chronic obstructive pulmonary disease. All medical patients scored lower than the population norms, but in this sample of patients with well-controlled epilepsy, health-related quality of life was better

than in the other medically ill groups. Predictors of quality of life have been examined in 435 patients recruited from the Jefferson Comprehensive Epilepsy Center in Philadelphia (Johnson et al 2002). The Beck Depression Inventory-II (BDI-II) was the strongest predictor of quality of life, with a lesser contribution from seizure frequency, medication, the Beck Anxiety Inventory, and driving status.

Schrag et al (2000), at the Institute of Neurology, examined the factors that influence quality of life in Parkinson's disease. The factor most closely associated with quality of life was the presence of depression, but disability, postural instability and cognitive impairment also contributed to poor quality of life The prominent role of depression in determining quality of life in Parkinson's disease has been replicated in several other studies (Chrischilles et al 2002, Global Parkinson's Disease Survey Steering Group 2002, Kuopio et al 2000). In Parkinson's disease, neuropsychiatric complications impair not just the quality of life of the patient, but also those of the main carers (Aarsland et al 1999). One mechanism

Table 82.1 Frequency of concerns expressed by people with epilepsy

Concern	Frequency (%)
Driving	64
Independence	54
Employment	51
Social embarrassment	36
Dependence on medication	33
Mood	32
Safety	31

After Gillam et al (1997)

could be the accelerated functional and motor decline that is caused by depression (Starkstein et al 1992). In multiple sclerosis, cognitive impairment has been related to quality of life and carer distress, as has depression, anxiety and fatigue (Amato et al 2001, Chipcase & Lincoln 2001, Cutajar et al 2000, Fruehwald et al 2001, Rao et al 1991). Each factor may contribute to health-related quality of life in a complex way (Benito-Léon et al 2002). At least five studies have examined neuropsychiatric predictors of quality of life in stroke. Infarct volume, aphasia, impaired motor function and impaired cognitive function were linked with poorer quality of life, but depression (when measured) was the most significant (Kauhanen 1999, Kauhanen et al 2000). The same association between either cognitive impairment or depression and reduced quality of life is present in sufferers of subarachnoid haemorrhage, motor neurone disease, CNS tumours and HIV infection (Giovagnoli 1999, Lou et al 2002, Mayer et al 2001, Sherbourne et al 2000).

Low self-blame and family support are factors in quality of life after head injury (Webb et al 1995). Quality of life in alcoholics is also associated with stability in the social environment, psychiatric comorbidity and physical symptoms (Foster et al 1999).

FINAL WORDS

What have we learned from this short exploration of neuropsychiatry? The brain is vulnerable to a wide range of insults, the mysteries of which are gradually being unravelled. There is now a better understanding of the way in which neurological diseases manifest as psychological, psychiatric and behavioural features. Not uncommonly, these features are the first indication of a pathological process involving the CNS. Disturbances in higher function are more closely affiliated with general well-being than is any other complication and can powerfully influence disease outcome. Predicting the exact nature of the neuropsychiatric complication can only be achieved by a better understanding of this brain disease–host interaction. Recognizing that in most cases neurological factors and psychological factors interact will help to reduce erroneous explanations of cause or outcome in individual clinical cases.

Social advances in the 20th century helped us to beat the old enemy of infectious disease, only to leave us vulnerable to the diseases influenced by lifestyle and neurodegeneration. Vascular disease is probably the single most important pathological process affecting the brain, because it is extremely common and potentially preventable. However, a significant change in the daily habits of the population is required in order to have a major impact on vascular disease. Whether the drugs of the 21st century will provide a significant effect on the progression of common neurodegenerative conditions is uncertain, but I believe this is a realistic goal. Beyond this, the ability of pharmaceuticals or genetic intervention to cure these diseases will, I fear, remain tantalizingly out of reach for many years to come.

REFERENCES AND FURTHER READING

Aarsland D, Larsen JP, Karlsen K et al 1999 Mental symptoms in Parkinson's disease are important contributors to caregiver distress. International Journal of Geriatric Psychiatry 14:866–874

Amato MP, Ponziani G, Stracusa G et al 2001 Cognitive dysfunction in early-onset multiple sclerosis. Archives of Neurology 58:1602–1606

Artero S, Touchon J, Ritchie K 2001 Disability and mild cognitive impairment: a longitudinal population-based study. International Journal of Geriatric Psychiatry 16:1092–1097

Astrom M, Olsson T, Asplund K 1993 Different linkage of depression to hypercortisolism early versus late after stroke. A three year longitudinal study. Stroke 24:52–57

Bachoud-Levi AC, Maison P, Bartolomeo P et al 2001 Retest effects and cognitive decline in longitudinal follow-up of patients with early HD. Neurology 56:1052–1058

Balestrieri M, Bisoffi G, Tansella M et al 2002 Identification of depression by medical and surgical general hospital physicians. General Hospital Psychiatry 24:4–11

Benito-Léon J, Morales JM, Rivera-Navario J 2002 Health-related quality of life and its relationship to cognitive and emotional functioning in multiple sclerosis patients. European Journal of Neurology 9:497–502

Callahan CM, Hendrie HC, Tierney WM 1995 Documentation and evaluation of cognitive impairment in elderly primary-care patients. Annals of Internal Medicine 122:422–429

Chipchase SY, Lincoln NB 2001 Factors associated with carer strain in carers of people with multiple sclerosis. Disability and Rehabilitation 23:768–776

Chrischilles EA, Rubenstein LM, Voelker MD et al 2002 Linking clinical variables to health-related quality of life in Parkinson's disease. Parkinsonism & Related Disorders 8:199–209

Chwastiak L, Ehde DM, Gibbons LE et al 2002 Depressive symptoms and severity of illness in multiple sclerosis: epidemiologic study of a large community sample. American Journal of Psychiatry 159:1862–1868

Cutajar R, Ferriani E, Scandellari C et al 2000 Cognitive function and quality of life in multiple sclerosis patients. Journal of Neurovirology 6(suppl):S186–S190

Dening TR, Berrios GE 1989 Wilson's disease. Psychiatric symptoms in 195 cases. Archives of General Psychiatry 46:1126–1134

Elliot AJ, Uldall KK, Bergam K et al 1998 Randomized, placebo-controlled trial of paroxetine versus imipramine in depressed HIV-positive outpatients. American Journal of Psychiatry 155:367–372

Espiritu DAV, Rashid H, Mast BT et al 2001 Depression, cognitive impairment and function in Alzheimer's disease. International Journal of Geriatric Psychiatry 16:1098–1103

Fallowfield L, Ratcliffe D, Jenkins V et al 2001 Psychiatric morbidity and its recognition by doctors in patients with cancer. British Journal of Cancer 84:1011–1015

Foster JH, Powell JE, Marshall EJ et al 1999 Quality of life in alcohol-dependent subjects: a review. Quality of Life Research 8:255–261

Fruehwald S, Loeffler-Stastka H, Eher R et al 2001 Depression and quality of life in multiple sclerosis. Acta Neurologica Scandinavica 104:257–261

Gilchrist AC, Creed FH 1994 Depression, cognitive impairment and social stress in multiple sclerosis. Journal of Psychosomatic Research 38:193–201

Gilliam F, Kuzniecky R, Faught E et al 1997 Patient-validated content of epilepsy-specific quality-of-life measurement. Epilepsia 38:233–236

Giovagnoli AR 1999 Quality of life in patients with stable disease after surgery, radiotherapy and chemotherapy for malignant brain tumour. Journal of Neurology and Psychiatry 67:358–363

Global Parkinson's Disease Survey Steering Committee 2002 Factors impacting on quality of life in Parkinson's disease: results from an international survey. Movement Disorders 17:60–76

Goetz C, Stebbins G 1995 Mortality and hallucinations in nursing home patients with advanced Parkinson's disease. Neurology 45:669–671

Griffin KW, Rabkin JG, Remien RH et al 1998 Disease severity, physical limitations and depression in HIV-infected men. Journal of Psychosomatics Research 44:219–227

Hansen SS, Munk-Jorgensen P, Guldbaek B et al 2000 Psychoactive substance use diagnoses among psychiatric in-patients. Acta Psychiatrica Scandinavica 102:432–438

Hansen MS, Fink P, Frydenberg M et al 2001 Mental disorders among internal medical inpatients. Prevalence, detection, and treatment status. Journal of Psychosomatics Research 50:199–204

Henderson R, Kurlan R, Kersun JM 1992 Preliminary examination of the comorbidity of anxiety and depression in Parkinson's disease. Journal of Neuropsychiatry and Clinical Neuroscience 4:257–264

Hughes TA 2000 A controlled study of dementia and mortality in Parkinson's disease. MD thesis, University of Leeds

Inouye SK, Foreman MD, Mion LC et al 2001 Nurses' recognition of delirium and its symptoms: comparison of nurse and researcher ratings. Archives of Internal Medicine 161:2467–2473

Johnson V, Cho R, Tracy JI et al 2002 Determinants of quality of life in epilepsy. Presented at the American Academy of Neurology 54th Annual Meeting, Denver, 13–20 April

Kauhanen ML 1999 Quality of life after stroke clinical, functional, psychosocial and cognitive correlates. Dissertation, Oulu University

Kauhanen ML, Korpelainen JT, Hiltunen P et al 2000 Domains and determinants of quality of life after stroke caused by brain infarction. Archives of Physical Medicine and Rehabilitation 81:1541–1546

Kuopio AM, Marttila RJ, Helenius H et al 2000 The quality of life in Parkinson's disease. Movement Disorders 15:216–223

Lesserman J, Petitto JM, Gu H et al 2002 Progression to AIDS, a clinical AIDS condition and mortality: psychosocial and physiological predictors. Psychological Medicine 32:1059–1073

Lou J-S, Reeves A, Benice T 2002 Factors affecting quality of life in patients with amyotrophic lateral sclerosis. Presented at the American Academy of Neurology 54th Annual Meeting, Denver, April 13–20

Magni E, Binetti G, Bianchetti A et al 1996 Risk of mortality and institutionalization in demented patients with delusions. Journal of Geriatric Psychiatry and Neurology 9:123–126

Margallo-Lana M, Swann A, O'Brien J et al 2001 Prevalence and pharmacological management of behavioural and psychological symptoms amongst dementia sufferers living in care environments. International Journal of Geriatric Psychiatry 16:39–44

Mayberg HS, Starkstein SE, Jeffrey PJ et al 1992 Limbic cortex hypometabolism in depression: similarities among patients with primary and secondary mood disorders. Neurology 42(suppl 3):181

Mayer SA, Kreiter KT, Ostapkovich N et al 2001 Cognitive dysfunction and quality of life after subarachnoid haemorrhage. Annals of Neurology 50(suppl 1):s78

Mayeux R, Stern Y, Cote L et al 1984 Altered serotonin metabolism in depressed patients with Parkinson's disease. Neurology 34:642–646

Minden SL, Orav J, Reich P 1989 Depression in multiple

sclerosis. General Hospital Psychiatry 9:426–434

Mintz M 1994 Clinical comparison of adult and pediatric neuroaids. Advances in Neuroimmunology 4:207–221

Moellentine C, Rummans T, Ahlskog JE et al 1998 Effectiveness of ECT in patients with parkinsonism. Journal of Neuropsychiatry and Clinical Neuroscience 10:187–193

Morris PLP, Robinson RG, Andrzejewski P et al 1993 Association of depression with 10-year poststroke mortality. American Journal of Psychiatry 150:124–129

Pohjasvaara T, Vataja R, Leppavuori et al 2001 Depression is an independent predictor of poor long-term functional outcome post-stroke. European Journal of Neurology 8:315–319

Rao SM, Leo GJ, Ellington L et al 1991 Cognitive dysfunction in multiple sclerosis. 2. Impact on employment and social functioning. Neurology 41:692–696

Rapoport MJ, Van Reekum R, Freedman M et al 2001 Relationship of psychosis to aggression, apathy and function in dementia. International Journal of Geriatric Psychiatry 16:123–130

Ring HA, Bench CJ, Trimble MR et al 1994 Depression in Parkinson's disease: a positron emission study. British Journal of Psychiatry 165:333–339

Rumpf HJ, Bohlmann J, Hill A et al 2001 Physicians' low detection rates of alcohol dependence or abuse: a matter of methodological shortcomings? General Hospital Psychiatry 233:133–137

Satz P, Forney DL, Zaucha K et al 1998 Depression, cognition, and functional correlates of recovery outcome after traumatic brain injury. Brain Injury 12:537–553

Schiffer RB, Caine ED, Bamford KA 1983 Depressive episodes in patients with multiple sclerosis. American Journal of Psychiatry 140:1498–1500

Schneekloth TD, Morse RM, Herrick LM et al 2001 Point prevalence of alcoholism in hospitalized patients: continuing challenges of detection, assessment, and diagnosis. Mayo Clinic Proceedings 76:460–466

Schrag A, Jahanshahi M, Quinn NJ 2000 What contributes to quality of life in patients with Parkinson's disease? Journal of Neurology, Neurosurgery and Psychiatry 69:308–312

Schrag A, Jahanshahi M, Quinn NP 2001 What contributes to depression in Parkinson's disease? Psychological Medicine 31:655–673

Sherbourne CD, Hays RD, Fleishman JA et al 2000 Impact of psychiatric conditions on health-related quality of life in persons with HIV infection. American Journal of Psychiatry 157:248–254

Shiba M, Bower JH, Maraganore DM et al 2000 Anxiety disorders and depressive disorders preceding Parkinson's disease: a case–control study. Movement Disorders 15:669–677

Shulman LM, Taback RL, Rabinstein AA et al 2002 Non-recognition of depression and other non-motor symptoms in Parkinson's disease. Parkinsonism & Related Disorders 8:193–197

Starkstein SE, Mayberg HS, Preziosi TJ et al 1992 A prospective longitudinal study of depression, cognitive decline, and physical impairments in patients with Parkinson's disease. Journal of Neurology, Neurosurgery and Psychiatry 55:377–382

Stavem K, Lossius MI, Kvien TK et al 2000 The health-related quality of life of patients with epilepsy compared with angina pectoris, rheumatoid arthritis, asthma and chronic obstructive pulmonary disease. Quality of Life Research 9:865–871

Steinlin MI, Blaser SI, Gilday DL et al 1995 Neurologic manifestations of pediatric systemic lupus erythematosus. Pediatric Neurology 13:191–197

Thomas VS 2001 Excess functional disability among demented subjects? Findings from the Canadian Study of Health and Aging. Dementia, Geriatrics and Cognitive Disorders 12:206–210

Wancata J, Windhaber J, Bach M, Meise U 2000 Recognition of psychiatric disorders in nonpsychiatric hospital wards. Journal of Psychosomatics Research 48:149–155

Webb CR, Wrigley M, Yoels W et al 1995 Explaining quality-of-life for persons with traumatic brain injuries 2 years after injury. Archives of Physical Medicine and Rehabilitation 76:1113–1119

Wiegartz P, Seidenberg M, Woodard A et al 1999 Co-morbid psychiatric disorder in chronic epilepsy: recognition and etiology of depression. Neurology 53(suppl 2):S3–S8

Appendices

Appendix I Historical landmarks in neuropsychiatry

Date	Event	Field*
1492	Christopher Columbus brought back tobacco from the Bahamas	Ψ
1518	King Henry VIII, on the advice of his court physician, founded the Royal College of Physicians, London	Θ
1641	French philosopher René Descartes (1596–1650) discussed the metaphysical split between mind and body in the publication *Meditationes*	Ψ
1760	Swiss philosopher Charles Bonnet described his grandfather who, after developing cataracts, started to experience 'amusing and magical' visions	Ψ
1806	Morphine was first extracted from opium by the German chemist Friedrich AW Serturner	℞
1816	French physician Rene TH Laennec (1781–1826) invented the stethoscope	Θ
1817	English physician James Parkinson (1755–1824) described 'shaking palsy', or *Parkinson's disease*	PD
1817	Lithium was discovered by the Swedish chemist Johan August Arfvedson during an analysis of petalite ore taken from the Swedish island of Utö	℞
1825	Jean E Esquirol (1772–1840) distinguished between delusions and hallucinations	Ψ
1848	Railway foreman Phineas Gage (1823–1860) suffered a frontal lobe injury from a tamping iron, during work on the Rutland and Burlington Railroad near Cavendish, Vermont	Ψ
1851	Pierre Louis Alphée Cazenave (1795–1877) named the long-recognised disease *lupus erythematosus*	Ψ
1851	Hermann von Helmholtz (1821–1894) invented the ophthalmoscope	Θ
1853	Bell and Cruveilhier noted the thinness of the anterior spinal roots in motor neurone disease	MND
1854	Louis P Gratiolet (1815–1865) described the convolutions of the cerebral cortex	Ψ
1855	Bartolomeo Panizza (1785–1867) showed that the occipital lobe is essential for vision	Ψ
1857	Sir Charles Locock (1799–1875) found that potassium bromide was an effective treatment for epilepsy	℞
1859	Paul Briquet (1796–1881) described what is now called 'somatization disorder'	Ψ
1859	Charles Darwin (1809–1882) published *The Origin of Species*	Θ
1861	French neurologist and pathologist Pierre Paul Broca (1824–1880) discussed cortical localization after describing the case of patient Tan	Ψ
1864	Barbiturates were first synthesised in Germany, by Adolf von Baeyer (1835–1917)	℞
1865	Gregor Mendel (1822–1884), an Augustinian monk, presented his laws of heredity to the Natural Science Society in Brunn, Austria	Θ
1866	John Langdon Haydon Down (1828–1896) published work on congenital 'idiots'	Ψ
1869	Charcot (1825–1893) studied the involvement of the corticospinal tracts and suggested the term *amyotrophic lateral sclerosis*	MND

Contd

Appendix I   Cont'd

Date	Event	Field*
1869	Otto Liebreich, Professor of Pharmacology in Berlin, determined that chloral hydrate was a hypnotic	℞
1872	George Sumner Huntington (1850–1916) first described an inherited form of chorea as a discrete clinical entity	HD
1873	Norwegian physician Dr Gerhard Henrick Armauer Hansen (1841–1912) discovered *Mycobacterium leprae* (published in 1874)	Θ
1874	Carl Wernicke (1848–1904) Professor of Neurology in Breslau, published *Der Aphasische Symptomencomplex* on aphasias	Ψ
1875	The electroencephalogram was invented in Liverpool by Dr Richard Caton (1842–1926)	Θ
1877	Theodor Hermann Meynert (1833–1892) attributed chorea in Huntington's disease to lesions in the corpus striatum	HD
1878	Pierre Paul Broca (1824–1880) described the limbic area	Ψ
1880	Jean Baptiste Edouard Gelineau introduced the word 'narcolepsy'	Ψ
1880	Sommer linked epilepsy with sclerosis in Ammon's horn (neuronal loss in the cornu ammonis 1 sector)	Ψ
1882	A link between progressive bulbar palsy and motor neurone disease was established by the French neurologist Joseph Jules Déjerine (1849–1917)	MND
1882	Cervello used paraldehyde (a polymer of acetaldehyde) for the first time	℞
1883	Brain introduced the term 'motor neurone disease' linking amyotrophic lateral sclerosis, progressive bulbar palsy and progressive muscular atrophy	MND
1883	German psychiatrist and neurologist Karl Friedrich Otto Westphal (1833–1890) offered the first description of Westphal–Strümpell's pseudosclerosis (Wilson's disease)	Ψ
1883	Emil Kraepelin (1856–1926) coined the terms 'neuroses' and 'psychosis'	Ψ
1884	French neurologist Georges Albert Édouard Brutus Gilles de la Tourette (1857–1904) described several movement disorders	Ψ
1884	Robert Koch (1843–1910) stated his 'postulates' for testing whether a microbe is the causal agent of a disease	Θ
1885	Louis Pasteur (1822–1895) tested his rabies treatment on Joseph Meister	℞
1887	Russian neuropsychiatrist Sergei Sergeievich Korsakoff (1853–1900) described symptoms characteristic in alcoholics	Ψ
1891	German physician Heinrich Irenaeus Quincke (1842–1922) introduced the lumbar puncture	Ψ
1891	German anatomist Heinrich Wilhelm Gottfried Waldeyer (1836–1921) coined the term 'neurone'	Ψ
1892	Blocq and Marinesco described senile plaques	AD
1892	Czechoslovakian neurologist and psychiatrist Arnold Pick (1851–1924) described a patient with aphasia and dementia associated with frontal and temporal lobe atrophy	Ψ
1894	At a conference in Dresden, Otto Binswanger (1852–1929) described arteriosclerotic brain degeneration, differentiating it from syphilitic paralysis	Ψ
1895	Wilhelm Konrad Roentgen (1845–1923) invented the X-ray	Θ

1897	Charles Scott Sherrington (1857–1952) coined the term 'synapse'	Ψ
1899	Austrian psychiatrist and neurologist Gabriel Anton (1858–1933) described cortical deafness and cortical blindness	Ψ
1900	Karl Landsteiner (1868–1943) discovered the first human blood groups (O, A and B)	Θ
1900	Walter Reed established that yellow fever is transmitted by mosquitoes, the first time a human disease had been shown to be caused by a virus	Θ
1900	Hugo Liepmann (1863–1925) described apraxia	Ψ
1902	German neuropathologist Max Bielschowsky (1869–1940) developed staining and silver impregnation techniques for histological study of the nervous system	Ψ
1903	Adelchi Negri (1876–1912) described intracytoplasmic inclusion bodies in brains of rabies victims	Ψ
1903	French neurologist Joseph Francois Felix Babinski (1857–1932) described the Babinski sign	Ψ
1903	German chemist Emil Fischer and collaborator Joseph von Mering modified diethyl barbituric acid (barbital). Phenobarbitone was marketed in 1912	Ψ
1903	Willem Einthoven (1860–1927), a Dutch physiologist, developed the electrocardiograph	Θ
1904	Friedrich Stolz synthesised adrenaline (epinephrine) and noradrenaline (norepinephrine)	Θ
1906	German neuropathologist Alois Alzheimer (1864–1915) described the pathological appearance of neuritic plaques and neurofibrillary tangles	AD
1906	Paul Erlich (1854–1915) investigated atoxyl/arsenic compounds and discovered Salvarsan, the first treatment for syphilis	ℜ
1908	Punnett proposed a dominant Mendelian pattern of inheritance in Huntington's disease	HD
1908	Albert Calmette and Camille Guerin developed a vaccine against tuberculosis (BCG) from live bovine tubercle bacilli, although it was not used until 1921 (1927 in the UK)	ℜ
1909	American neurosurgeon Harvey Williams Cushing (1869–1939) electrically stimulated the human sensory cortex	Ψ
1909	German neurologist Korbinian Brodmann (1868–1918) described 52 cortical areas	Ψ
1910	Kraeplin (1856–1926) introduced the term 'Alzheimer's disease' after his student's early descriptions	AD
1911	Alois Alzheimer (1864–1915) described the histological findings of Pick bodies and Pick cells associated with Pick's disease	Ψ
1911	Nicotinic acid was isolated from rice polishings by Polish born chemist Casimir Funk, leading to a dramatic reduction in cerebral pellagra	Ψ
1912	Frederich Heinrich Lewy (1885–1950) described 'Lewy body' inclusions in the basal forebrain in Parkinson's disease	PD
1912	British neurologist Samuel Alexander Kinnier Wilson (1878–1937) fully described Wilson's disease in a doctoral thesis	Ψ
1913	Santiago Ramon y Cajal (1852–1934) developed gold chloride–mercury stain to show astrocytes	Ψ
1914	Henry H Dale (1875–1968) isolated acetylcholine	Θ

Contd

Appendix 1 *Contd*

Date	Event	Field*
1915	The first aspirin tablets were made by German chemist Felix Hoffmann, who rediscovered French chemist Charles Frederic Gerhardt's 1853 formula	ℜ
1916	Richard Henneberg (1868–1962) coined the term 'cataplexy'	Ψ
1919	Tretiakoff identified the loss of pigmented cells in the substantia nigra in Parkinson's disease	PD
1919	Cushing's student Walter E Dandy (1886–1946) introduced air encephalography	Ψ
1920	German neuropathologist Hans Gerhard Creutzfeldt (1885–1964) described a case of what is now thought to be Creutzfeldt–Jakob disease	CJD
1921	German neurologist Alfons Maria Jakob (1884–1931) described a similar case of Creutzfeldt–Jakob disease	CJD
1921	An accidental discovery led to the development of the anticonvulsant phenobarbital	ℜ
1922	Walther Spielmeyer (1879–1935) brought together the two cases described previously and introduced the term *Creutzfeldt–Jakob disease*	CJD
1922	Canadian surgeon Frederick Banting (1891–1941) and research assistant Charles Best (1899–1978) discovered insulin	Θ
1924	Walter Kirschbaum identified the first case of familial Creutzfeldt–Jakob disease	CJD
1926	Onari and Spatz named Pick's disease	Ψ
1928	Harrison Stanford Martland (1883–1954) described dementia pugilistica	Ψ
1928	Alexander Fleming (1881–1955) discovered penicillin	Θ
1930	German pathologist Theodor Fahr (1877–1945) described Fahr's disease	Ψ
1932	Walter B Cannon (1871–1945) coined the term 'homeostasis'	Ψ
1935	Percy Lavon Julian (1899–1975) synthesized physostigmine from the calabar bean	ℜ
1935	Prinzmetal and Bloomberg introduced racemic amphetamine for the treatment of narcolepsy	ℜ
1936	Antonio Caetano de Abreu Freire Egas Moniz (1874–1955) published work on the first human frontal lobotomy	Θ
1937	James Enceslas Papez (1898–1982), neuroanatomist at Cornell Medical School, published work on the limbic circuit	Ψ
1937	American neurologists Heinrich Klüver (1897–1979) and Paul Clancy Bucy (b. 1904) published work on bilateral temporal lobectomies	Ψ
1937	Bradley used dextroamphetamine to calm excitable children (attention deficit hyperactivity disorder)	ℜ
1937	Electroconvulsive shock therapy was discovered by Ugo Cerletti and Lucio Bini in Rome	ℜ
1938	Albert Hoffman, a Swiss chemist, began synthesizing various derivatives of lysergic acid	Ψ
1938	Phenytoin first used as an antiepileptic, having been synthesised from urea and phenol by Putnam and Merritt	ℜ
1939	David Weschler (1896–1981), Chief Psychologist at Bellevue Psychiatric Hospital, introduced the Wechsler Adult Intelligence Scale	Ψ

1940	Alexander highlighted a link between Wernicke's encephalopathy and thiamine by experimentally reproducing the syndrome in pigeons	Ψ
1948	The National Health Service Act came into operation	Θ
1949	Australian psychiatrist John Cade used lithium	℞
1950	Eugene Roberts and J Awapara independently identified GABA in the brain	Ψ
1950	Chlorpromazine was first synthesized at the Laboratoires Rhone-Poulenc/Specia by the chemist Paul Charpentier	℞
1952	Jonas Salk (1914–1995) refined a vaccine for polio	Θ
1953	James Watson and Francis Crick discovered the structure of DNA	Θ
1953	Murray Falconer developed the temporal lobectomy for refractory temporal lobe seizures	Ψ
1953	Eugene Aserinski and Nathaniel Kleitman described rapid eye movement (REM) during sleep	Θ
1954	Edward Freis reported on reserpine-induced depression	℞
1954	First kidney transplant was performed in Boston on Richard and Ronald Herrick	Θ
1957	Swiss psychiatrist Roland Khun reported success with imipramine (first trialed in 1955)	℞
1957	The antidepressant effects of the monoamine oxidase inhibitor iproniazid (Marsilid) were first announced by Harry Loomer at a meeting in Syracuse, New York	℞
1957	British researchers Alick Isaacs and J Lindenman, of the National Institute for Medical Research, London, discovered interferon	℞
1958	Haloperidol was introduced	℞
1959	Sternbach synthesized diazepam (Valium)	℞
1959	The radioimmunoassay was developed by Rosalyn Yalow and Solomon Berson	Θ
1960	Ehringer and Hornykiewicz identified dopamine loss in post-mortem studies of patients with Parkinson's disease	PD
1961	Birkmeyer and Hornykiewicz first treated Parkinson's disease patients with levodopa	PD
1961	Chlordiazepoxide was marketed, 6 years after its invention by Sternbach in 1955	℞
1962	Carbamazepine was introduced (it had been developed by Schindler at Geigy Labs in Europe in the 1950s), initially for the treatment of trigeminal neuralgia	℞
1963	M Kidd described paired helical filaments	AD
1963	Drs John C Steele (neurology resident) and J Clifford Richardson (Chief of Neurology), at the Toronto General Hospital, and Jerzy Olszewski, Professor of Neuropathology at the Banting Institute, described *progressive supranuclear palsy*	Ψ
1963	Roche Laboratory marketed diazepam	℞

Contd

Appendix I Contd

Date	Event	Field*
1964	Leschal Nyhan described a familial disorder of abnormal uric acid metabolism in two brothers	Ψ
1964	Hakim described normal pressure hydrocephalus while working at the Massachusetts General Hospital	Ψ
1966	Cotzias and colleagues introduced soluble levodopa/carbidopa as a treatment for Parkinson's disease	PD
1967	Sir Martin Roth provided evidence that a decline in mental test scores in life correlates with plaque and tangle pathology at post mortem	AD
1967	Griffith proposed that the infective agent in Creutzfeldt–Jakob disease was some form of protein	CJD
1967	Christiaan Barnard, a South African surgeon, performed the first whole heart transplant from one person to another	Θ
1968	Gibbs and colleagues showed that Creutzfeldt–Jakob disease is transmissible	CJD
1968	Rebitz and colleagues described corticobasal degeneration	Ψ
1969	Graham and Oppenheimer united olivopontocerebellar atrophy, Shy–Drager syndrome and striatonigral degeneration in the term *multiple system atrophy*	Ψ
1971	Lorazepam (Ativan), or 2'-chloro substituted oxazepam, was synthesized	ℜ
1972	Fluoxetine was discovered by Lilly scientists Drs Bryan B Molloy, David T Wong and the late Ray W Fuller	ℜ
1974	The first case of iatrogenic Creutzfeldt–Jakob disease was recorded in a woman receiving a corneal graft from an infected donor	CJD
1975	Warrington reported what she termed 'selective impairment of semantic memory', later referred to as *semantic dementia*	Ψ
1975	On 25 November, Robert S Ledley was granted Patent No. 3,922,552 for the computerized tomographic scanner	Θ
1976	Several groups, including P Davies and AJF Maloney, demonstrated a decline in cholinergic enzymes in the neocortex in Alzheimer's disease	AD
1976	Gunnar Husby and Ralph Williams used an immunofluorescent antibody staining technique to show specific cross-reactivity of immunoglobulin G to shared amino acid sequences in group A streptococcal M protein and neuronal cytoplasmic antigens in the basal ganglia in Sydenham's chorea	Ψ
1977	The use of positron emission tomography (PET) to obtain images of the brain was demonstrated	Θ
1978	Sodium valproate was approved for use in epilepsy, although it had been synthesized almost a hundred years earlier in 1881 by Burton	ℜ
1981	Langston described a parkinsonian syndrome associated with MPTP	PD
1981	Whitehouse demonstrated a loss of cholinergic neurones in basal forebrain in Alzheimer's disease	AD
1981	Transmission of the familial form of Creutzfeldt–Jakob disease (Gerstmann–Sträussler disease) was demonstrated by Masters and colleagues	CJD
1982	Prusiner introduced the term 'prion' in the field of Creutzfeldt–Jakob disease research (he later received a Nobel Prize)	CJD
1983	Backlund and Olson first reported human neural transplantation in Parkinson's disease	PD
1983	James Gusella and Nancy Wexler localized the Huntington's disease locus to the tip of the short arm of chromosome 4	HD

1984	Kosoka, from the Yokohama City University, Japan, proposed that cortical Lewy bodies are a specific cause of dementia	Ψ
1984	Glenner and Wong isolated and then sequenced perivascular β-amyloid from the brain of Alzheimer's disease sufferers	AD
1985	Crowther and Wischik described the paired helical filament structure of neurofibrillary tangles	AD
1986	Fluoxetine was introduced in Belgium	ℜ
1987	Kang and colleagues sequenced the amyloid precursor protein	AD
1988	Goedert and colleagues cloned and sequenced tau, the main constituent of paired helical filaments	AD
1989	Owen and colleagues identified the first mutation in Gerstmann–Sträussler disease in codon 144 of the human prion gene	CJD
1989	The National Centre for Human Genome Research and, shortly after, the Human Genome Project were created in an effort to map all human DNA by 2005	Θ
1990	Lindvall and colleagues showed the therapeutic benefit of substantia nigra grafts in Parkinson's disease patients	PD
1991	Siddique and colleagues linked motor neurone disease to chromosome 21	MND
1993	Rosen and colleagues discovered that mutations in the superoxide dismutase gene are an important cause of familial motor neurone disease	MND
1993	The Huntington's Disease Study Group identified the expanded CAG repeat in the IT15 gene. The gene encodes a protein, designated 'huntingtin'	HD
1993	The Food and Drug Administration approved the application from the Warner-Lambert Company, and tacrine became the first drug available in the USA for the treatment of Alzheimer's disease	ℜ
1993	Felbamate, first synthesized in 1954, was launched in the USA for partial seizures and the Lennox–Gastaut syndrome	ℜ
1995	Britton, Bateman and colleagues described two cases of Creutzfeldt–Jakob disease in the UK, which were also unusual in having Kuru-type plaques	CJD
1996	Mangiarini, Bates and colleagues described the first Huntington's disease transgenic mouse with a dyskinetic phenotype	HD
1996	Will and colleagues suggested a link between new variant Creutzfeldt–Jakob disease affecting young adults and bovine spongiform encephalopathy	CJD
1997	Polymeropoulos and colleagues, at the Center for Human Genome Research, Bethesda, MD, reported the α-synuclein gene in Parkinson's disease	PD

*Θ, Historical landmark; Ψ, treatment related; ℜ, general neuropsychiatric event; CJD, Creutzfeldt–Jakob disease; HD, Huntington's disease; MND, motor neurone disease; PD, Parkinson's disease

Appendix II Professional agencies and support groups

Disorder	Agency in the USA	Agency in the UK
Ageing	National Institute on Aging (NIA) National Institutes of Health, Building 31, Room 5C27, Bethesda, MD 20892 2292 Tel.: 301 496 1752; 800 222 2225 TTY: 800 222 4225 http://www.nih.gov/nia	Age Concern Astral House, 1268 London Road, London SW16 4ER Tel.: 020 8765 7200 http://www.ace.org.uk
AIDS	National Association of People with AIDS 1413 K Street, NW, 7th Floor, Washington, DC 20005 3442 Tel.: 202 898 0414, ext. 124 Fax: 202 898 0435 E-mail: jmbrevelle@napwa.org http://www.napwa.org	Terrence Higgins Trust 52–54 Grays Inn Road, London WC1 8JU Tel.: helpline 020 7242 1010 (noon to10 p.m. daily) http://www.chaps.org.uk
Alzheimer's disease	Alzheimer's Association 919 North Michigan Avenue, Suite 1100, Chicago, IL 60611 1676 Tel.: 800 272 3900 Fax: 312 335 1110 E-mail: info@alz.org http://www.alz.org	The Alzheimer's Society Gordon House, 10 Greencoat Place, London SW1P 1PH Tel.: 0207 306 0606; helpline 0845 300 0336 Fax: 0207 306 0808 http://www.alzheimers.org.uk
Ataxia	National Ataxia Foundation (NAF) 2600 Fernbrook Lane, Suite 119, Minneapolis, MN 55447 4752 Tel.: 763 553 0020 Fax: 763 553 0167 E-mail: naf@ataxia.org http://www.ataxia.org	National Ataxia and Friedreich's Ataxia Group Room 10, Winchester House, Kennington Park, Cranmer Road, London SW9 6EJ Tel.: 020 7582 1444 Fax: 020 7582 9444 http://www.ataxia.org.uk
Creutzfeldt–Jakob disease	Creutzfeldt–Jakob (CJD) Foundation Inc. PO Box 5312, Akron, OH 44334 Tel.: 800 659 1991 Fax: 330 668 2474 E-mail: crjakob@aol.com http://cjdfoundation.org http://www.spinalcord.org	CJD Support Network Birchwood, Heath Top, Ashley Heath, Market Drayton, Shropshire Tel.: 01630 673 993 http://www.alzheimers.org.uk/cjd/index.html

Depression	Depression Alliance 35 Westminster Bridge Road, London SE1 7JB Tel.: administration 020 7633 0557 Fax: administration 020 7633 0559 http://www.depressionalliance.org
	National Depressive and Manic-Depressive Association NDMDA, 730 N. Franklin, Suite 501, Chicago, IL 60610 7204 Tel.: 800 826 3632; 312 642 0049 Fax: 312 642 7243 http://www.ndmda.org
Epilepsy	British Epilepsy Association New Anstey House, Gate Way Drive, Yeadon, Leeds LS19 7XY Tel.: 0113 210 8800 Fax: 0113 391 0300 E-mail: epilepsy@bea.org.uk http://www.epilepsy.org.uk
	Epilepsy Foundation 4351 Garden City Drive, Suite 406, Landover, MD 20785 2267 Tel.: 301 459 3700; 800-EFA-1000 (332 1000) Fax: 301 577 2684 E-mail: postmaster@efa.org http://www.epilepsyfoundation.org
General and miscellaneous	Pick's Disease Support Group Carol Jennings, 8 Brooksby Close, Oadby, Leicester LE2 5AB E-mail: mailto:carol@pdsg.org.uk
	National Organization for Rare Disorders (NORD) 55 Kenosia Avenue, PO Box 1968, Danbury, CT 06813 1968 Tel.: 800 999-NORD (6673) Fax: 203 798 2291 E-mail: orphan@rarediseases.org http://www.rarediseases.org
Head injury	Headway 4 King Edward Court, King Edward Street, Nottingham NG1 1EW Tel.: 0115 9240800 Fax: 0115 9240432 http://www.headway.org.uk
	Brain Injury Association of America 105 North Alfred Street, Alexandria, VA 22314 Tel.: 703 236 6000; 800 444 6443 Fax: 703 236 6001 E-mail: publicrelations@biausa.org http://www.biausa.org
Huntington's disease	Huntington's Disease Association 108 Battersea High Street, London SW11 3HP Tel.: 020 7223 7000 Fax: 020 7223 9489 http://www.hda.org.uk
	Huntington's Disease Society of America 158 West 29th Street, 7th Floor, New York, NY 10001 5300 Tel.: 212 242 1968; 800 345-HDSA (4372) Fax: 212 239 3430 E-mail: hdsainfo@hdsa.org http://www.hdsa.org
Motor neurone disease	Motor Neuron Disease Association National Office, Sharon Barker, MND Association UK, PO Box 246, Northamptonshire NN1 2PR Tel.: 01604 250505 Fax: 01604 638289 http://www.mndassociation.org/home.htm
	ALS Association of America (ALSA) 27001 Agoura Road, Suite 150, Calabasas Hills, CA 91301 5104 Tel.: 818 880 9007; 800 782 4747 Fax: 818 880 9006 http://www.alsa.org

Contd

Appendix II Contd

Disorder	Agency in the USA	Agency in the UK
Multiple sclerosis	The National Multiple Sclerosis Society 733 Third Avenue, New York, NY 10017 Tel.: 1212 986 3240 Fax: 1212 986 7981 E-mail: info@nmss.org http://www.nationalmssociety.org	Multiple Sclerosis Society MS National Centre, 375 Edgware Road, London NW2 6ND Tel.: 020 8438 0700; helpline 0808 800 8000 (free phone) Fax: 020 8438 0701 http://www.mssociety.org.uk
Parkinson's disease	American Parkinson Disease Association 1250 Hylan Boulevard, Suite 4B, Staten Island, NY 10305 1946 Tel.:800 223 2732 Fax: 718 981 4399 E-mail: info@apdaparkinson.org http://www.apdaparkinson.org	Parkinson's Disease Society United Scientific House, 215 Vauxhall Bridge Road, London SW1V 1EJ Tel.: 020 7931 8080; helpline 0808 800 0303 (free phone) Fax: 020 723 39908 E-mail: helpline@parkinsons.org.uk (helpline) http://www.parkinsons.org.uk
Progressive supranuclear palsy	Society for Progressive Supranuclear Palsy Woodholme Medical Building, 1838 Greene Tree Road, #515 Baltimore, MD 21208 Tel.: 800 457 4777 Fax: 410 486 4283 E-mail: spsp@psp.org http://www.psp.org	PSP (Europe) Association The Old Rectory, Wappenham, Towcester, Northamptonshire NN12 8SQ Tel.: 01327 860299 Fax: 01327 861007 E-mail: psp.eur@virgin.net
Systemic lupus erythematosus	Lupus Foundation of America 1300 Piccard Drive, Suite 200, Rockville, MD 20850 4303 Tel.: 301 670 9292 Fax: 301 670 9486 E-mail: info@lupus.org http://www.lupus.org	Lupus UK St. James House, Eastern Road, Romford Essex RM1 3NH Tel.: 01708 731251
Sleep disorders	Narcolepsy and Sleep Disorders: A Newsletter American Narcolepsy Foundation 528 Abrego Street, PMB, 149 Monterey, CA 93940 Tel.: 831 646 2055 Fax: 831 646 2051 http://www.narcolepsy.com	Narcolepsy Association (UK) 1st Floor, Craven House, 121 Kingsway, London WC2B 6PA http://www.narcolepsy.org.uk

Spinal injuries

National Spinal Cord Injury Association
6701 Democracy Boulevard, Suite 300-9, Bethesda, MD 20817
Tel.: 301 588 6958
Fax: 301 588 9414
http://www.spinalcord.org

Spinal Injuries Association
76 St. James's Lane, Muswell Hill, London N10 3DF
Tel.: 020 84442121; 0800 980 0501
Fax: 020 84443761
E-mail: sia@spinal.co.uk
http://www.spinal.co.uk

Stroke

National Stroke Association
9707 East Easter Lane, Englewood, CO 80112 3747
Tel.: 800-STROKES (787 6537)
Fax: 303 649 1328
E-mail: info@stroke.org
http://www.stroke.org

The Stroke Association
Stroke House, Whitecross Street, London EC1Y 8JJ
Tel.: helpline 0845 30 33 100; administration 020 7566 0300
Fax: 020 7490 2686
http://www.stroke.org.uk

Tourette syndrome

Tourette Syndrome Association
42 40 Bell Boulevard, Suite 205, Bayside, NY 11361 2820
Tel.: 718 224 2999; 888 4-TOURET (486 8738)
Fax: 718 279 9596
E-mail: tsa@tsa-usa.org
http://www.tsa-usa.org

Tourette's Syndrome Association
1st Floor Offices, Old Bank Chambers, London Road, Crowborough,
East Sussex TN6 2TT
Tel.: helpline 01892 669151
Fax: 01892 663649
E-mail: 101667.3131@compuserve.com
http://www.tsa.org.uk

CNS tumours

American Brain Tumor Association
2720 River Road, Suite 146, Des Plaines, IL 60018 4110
Tel.: 0708 827 9910; patient line 800 886 2282
Fax: 0708 827 9918
E-mail: info@abta.org
http://www.abta.org

British Brain Tumour Association
2 Oakfield Road, Hightown, Merseyside L38 9GQ
Tel.: 0151 929 3229

Wilson's disease

Wilson's Disease Association, International
Executive Director, Wilson's Disease Association,
1802 Brookside Drive, Wooster, OH 44691
Tel.: 800 399 0266
Fax: 509 757 6418
E-mail: wilsonsdiseaseassoc@yahoo.com
http://www.wilsonsdisease.org

Wilson's Disease UK
Dr Caroline Simms, 36 Sunningdale Drive, Woodborough,
Nottingham. NG14 6EQ
http://www.wilsons-disease.org.uk

Appendix III   Useful web addresses

Subject	Web address
Ageing	http://www.library.miami.edu/netguides/socage.html
Alzheimer's disease	http://www.neuro.med.cornell.edu
Assessments and algorithms	http://www.medal.org
CNS tumours	http://www.neuro.psyc.memphis.edu/NeuroPsyc/np-dx-tumor.htm
Community medicine	http://www.aafp.org
Delirium	http://www.emedicine.com/med/topic3006.htm
Drug–drug interactions	http://www.drug-interactions.com
Early dementia	http://www.cma.ca/cmaj/vol-160/issue-12/dementia/diagnosis.htm
Evidence-based medicine	http://www.evidence.org
Genetics	http://www.ncbi.nlm.nih.gov/genome/guide/human
Head injury	http://www.headinjury.com
History of medicine	http://www.mic.ki.se/HistDis.html
Hospital medicine	http://www.emedicine.com
HIV and AIDS	http://www.hnrc.ucsd.edu
Huntington's disease	http://www.geneclinics.org/profiles/huntington/details.html
Infectious diseases	http://www.geocities.com/CapeCanaveral/3504
Lewy body dementia	http://www.nottingham.ac.uk/pathology/lewy/lewyhome.html
Medical revision	http://www.fpnotebook.com
Neuroanatomy	http://www.placidity.net/neuro/page/outline.shtml
Neurology	http://www.neuroland.com/default_old.htm
Neuropsychology	http://www.biols.susx.ac.uk/ugteach/cws/iin/teach.html
Neuroradiology	http://www.med.harvard.edu/AANLIB/home.html
Neurosciences	http://www.neuro.med.cornell.edu
Parkinson's disease	http://www.parkinson.org
Pathology	http://www-medlib.med.utah.edu/WebPath/TUTORIAL/CNS/CNSDG.html
Patient information	http://www.ninds.nih.gov/health_and_medical/disorder_index.htm
Physical examination	http://www.neuropat.dote.hu/neurology.htm
Psychiatry	http://www.mentalhealth.com
Psychology	http://www.mrc-cbu.cam.ac.uk/psychology.links.netscape.html
Quality of life	http://www.qlmed.org/fpage_neur.htm
Young people	http://www.faculty.washington.edu/chudler/neurok.html
Sleep	http://www.sleepquest.com
Support groups	http://www.netdoctor.co.uk/directory/support_groups/showlist.asp
Tourette's syndrome	http://www.mentalhealth.com/book/p40-gtor.html
Toxicology	http://www.swosu.edu/~longs/txcl/txclindx.htm
Treatment	http://www.merck.com/pubs/mmanual/section14/sec14.htm

Appendix IV   Recommended reference books of relevance to neuropsychiatry

Topic	Book
Alzheimer's disease	Gauthier S 1999 Clinical diagnosis and management of Alzheimer's disease, 2nd edn. Martin Dunitz, London
Biological psychiatry	D'Haenen H, den Boer JA, Willner P 2002 Biological psychiatry, vols 1 & 2. Wiley, Chichester
Child neuropsychiatry	Coffey CE, Brumback RA 1998 Textbook of pediatric neuropsychiatry. American Psychiatric Press, Washington, DC
Clinical examination	Kaufman DM 2001 Clinical neurology for psychiatrists, 5th edn. WB Saunders, Philadelphia
Consultation–liaison psychiatry	Stoudemire A, Fogel BS, Greenberg DB 2000 Psychiatric care of the medical patient, 2nd edn. Oxford University Press, Oxford
Delirium	Lindesay J, Rockwood K, MacDonald A 2002 Delirium in old age. Oxford University Press, Oxford
Dementia	O'Brien J, Ames D, Burns A 2000 Dementia. Edward Arnold, London
Depression	Starkstein SE, Robinson RG 1993 Depression in neurological disease. Johns Hopkins University Press, Baltimore
Epilepsy	Trimble MR, Bettina Schmitz E 2002 The neuropsychiatry of epilepsy. Cambridge University Press, Cambridge
Head injury	Richardson JTE 2000 Clinical and neuropsychological aspects of closed head injury. Psychology Press, London
Learning disability	Gaddes WH, Edgell D 1996 Learning disabilities and brain function: a neuropsychological approach, 3rd edn. Springer-Verlag, New York
Movement disorders	Joseph AB, Young RR 1999 Movement disorders in neurology and neuropsychiatry. Blackwell Science, Oxford
Neuroanatomy	Clark DL, Boutros NN 1999 The brain and behavior: an introduction to behavioural neuroanatomy. Blackwell Science, Oxford
Neuropathology	Markesbery WR 1998 Neuropathology of dementing disorders. Edward Arnold, London
Neuropsychiatry	Moore D 2000 Textbook of clinical neuropsychiatry. Edward Arnold, London
Neuropsychology	Heilman KM, Valenstein E 2003 Clinical neuropsychology. Oxford University Press, New York
Old age psychiatry	Copeland J, Abou-Saleh M, Blazer D 2002 Principles and practice of geriatric psychiatry, 2nd edn. Wiley, New York
Psychiatric treatment	Yudofsky SC, Hales RE 2002 Neuropsychiatry and clinical neurosciences, 4th edn. American Psychiatric Press, Arlington
Psychopharmacology	Davis KL, Charney D, Coyle JT et al 2002 Neuropsychopharmacology. The fifth generation of progress. Lippincott Williams & Wilkins, Philadelphia
Stroke	Warlow C 2000 Stroke. Blackwell Science, Oxford
Wilson's disease	Hoogenraad T 2001 Wilson's disease. Baillière Tindall, London

Appendix V   Recommended assessment scales

Disorder/presentation/domain	Assessment scale

Neuropsychiatric symptoms and syndromes

Abnormal movements
Abnormal Involuntary Movements Scale (AIMS)
Guy W 1976 ECDEU Assessment manual for psychopharmacology. US Department of Health, Education and Welfare, Washington, DC

Agitation
Cohen-Mansfield Agitation Inventory (CMAI)
Cohen-Mansfield J, Marx MS, Rosenthal AS 1989 A description of agitation in a nursing home. Journal of Gerontology 44:M77–M84

Anger
Rating Scale for Aggressive Behaviour in the Elderly (RAGE)
Patel V, Hope RA 1992 A rating scale for aggressive behaviour in the elderly. The RAGE. Psychological Medicine 22:211–221

Anxiety
Beck Anxiety Inventory
Beck AT, Epstein N, Brown G et al 1988 An inventory for measuring clinical anxiety: psychometric properties. Journal of Consulting and Clinical Psychology 56:893–897

Apathy
Marin's Apathy Evaluation Scale (AES)
Marin RS, Biedrzycki, RC, Firinciogullari S 1991 Reliability and validity of the Apathy Evaluation Scale. Psychiatry Research 38:143–162

Ataxia
International Cooperative Ataxia Rating Scale
Trouillas P, Takayanagi T, Hallett M 1997 International Cooperative Ataxia Rating Scale for pharmacological assessment of the cerebellar syndrome. The Ataxia Neuropharmacology Committee of the World Federation of Neurology. Journal of Neurological Science 145:205–211

Coma
Glasgow Coma Scale
Teasdale G, Jennett B 1974 Assessment of coma and impaired consciousness: a practical scale. Lancet ii:81–84

Depression
Montgomery–Asberg Depression Rating Scale (MADRS)
Montgomery SA, Asberg M 1979 A new depression scale designed to be sensitive to change. British Journal of Psychiatry 134:382–389

Function
Instrumental Activities of Daily Living
Lawton MP, Brody EM 1969 Assessment of older people: self-maintaining and instrumental activities of daily living. The Gerontologist 9:179–186

Health anxiety
Health Anxiety Questionnaire
Lucock MP, Morley S, White C et al 1997 Responses of consecutive patients to reassurance after gastroscopy: results of a self-administered questionnaire survey. BMJ 315:572–575

Neuropsychiatry screening
The Neuropsychiatric Inventory
Cummings JL, Mega M, Gray K et al 1994 The Neuropsychiatric Inventory – comprehensive assessment of psychopathology in dementia. Neurology 44:2308–2314

Pain
West Haven–Yale Multidimensional Pain Inventory
Kerns RD, Turk DC, Rudy TE 1985 The West Haven–Yale Multidimensional Pain Inventory (WHYMPI). Pain 23:345–356

Psychotic symptoms
Positive and Negative Syndrome Scale (PANSS)
Kay SR, Fiszbein A, Opler LA 1987 The positive and negative syndrome scale (PANSS) for schizophrenia. Schizophrenia Bulletin 13:261–276

Sleep
Epworth Sleepiness Scale (ESS)
Johns MW 1991 A new method for measuring daytime sleepiness: the Epworth Sleepiness Scale. Sleep 14:540–545

Appendix V *Contd*

Disorder/presentation/ domain	Assessment scale
Soft signs	Cambridge Neurological Inventory *Chen EYH, Shapleske J, Luque R et al 1995 The Cambridge Neurological Inventory – a clinical instrument for assessment of soft neurological signs in psychiatric patients. Psychological Research 56:183–204*
Somatization complaints	Somatoform Disorders Symptom Checklist *Janca A, Isaac M, Costa e Silva JA 1995 World Health Organization International Study of Somatoform Disorders: background and rationale. European Journal of Psychiatry 9:100–110*
Suicide intent	Suicide Intent Scale (SIS) *Beck AT, Schuyler D,Herman I 1974 Development of suicidal intent scales. In: Beck AT, Resnik HLP, Lettieri D (eds) The prediction of suicide. Charles Press, Baltimore, MD, p 45–56*
Well-being	Sickness Impact Profile (SIP) *Bergner M, Bobbitt RA, Carter WB et al 1981 The Sickness Impact Profile: development and final revision of a health status measure. Medical Care 19:787–805*

Neuropsychiatric diseases

Alzheimer's disease	Alzheimer's Disease Assessment Scale (ADAS) *Rosen WG, Mohs RC, Davis KL 1984 A new rating scale for Alzheimer's disease. American Journal of Psychiatry 141:1356–1364*
Huntington's disease	Unified Huntington's disease Rating Scale *Huntington Study Group 1996 Unified Huntington's disease rating scale: reliability and consistency. Movement Disorders 11:136–142*
Behaviour in dementia	Behavioral Pathology in Alzheimer's Disease Rating Scale (BEHAVE-AD) *Reisberg B, Borenstein J, Salob SP et al 1987 Behavioral symptoms in Alzheimers disease: phenomenology and treatment. Journal of Clinical Psychiatry 48(suppl):9–15*
Delirium	Delirium Rating Scale *Trzepacz PT, Baker RW, Greenhouse J 1988 A symptom rating scale for delirium. Psychiatry Research 23:89–97*
Emotionalism	The Pathological Laughing and Crying Scale *Robinson RG, Parikh RM, Lipsey JR et al 1993 Pathological laughing and crying following stroke – validation of a measurement scale and a double-blind treatment study. American Journal of Psychiatry 150:286–293*
Mania	Mania Rating Scale *Bech P, Rafaelsen OJ, Kramp P et al 1978 The mania rating scale: scale construction and inter-observer agreement. Neuropharmacology 17:430–431*
Motor neurone disease disability	The Amyotrophic Lateral Sclerosis Functional Rating Scale *The ALS CNTF Treatment Study (ACTS) Phase I–II Study Group 1996 The Amyotrophic Lateral Sclerosis Functional Rating Scale. Archives of Neurology 53:141–147*
Multiple sclerosis disability	Expanded Disability Status Scale *Kurtzke JF 1983 Rating neurologic impairment in multiple sclerosis: an expanded disability status scale (EDSS). Neurology 33:1444–1452*
Parkinson's disease	Unified Parkinson's Disease Rating Scale *Fahn S, Marsden CD, Calne DB et al (eds) 1987 Recent developments in Parkinson's disease, vol 2. Macmillan Health Care Information, Florham Park, NJ, p 153–163, 293–304*
Subarachnoid haemorrhage	Hunt and Hess SAH Grading System *Hunt WE, Hess RM 1968 Surgical risk as related to time of intervention in the repair of intracranial aneurysms. Journal of Neurosurgery 28:14–20*

Appendix V *Contd*

Disorder/presentation/ domain	Assessment scale
Stroke disability	Stroke Impact Scale *Duncan PW, Wallace D, Lai SM et al 1999 The stroke impact scale version 2.0: evaluation of reliability, validity, and sensitivity to change. Stroke 30:2131–2140*
Tourette's syndrome	Tourette's Syndrome Global Scale (TSGS) *Harcherik DF, Leckman JF, Detlor J et al 1984 A new instrument for clinical studies of Tourette's syndrome. Journal of the American Academy of Child Psychiatry 23:153–160*
Vascular dementia	Hachinski Ischemic Score *Hachinski VC, Iliff LD, Zilkha E et al 1975 Cerebral blood flow in dementia. Archives of Neurology 32:632–637*

Cognitive assessment tools

1 minute screening	Clock Drawing Test *Tuokko H, Hadjistavropoulos T, Miller JA et al 1995 The Clock Drawing Test: administration and scoring manual. Multi-health Systems, Toronto*
5-minute screening	Mini-Mental State Examination *Folstein MF, Folstein SE, McHugh PR 1975 Mini-mental state: a practical method for grading the cognitive state of patients for the clinician. Journal of Psychiatric Research 12:189–198*
Premorbid ability	Wechsler Test of Adult Reading (WTAR) *The Psychological Corporation (Harcourt Education), Halley Court, Jordan Hill, Oxford OX2 8EJ, UK*
General intelligence	Wechsler Adult Intelligence Scale, Third Edition (WAIS-III) *The Psychological Corporation (Harcourt Education), Halley Court, Jordan Hill, Oxford OX2 8EJ, UK*
Clinic battery	CAMDEX-R The Revised Cambridge Examination for Mental Disorders of the Elderly *Cambridge University Press, The Edinburgh Building, Shaftesbury Road, Cambridge CB2 2RU, UK*
Computerized battery	CANTAB – Cambridge Neuropsychological Test Automated Battery *Robbins TW, James M, Owen AM et al 1995 Cambridge Neuropsychological Test Automated Battery (CANTAB): a factor analytic study of a large sample of normal elderly volunteers. Dementia 5:266–281*
Memory	Wechsler Memory Scale, Third Edition *Wechsler D 1997 Wechsler Memory Scale – Third Edition. The Psychological Corp., San Antonio, TX*
Executive function	Behavioural Assessment of the Dysexecutive Syndrome (BADS) *Thames Valley Test Company, Unit 22, Thurston Granary, Station Hill, Thurston, Suffolk IP31 3QU, UK*

Appendix VI Finding the evidence in neuropsychiatry

In order to justify the statement that this text is evidence based, it is necessary to list the sources and methodology used to collate the information. The main source of information was the Science Citation Index. This excellent database is updated with 17,750 new records and 362,000 new cited references every week. Additional material was sourced from the Internet (see Appendix III) and reference books (see Appendix IV). Conference proceedings and many journals were also hand-searched to find articles not adequately referenced in electronic databases.

Databases
CINAHL (1982 to March 2003) Cumulative Index to Nursing & Allied Health, lists more than 500 journals

Cochrane Database of Systematic Reviews, Issue 1 (2003) A database of 1000 selected reviews of treatment interventions in a critically appraised form

Dissertation Abstracts International (1861–2003) ProQuest Digital database, contains 1.6 million dissertation titles

EMBASE (1980 to 3 week 13, 2003) EMBASE Psychiatry provides 297,000 citations from the parent EMBASE database from Elsevier Science

INSIDE (1993 to June 2000) A British Library database of conference proceedings and journals, provides access to over 15 million article titles

MEDLINE (1966 to March 2003) The National Library of Medicine's main database, contains over 10 million references

PsycINFO (PsycLIT) (1887 to March 2003) Catalogues 2 million references to psychological literature from 1887 to the present, including book chapters and dissertations

Web of Science (1981 to March 2003)* An interface that searches the Science Citation Index, updated with 17,750 new records and 362,000 new cited references every week. Total contents are approximately 17 million records

Hand-searched conference proceedings
6th World Congress of Biological Psychiatry, Nice, 1997

XIV International Congress of Neuropathology, Birmingham, 2000

31st Annual Meeting of the Society for Neuroscience, San Diego, CA, 2001

7th World Congress of Biological Psychiatry, Berlin, 2001

XVII World Congress of Neurology, London, 2001

2nd International Congress on Vascular Dementia, Salzburg, 2002

54th Annual Meeting of the American Academy of Neurology, Denver, CO, 13–20 April 2002*

8th International Conference on Alzheimer's Disease and Related Disorders, Stockholm, 20–25 July 2002

32nd Annual Meeting of the Society of Neuroscience, Orlando, FL, 2–7 November 2002

55th Annual Meeting of the American Academy of Neurology, Honolulu, Hawaii, 29 March to 5 April 2003

2003 American Psychiatric Association Annual Meeting, San Francisco, CA, 17–22 May 2003

Hand-searched journals
Acta Neurologica Scandinavica
Acta Neuropathologica
Acta Psychiatrica Scandinavica
Advances in Psychiatric Treatment
Alzheimer's Disease and Related Disorders
*American Journal of Geriatric Psychiatry**
American Journal of Physical Medicine and Rehabilitation
American Journal of Psychiatry
Annals of Neurology
Archives of Clinical Neuropsychology

*Archives of General Psychiatry**
*Archives of Neurology**
Biological Psychiatry
Brain
Brain Injury
Brain Research Reviews
Brain Pathology
British Journal of Psychiatry
Clinical Neurology and Neurosurgery
Clinical Neuropsychopharmacology

Contd

Appendix VI *Contd*

Hand-searched journals – *Contd*

Clinical Neuroscience Research
Clinical Rehabilitation
Current Opinion in Neurology
Disability and Rehabilitation
Epilepsia
Epilepsy and Behaviour
Epilepsy Research
European Archives of Psychiatry & Clinical Neuroscience
European Journal of Neurology
European Neuropsychopharmacology
European Psychiatry
General Hospital Psychiatry
HIV Medicine
International Journal of Geriatric Psychiatry
JAMA
Journal of Affective Disorders
Journal of Nervous and Mental Disease
Journal of Neural Transmission
Journal of Neurology
Journal of Neurology, Neurosurgery and Psychiatry*
Journal of Neuropathology and Experimental Neurology
Journal of Neuropsychiatry and Clinical Neuroscience*
Journal of Psychiatric Research
Journal of Psychosomatic Research
Journal of the Neurological Sciences

Lancet Neurology*
Movement Disorders
Nature Neuroscience
Neurobiology of Aging
Neurological Sciences
Neurologist
Neuropathology and Applied Neurobiology
Neuropsychiatry, Neuropsychology and Behavioral Neurology
Neurology*
Neuropsychologica
Neuroscience and Biobehavioral Reviews
New England Journal of Medicine
Parkinsonism and Related Disorders
Practical Neurology
Progress in Neuro-Psychopharmacology and Biological Psychiatry
Psychiatry and Clinical Neurosciences
Psychiatry Research
Psychological Medicine
Psychosomatic Medicine
Psychosomatics
Sleep Medicine
Stroke

*Highly recommended for neuropsychiatry primary research

Index